Shaping for Cleaning the Root Canals

Gustavo De Deus • Emmanuel J. N. L. Silva
Erick Souza • Marco A. Versiani
Mario Zuolo
Editors

Shaping for Cleaning the Root Canals

A Clinical-Based Strategy

Springer

Editors
Gustavo De Deus
Fluminense Federal University
Niterói, Brazil

Emmanuel J. N. L. Silva
Fluminense Federal University, Grande Rio University, Rio de Janeiro State University
Niterói, Brazil

Erick Souza
Federal University of Maranhão
São Luis, Brazil

Marco A. Versiani
Dental Specialty Center
Brazilian Military Police
Minas Gerais, Brazil

Mario Zuolo
Dental School of APCD – FAOA
São Paulo, Brazil

ISBN 978-3-030-84616-9 ISBN 978-3-030-84617-6 (eBook)
https://doi.org/10.1007/978-3-030-84617-6

This Springer imprint is published by the registered company Springer Nature Switzerland AG
The registered company address is: Gewerbestrasse 11, 6330 Cham, Switzerland

Nobody likes scientists. They like what science gives them, but not the questions, no. Not the questions that science asks.

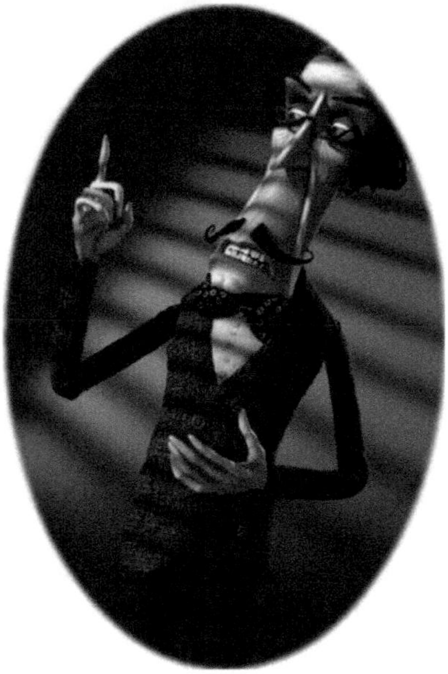

Actually, I have a question.

He, he. That is why you are a scientist.

I was doing my experiment, my project, and the first time it worked great, but the next time it didn't. I mean, it sort of worked, but then it didn't. And I don't know why.

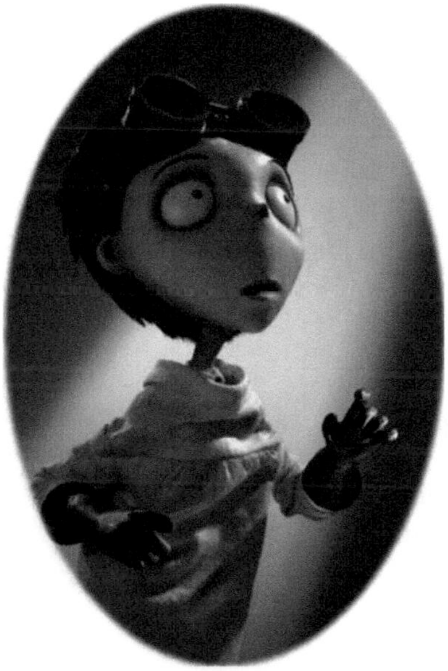

Then maybe you never really understood it the first time. People think science is here, but it is also here. The first time, did you love your experiment?

Yes.

And the second time?

No. I just wanted it over.

Then you changed the variables.

I was doing it for the wrong reason.

Science is not good or bad, Victor. But it can be used both ways. That is why you must always be careful.[1]

[1] Dialogue about the scientific method between Victor (the student) and Mr. Rzykruski (the science teacher), characters from Tim Burton's 2012 film Frankenweenie©.

Preface

In a world of fast-paced technological advancements, the task of writing a book is challenging considering the risk of being immediately outdated at the moment it is released. This is even more sensitive when exploring root canal preparation, one of the topics in endodontics that received the highest amount of technological improvements in the last decade. In this regard, during the brainstorming phase to conceive this book, we agreed that this subject should not be explored from an ordinary way, using mere analytical descriptions of these advancements that usually convey into a simple comparative analysis about the performance of instruments and techniques. Our idea was to go beyond, by synthesizing all knowledge acquired by our large clinical and laboratory experiences, aiming to provide an update on the Cleaning & Shaping concept, coined by Dr. Schilder back in the 1970s. This paradigm consolidated itself as the main guide for root canal preparation and disinfection, grounded on simultaneously performing the cleaning and shaping procedures to achieve disinfection while enlarging the root canal. However, with the advent of nickel-titanium rotary systems in the early 2000s, a new challenge for the Schilder's concept arose, inasmuch as a clear discompass became evident between the preparation speed resulting from these overfast mechanical systems and the effective infection control. Therefore, as overfast preparation was an undeniable technical advance that ultimately made canal shaping easier and safer, an update on the Cleaning & Shaping concept is now required. In fact, as cleaning and disinfection requires time to be accomplished, it shall not be considered to sidewalk with overfast shaping, as Schilder has theorized. In this sense, Shaping for Cleaning fits well enough into the current standard of root canal preparation, which is our desire not to be a simple semantic change, but also a road to enlighten clinicians to maximize specific efforts to grant disinfection after accomplishing canal shaping.

To synthesize the ideas around the Shaping for Cleaning concept, the authors of the present textbook explored the recent evolution of root canal preparation through an in-depth discussion of the impact of the technological revolution over each phase of the root canal treatment, including scouting, glide path, patency, coronal enlargement, irrigation, shaping and re-shaping, grounded on the best available knowledge supported by cutting-edge scientific evidence. Moreover, a flawless view of the current limitations to achieve disinfection in endodontics is presented and debated. The milestone of this textbook is the pristine combination of clinical, scientific, and educational expertise, gathered to provide the reader a pleasant and meaningful learning process. We hope it becomes an important source of reliable information for any professional interested in the field of Endodontology.

Niterói, Brazil — Gustavo De Deus
Niterói, Brazil — Emmanuel J. N. L. Silva
São Luis, Brazil — Erick Souza
Minas Gerais, Brazil — Marco A. Versiani
São Paulo, Brazil — Mario Zuolo

Contents

Classical Cleaning & Shaping: Historical Cornerstones

1

Gustavo De Deus, Emmanuel J. N. L. Silva, Erick Souza,
Marco A. Versiani, and Mario Zuolo

1.1 Historical Development of Shaping Concepts

The mechanical shaping of root canals embraces a set of transoperative procedures with the core purpose of acting against microbial intracanal infection, with tooth retention as the ultimate target. Such procedures are based on technical, scientific and philosophical concepts that have evolved, developed and been tested since the seventeenth century. At this point, it becomes important to scrutinize and review the theoretical historical grounds of mechanical canal preparation. Understanding how instrumentation evolved during the twentieth century is necessary to pave the thinking route required to comprehend the current status of mechanical shaping.

The Standardized Technique was the first systematic approach used for the mechanical canal preparation, formally described by Ingle in 1961 [1]. Actually, it represents the simplest approach for enlarging the canal space, classified as parallel or non-tapering shaping. The Standardized Technique employs the working length as a reference point using a series of sequential instruments. Thus, it relies exclusively on the own design of the instruments to create the desired canal shape.

G. De Deus
Fluminense Federal University, Niterói, Brazil

E. J. N. L. Silva
Fluminense Federal University, Grande Rio University, Rio de Janeiro State University, Niterói, Brazil

E. Souza
Federal University of Maranhão, São Luis, Brazil

M. A. Versiani (✉)
Dental Specialty Center, Brazilian Military Police, Minas Gerais, Brazil
e-mail: marcoversiani@yahoo.com

M. Zuolo
Dental School of APCD – FAOA, São Paulo, Brazil

G. De Deus et al. (eds.), *Shaping for Cleaning the Root Canals*,
https://doi.org/10.1007/978-3-030-84617-6_1

Ingle described the sequential usage of standardized reamers of increasing sizes focused on the mechanical enlargement of the apical third, but later the use of K-files replaced reamers. In this way, the direct ascending order of hand files lies on the central logic of the Standardized Technique: if a K-file size 15 penetrates tightly in relatively narrow canals and, after a sequential usage of few instruments, a K-file size 25 is loose at the full working length, contemporary thinking at that time believed that the canal was clean, disinfected and thus enlarged enough for filling. To better understand this rationale, before considering the size of the canal enlargement, it is necessary to remember the quality of the endodontic instruments in those days, still manufactured in carbon steel and without standardization (Fig. 1.1).

As time went by, it was figured out that the dimensions of a shaped canal up to a K-file size 25 loose at the working length would not be enough to assure adequate conditions for root canal filling; furthermore, this enlarment size hardly produce a minimally acceptable intracanal disinfection pattern. As a consequence, the Standardized Technique was further improved by Clem [2] and Weine [3], who implemented a complementary step in order to render the canal space more tapered, thus facilitating the cleaning and filling procedures. In fact, Clem [2], Weine [3] and afterwards Walton [4] observed that the final canal shape was defined by the interplay between the size and the sequence of the endodontic instruments.

Similarly simple in its essence, the Step-back Technique, also known as telescopic or serial root canal preparation, became commonplace on a worldwide scale

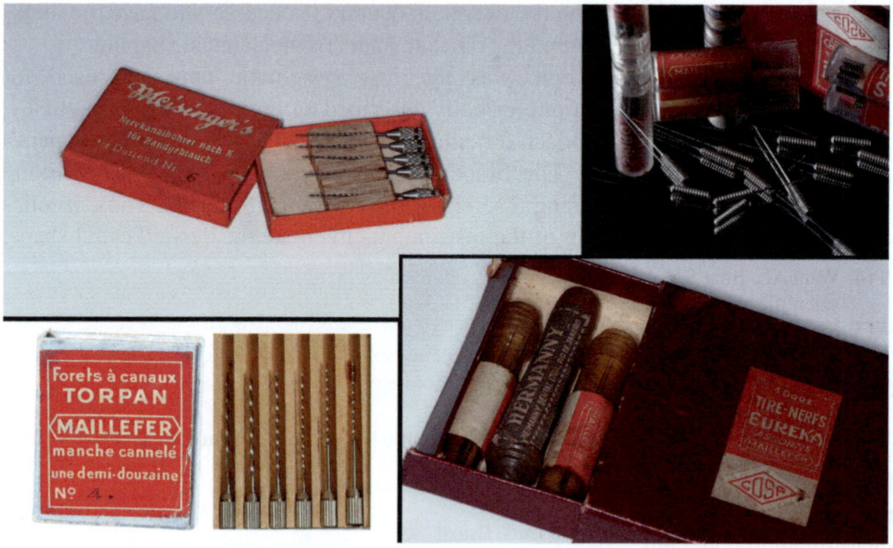

Fig. 1.1 Carbon steel endodontic instruments developed at the beginning of the twentieth century before ISO norm. It seems unimaginable that it was possible to perform a root canal treatment with such instruments, but certainly, their limitations explain the technical difficulties faced by clinicians at that time

from the early 1970s onward. The first stage of the Step-back Technique is precisely Ingle's Standardized Technique, which means the apical sequential usage of instruments, in general, until a K-file size 25 is loosen at the working length. At this moment, a premeditated step back is performed in which working lengths stepwise decrease by instrument size increase. As larger instruments are less flexible, they are moved back millimeter by millimeter to the coronal direction, thus mechanically working only in the larger and straighter parts of the canal of the middle and coronal thirds. In short, the sequential use of instruments from the smallest to the largest provides a more tapered and thus appropriate canal shape. As larger instruments work away from the apical third, the risk of iatrogenic occurrences and procedural accidents is better controlled. Moreover, the Step-back Technique is more efficient in managing curved root canals. Inevitably, the development of the Step-back Technique is considered a sharp advance over the elementary Standardized Technique.

There are two critical differences between the Standardized and Step-back Techniques. While the former produces a more parallel shape (non-tapering), the Step-back Technique results in a conical-shaped canal (tapering). The latter refers to the fact that while Standardized is a single operative procedure, the Step-back Technique can be naturally divided into two separate phases. We believe that it is essential that our readers understand the rationale that led Clem [2] and Weine [3] to split the Step-back Technique into two distinct phases:

1. The first phase is actually the Standardized Technique. The working length is established and then the canal enlargement is performed using instruments in a serial increasing sequence. Similarly to the Standardized Technique, the first phase is in charge of intracanal cleaning-disinfection process.
2. The second step is the innovative aspect of the technique; working lengths decrease in a stepwise manner by increments of 1 mm using larger instruments; this way, a relatively continuous taper is created to favor the filling procedure.

In summary, the first mechanical phase is responsible for disinfection. The task then is to overcome the canal curvature by being able to produce a tapered canal. Then, a proper shape for the filling procedures is obtained in the second phase (Fig. 1.2).

Conceptually, the intentional and thoughtful division of the Step-back Technique in two operative phases rendered it more sophisticated. Realistically, it created the first effective instrumentation technique for typical molar anatomies. On account of this, the Step-back Technique is appointed as the most universally learned and used instrumentation technique worldwide. Actually, it is still considered the standard for manual shaping. As Scianamblo [5] summarized so well, "*Step-back methodology has been the core of most instrumentation techniques for decades and will probably remains an integral part of most modern procedures.*"

Cleaning & Shaping approach onward, a radical conceptual break was proposed where cleaning and shaping were a concomitant and synchronized single process. From the strength of its efficacy, Dr. Herbert Schilder's methodical and efficient Cleaning & Shaping regimen emerged as a universally accepted and widely used philosophy for root canal preparation.

1.3 From the 1980s to the 1990s

Several technical modifications, operative maneuvers and new techniques and concepts were proposed to be used with stainless steel files between the 1980s and 2000s and integrated in endodontic practice worldwide. The most important were:

1. Crown-down technique [8]
2. Anti-curvature filing [9]
3. Balanced force technique [10]
4. Oscillatory movement technique [11]

In clinical practice, all these preparation methodologies and operative maneuvers somehow incorporated the main principles of the classical Cleaning & Shaping concept [6]. Real-life contemporary clinical endodontics happen somewhere along this range of mechanical canal preparation strategies. For instance, most conventional rotary techniques take advantage of the crown-down approach; thus, a better control of torsional stress is achieved and the risk of instrument separation is minimized. In general, the trained and experienced dentist combines some of these concepts and operative maneuvers into a hybrid technique, but usually keeping the Cleaning & Shaping regimen as its basis. This means that Dr. Schilder's Cleaning & Shaping concept has been the paragon of clinical endodontic practice from the mid-1970s onward.

1.4 Overfast Mechanical Shaping: An Undeniable Current Reality

Current mechanical shaping is mostly produced by engine-driven instruments and can be done in a fast and rather predictable way. This scenario took place in the mid-2000s with the evolution of the rotary systems [12]. Moreover, since 2011, due to clinical experience and research information, reciprocating instruments have expedited the shaping process even more. A micro-computed tomographic (micro-CT) study in lower molars concluded that reciprocating motion is about 40% faster than rotaty [13]. In another study, Bürklein et al. [14] reported that rotary systems (ProTaper and MTwo) demanded about 200 s to complete the mechanical preparation, while reciprocating systems (WaveOne and Reciproc) completed it in less than half that time (Fig. 1.4).

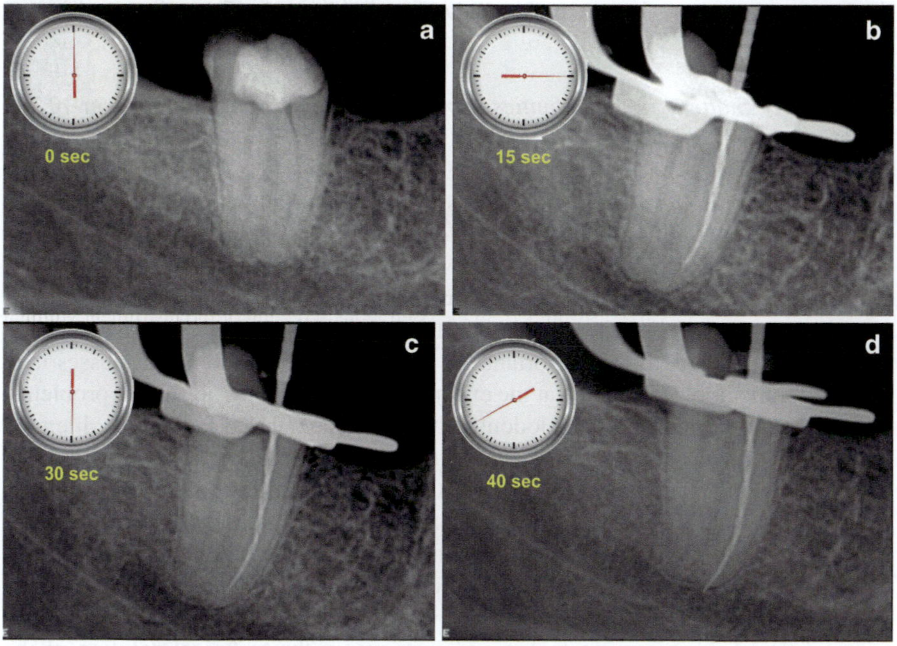

Fig. 1.4 Clinical case of a mandibular molar with a common internal anatomy demonstrating how fast the canal shape can be nowadays. (**a**) Intact root canal; (**b**) In few seconds it is possible to prepare the coronal and middle thirds and (**c**) advance to the apical third; (**d**) In less than one minute the root canal is mechanically shaped in an easy and predicable way

The competence in producing overfast mechanical canal preparations is a direct result of the impressive shaping ability of reciprocating instruments. Over the last decade, everyday practice revealed that reciprocating instruments are a very efficient way of cutting dentin, allowing us to reach the apex faster than with conventional rotary systems. Thus, the message is that the development of the reciprocation movement has expedited even more the speed of the mechanical canal preparation.

The ongoing scenario, where canal shaping often requires only a few minutes to be completed, has led us to ponder the further possible consequences on the operative sequence of canal irrigation and disinfection procedures. This is based on the ever-close relationship between mechanical canal enlargement and irrigation and this will be methodically explored in the next chapter.

1.5 What Should Be the Main Target in Endodontics? Speed or Quality?

It is of note that several manufacturers broadly advertised overfast canal shaping as a highly positive aspect of the NiTi systems, which indirectly means that speed matters for the practice. However, a dangerous mainstream is potentially created taking the focus away from what the real agenda of endodontics is. Thus, we can ask ourselves quite frankly:

What really matters in endodontics: speed or an effective management of the infection?

Very usually in life, speed and quality are two important variables for countless processes and situations and it is not rare to witness a tug of war. In fact, we all trade off quality and time, every day. We can say that speed versus quality stands for a well-known dilemma of contemporary times. Unfortunately, prioritizing one often comes at the cost of the other, leaving professionals (clinicians) to make a decision as to which is indeed more important. As a general rule, different businesses may put a different emphasis on one at the expense of the other with no further problems. Yet within the framework of endodontics, the clinician started facing this dilemma when overfast canal shaping became a day-to-day reality. There is an interesting decision-making mental model developed to help in determining a trade-off between speed and quality, when building products, that can be employed in the context of endodontics. Since at a given point the clinician needs to push the button and make a choice between speed or quality, the following rationale may be useful. The decision to prioritize speed or quality should be based on our confidence in the importance of the problem we are facing and certainty in the technical solution of the problem. Contextualizing the above points to the endodontics scenario, two basic questions appear:

1. Is endodontic disease really significant for your patient's care?
2. What is the efficiency of the currently available methods for shaping, cleaning and disinfecting?

Before starting, make sure that your confidence is based on scientific evidence rather than subjective views. There are three basic possible outcomes for these questions:

1. Do you have little confidence in the significance of the problem? If so, focus on speed. If you are unsure of the significance of the problem, it is unlikely to be a case of endodontics, which is on a gradual journey to becoming an evidence-based and patient-centered clinical discipline.
2. Is your confidence in the problem and in the solution high? If so, again focus on speed. Here, we can state with confidence that this is not the case in root canal treatment in general due to its well-known inherent technical limitations and complex root canal anatomy. However, this can be an option for cases with simple anatomy and large straight canals where an expedited mechanical shaping is often able to provide a proper degree of intracanal cleaning and disinfection. Note that this is not the prevalent scenario in endodontics as, very often, root canal anatomy is a real technical challenge.

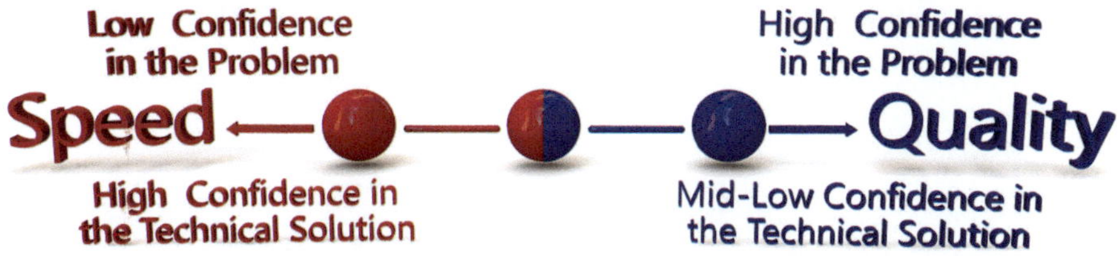

Fig. 1.5 Illustrative representation of Quality vs. Speed as a function of Confidence theory

3. Is your confidence in the problem high, but only average in the solution? Always focus on quality. We believe that this is the most frequent case in endodontics due to the interplay between the well-described anatomical challenges and technical limitations of root canal treatment.

Therefore, the message is rather clear: a speed-ruled canal shaping comes at the expense of the quality of the NaOCl-based cleaning and disinfection process (Fig. 1.5), which may compromise the main target of the treatment, and this is methodically addressed in the next chapter.

References

1. Ingle JI. A standardized endodontic technique utilizing newly designed instruments and filling materials. Oral Surg Oral Med Oral Pathol. 1961;14:83–91.
2. Clem WH. Endodontics: the adolescent patient. Dent Clin N Am. 1969;13:482–93.
3. Weine F. Endodontic therapy. 1st ed. St. Louis: Mosby; 1972.
4. Walton RE. Histologic evaluation of different methods of enlarging the pulp canal space. J Endod. 1976;2:304–11.
5. Scianamblo MJ. A contemporary approach to cleaning and shaping of the root canal system emphatizing "early coronal enlargement". In: Castelucci A, editor. Endodontics. Florence: Edizioni Odontoiatriche Il Tridente; 2005. p. 470–501.
6. Schilder H. Cleaning and shaping the root canal. Dent Clin N Am. 1974;18:269–96.
7. Berutti E, Castelucci A. Cleaning and shaping the root canal system. In: Castelucci A, editor. Endodontics. Florence: Edizioni Odontoiatriche Il Tridente; 2005. p. 396–437.
8. Marshall FJ, Pappin JA. A crown-down pressureless preparation root canal enlargement technique. Portland: Oregon Health Sciences University; 1980.
9. Abou-Rass M, Frank AL, Glick DH. The anticurvature filing method to prepare the curved root canal. J Am Dent Assoc. 1980;101:792–4.
10. Roane JB, Sabala CL, Duncanson MG Jr. The "balanced force" concept for instrumentation of curved canals. J Endod. 1985;11:203–11.
11. De Deus QD. Endodontia. 5th ed. Rio de Janeiro: MEDSI; 1992.
12. Thompson SA. An overview of nickel-titanium alloys used in dentistry. Int Endod J. 2000;33:297–310.
13. Paqué F, Zehnder M, De-Deus G. Microtomography-based comparison of reciprocating single-file F2 ProTaper technique versus rotary full sequence. J Endod. 2011;37:1394–7.
14. Bürklein S, Hinschitza K, Dammaschke T, Schäfer E. Shaping ability and cleaning effectiveness of two single-file systems in severely curved root canals of extracted teeth: Reciproc and WaveOne versus Mtwo and ProTaper. Int Endod J. 2012;45:449–61.

Shaping for Cleaning: Reconsidering Root Canal Debridement

2

Gustavo De Deus, Emmanuel J. N. L. Silva, Erick Souza, Marco A. Versiani, Matthias Zehnder, and Mario Zuolo

2.1 How Effectively Can We Debride?

2.1.1 The "Fake Iceberg Illusion"

In order to describe and discuss the limitations of the current technology for engine-driven NiTi mechanical shaping, a rationale is developed by making an analogy with the "Iceberg Illusion," which is not normally used in that context. However, calling modern shaping concepts a "Trojan Horse" or "Fools Gold" would be stretching the limit a bit, because nobody will argue that these tools do not have their merits. Nevertheless, this section addresses the drawbacks behind current shaping methods.

As we learned in primary school, only a fraction of an iceberg's volume mass is evident above the water, with 90% being hidden beneath the sea surface and thus not

G. De Deus (✉)
Fluminense Federal University, Niterói, Brazil
e-mail: endogus@gmail.com

E. J. N. L. Silva
Fluminense Federal University, Grande Rio University, Rio de Janeiro State University, Niterói, Brazil

E. Souza
Federal University of Maranhão, São Luis, Brazil

M. A. Versiani
Dental Specialty Center, Brazilian Military Police, Minas Gerais, Brazil

M. Zehnder
Division of Endodontology, Clinic of Conservative and Preventive Dentistry, University of Zürich, Zürich, Switzerland

M. Zuolo
Dental School of APCD – FAOA, São Paulo, Brazil

G. De Deus et al. (eds.), *Shaping for Cleaning the Root Canals*,
https://doi.org/10.1007/978-3-030-84617-6_2

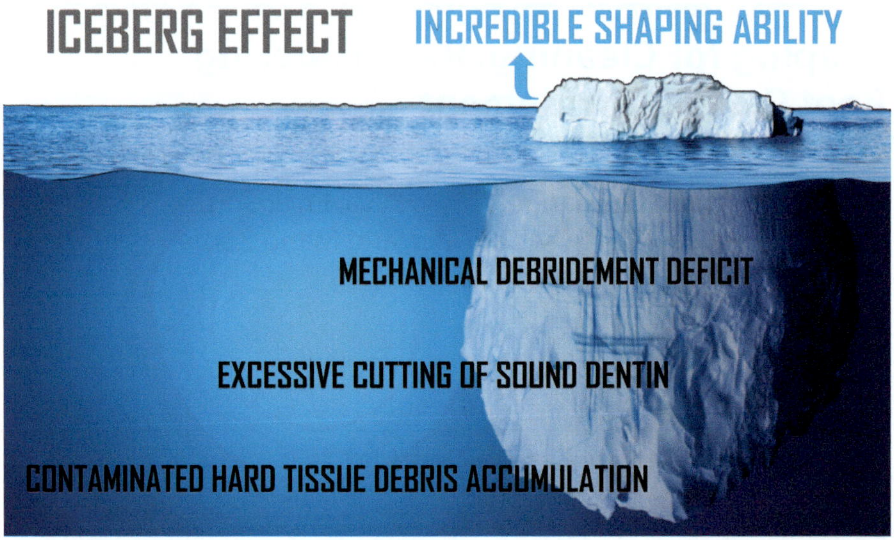

Fig. 2.1 Iceberg illusion analogy to illustrate the limitations of the current technology for engine-driven NiTi mechanical shaping. The visible 10% of the iceberg's volume is the amazing shaping ability and safety degree of the NiTi instruments available today. These are features possible to be observed in clinical practice. However, going below the sea's surface, the undesired side effects of the current shaping methods, which are usually hidden in clinical practice, start to appear, which are (1) the debridement deficit, (2) the unnecessary root dentin removal, and (3) the accumulation of hard-tissue debris in irregular areas of the canal space

visible. The iceberg is frequently used as a metaphor for success, in the sense that what people do not see is how hard an individual worked and which sacrifices he or she made to reach that state of success. Translating this to the context of mechanical preparation in endodontics, the visible 10% of the iceberg's volume is the amazing shaping ability and safety degree of the NiTi instruments available today (Fig. 2.1). These are features possible to be observed in clinical practice, and make clinicians and sales people happy, as they can be appreciated by the multitude of cases proudly presented on social media. However, shaping and filling a root canal to the apical area and proving that on a radiograph are mere surrogate outcomes, and are only related to clinical success within a given shaping protocol [1]. Going below the surface of the iceberg, the undesired side effects of the current shaping methods, which are usually hidden in clinical practice, start to appear. Let us take a moment to reflect on those hidden side effects of shaping procedures, which can be summarized as:

1. Debridement deficit;
2. Unnecessary root dentin removal;
3. Accumulated hard-tissue debris in irregular areas of the canal space.

2.1.2 Debridement Deficit

This first side effect is a limitation of the current technology for canal shaping. Proper mechanical preparation should uniformly debride and plane the entire root canal perimeter—a kind of scrubbing action on the canal walls. This, in turn, would ensure an effective removal of as much of the remaining soft tissue and heavily biofilm-contaminated dentin as possible which may cause or maintain the perirradicular disease, influencing the outcome of treatment [2–4]. Nowadays, however, there is a considerable body of evidence—mainly based on histological slicing and micro-CT studies—attesting the suboptimal canal preparation by either rotary or reciprocating NiTi instruments. In fact, this is an ever-present condition in endodontic practice. Hatton et al. [5] were the first to demonstrate that the canal was only superficially cleaned and much of the pulp tissue was not removed after preparation with stainless steel instruments, but it was only after the seminal study by Walton [6], in the mid-1970s, that awareness of the limitations of cleaning and shaping procedures started to find its way into the endodontic community. Over the last decades, however, the establishment of nondestructive micro-CT imaging technology as a gold standard analytical tool to evaluate endodontic procedures consolidate the evidence of this suboptimal quality of mechanical preparation reported in previous studies. Overall, studies using micro-CT revealed that more than half of the dentinal walls in oval-shaped canals (ranging from 59.6 to 79.9%) remain unprepared after mechanical preparation with NiTi instruments [7–10] (Fig. 2.2).

Micro-CT allows the identification and quantification of root canal areas affected by the mechanical preparation (hard mineralized tissues), while the remaining pulp tissue is usually assessed in histological sections, both confirming the inability of shaping protocols to promote an efficient mechanical debridement. Recently, a sophisticated nondestructive longitudinal 3D contrast-enhanced micro-CT method (CE-CT) was introduced in the endodontic research to assess the quality and quantity of soft and hard tissues simultaneously [11]. And again, the suboptimal condition of the chemomechanical canal preparation was confirmed (Fig. 2.3).

Worthy of note is that, oddly enough, from a strictly clinical point of view, the importance of this phenomenon has been mitigated over time as it cannot be directly observed in two-dimensional periapical radiographs, usually used to evaluate the overall quality of root canal treatment. Senia [12] defined the root canal diameter as "the forgotten dimension" because research and dental practitioners mostly ignore it, while Jou et al. [13] stated that the canal "working widths" is typically underestimated and not only more complicated than the vertical dimension (working length) but also more difficult to assess because the horizontal dimension varies significantly along the root length (Fig. 2.4).

The explanation for this limited debridement ability previously described is simple and related to the geometry of current NiTi engine-driven instruments. Even the ones with innovative designs such as the Self-Adjusting File or XP-endo Shaper (discussed later in this chapter) are unable to adapt to the irregular cross-sectional shape of the root canals. The designs of the NiTi instruments are basically similar among different manufacturers: aside from differences in taper, cutting blades and

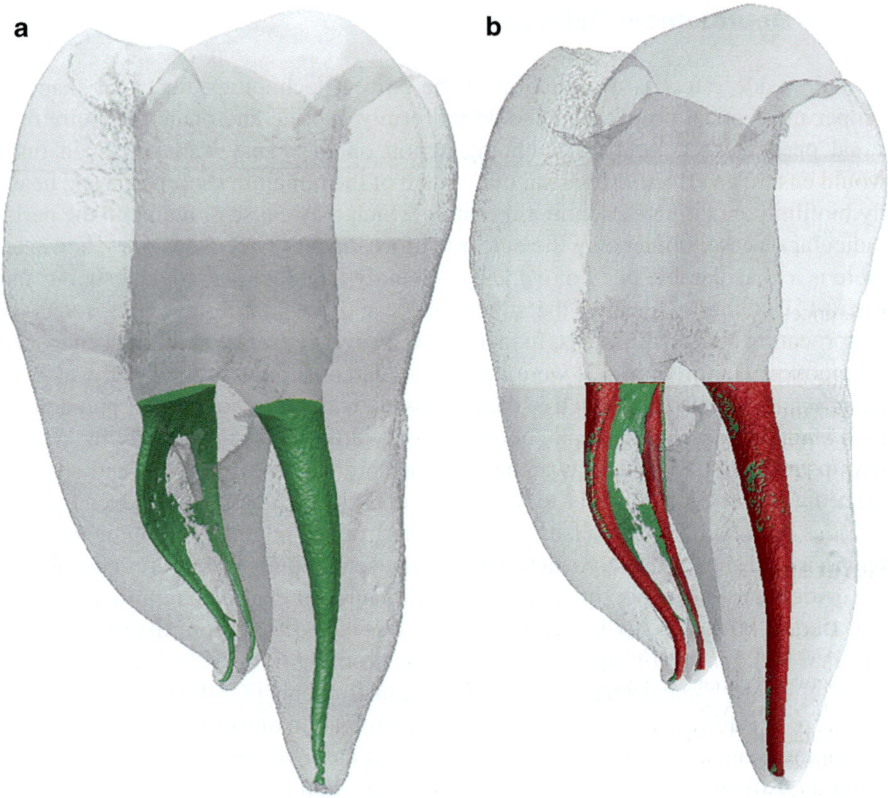

Fig. 2.2 A representative three-dimensional model of typical mandibular molar (**a**) before (in green) and (**b**) after (in red) root canal preparation in which is possible to observe the significant amount of dentinal walls (green areas in **b**) that was not touched by the mechanical instruments

cross sections, essentially they are manufactured from straight metal blanks, but always resulting in a round cross section able to prepare only the main root canal space into a circular shape, leaving unprepared buccal and lingual extensions of the canal, which means a substantial amount of untouched dentin surface [7–9] (Figs. 2.5 and 2.6).

As a consequence, the contribution of the mechanical preparation to the infection control and debridement of the organic tissue is indeed limited, being aggravated in curved or narrow canals [14–16]. Hence, microorganisms that remain in unprepared dentinal walls may have the opportunity to recolonize the insufficiently filled canal system, thus compromising the treatment outcome [17, 18].

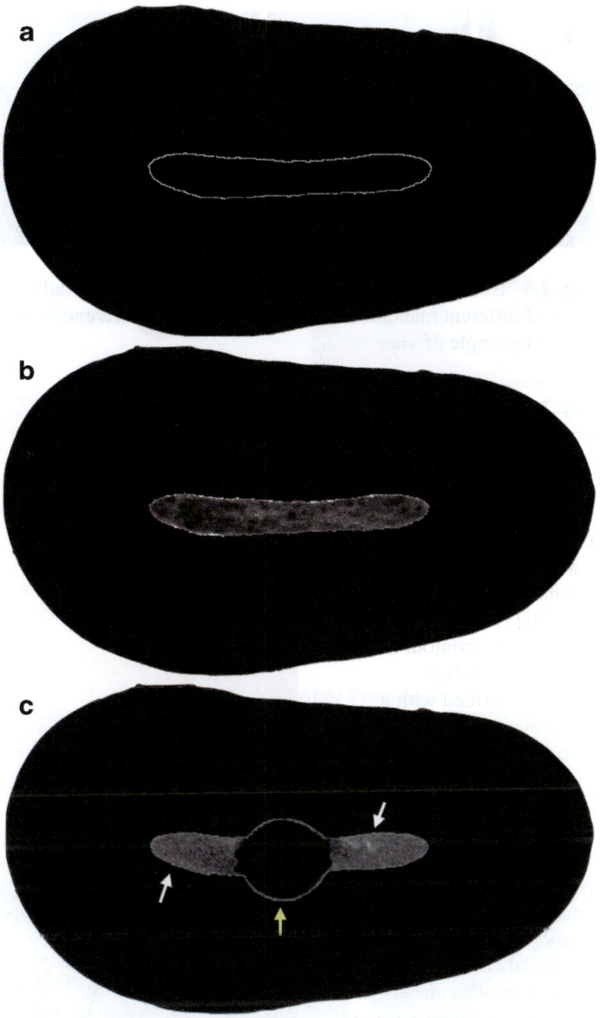

Fig. 2.3 (**a**) Typical cross-sectional micro-CT images of a non-stained long oval-shaped canal (outlined in white) in which is not possible to observe the dental pulp tissue. (**b**) After applying the Lugol-based staining protocol, it is possible to see the root canal space completely filled with the pulp tissue. The impregnation of Lugol's solution renders the dental pulp tissue able to absorb the X-rays and thus create a density map of the tissue. (**c**) After the mechanical preparation, in the central area of the canal, the NiTi instrument created a round preparation (yellow arrow) leaving unprepared buccal and lingual extensions (white arrows)

2.1.3 Unnecessary Root Dentin Removal

Mechanical canal preparation is invasive in nature and different degrees of dentin removal may occur as distinct instrumentation techniques and systems are used, which may alter the biomechanical response of teeth [19]. One of the critical points of mechanical damage is normally caused by overinstrumentation against an already thin dentinal wall (Fig. 2.7), which may seriously compromise the long-term outcome of root canal treatment [20] (Figs. 2.8, 2.9, and 2.10).

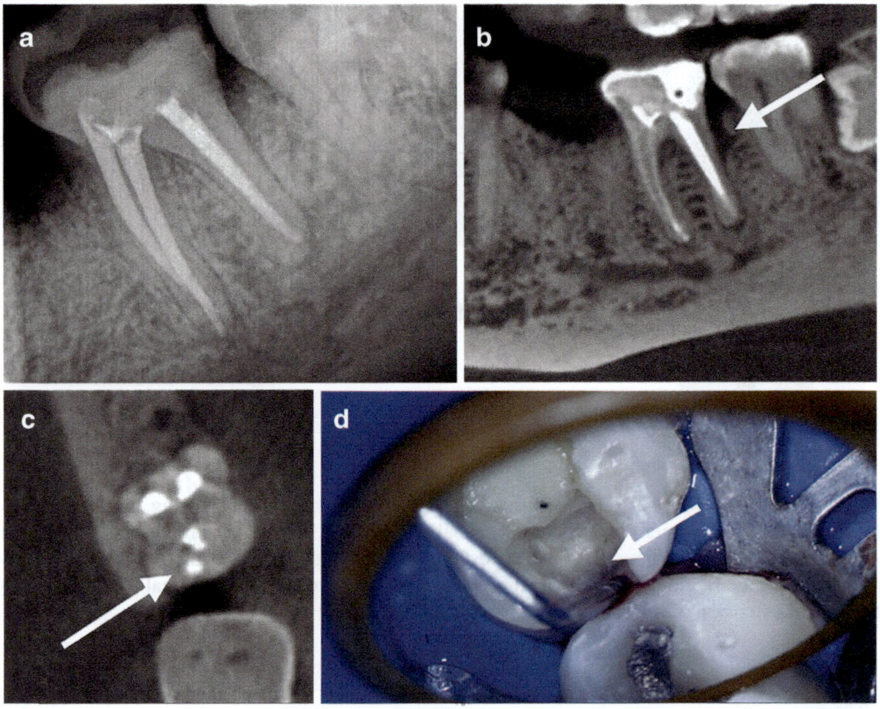

Fig. 2.8 (**a**) Periapical radiograph of endodontically treated teeth with a large tapered root canal preparation with an excessive removal of dentinal tissue especially at the coronal level. (**b**) Sagittal CBCT image showing a bone defect at the distal bone crest possible associated with a vertical fracture (arrow). (**c**, **d**) Axial CBCT cross-section and clinical image depicting the fracture line at the distal aspect of the crown (arrows)

The performance of the mechanical shaping is determined by the preoperative dimensions of the root canal, the filling technique and the restorative treatment plan. However, the greatest focus today is being able to clean the canal space while preserving the maximum of the sound structure of the tooth (Figs. 2.11, 2.12, and 2.13). Within this framework, one may argue that current mechanical preparations should keep the canal dimensions as small as possible, since instrumentation per se is ineffective in cleaning and disinfecting the inner dentinal walls in irregular and hard-to-reach areas, such as fins and isthmuses [21–23]. On the other hand, the mechanical enlargement must be enough to create an operational pathway to irrigate the root canal space. For that, it is necessary a minimal but optimal size/taper to be set, which is not currently supported by reliable evidence. As previously discussed in this chapter, this problem exists because current endodontic instruments are not able to perfectly adapt to the root canal anatomy. Faced with the need to perform a better debridement of attached biofilm by mechanically reaching all root canal walls, an unnecessary removal of dentin tissue, often healthy, is the result of any preparation protocol available today. This problem is aggravated with the current concepts of root canal disinfection, based on the enlargement of the root canal space, especially in the apical portion, to optimize the intracanal disinfection [24].

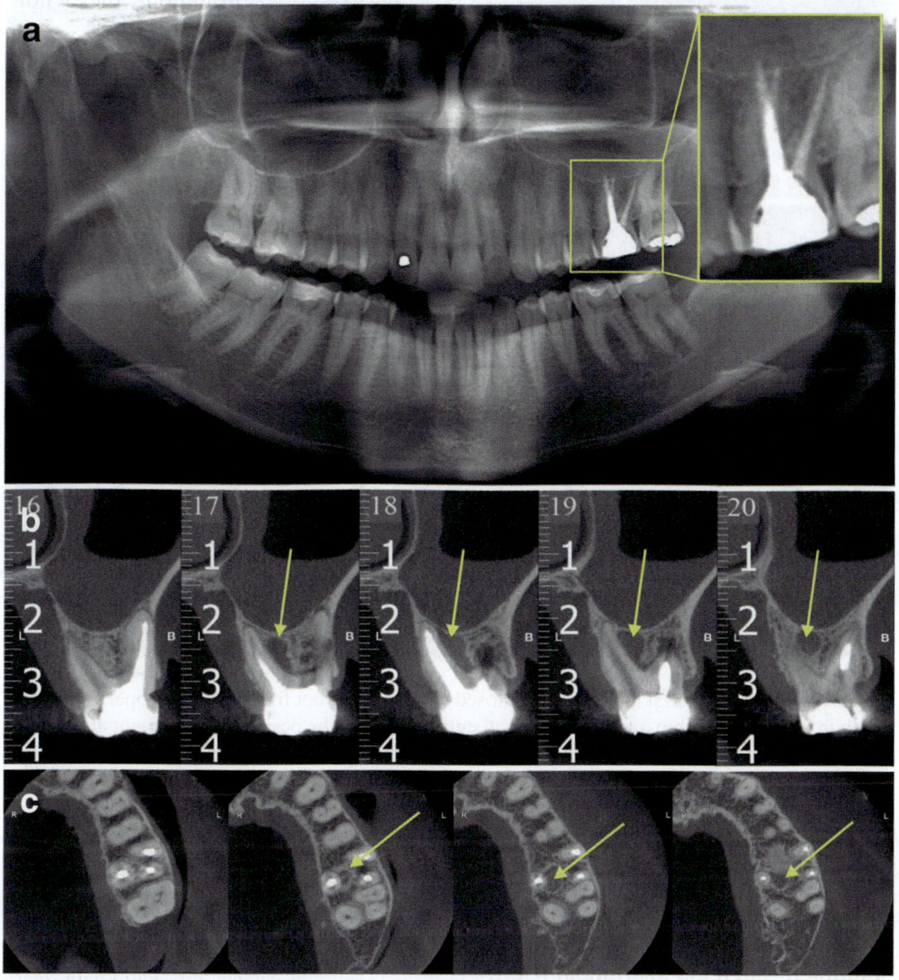

Fig. 2.9 (**a**) Panoramic radiograph showing a maxillary first left molar which was endodontically treated in 1998. Patient returned in 2020 showing an abscess at the buccal aspect of the gingiva related to this tooth. (**b**) Transaxial and (**c**) axial tomographic images of the tooth demonstrated a huge radiolucency (arrows) involving the coronal and middle thirds of the palatal root

New instruments with different thermomechanical treatments and geometric designs are being constantly developed in pursuance of achieving better performances regarding root canal preparation and minimum removal of dentin.

The Self-Adjusting File (SAF) (ReDent Nova, Ra'anana, Israel) system was launched in 2009 as an innovative proposal against the conventional NiTi rotary instruments. SAF is a hollow cylindrical instrument derived from a nickel-titanium stent, i.e., a lattice with compressible walls. In theory (and according to the manufacturer), when a root canal is prepared, the compressible walls allow the instrument to adapt to the root canal shape both longitudinally and along its cross section. In other words, the SAF instrument conforms three-dimensionally to root canals with

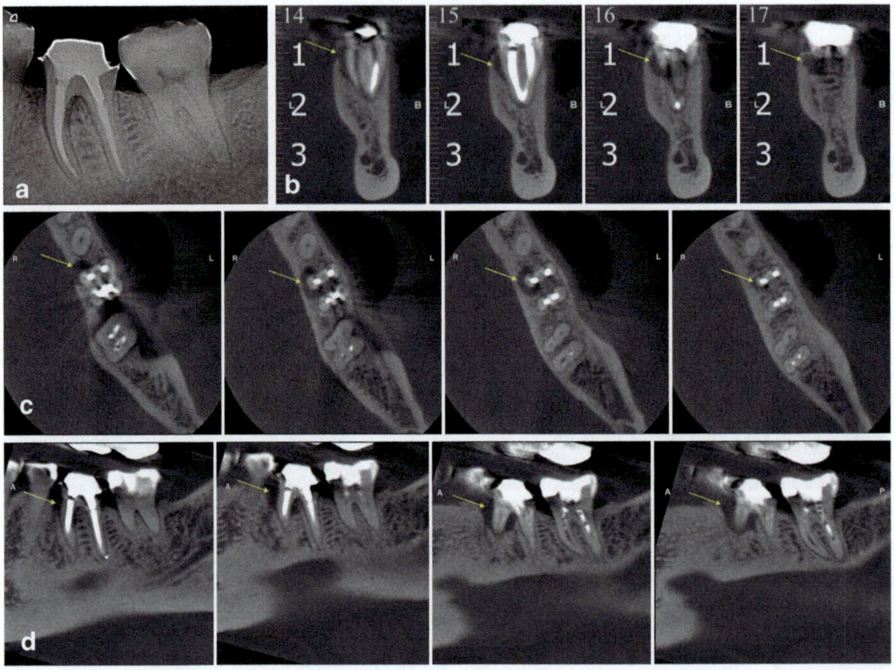

Fig. 2.10 Mandibular first left molar diagnosed with vertical root fracture. (**a**) Preoperative radiograph in which is possible to note an atypical enlargement of the periodontal ligament at the coronal and middle portions of the mesial root. (**b**) Transaxial and (**c**) axial tomography images showing bone loss at the lingual aspect of the mesial root. (**d**) Parasagittal image view of the mesial root showing bone loss at the furcation area

circular, oval, or flat-oval cross sections, maintaining its original shape, while removing the minimum amount of dentin tissue (Fig. 2.14). Moreover, and in contrast to all other instrumentation systems on the market, the SAF delivers the irrigate solution through the instrument itself.

The XP-endo Shaper system (FKG Dentaire, La Chaux-de-Fonds, Switzerland) is made with the MaxWire alloy and, according to the manufacturer, it contracts and expands depending on the temperature, reaching areas that conventional NiTi instruments cannot reach, while better preserving the dentin (Fig. 2.15).

Another proposal to improve root canal debridement is the GentleWave system (Sonendo, Laguna Hills, USA). This device aims to clean the root canal through different physicochemical mechanisms, including a broad spectrum of sound waves. Multisonic waves are initiated at the tip of the GentleWave handpiece positioned inside the pulp chamber. It delivers a stream of treatment solution into the pulp chamber, while the excess of fluid is simultaneously removed by the built-in vented suction through the handpiece. Upon initiation of flow through the tip of the handpiece, the stream of the fluid interacts with the stationary fluid inside the pulp chamber, generating shock waves that create a hydrodynamic cavitation. The continuous formation of microbubbles inside a cavitation cloud generates an acoustic field with a broadband

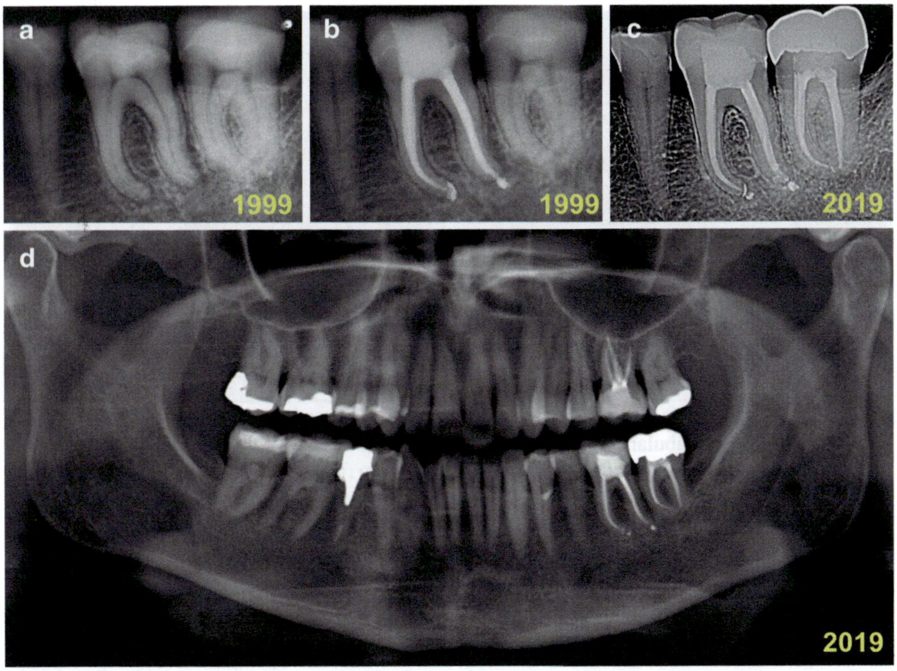

Fig. 2.11 (**a**, **b**) Mandibular first left molar diagnosed with pulp necrosis and chronic apical periodontitis treated in 1999. At that time, the chief complaint of the patient was pain on biting. (**c**, **d**) Radiographic follow up after 20 years showing the final restoration in position and complete healing in a functional tooth

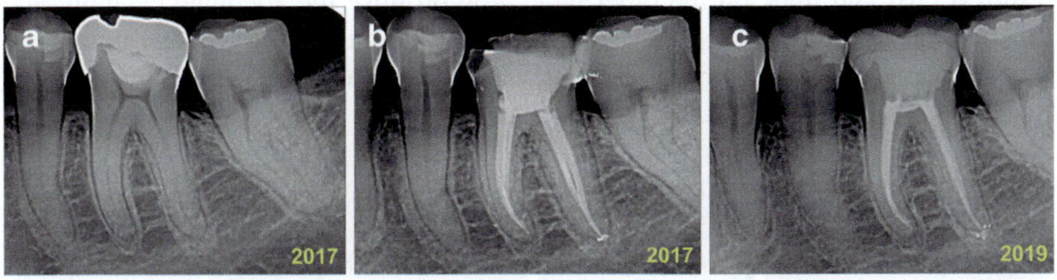

Fig. 2.12 (**a**) Mandibular first left molar diagnosed with pulp necrosis and chronic apical periodontitis. Patient's chief complaint was spontaneous pain. (**b**) Root canal treatment was performed in 2017. Canal preparation was done using Reciproc 25 followed by apical enlargement with instruments sizes 35/0.02 in the mesial canals and 45/0.02 in the distal canals. (**c**) A 24-month follow up radiographic exam showed this tooth presenting a normal periodontal ligament space and proper restoration

frequency spectrum that travels through the fluid into the entire canal, without the need for excessive root canal enlargement to promote disinfection (Fig. 2.16).

All the aforementioned innovative systems, however, still run into the same problem: the unnecessary removal of some amount of sound dentin tissue. For

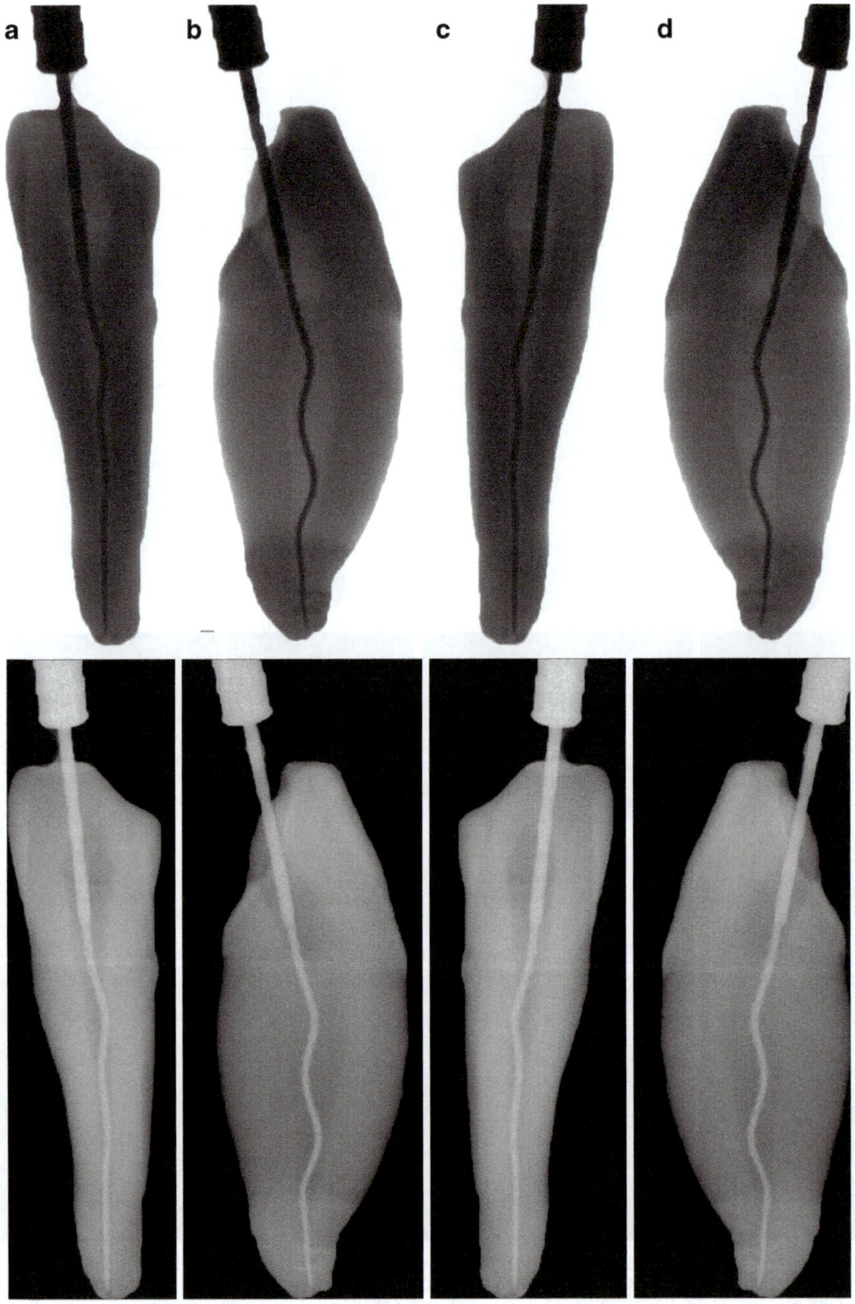

Fig. 2.15 Micro-CT projection images taken from the buccolingual (**a** and **c**) and mesiodistal (**b** and **d**) directions of a mandibular canine with a XP-endo Shaper instrument inserted within its oval-shaped canal. XP-endo Shaper was developed with a new NiTi alloy technology named MaxWire. It is a snake-shaped instrument with a triangular booster tip cross-sectional design that works in an eccentric rotary motion by taking a semicircular shape. The change in its shape results from the molecular memory of the NiTi austenitic phase

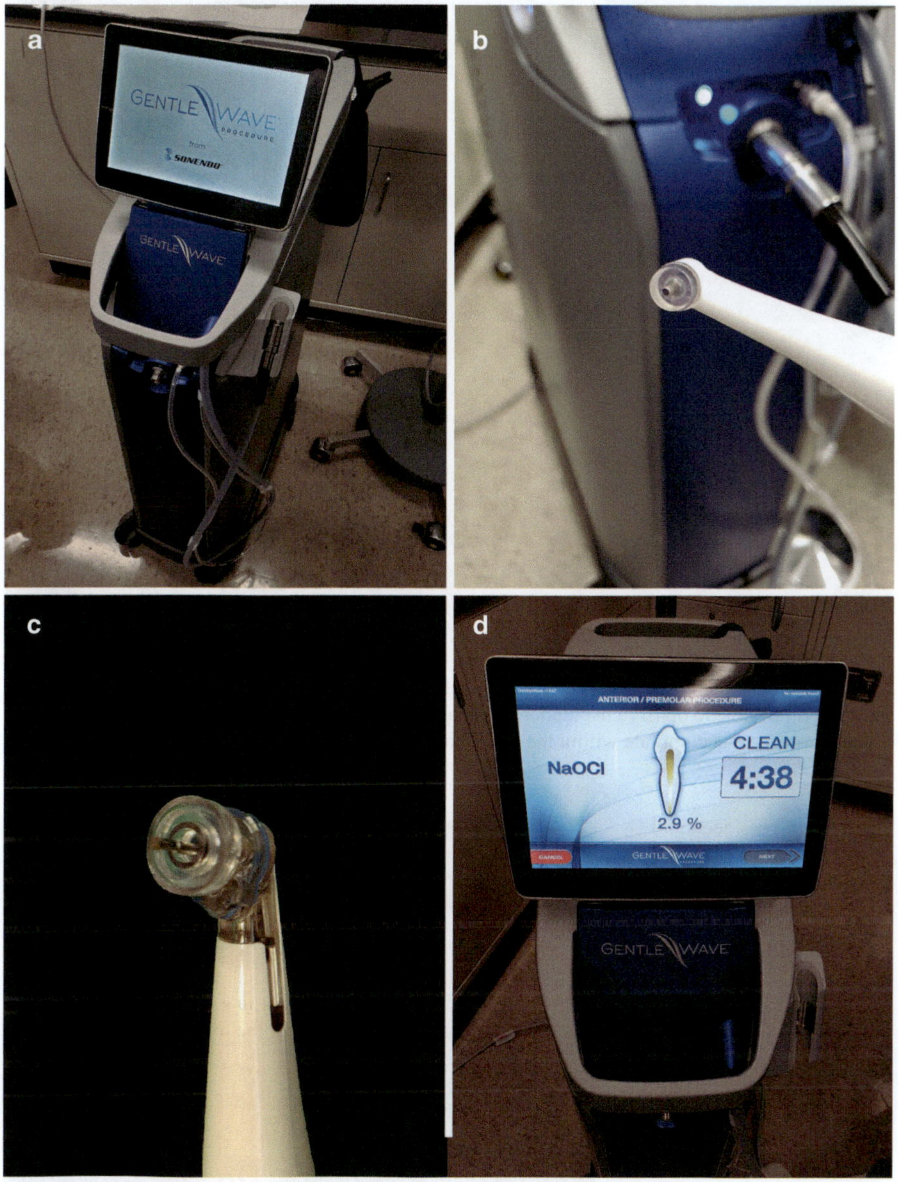

Fig. 2.16 (**a–d**) Multisonic ultraclean system or GentleWave system (Sonendo Inc., USA). This device consists of a console (**a**), a procedure instrument which is a single-use tip attached to a handpiece (**b**, **c**), and a central unit that contains three individual irrigation solution containers, one waste canister, a degassing system and a pressure generator. (**d**) The programmed irrigation regimen begins with 3% NaOCl followed by 8% EDTA, with a rinse of distilled water in between and at completion. The spray is released at approximately 45 mL/min and at a pressure of 9000 psi. The fluid within the root canal space is continuously removed from the chamber through a five-point vented suction system built in the sealing lid of the procedural instrument. (Courtesy of Dr. Ordinola-Zapata, USA)

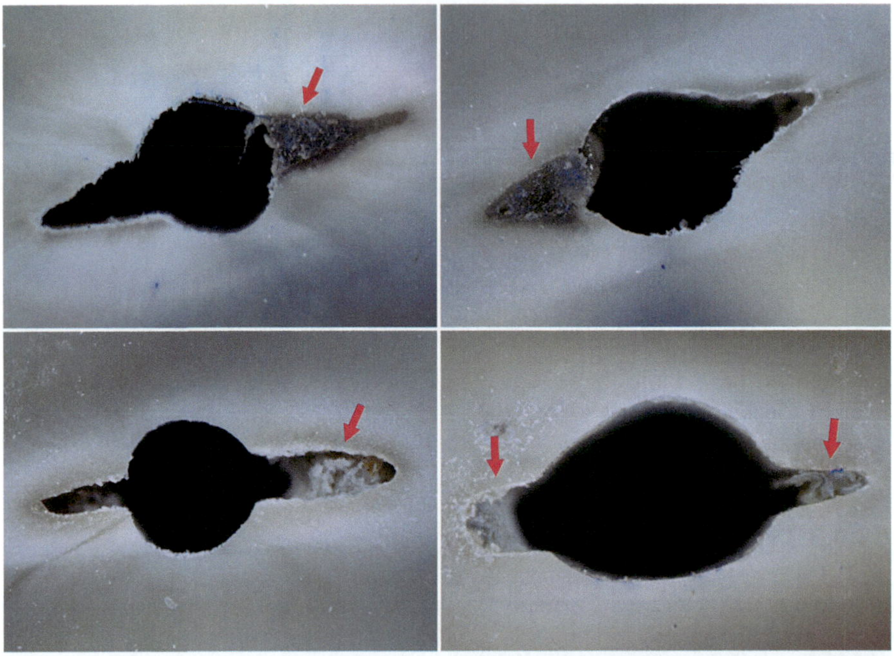

Fig. 2.17 Cross-sectional images of four oval-shaped canals after chemomechanical preparation in which is possible to observe the tendency of hard-tissue debris created by the mechanical instruments (arrows) to accumulate within the irregularities of the canal space

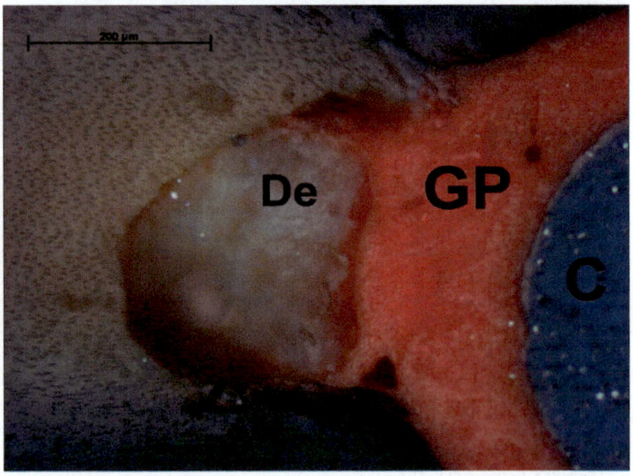

Fig. 2.18 Cross-sectional image of an oval-shaped canal after chemomechanical preparation showing hard-tissue debris (De) blocking the thermoplasticized gutta-percha (GP) to flow into an irregular area of the canal space

co-registered, i.e., different sets of data can be transformed and integrated into one coordinate system [32]. This procedure allows the detection of dentinal debris that were packed into the original root canal space after preparation by identifying "pixels that were occupied by air and then became dentin must be debris" [30, 31] (Figs. 2.19 and 2.20).

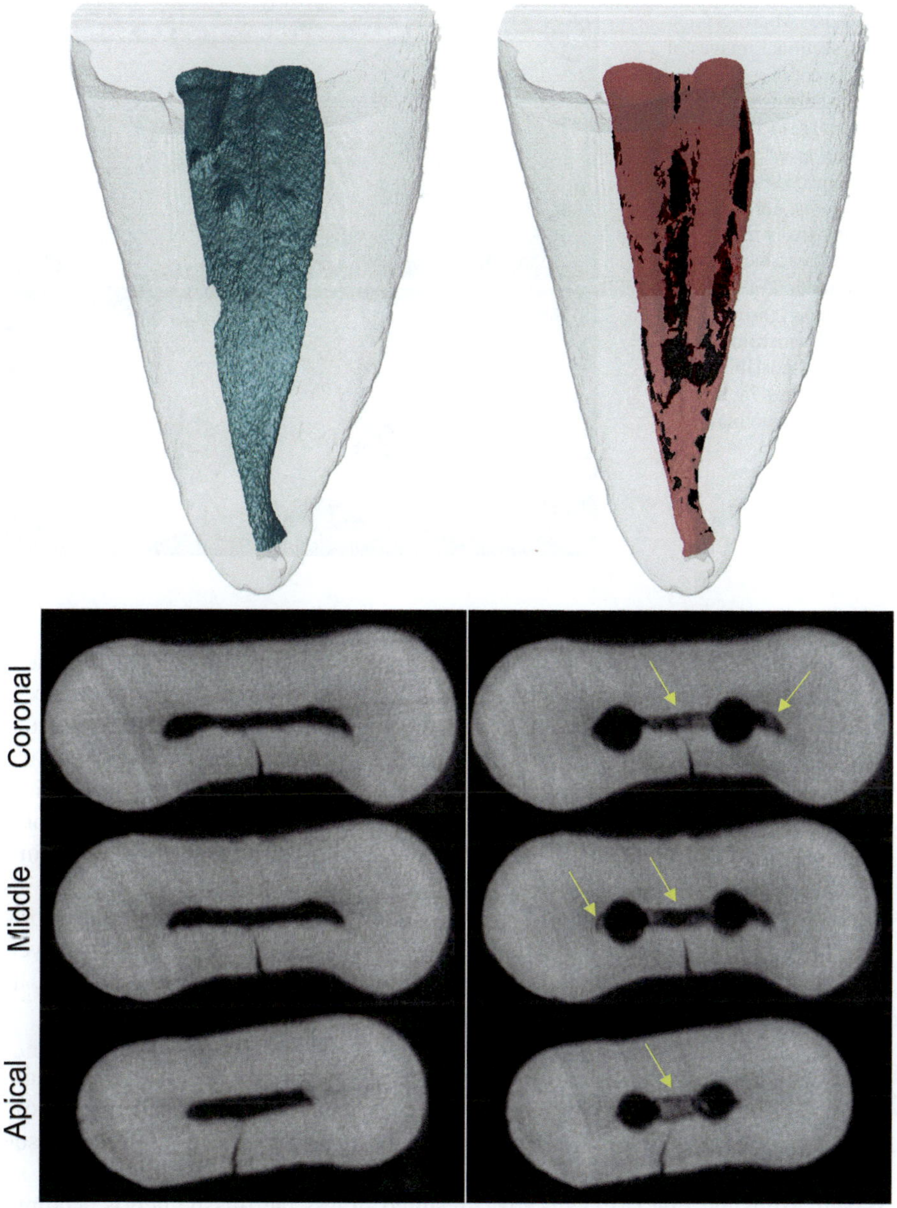

Fig. 2.19 3D models (top) and cross-sectional images (bottom) of a mesial root of a mandibular molar before (green) and after (red) preparation with a reciprocating instrument showing the accumulation of hard-tissue debris (in black) within the anatomical irregularities of the canal system at the coronal, middle and apical thirds (arrows)

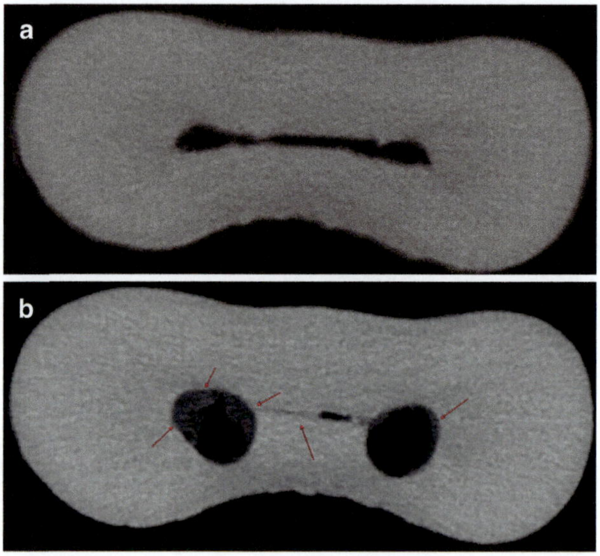

Fig. 2.20 Micro-CT cross-sectional images of a mesial root of a mandibular molar showing a large isthmus area (**a**) before and (**b**) after preparation. After chemomechanical procedures, not only the isthmus area was drastically reduced by the accumulation of hard-tissue debris (arrows) created by instruments, but also it was possible to observe debris in the lumen of the prepared canal (arrows)

Hard-tissue debris accumulation is a side effect of the mechanical preparation [32] and carries the likelihood of being more clinically relevant than the smear layer, which used to be an ever-present topic in the endodontic irrigation research. The rationale behind this assumption is that contaminated hard-tissue debris could easily harbor bacteria biofilm from the disinfection procedures and/or reduce the antiseptic activity of the irrigating solution [33–35]. As reported in a histological assessment of prepared mesial root canals of mandibular molars, the bacteria biofilm was apparently embedded in hard-tissue debris, reinforcing the potential clinical relevance of this phenomenon.

From the first studies on hard-tissue debris using micro-CT, scientific efforts were directed toward providing a better understanding of this phenomenon, as well as to develop effective anti-debris strategies. Interesting findings were reported, as follows:

1. EDTA and passive ultrasonic irrigation reduced hard-tissue debris accumulation, but approximately 50% of the debris still remained in the root canal space [36];
2. The use of a hypochlorite-compatible chelator enabled reduction of hard-tissue debris [37];
3. Self-Adjusting File (ReDent Nova) resulted in less hard-tissue debris accumulated in isthmus-containing canal systems than conventional rotary instrumentation and needle/syringe irrigation [38].

These findings need to be underscored because they were provided by methodologically sound experiments using the combination of micro-CT technology and image analysis. Additionally, the ability to independently assess the debris either in the non-instrumented isthmus or in the instrumented canal space is suitable as it enables the understanding of the effect of a given preparation technique or irrigating protocol not only in each one of these areas, but in the canal system as a whole. As a closing comment, we would like to emphasize that the current technology for canal shaping has been proven to be satisfactory from a technical point of view, but is still limited from a biological standpoint.

2.2 The Overload on the Shoulders of Irrigation

The suboptimal performance of the canal shaping methods reported in several studies using different methodologies ultimately lays too much responsibility on the shoulders of canal irrigation, which means that the final intracanal disinfection is largely dependent upon the physicochemical action of irrigation. Root canal irrigation, however, has its own limitations and is indeed overcharged by the technical restrictions of mechanical preparation.

Recent in vitro experiments demonstrated that, on the dentinal wall surfaces untouched by the instruments during mechanical preparation, biofilm can remain attached and probably covered with hard-tissue debris [25]. Thus, when instruments fail to prepare the canal walls in complex canal systems, like molar teeth, or even in ordinary oval-shaped canals, it is necessary to reach such unprepared areas with the NaOCl solution in order to dissolve the biofilm and remaining necrotic tissues. From that context arises the main challenge of canal irrigation, which is for the NaOCl solution to reach these unprepared canal areas at an effective concentration of free chlorine (its active component), with adequate volume and shear forces, as well as to stay in contact long enough to affect the target substrate. Thus, a question naturally arises:

To what extent is conventional irrigation effective in the cleaning and disinfection of unprepared canal areas?

Even though micro-CT technology can provide valuable and accurate measurements regarding the position and the amount of dentinal tissues affected or not by the shaping procedures, until recently no information could be given about the conditions of the pulp tissue or biofilm that remained attached to the canal walls. Thus, the rationale for a micro-CT assessment of shaping procedures is based on the assumption that if dentin was mechanically removed, consequently attached pulp tissue and/or biofilm were also displaced. However, an uncertainty remains as to whether the area unaffected by the mechanical procedure was properly cleaned by the irrigants (Fig. 2.21). Recently, a correlative approach using histology as a complementary method for micro-CT assessment was employed in two studies to evaluate different chemomechanical irrigating protocols [25, 39]. Both studies demonstrated, by histological examination, the presence of pulp tissue remnants attached to untouched canal walls previously identified by micro-CT analysis. In other words, unprepared canal areas were not predictably debrided, and this underlines the limited ability of conventional canal irrigation in compensating the limited performance of the shaping method itself. Therefore, it seems that the common belief that "the file shapes; the irrigant cleans" is based more on wishful thinking rather than on experimental evidence.

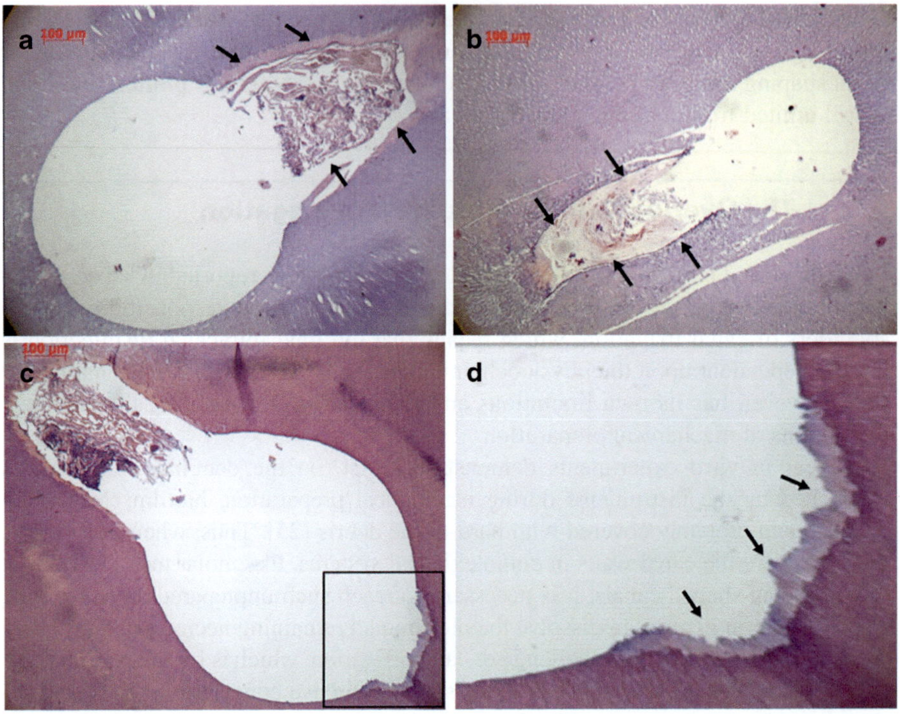

Fig. 2.21 (**a–c**) Histological cross sections of oval-shaped root canals after chemomechanical preparation showing the central area of the main canals were enlarged to a round shape after preparation with NiTi instruments leaving untouched their buccal and lingual extensions (black arrows). (**d**) High magnification of the square area in (**c**) showing the predentin layer in a slight irregularity of the root canal space which was not mechanically prepared by the NiTi instrument. Even small areas like this can contain infected tissue that may compromise the long-term outcome of the root canal preparation

2.3 The Shaping for Cleaning Concept

One co-author of this chapter (MZ), in his review on root canal irrigation from 2006, formally raised concerns regarding the potential consequences of overly quick mechanical canal preparation, stating that: "*Even fast-acting biocides like sodium hypochlorite require an adequate working time to reach their potential. This should be specially considered in view of the fact that rotary canal preparation techniques have expedited the shaping process*" [40]. However, some years before, Berutti and Castellucci [41] had already suggested that the operative sequence of cleaning and shaping should be reversed:

> …today, it is preferred to speak in terms of "shaping" first and "cleaning" later. Furthermore, taking into consideration the results obtained with the new NiTi instruments, which allow ideally shaped canals sometimes in just a few minutes while the cleaning of the same system needs much more time, today it is considered more appropriate to speak in terms of shaping and cleaning, since in chronological order the root canal system is first shaped and then later becomes adequately cleaned, if irrigation protocols are followed.

Seven years later, Peters [42] also mentioned that: "*Although the terms cleaning and shaping are often used to describe root canal treatment procedures, reversing the order to shaping and cleaning more correctly reflects the fact that enlarged canals direct and facilitate the cleaning action of irrigants and removal of infected dentin.*" Using other words, Haapasalo [33] followed the same train of thought: "*In teeth with simple root canal anatomy and large canals where instrumentation may be finished quickly, NaOCl irrigation should be continued following instrumentation to provide enough time for the tissue dissolution and antibacterial effects.*"

As noticed, some researchers had foreseen the new scenario created by overfast canal shaping. Yet, despite the word of warning from these authors, attention was not given to a crucial point: the traditional Cleaning & Shaping concept is grounded on a slow shaping procedure in which the time necessary for the NaOCl reaches its full potential is naturally achieved. As long as contemporary endodontics is conceptual and evidence-based driven by principle, it is natural to question the impact of the expedited shaping on treatment outcome and, therefore, to critically decode the clinical impact of this overfast canal shaping. This understanding affects the dynamic of the traditional Cleaning & Shaping concept and is a prerequisite to guide us toward a predictable improvement of the cleaning and disinfection procedures. Considering the limits of NaOCl-based irrigation, the following sentence aimed to start trying to eradicate the idea that overfast canal shaping is the effective way of saving time: the intracanal cleaning and disinfection process using chlorine solutions is a function of time and is the point at which the current problems emerge. Thus, a paradox is created: on one hand, canal shaping techniques have undergone an unprecedented evolution with the development of NiTi instruments able to cut significant amounts of dentin in short periods of time, while on the other hand, the universally accepted irrigating solution for more than one century—the sodium hypochlorite—demands a long period of time to reach its full potential. In practice, this means that the root canal is shaped, but not yet properly cleaned and disinfected. Thus, we consider that, in contemporary endodontic practice, the term "**Shaping for Cleaning**" must replace the classical "**Cleaning & Shaping**" concept; in this sense, when we shape to clean, we are incidentally saying that the canal shaping will save operative time that can be used wisely for increasing the efficacy of subsequent cleaning and disinfection procedures.

In this new concept, it is important to identify cleaning and shaping as isolated procedures from both operative and temporal aspects. The Shaping for Cleaning approach is based on undertaking an irrigation method capable of reaping the benefits of the shaped and enlarged condition of the root canal space by:

1. Optimizing the irrigation process as much as possible once it is running smoothly to operate the traditional syringe–needle irrigation process and also to employ further irrigation methods in a larger canal space. Effective irrigation demands a high flow rate and turbulence of the irrigation solution as well as placing the needle tip close to the WL (Figs. 2.22 and 2.23). These conditions are more predictably achieved in a shaped and enlarged canal space because, at least theoretically, it facilitates the NaOCl solution to reach the unprepared dentinal walls at

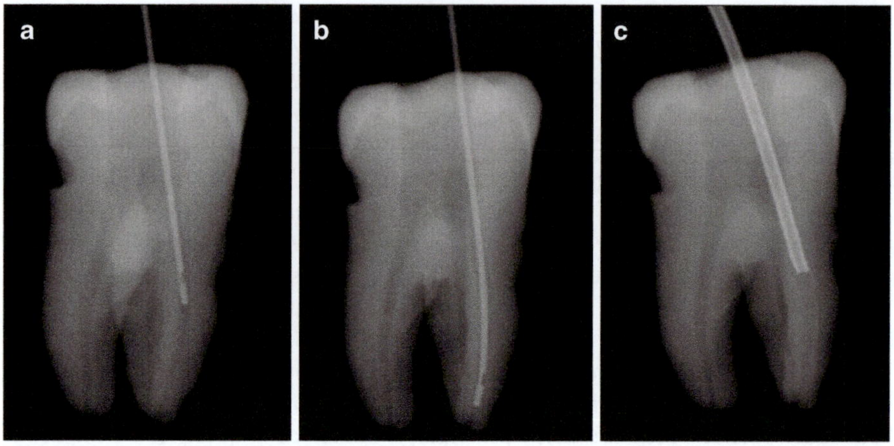

Fig. 2.22 Radiographic images showing (**a**) a 30-G close-ended side-vented needle before and (**b**) after canal preparation of a mandibular molar. (**c**) It is important to highlight that even after preparation, a 25-G open-ended flat needle is unable to reach the apical portion of the root canal

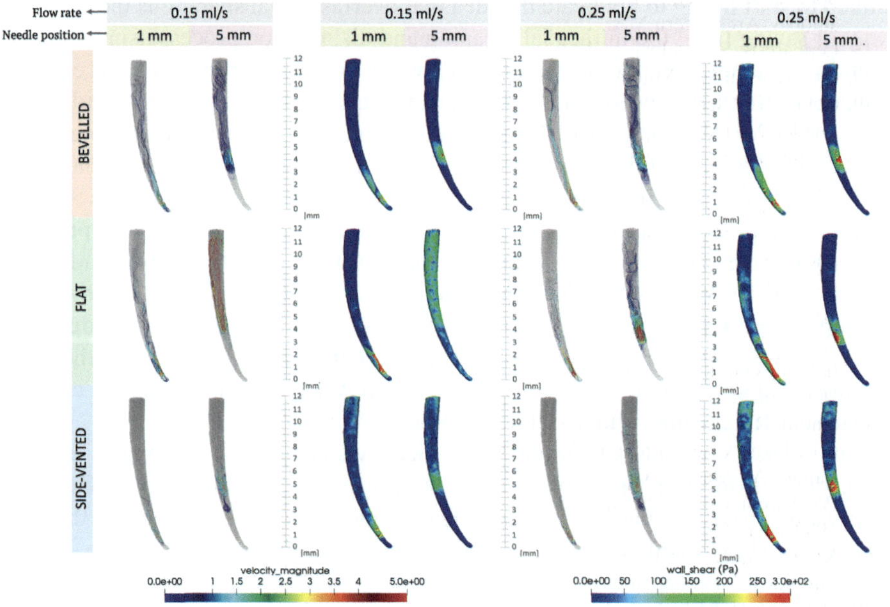

Fig. 2.23 Flow pattern, irrigant velocity, and shear stress produced by positive pressure irrigation with different needle types (beveled, flat and side-vented), insertion depths (1 and 5 mm), flow rates (0.15 and 0.25 m/s) using the Computational Fluid Dynamics method applied to 3D models of real mesial curved canals of mandibular molars obtained through micro-CT technology after canal enlargement with a size 25, 0.08v large-tapered instrument. Color-coded images show that turbulence of the irrigating solution is more effective closest to the needle tip and that the apical region is only affected when the needle tip is positioned 1 mm from the working length

an effective concentration of its active component, with adequate volume, flush and contact time to reach its full potential.

2. Timesaving with the overfast shaping may turn into a profitable transoperative condition when all the efforts focus on maximizing the intracanal contact time of the NaOCl with the dentinal walls. Irrigation is divided into two well-separated phases: a flow phase, when there is a flow movement throughout the full extent of the canal, and the resting phase, when the irrigant solution is placed and kept standstill. The enlarged-shaped condition of the canal simplifies and optimizes both phases (Figs. 2.24 and 2.25).

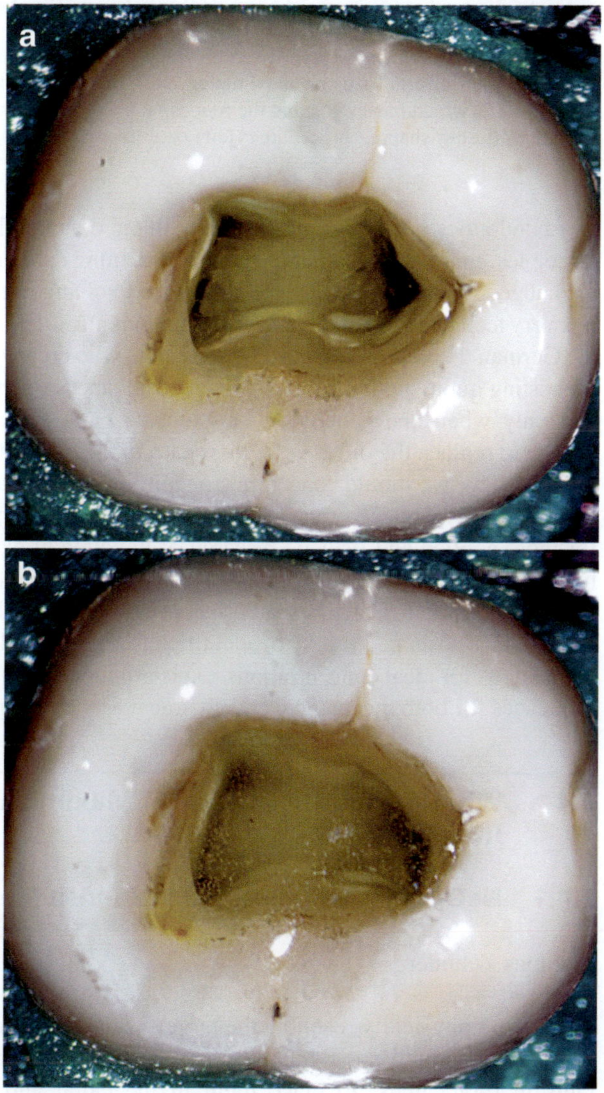

Fig. 2.24 (**a**) Resting phase in the Shaping for Cleaning protocol. The resting phase takes place when the canal is filled with the irrigant solution and kept standstill. The enlarged-shaped condition of the canal simplifies and optimizes this important phase of the cleaning-disinfection process. (**b**) The formation of bubbles during the resting phase (which can be seen through a dental microscope) indicates that NaOCl solution is still acting over the organic matter within the canal space

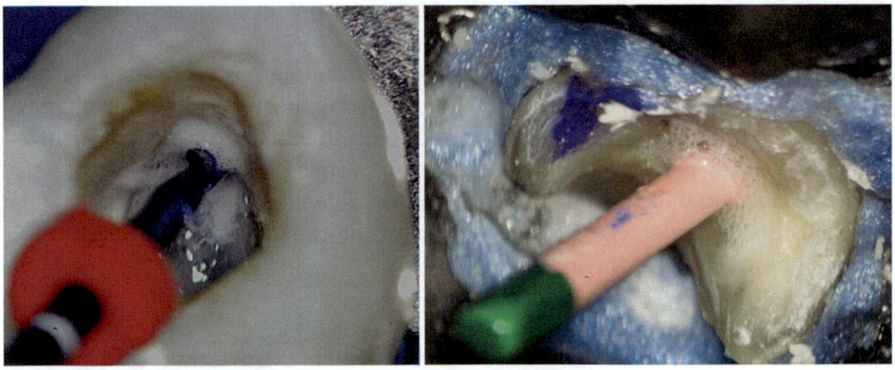

Fig. 2.25 The timesaving with the overfast shaping may turn into a profitable transoperative condition when all efforts focus on maximizing the intracanal contact time of the NaOCl with the dentinal walls which means keeping the root canal flooded with irrigant solution in all transoperative steps, during shaping procedures (left) or even when testing the gutta-percha master cone fit (right)

Endodontics is a traditional specialty in the dental field in which some of its core principles, such as the classical Schilder's Cleaning & Shaping concept, have remained unchanged for decades. Thus, the resistance to changes is understandable, even more in a very technical and clinical area like endodontics. The famous Nobel-prize winner, the German theoretical physicist Max Planck, who created the quantum theory, had an interesting quote on that subject: "Science advances one funeral at a time." He meant that only when one generation of scientists passes away, do new theories have a chance to replace the old ones. With regard to the topic of this section, from a clinical point of view, we should concentrate on putting into operation shaping first and cleaning afterwards while, from a scientific perspective, it is necessary to move the target for more applied and realistic research of the already-existing irrigation models and methods. As Haapasalo [43] precisely observed, throughout the years, much of the focus in irrigation-related research has been placed on the study of the smear layer. For instance, it is necessary to scientifically establish clinical guidance and recommendations for ideal concentrations, exposure times, flow rates, and optimal operative sequences for both mechanical and chemical aspects of irrigation.

2.4 What to Do After Shaping? Maximizing the NaOCl Intracanal Time

2.4.1 NaOCl as a Non-agitated Intra-Visit Medication

Matthias Zehnder

Apart from physically reaching the target, which in our context is intracanal biofilm and necrotic pulp tissue remnants, there is a second route to administering disinfectants in root canals: to place them in the canal and let them passively act by diffusion. According to Fick's second law of diffusion, in any liquid-filled closed space dissolved molecules flow in a gradient of concentration until a state of equilibrium is reached. Root canals are intrinsically wet [44], and therefore aqueous carriers for the disinfecting/cleansing chemicals to be administered are the best choice. The classical "passive" intracanal antimicrobial agent is calcium hydroxide ($Ca(OH)_2$), which is prepared as a suspension from the pure chemical powder. Some commercial products contain up to 50 wt% of a radiopacifier, which, in the eyes of the authors, is not necessary. Calcium hydroxide is not very soluble in water [45], and therefore the suspension acts as a depot for alkali (OH-), creating an environment that is not tolerated well by bacteria. Because of the above-described chemistry of calcium hydroxide suspensions, thin slurries disinfect better than counterparts with too much powder and little liquid [46]. Moreover, a calcium hydroxide suspension requires time to act, and is best administered as an interim dressing with at least 1–2 weeks between visits [47]. Apart from its antimicrobial effect, a calcium hydroxide suspension also cleans out necrotic tissue remnants [48, 49] and dissolves biofilms including their matrix (unpublished observations).

Another way to chemically clean the root canal has not been investigated in depth, but is used in many endodontic practices: leaving a fast-acting antimicrobial agent passively in the canal system during the treatment session. Depending on the practice environment, this can be advantageous when, for example, another patient can be tended to and the goal is to finish the root canal treatment in one single visit. The only scientifically sound clinical study with a proper design on this topic was performed in Sweden, using 5% iodine potassium iodide as the "intra-visit medicament" [50]. Disinfection was similar to that achieved by an inter-visit calcium hydroxide dressing. However, in the opinion of the authors of this chapter, root canal cleaning goes beyond mere disinfection. Using an agent that only disinfects but does not clean, such as iodine potassium iodide, makes little sense in that context. As an example, a recent case series showed that vital cases treated in one visit with a chlorhexidine solution and no NaOCl as the disinfectant in combination with EDTA to remove the smear layer showed a remarkably low success rate, which was no higher than that of necrotic or retreatment cases [51]. This may be explained by the fact that root canal instrumentation leaves formerly vital pulp tissue behind [14], which will then turn necrotic and can act as a pathway for invading microorganisms. It appears obvious that if the concept is to seal the root canal as tightly as possible using gutta-percha and a sealer, then pulp tissue remnants should be removed. In the context of intra-visit medication, it may thus be a good idea to use an NaOCl solution, which is the only root canal irrigant with any soft-tissue-dissolving effect [52].

The concept of placing a NaOCl solution passively in the root canal system during the treatment visit has not been studied in clinics. However, some useful information from ex vivo experiments in extracted human teeth is available. When placed passively in the root canal system, a NaOCl solution of between 1 and 5.5% remains active for about 1 h, i.e. above a concentration of 0.1%, which is still strongly antiseptic [53]. One more advantage of placing an NaOCl solution passively into an instrumented root canal system is its diagnostic value. As long as there are organic remnants from biofilm and/or pulp tissue in the root canals, the NaOCl will react and form carbon dioxide (and also oxygen), that rise to the surface of the solution. This means that more cleaning is necessary before the root canal system can be filled.

If a two-visit approach is favored or indicated, then the calcium hydroxide dressing can be mixed (in the case of commercial $Ca(OH)_2$ pastes) or the powder can be directly suspended in the NaOCl solution used for root canal irrigation [49]. This will provide a double effect: the NaOCl will be active for about 1 h beyond the treatment visit, and suspended $Ca(OH)_2$ will then still be there to create a long-term environment in the root canal system that is not well tolerated by microorganisms. In this context, it should be mentioned that both NaOCl and $Ca(OH)_2$ are proteolytic agents, and could thus make teeth more prone to fracture based on their effects on the collagen in the dentin [54]. The effects of the NaOCl, especially in concentrated solutions of more than 3%, are much higher, though, than those of the calcium hydroxide [55, 56]. Therefore, the authors of this chapter would advise against using a NaOCl solution of more than 3% in clinical endodontics, as there is no clinical data supporting the usage of such concentrated solutions [57, 58], and ample in vitro data showing that it can affect tooth integrity [59]. One core aspect, which is sometimes forgotten by keen endodontists, should be kept in mind: Preserving teeth should be our main goal. Root canal-treated teeth of patients with good oral hygiene are lost as a result of vertical root fractures much more often than for any other reason [60].

2.4.2 Updated Syringe-Needle Irrigation: A Close-to-WL Approach

Despite the extensive amount of publications and the long tradition in research on irrigation and agitation techniques, the conventional delivery of the irrigant solution by a syringe-needle system is still the most commonly used irrigation method [61, 62] either used exclusively or alternating with other techniques [63]. Irrigants are fundamentally delivered into the canal space through a needle connected to a syringe by a traditional luer-lock connection (Fig. 2.26). The use of the simple syringe-needle system has a long history in endodontics and its role was precisely highlighted by Boutsioukis and van der Sluis et al. [64]: "It seems rather unlikely that syringe irrigation will be totally replaced by other delivery system techniques any time soon." By itself, this perspective justifies the renewed research interest in better protocols for syringe-needle-based irrigation.

Although essentially simple, the operation of the syringe is difficult to control and standardize among clinicians. The professional applies finger pressure on the syringe plunger, which pushes the irrigant solution through the needle and into the canal space, a technique which is usually referred to as the so-called "positive pressure irrigation technique" or simply "direct injection."

As a rule of thumb, the irrigant should never be forced into the canal, and therefore forefinger pressure as opposed to thumb pressure is the highest pressure suggested. Yet, this is a quite subjective recommendation since it creates difficulties for

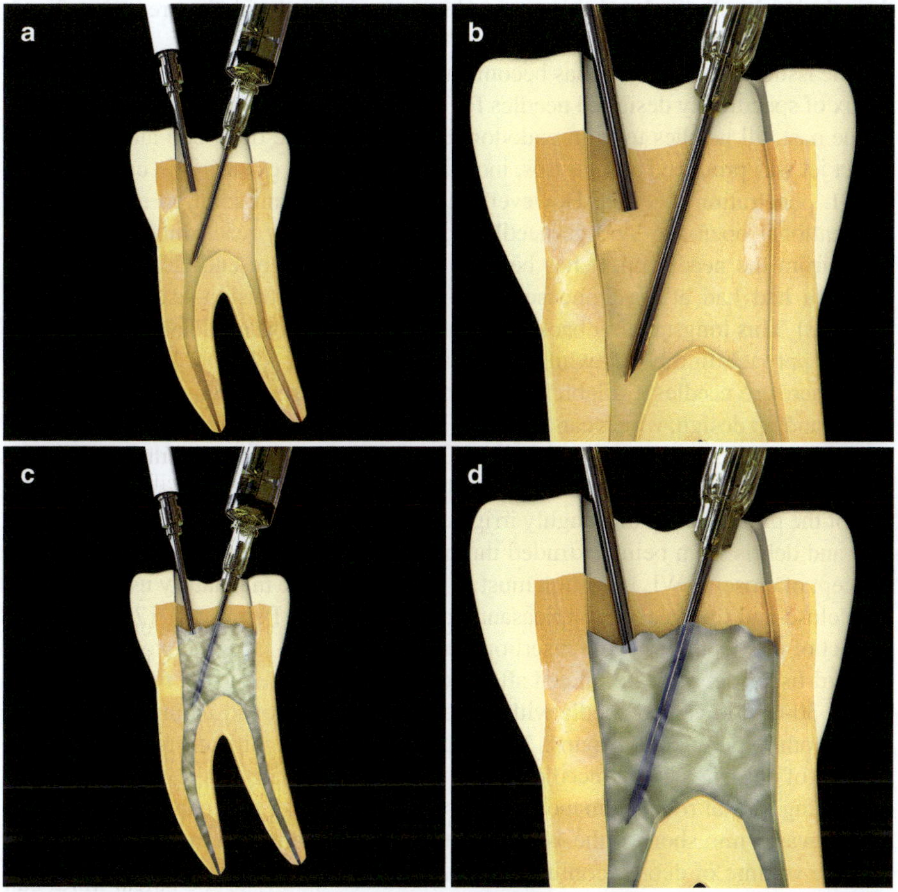

Fig. 2.26 Positive pressure irrigation technique. (**a, b**) Syringe-needle and suction cannula routinely used for positive pressure irrigation. (**c, d**) The clinician applies finger pressure on the syringe plunger, which pushes the irrigant solution through the needle into the canal space by directly injecting the solution while it is simultaneously aspirated by the suction cannula

a more reproducible clinical guideline. Moreover, it is necessary to prevent the binding of the needle to the canal walls, as it can act like a piston, forcing the solution beyond the apex, requiring constant attention during the irrigation process.

Dr. Louis Grossman [65] was the first to provide detailed and specific guidelines for canal irrigation with the syringe-needle method, and his orientations have been used by clinicians worldwide for decades [64]. At that period, only inappropriately large needles (21–25G) were available resulting in partial or even no penetration of the irrigant into the whole canal space. While part-way penetration of the needle into the canal provides only very limited circulation of the irrigant, it also controls the risk of NaOCl extrusion. The endpoint of using large needles is the well-known inability to irrigate the apical region given the difficulty of spreading and flushing the solution in a limited and narrow canal space combined with the presence of back pressure and/or gas entrapment.

The issue around needles has become more complex since the rapid development influx of specifically designed needles for endodontic irrigation over the last decade. In the past, all needles used in endodontic treatment were open-end and an intense direct jet was produced at their tips, increasing the risk of extrusion in case of close-to-WL penetration [66, 67]. However, although the irrigant solution used with the conventional open-end syringe-needle technique does not reach more than 1 mm away from the needle tip, it has been reported that 42% of endodontists in North America had had at least one accident with NaOCl extrusion using this procedure [68]. This longstanding background explains why most clinicians often avoid a closer approach to the WL while irrigating with NaOCl solution. However, nowadays, there are needles available on the international market varying in size (gauge), length and tip design, which can be placed 1 mm from the WL, and to rinse the apical third in an effective and safe way (Fig. 2.22). The jet created by the side-vented needle, for example, produces an upward turbulent motion around and beyond the end of the probe, which thoroughly irrigates the root canal system and prevents solution and debris from being extruded through the apical foramen [69, 70]. Thus, the concept of close-to-WL irrigation must be followed by the mandatory use of needles with close-end tips to avoid unpleasant NaOCl incidents. Perez et al. [71] tested the impact of the depth of needle insertion (at 1 mm or 5 mm from the working length) on hard-tissue debris accumulated after root canal preparation using micro-CT. They used a 30-G side-vented needle with a lateral lumen positioned 2 mm from its blunt tip in both experimental groups. The results showed a significant reduction in the volume of debris when the needle tip was placed 1 mm short of the WL in isthmus-containing mesial roots of mandibular molars. In contrast, root canals in which the needle was 5 mm short of the WL exhibited almost a threefold increase in the percentage volume of debris, confirming that the optimization of the cleaning process using conventional syringe–needle irrigation is related to the depth of needle penetration.

Side-vented fine-diameter needles (30 or 31G) easily outperform the ordinary open-ended larger needles (21–25G) and the most likely explanation for this is that they improve the irrigant exchange by the interplay of two factors: (1) the larger escape area around the needle for the reverse flow of the solution toward the canal orifice; and (2) the better irrigant flow and refreshment in the apical third. The physical effect promoted by the reverse flow is important to carry out planktonic bacteria, biofilm, soft- and hard-tissue debris detached or washed out from the irregular areas by the frictional forces between the flowing solution and the dentinal walls [72, 73]. Moreover, small-sized flexible needles do not demand an over enlargement of the canal to reach the WL, even if it is curved (Figs. 2.27 and 2.28). A significant development in this context can be seen in the recently launched side-vented polypropylene tips by Produits Dentaires (Vevey, Switzerland). These tips, if equipped with a rubber stopper, allow for the controlled delivery of the irrigant to working length even in severely curved and narrowly prepared root canals. Nowadays, different types of needles for root canal irrigation are available in the market (Fig. 2.29).

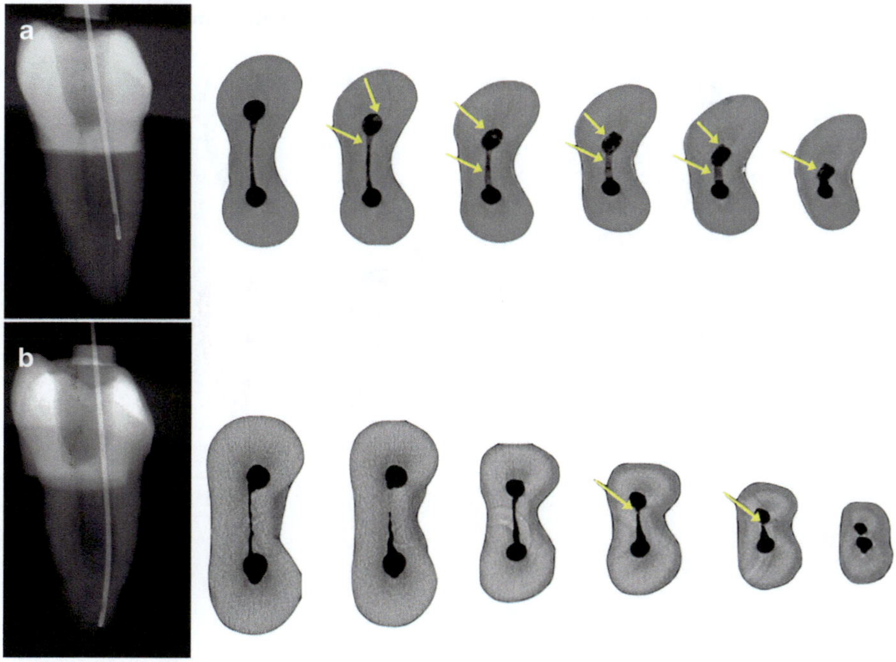

Fig. 2.27 Radiography (on the left) and cross-sectional micro-CT images of mesial roots of mandibular molars showing the use of a 30-G close-ended side-vented needle at (**a**) 5 mm and (**b**) 1 mm from the working length. Irrigation at 5 mm (**a**) allowed for the accumulation of debris in the isthmus area and the lumen of the prepared canal (arrows). However, when the needle was placed 1 mm from the working length (**b**), no accumulated debris could be observed

Regarding its size, a 5 mL irrigation syringe has been recommended as it presents a good balance between the refilling rate and operating, allowing proper flow rates of around 0.20–25 mL/s to be reached. As a good example of a syringe designed for endodontic irrigation, the Ultradent (South Jordan, USA) 5-mL syringe barrels has its walls (with precise internal diameters) treated by a proprietary process able to maintain an airtight seal with pistons, thus allowing a smoother delivery flow. In summary, a combination of a 5 mL syringe with small-sized close-end side-vented needles (30 or 31G) is able to provide close-to-optimal flow rates (~0.25 mL/s), affording an effective refreshment of the solution at the apical third [74].

Within the context of the Shaping for Cleaning concept, a close-to-WL syringe-needle irrigation can be considered as a great strategy to optimize the cleaning and disinfection process. Syringe-needle irrigation is the right tool for the stagnation phase of the irrigation (later discussed in this chapter), which is a crucial aspect of the Shaping for Cleaning concept.

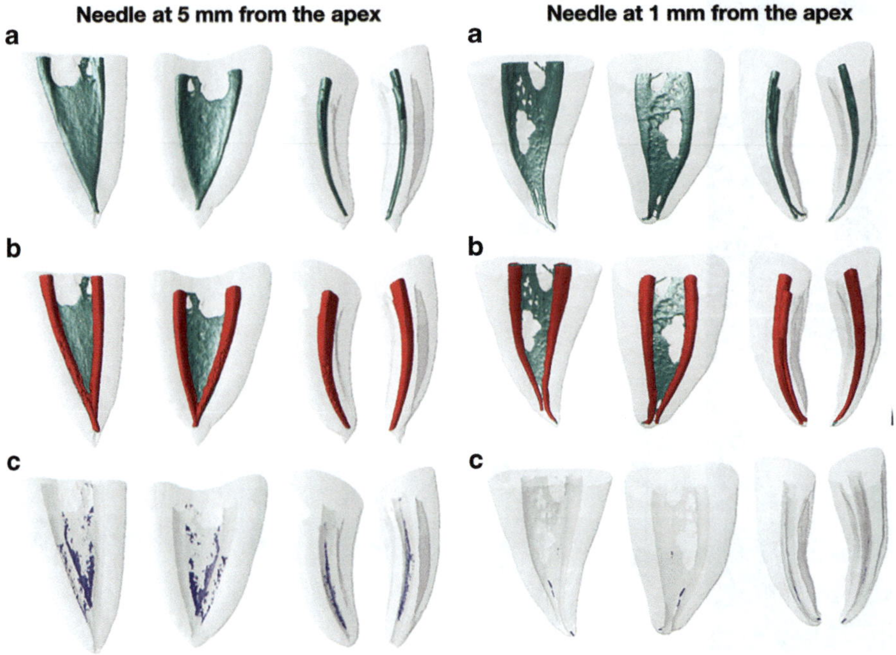

Fig. 2.28 Different views of 3D models of 2 mesial roots of mandibular molars (**a**) before (in green) and (**b**) after (in red) shaping procedures with Reciproc R25 instrument. During preparation, canals were irrigated with the needle positioned at 5 (on the left) or 1 mm (on the right) short of the working length. (**c**) Superimposition of the micro-CT models allowed to observe large amounts of hard-tissue debris (in blue) accumulated in the root canal space (in blue) when the needle was placed at 5 mm from the working length, compared to the 1 mm level

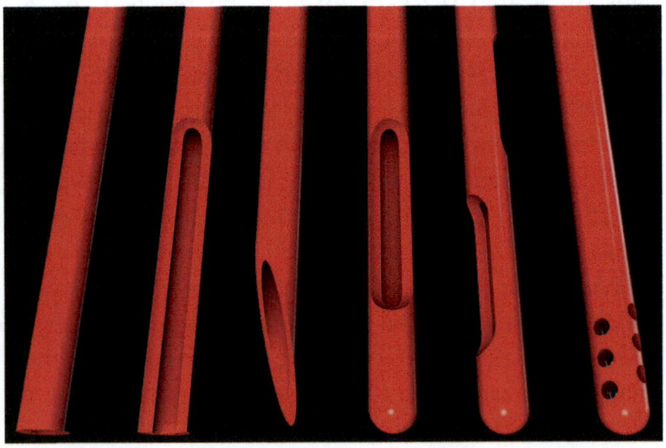

Fig. 2.29 Types of needles for root canal irrigation. From left to right, the open-ended (flat, notched, and beveled) and closed-ended (side-vented, double-side-vented, and multi-vented) needles

2.4.3 Handling the Vapor Lock Phenomenon

Syringe-based irrigation has limitations mainly when traditionally open-ended needles are used far from the apex. Because of its predominant laminar flow, it is well documented that a dead-water or stagnation zone is produced in between the tip of the close-ended needle and the apex, where no irrigant flux occurs [75–77], resulting in gross debris accumulation in this region [78].

Since the late 2010s, studies have demonstrated the creation of air bubbles at the apical canal end during syringe irrigation (Figs. 2.30 and 2.31). Gas bubbles occur because the root canal behaves as a close-ended system [79] once roots are

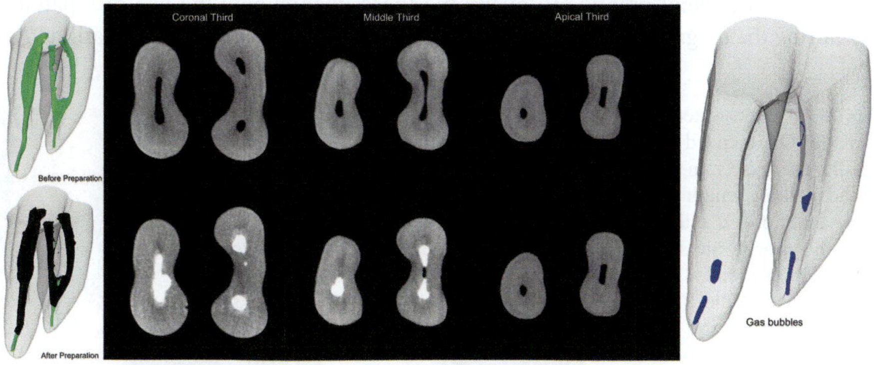

Fig. 2.30 Root canal system of a mandibular molar tooth showing the three-dimensional morphology (on the left) and cross sections of the original canal (in green) before (top) and after (bottom) chemomechanical preparation depicting the irrigant solution in black (3D models) and white (cross sections), as well as, apical gas bubbles (in blue) in irrigant-free areas (on the right)

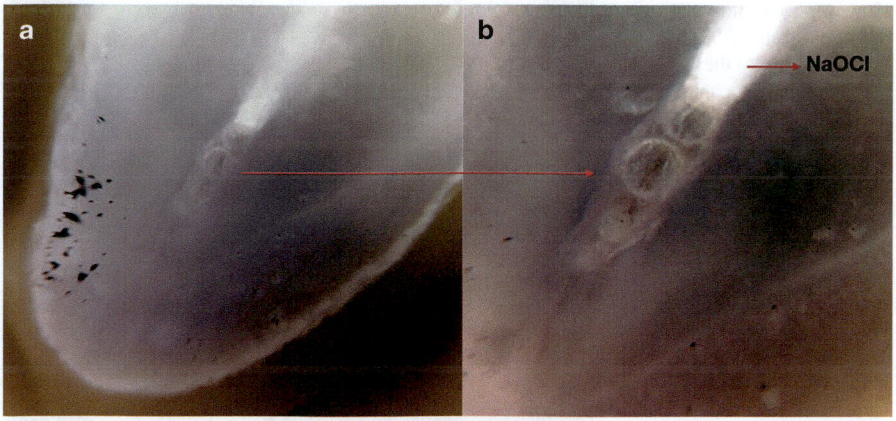

Fig. 2.31 The vapor lock phenomenon. (**a**, **b**) Apical third of a mandibular molar irrigated with NaOCl solution showing the presence of apical gas bubbles (arrow) blocking the penetration of the NaOCl solution. (Courtesy of Prof. Alfredo Landolo, Italy)

surrounded by the periodontal ligament and bone. This phenomenon, known as an "apical vapor lock" was confirmed not only by a series of laboratory experiments using simulated closed-end root canal systems, but also in the clinical setting [78, 80]. Its origin is attributed to the interplay between the air bubble entrapment originated by the irrigation delivery (positive pressure) and gas production created by the chemical reaction of the NaOCl with organic tissues. As a result, the vapor lock can theoretically block the irrigant from flowing toward the apical third. It must be conceded here, however, that this was propagated and, the name "vapor lock", created by the developer of the first negative pressure irrigation device, John Schoeffel. Nevertheless, vapor lock and dead-water zone phenomena (Fig. 2.32) have a negative impact in the apical cleaning and disinfection [78]. Two approaches have been suggested in clinical practice to overcome these phenomena: the use of a patency file during the irrigation process [80–82] and apical negative pressure irrigation [78].

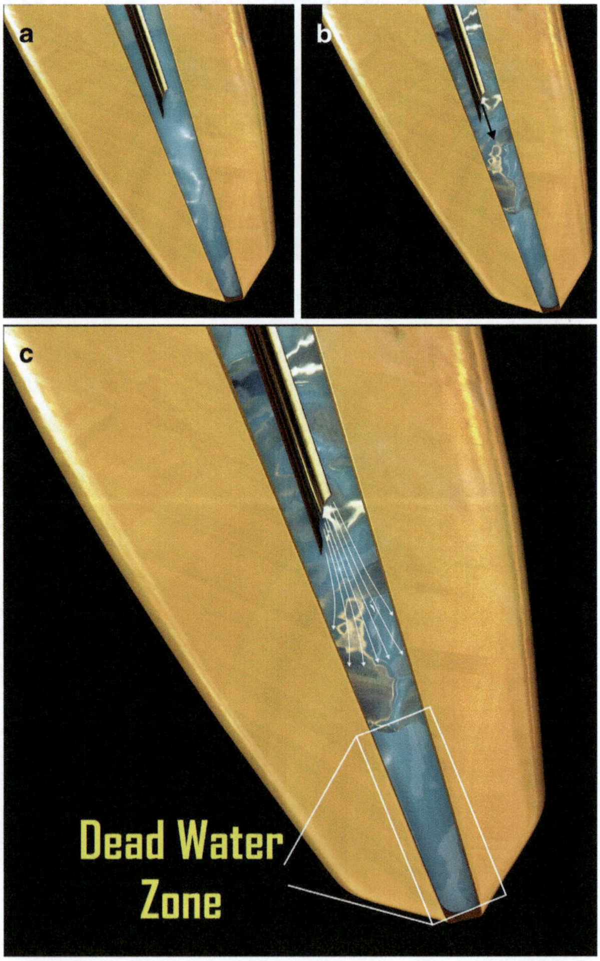

Fig. 2.32 Dead-water zone. (**a**) Open-ended needle inserted 3 mm short of the working length in a root canal flooded with sodium hypochlorite. (**b**) Although open-ended needles create a more intense jet of irrigant apically, which is a clear advantage in terms of irrigant penetration in the main root canal, jet penetration is dependent on the size and taper after apical enlargement as well as on the irrigant flow rate. However, irrigant usually does not reach farther than 1 mm apically to the needle tip in root canals having an apical size less than 30. (**c**) Considering the predominant laminar flow of syringe-based irrigation, it is well documented that a dead-water or stagnation zone is produced in between the tip of needle and the apex, where no irrigant flux occurs

2.4.4 The Role of the Patency File

In three important clinical studies, Vera et al. [80–82] demonstrated that the apical patency is able to optimize the distribution of the irrigation solution in the apical third by overcoming the vapor lock phenomenon (Fig. 2.33). Authors reported that the phenomenon of gas bubble trapping occurred in 40% of non-patent root canal canals, while 25% of the cases showed gas bubbles when the apical patency was performed throughout the irrigation procedure. It was postulated that the gas or air bubbles move toward canal entrance by the action of the in-and-out movement of the patency file. The authors concluded that the presence of gas bubbles in the middle and cervical thirds is a common finding that does not depend on the use of a patency file, but they clarify that the maintenance of a patent foramen significantly minimizes its presence, improving the irrigant delivery into the apical zone. Unpublished observations by the authors strongly suggest that even in closed simulated canal systems, gas bubbles can be removed rather easily from the apical third using a slim irrigation needle close to working length. It is timely to highlight that the simple presence of the NaOCl within the root canal space does not assure a proper cleaning-disinfection process as it needs to stay in place long enough until it reaches its full potential by both disrupting the extracellular matrix of the biofilm and dissolving the remaining pulp tissue.

2.4.5 Negative Apical Pressure Irrigation

Traditionally, root canal irrigation has been based on positive apical pressure using the syringe-needle technique, however, currently, negative pressure irrigation is also proposed. The efficiency of this technique is dependent on positioning the suction cannula at the apical region of the canal, which aspirates the irrigating solution that is supplied in the pulp chamber. The first irrigation system using negative apical pressure (EndoVac; SybronEndo, USA) became commercially available in 2007. However, an earlier report on apical aspiration using negative pressure was made in 1980 by Alceu Berbert, Professor at Bauru School of Dentistry in Brazil [83] (Fig. 2.34). Even before that, a multitude of negative pressure devices have been described, especially in the German literature [84].

Currently, there is a considerable body of evidence showing that this approach is able to improve the cleaning and disinfection process as well as the overall safety of the irrigation procedure [85–90]. The EndoVac irrigation system is based on two distinct phases: macro-irrigation and micro-irrigation. A tip adapted to a conventional syringe promotes irrigation and aspiration simultaneously with the aid of the high-power suction of the equipment. The irrigation/aspiration tip delivers large amounts of irrigation solution into the pulp chamber while controlling its excessive flow. The macro-cannula is a small plastic tube with a final opening of 0.55 mm and a .02 taper and is responsible for the suction of excess irrigation solution. In its turn,

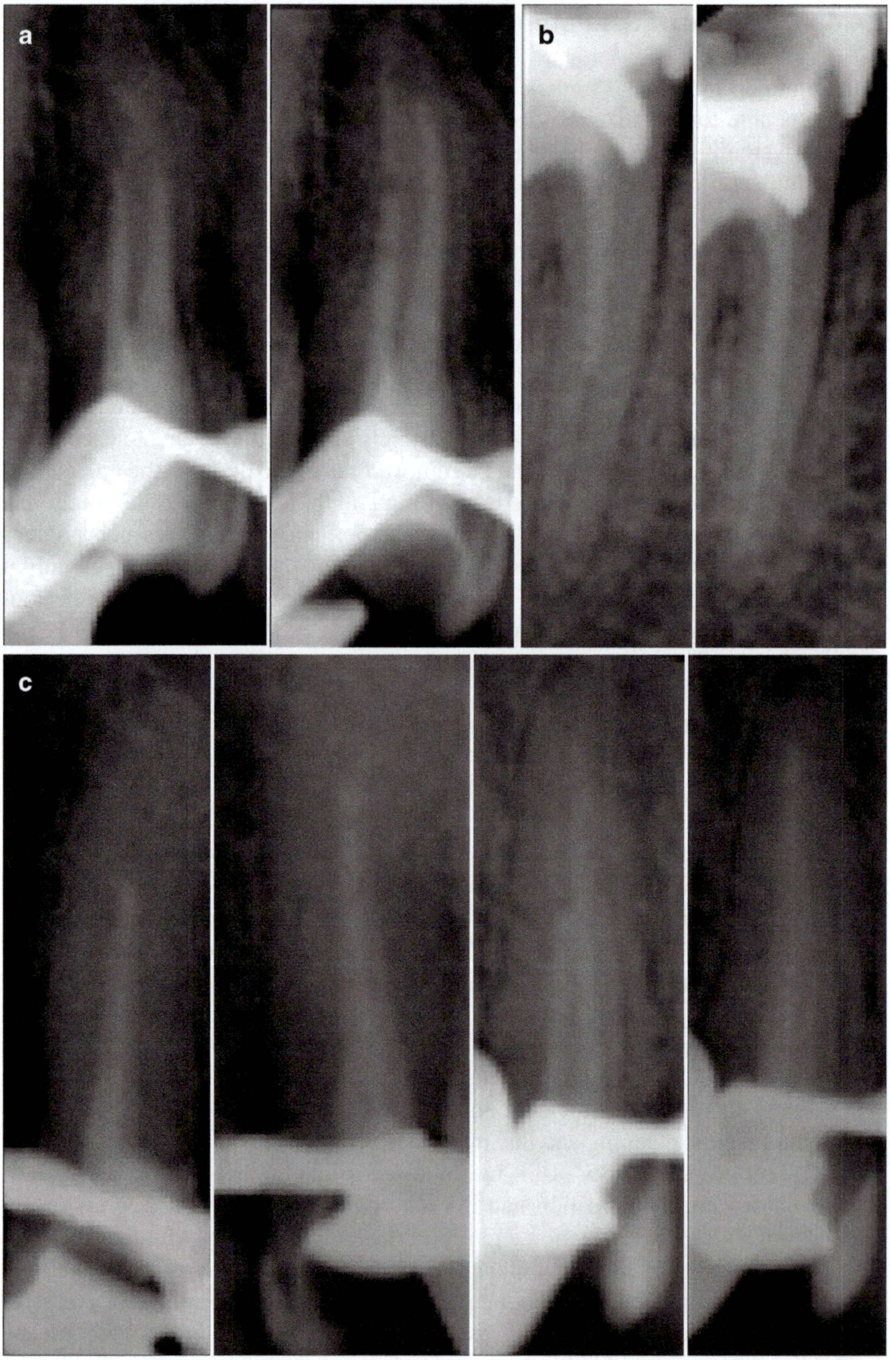

Fig. 2.33 (**a**–**c**) Three clinical cases demonstrating that apical patency can optimize the distribution of the irrigation solution (radiopaque solution within the root canal space) to the apical third, overcoming the vapor lock phenomenon. (Courtesy of Dr. Jorge Vera, USA)

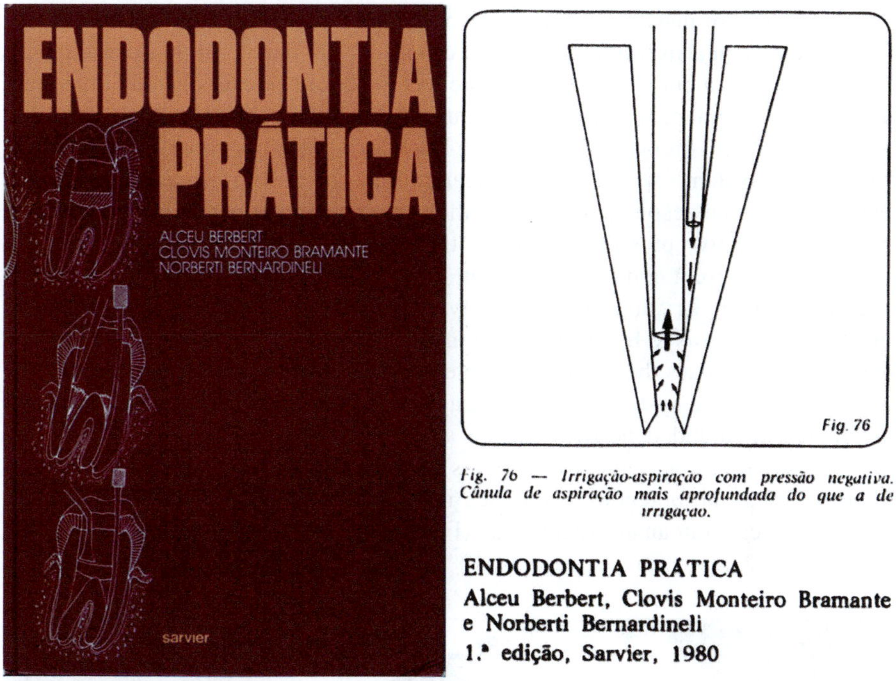

Fig. 2.34 The first irrigation system using negative apical pressure (EndoVac; SybronEndo, USA) became commercially available in 2007. However, the first report in the literature showing this technique was published by Dr. Alceu Berbert, Dr. Clóvis Bramante and Dr. Norberti Benardineli from the Bauru School of Dentistry in Brazil in 1980

the micro-cannula is a close-ended stainless steel piece (0.32 mm in diameter) containing 12 micro-holes positioned laterally and distributed in rows of 3 holes responsible for the aspiration and renewal of the irrigation solution at the apical third. Following the described dynamics, the irrigating solution circulates through the canal space by creating a negative apical pressure in the working length, which generates a kind of fast and turbulent cascade, allowing the use of a greater volume of solution compared to the conventional irrigation at the same time interval, as well as a better control of irrigant extrusion, even in teeth with incomplete apex formation [91]. Both cannulas are for individual use only and depend on a minimum apical enlargement to a size ISO 35 to be effective [89, 90, 92–96].

The literature is full of positive aspects regarding the use of the EndoVac system compared to the conventional positive pressure technique, including: better extrusion control of the irrigating solution [91, 97, 98]; being more effective in removing accumulated hard-tissue debris and supplying the irrigation solution at the working length [94, 95]; and no difference between the EndoVac system and the conventional positive pressure method was found in the cleaning quality at 1 mm from the apex [92, 99] with regards to the cleaning pattern of the root space and isthmus when similar volumes of irrigating solution were used. These findings indicated that the best results of negative pressure irrigation may be related to the fluid dynamics generated by apical aspiration in the root canal space or that it is only a consequence of using larger amounts of irrigant. Moreover, it should be cautioned that the main advertising argument for negative pressure irrigation is the avoidance of lawsuits when using "full-strength" Clorox (i.e., NaOCl of 5.25% or more) to irrigate the root canal system, which is a concentration not recommended by science. Nevertheless, and despite a possible conflict of interest by some authors of research papers on negative pressure irrigation, the concept highlighted a very important aspect in the current context, and that is *safety versus efficacy*. In summary, apical negative pressure irrigation is a relatively simple and very safe resource with sufficient scientific basis to be incorporated into routine clinical practice. There is however no doubt that the EndoVac represents a somewhat counterintuitive and energy-consuming system for daily usage. On the other hand, simple low-cost small-size open-ended needles can be adapted as an operative negative-suction device (no need for dedicated systems), enabling the negative apical pressure approach with the potential to produce more forceful currents inside an already-shaped root canal in an affordable way (Fig. 2.35).

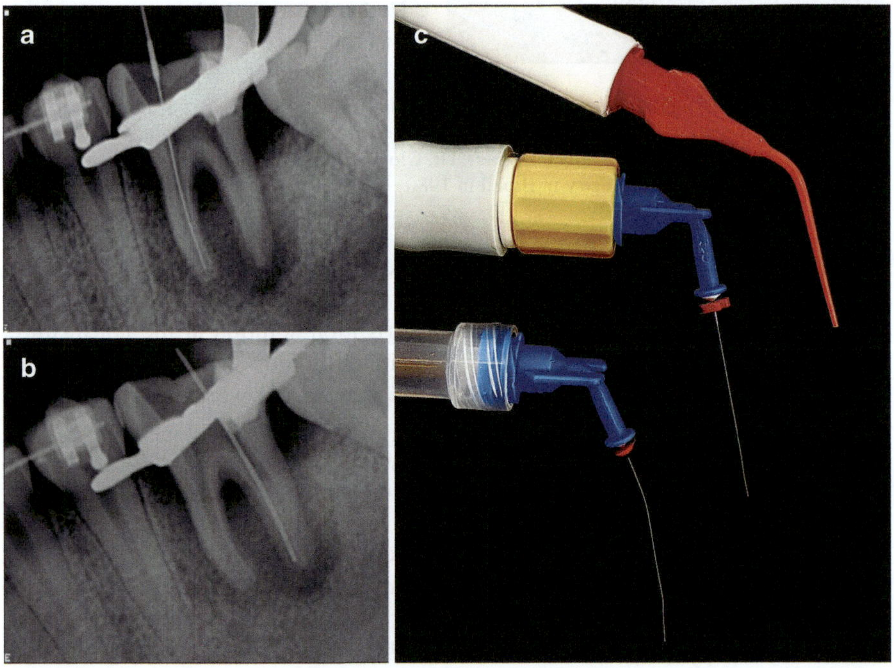

Fig. 2.35 (**a**, **b**) Irrigation of the root canal system of a mandibular molar using (**c**) different combinations of needles and cannulas adapted to work in a negative pressure approach

2.4.6 Is It Still Necessary to Agitate the NaOCl?

It is timely to recap the core philosophical approach of our line of thinking: Shaping is quick, but effective irrigation still demands time. Hence, the rationale proposed herein for canal irrigation must take advantage of the interplay between the already-shaped physical condition of the canal and the chair time saved with the expedited mechanical preparation. This purpose is unique and crystal clear: we must help the NaOCl to reach its maximum potential within the confined microenvironment of the canal space by taking advantage of the resting phase of the irrigation process, as well as the agitation of the irrigant. Nowadays, there are simple and affordable irrigation technologies and methodologies that are able to overcome the limitations of the laminar flow that characterizes traditional syringe-needle irrigation. Actually, the way in which energy is transferred to the irrigant establishes the specific flow, improving its delivery, mixing and influx refreshment.

2.4.6.1 Sonic and Ultrasonic Irrigation

Sonic and ultrasonic irrigation techniques are designed to induce agitation or streaming movements of the irrigants, increasing their efficiency [100–103] (Fig. 2.36). Sonic irrigation operates at a low frequency (1–6 kHz), high amplitude, and generates small shear stresses, which have been shown to be efficient for root canal debridement. The EndoActivator with attached polymer tips (Dentsply Tulsa Dental Specialties) and the Vibringe (Vibringe B.V.) systems are examples of devices specifically designed to perform sonic irrigation. Studies reported that sonic devices may contribute to the removal of the smear layer [104, 105] and intracanal medications [106], as well as better disinfection ability [107] when compared to conventional irrigation. However, there is still no clinical study evaluating their long-term influence on the endodontic outcome.

Ultrasound was introduced in endodontics by Richman in 1957 [108] and since then its use has been modified and applied to the irrigation procedure. Ultrasonic tips and inserts oscillate at frequencies of between 25 and 30 kHz, being beyond the limit of human hearing [76, 100]. One of the most used techniques is the so-called passive ultrasonic irrigation (PUI). PUI is based on the transmission of acoustic mechanical energy through the irrigation solution by the action of an energy source coupled to an insert or file. This energy is dissipated in the irrigating solution, usually sodium hypochlorite, through ultrasonic waves producing the phenomenon of cavitation and acoustic micro-current. The term PUI was firstly used in 1980 by Weller et al. [109] to outline a process of activation of the irrigating solution by ultrasonic energy without simultaneous mechanical preparation. Passive refers to the noncutting action of the tip or ultrasonic insert used in the procedure. PUI includes the irrigation procedures by means of the syringe-needle technique, with the subsequent ultrasonic activation, or the continuous release of the irrigant through an ultrasonic handpiece [76, 110]. PUI is considered a complementary approach, usually indicated after mechanical preparation, which is in line with the Shaping for Cleaning concept proposed in this chapter.

There is evidence demonstrating that PUI is able to optimize the final quality of cleaning and disinfection [28, 111–113], to work in areas not accessible to

a
b
c
d
e
f

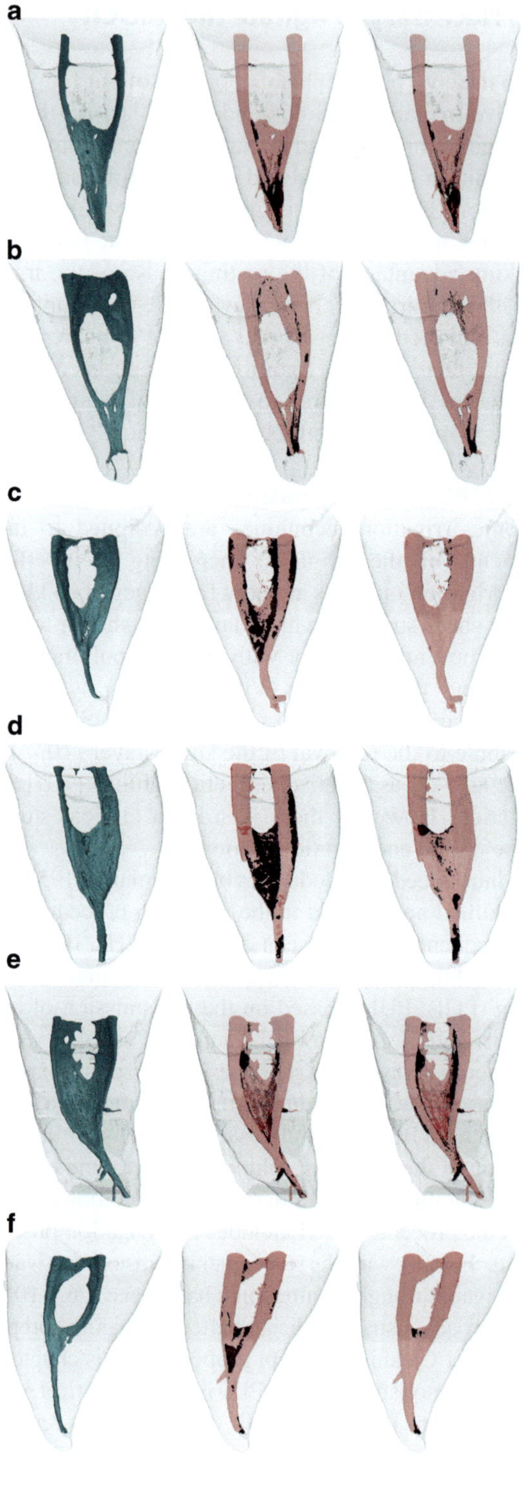

mechanical instrumentation [112, 114, 115], and to reduce the number of microorganisms when compared to conventional positive pressure needles [116]. In addition to these findings, ultrasound devices have undergone a drastic reduction in price over the last 10 years, mostly because of market competition created by the development of new brands from new companies worldwide, which make the equipment more affordable for the dentists. Likewise, the ultrasonic inserts specific to PUI have evolved in technology, acquiring efficiency and safety. It is important to emphasize that the aforementioned benefits of PUI over nonactivated irrigation are mostly based on laboratory studies [103, 116].

More recently, developments in dental laser technology resulted in new irrigating tips and pulse frequencies suitable for root canal cleaning by controlled cavitation: first the PIPS and now the SWEEPS technology by Fotona (Ljubljana, Slovenia). In essence, these clinical protocols employ a pulsed hard-tissue laser (Er:YAG), which absorbs water, creating shock waves and cavitation bubbles in the irrigant and negative pressure in the apical root canal aspects in a continuum filled with fluids, similar to the GentleWave system described before in this chapter [117]. However, these mentioned devices are not available worldwide, and are also not cheap. We therefore refrained from discussing them in further detail in this edition of the current publication.

Fig. 2.36 Mesial root canal systems (Vertucci Type IV) of 6 mandibular molars before (in green) and after (in red) preparation using reciprocating instruments to create hard-tissue debris (in black) and submitted to different supplementary irrigation protocols demonstrating that agitation techniques are efficient in the removal of debris; however, none of tested techniques were able to render root canals completely free of debris. Supplementary irrigation protocols: (**a**) Syringe and needle irrigation: canals were irrigated with 3 mL of 2.5% NaOCl using a 30-G notched needle (Appli-Vac Irrigating Needle Tip) adapted to a 3-mL syringe at a mean flow rate of 0.14 mL/s. (**b**) Ultrasonically activated irrigation: a noncutting, stainless steel size 20 wire (Irrisafe) driven by an ultrasonic device (Suprasson Pmax Newtron) was used in the root canals for 3 × 20 s at 45% of the maximum power. The wire was prebent in order to limit contact with the canal walls. (**c**) a noncutting, 200-mm stainless steel ultrasonic instrument (Irrisafe) driven by the P5 Newtron ultrasonic system (Acteon North America) at a power setting of 9 was placed at 2 mm from the working length and agitated in a 1–2 mm up-and-down motion. The final irrigation protocol began with 6% NaOCl for 3 × 20 s followed by 17% EDTA for 3 × 20 s and a final rinse with 6% sodium hypochlorite for 3 × 20 s. Irrigation was performed in a flow rate of 15 mL/min per canal. (**d**) a ProUltra PiezoFlow ultrasonic irrigation needle (ProUltra) was connected to the P5 Newtron ultrasonic system (Acteon North America) at a power setting of 9. The 500-mm ultrasonic irrigation needle was positioned 1 mm short of binding, no deeper than 75% of the working length, and agitated in a 1–2 mm up-and-down motion. The final irrigation protocol began with 6% NaOCl followed by 17% EDTA and a final rinse with 6% NaOCl. Irrigation was performed in a flow rate of 15 mL/min for 1 min per canal. (**e**) Sonically activated irrigation: a noncutting polyamide size 25, 0.04 tip (EDDY) operated by an air-driven handpiece (Proxeo) was used in each canal for 3 × 20 s at maximum intensity (frequency of 6000 Hz). (**f**) GentleWave: before the final irrigation protocol, an occlusal platform was fabricated of a resin material (SoundSeal) and a preformed plastic matrix to ensure an airtight seal between the access cavity and the procedural instrument. The final irrigation protocol began with 3% NaOCl for 5 min followed by distilled water for 30 s, 8% EDTA for 2 min, and a final rinse with distilled water for 15 s in a flow rate of 50 mL/min

2.4.6.2 Manual Dynamic Activation (MDA) Technique

The manual dynamic activation (MDA) can be performed with hand files, brushes or a well-fitting tapered gutta-percha point. The MDA starts when the first scouting hand file is placed inside the canal. The apical progression of the instrument moves the irrigant beyond the tip, and once the working length has been reached, the vertical and oscillatory movement of the file allows the solution to spread within the canal space. During canal shaping, the repeated use of a patency file after each active shaping instrument helps break up the gas bubbles and moves fresh irrigant into the last apical millimeters [82] mixing it with the stagnant solution of the "dead zone" [118, 119]. The frequency of replenishment of the coronal irrigant with the syringe along with the progressive shaping of the root canal and the repeated use of patency files are factors that allow the delivery of irrigant further and further apically (Fig. 2.37).

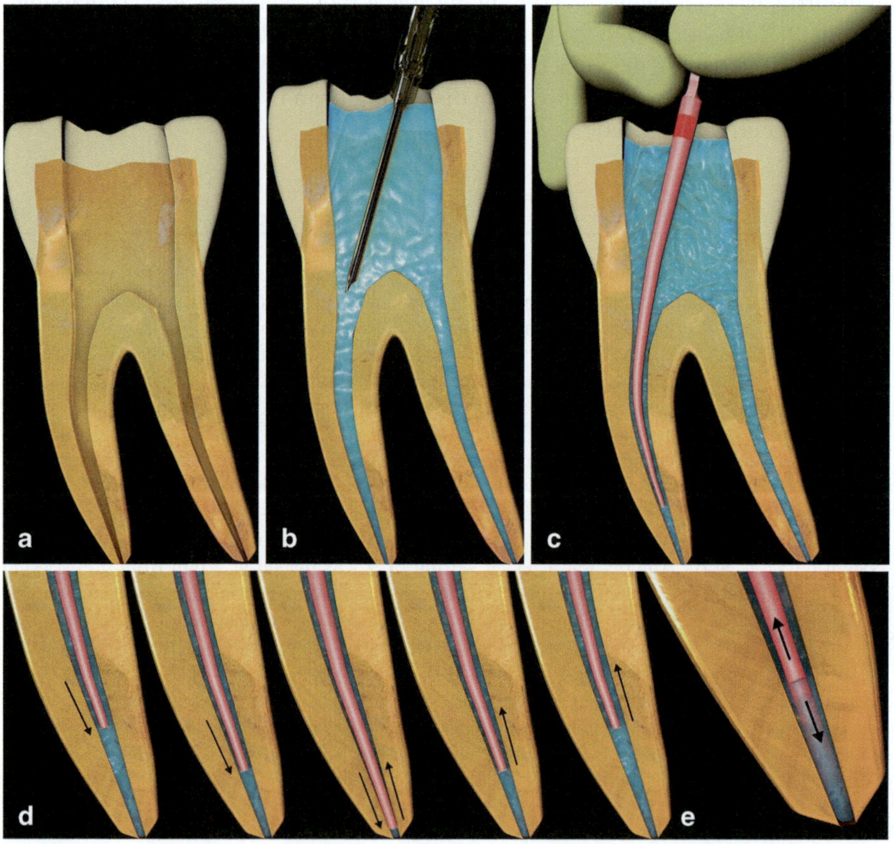

Fig. 2.37 Manual dynamic activation (MDA) technique in a mandibular molar tooth. (**a**) Following completion of shaping procedures, (**b**) the canal is filled with irrigant and (**c**) a gutta-percha master cone inserted close to the working length and then (**d**, **e**) rapidly "pumped" up and down in 3-mm length motions to promote the agitation of the irrigant

The use of a well-fitting tapered master cone at the end of the shaping procedure to agitate the irrigating solution and enable it to involve the entire length of the root canal was first proposed by Pierre Machtou at a point in time when slim irrigation needles for endodontic usage were not available [120]. MDA is a simple yet cost-effective way not only to help the irrigant to make contact with the canal walls and reach their apical portion, but also to dislodge the vapor lock effect and facilitate the mixing of fresh solution with the stagnant solution at the apical millimeters [118]. This procedure generates high intracanal pressure changes during the in-and-out movement of the gutta-percha cone, and the frequency of the strokes creates turbulence and enhances the diffusion of the irrigant solution by shear stresses. The presence of a thin reflux space between the cone and the canal walls is critical to allow the irrigant to flow back along the cone and induce an effective hydrodynamic effect. The efficiency of this technique was confirmed by several studies [121–123]. The main concern during irrigant activation is the risk of apical extrusion. According to available data [72, 124, 125], all tested devices, including MDA, appear to extrude some irrigant, except for apical negative pressure, which in fact should be seen more as a delivery device rather than an activation system. However, it is worth noting that, in clinics, the resistance of the periapical tissues plays a role in limiting the occurrence of extrusion. Therefore, irrigant extrusion can be prevented with an accurate use of the MDA technique.

2.4.6.3 Continuous Instrumentation and Irrigation: The Self-Adjusting File (SAF) System

The SAF system was developed to perform a continuous instrumentation and irrigation, removing a minimal amount of dentin from the root canal walls. While rotary and reciprocating instruments remove large amounts of dentin and fail to clean the buccal and lingual extensions of oval canals and isthmus [15, 34, 126], the SAF was designed to overcome these limitations (Fig. 2.38). Differing from the traditional instruments, the SAF does not have a solid metal core but consists of a hollow tube made from a thin nickel-titanium lattice that provides an extremely high compressibility [127–129]. As a result, this instrument adapts itself to the shape of root canals. For instance, in oval canals the SAF compresses and spreads itself in the buccolingual direction, adapting to the morphology of the root canal. Moreover, this instrument has an important mechanical scrubbing effect on the root canal walls, generated by the continuous movement of the metal over the dentinal surface, resulting in the removal of a uniform thin layer of the surrounding dentin (Fig. 2.39). This mechanical action, combined with the simultaneous irrigation, is important to remove tissue debris and biofilms [128].

The first generation of the SAF instruments was used with a special RDT handpiece and an irrigation pump [127–129]. This handpiece could be adapted to a wide variety of endodontic motors, and the SAF instrument operated at 5,000 rpm, with in-and-out vibrations of 0.4 mm amplitude. Before its use, however, it was necessary to perform a glide path, so that the instrument could reach the working length. For this purpose, the manufacturer also developed a specific rotary instrument: the pre-SAF glide path. SAF should be used for 4 min using pecking motions until it

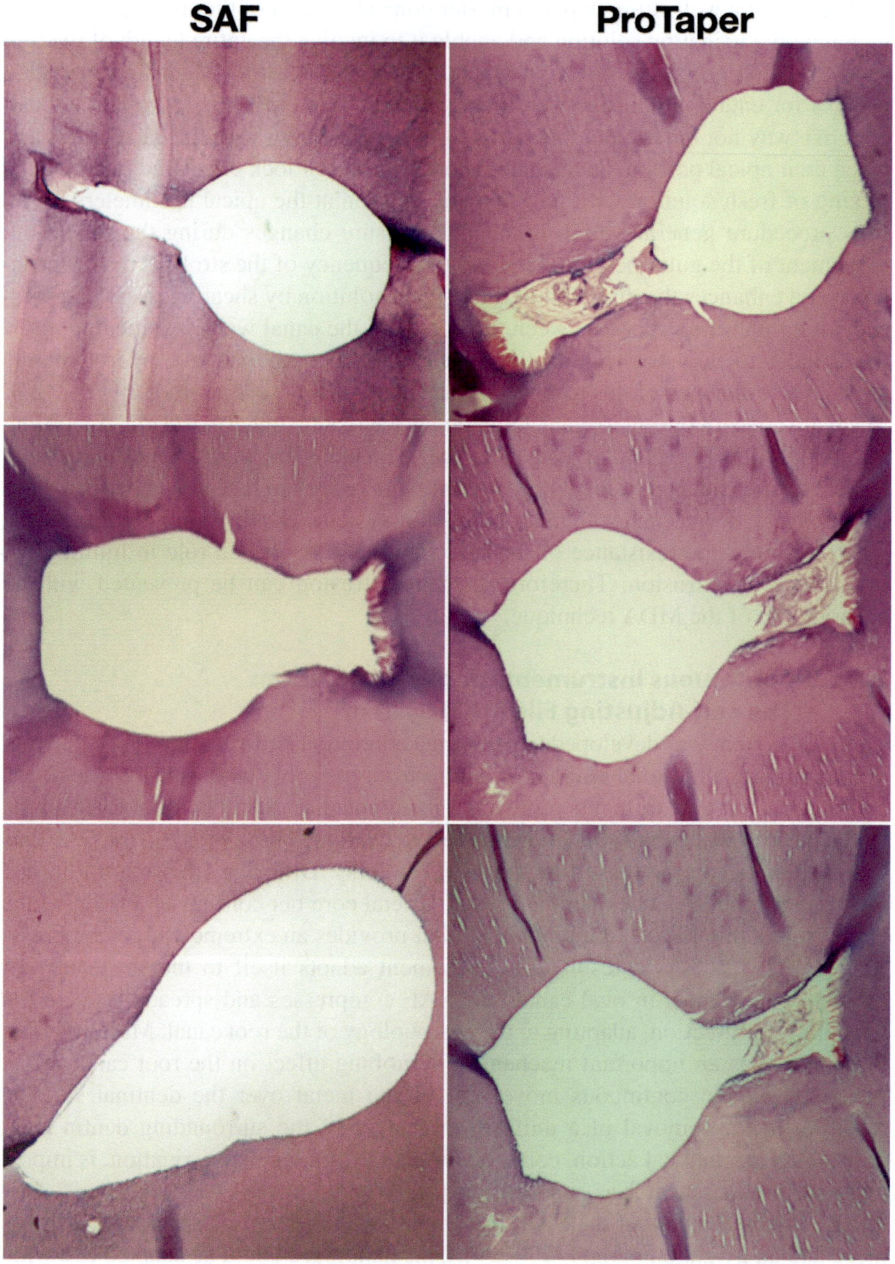

Fig. 2.38 Histological cross sections of oval-shaped canals after preparation with the Self-adjusting File (SAF; on the left) and ProTaper Universal (on the right) systems. While it is possible to observe almost all root canal space free of pulp tissue remnants after using the SAF system, root canals prepared with the ProTaper Universal instruments had a significant amount of pulp tissue within unprepared buccal and lingual canal extensions

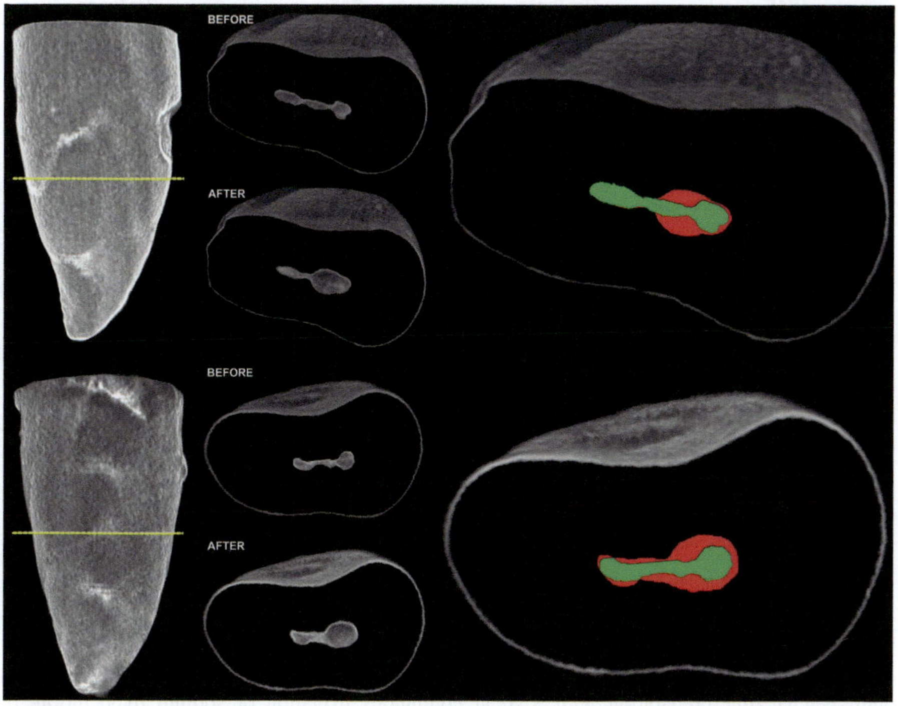

Fig. 2.39 Micro-CT models of two mandibular incisors with flat-shaped canals prepared with a rotary system (top) and the Self-adjusting File (bottom) showing cross sections of the middle level of the root (yellow line) before (in green) and after (in red) preparation. Root canal preparation with SAF (below) removed a uniform layer of dentin around the canal outline, while rotary instrumentation (above) resulted in substantial untouched areas (green areas on the right) after canal preparation

reaches the working length. This instrument has a rotating hub to which an irrigation tube is connected, delivering a continuous flow of fresh irrigant from the irrigation pump at an adjustable rate of 1–10 mL/min. Any pressure generated by the irrigation device is eliminated when the irrigant enters the instrument, thus it is also a non-pressure irrigation system [127–129].

Several studies were conducted to confirm the efficacy of the SAF system. Compared with rotary instruments, the use of the SAF resulted in a more effective removal of debris and smear layer from the apical canal [130, 131], reduction of bacterial biofilm [132, 133], removal of pulp tissue [15], better adaptation of the filling materials to the root canal walls [131, 134] (Fig. 2.40), and less remaining root filling after retreatment [135–137]. In addition, it has been suggested that the SAF would be beneficial to treat immature teeth, to effectively clean without affect the dentin thickness, and to avoid the overflow of the irrigant solutions beyond the apex. Nevertheless, despite these advantages, it was also demonstrated that there was no difference in the disinfection efficiency between the SAF system and rotary files in isthmus-containing canal systems of mandibular molars [138]. The SAF

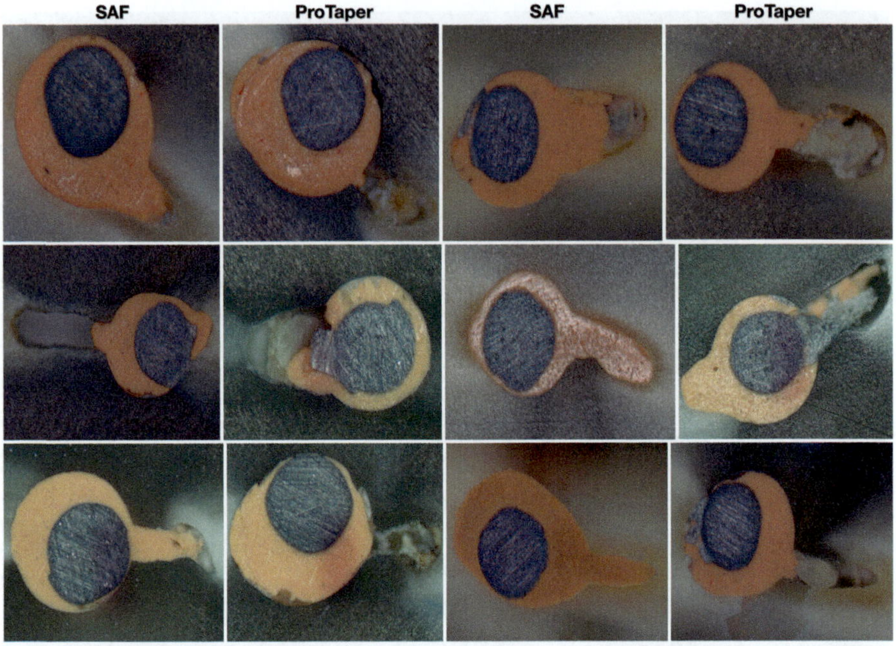

Fig. 2.40 Optical microscopy images from sections of root canals filled with thermoplasticized gutta-percha after preparation with SAF at continuous irrigation of sodium hypochlorite or ProTaper with syringe and needle irrigation. Preparation with ProTaper allowed the accumulation of debris that prevented the gutta-percha to flow into canal recesses. On the other hand, in the specimens prepared with SAF system, the buccal and lingual canal extensions were mostly devoided of debris, allowing the thermoplasticized gutta-percha and the sealer to flow and fill these areas

cannot enter isthmuses that are thinner than 0.2 mm and, because of this, narrow isthmuses are still a limitation for all available techniques. Besides, there is a lack of well-designed clinical studies to determine the role of the SAF in the long-term outcome of root canal treatment. Its main disadvantage, however, may be the fact that no achieved canal shape could be easily filled using a "system-based approach" with mold-injected gutta-percha. Such a system-based approach that links shaping with root filling has been developed by most manufacturers of rotary or reciprocating systems in recent years, and may be one of the reasons why these systems have a high sales rate, especially among general practitioners.

2.4.7 Chelating Agents: Washing out the Biofilm?

Matthias Zehnder

Because biofilms, by definition, consist of microorganisms embedded in a sticky matrix that adheres to a surface [139] (Fig. 2.41), chemical root canal debridement concepts can target biofilm adhesion and cohesion. However, the reader should realize

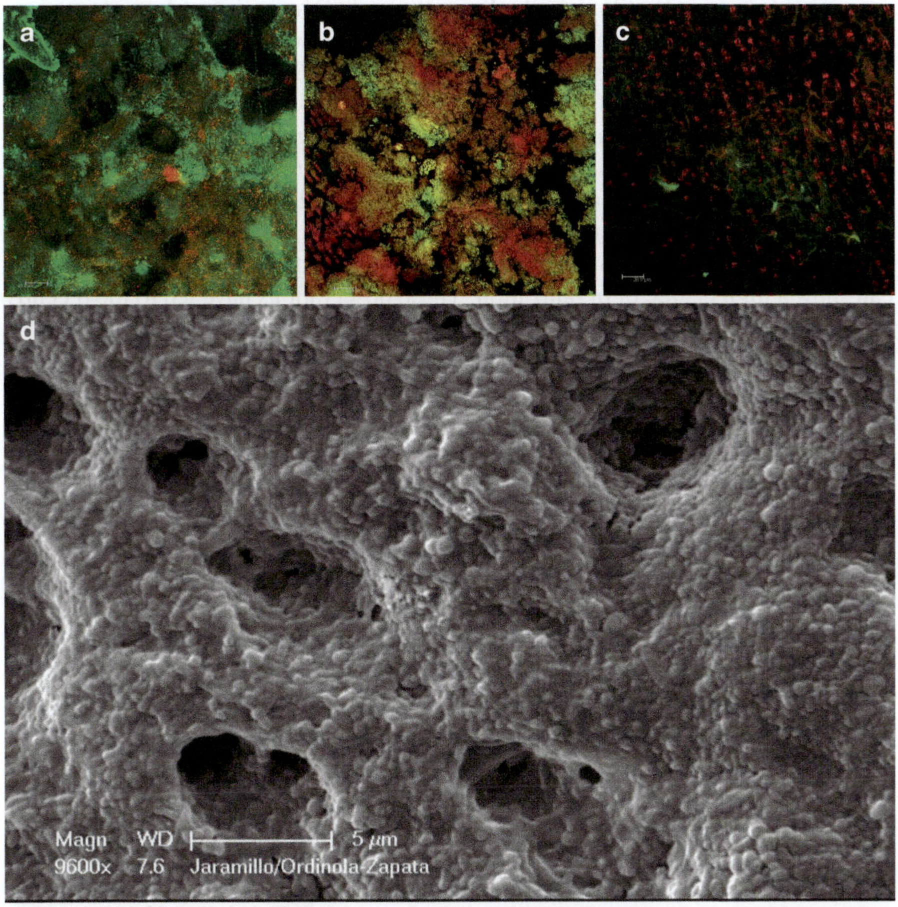

Fig. 2.41 Confocal laser scanning microscopy of biofilm-infected dentin after exposure to (**a**) distilled water, (**b**) chlorhexidine and (**c**) sodium hypochlorite for 15 min. Dentin was labeled with the live/dead fluorescence kit in which green and red colors represent live and dead cells, respectively. Biofilms exposed directly to (**a**) water or (**b**) chlorhexidine were not removed, although chlorhexidine was able to kill most of the bacteria (red color). On the other hand, biofilm was completely removed by exposure to sodium hypochlorite together with the most superficial bacterial cells located into the dentinal tubules. (Courtesy of Dr. Ordinola-Zapata, USA). (**d**) Scanning electron microscopy of the root canal wall surface showing the dentinal tubules covered by biofilm. (Courtesy of Dr. Ordinola-Zapata and Dr. Jaramillo USA)

that the term "biofilm" is derived from biological observations on how microorganisms are typically organized in nature. The original observations were made on inanimate objects under water, such as stones in rivers and underwater pipelines [140]. Hence, extrapolations to other spaces and disinfection concepts are not always straightforward. Root canal biofilms were originally described by Hansueli Luder and Ramachandran Nair in the *Swiss Dental Journal* as "adhering bacteria" in histology slides of roots with a clinical diagnosis of a necrotic pulp and symptomatic apical periodontitis [141]. How well these bacteria adhere to the canal wall, however, is currently not known. Biofilms as a biological concept form under ecological pressure. In liquids, bacteria have a natural tendency to adhere to solids such as the walls of the liquid container [142]. The strength of that adhesion is most likely dependent on the shear forces/fluid flow a biofilm is exposed to. It may be suspected that shear forces in the root canal are lower than, for example, on supragingival dental hard tissues, and hence the biofilm that forms therein adheres less than dental plaque.

The other unknown or uninvestigated issue is the matrix of endodontic biofilms [143]. Biofilm matrices can be composed of a multitude of elements, including polysaccharides, proteins, nucleic acids and lipids, in differing amounts [144]. They can show a high degree of organization. These observations have led to the recently proposed term "biofilm matrixome," [145]. Interestingly, minerals derived from biomineralization processes by the bacteria contained in the biofilm can be a stabilizing structural component in biofilms [145, 146]. Whether these mineralized matrix components exist in root canal biofilms is not known.

In summary, it should be acknowledged that, because the environmental stress factors that are present in a pulpless root canal system differ largely from those in, for example, supragingival plaque, it is questionable whether biofilms in root canals show consistent patterns of organization, or whether they should even be called biofilms, for that matter. Again, this has not yet been investigated and awaits further studies that go beyond simple histology.

Because of the above unknown issues in endodontic research, concepts of biofilm disruption and detachment are derived from in vitro experiments using artificial biofilms as model systems. While basic information can be gained from such studies under controlled experimental conditions, it is not necessarily clear whether observations made that way apply to clinics. Nevertheless, studies have unequivocally shown that NaOCl solutions at their concentration range used in endodontics (0.5–5% NaOCl) (Figs. 2.42 and 2.43) are unique in their ability to disrupt and dissolve simulated endodontic biofilms, including their matrix [147, 148]. However,

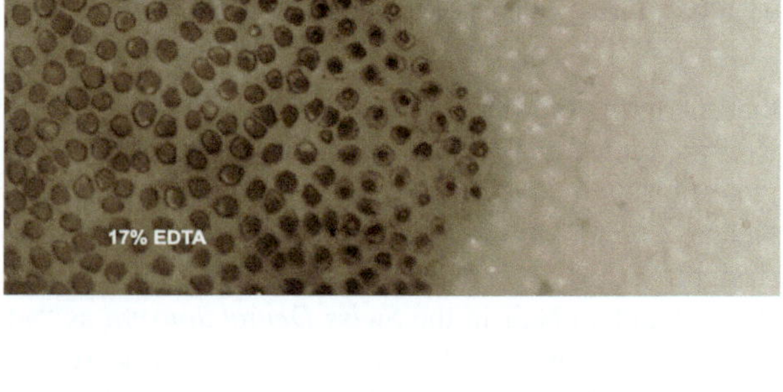

Fig. 2.42 Optical microscopy image showing the interface between masked and unmasked dentin after 600 s of EDTA etching. The boundary between etched and unetched regions is clear. EDTA etching not only removed the smear layer but also destroyed the peritubular dentin enlarging the dentinal tubules

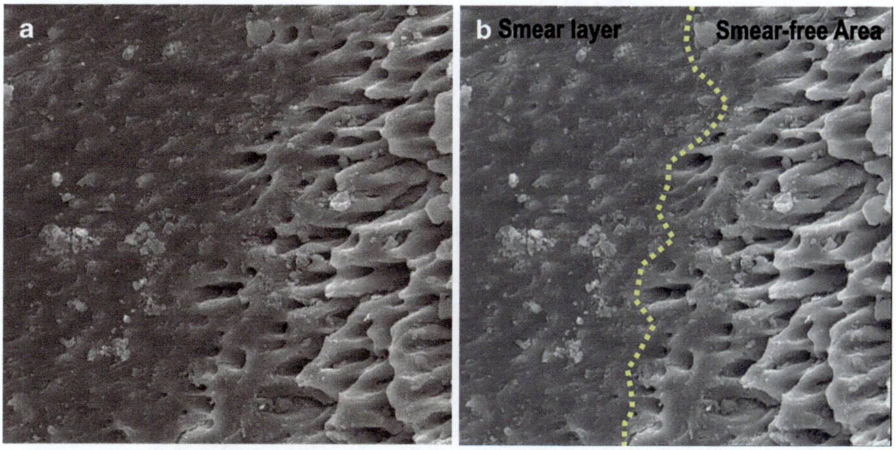

Fig. 2.43 (**a**, **b**) Optical microscopy image showing the interface (yellow line) between an area that was mechanically touched by the NiTi instrument—where dentinal tissue was cut and thus smear layer was created—blocking dentinal tubules, as well as, a smear free area in which the instrument did not act, depicting the presence of opened dentinal tubules

EDTA can also have an effect on certain biofilms by interfering with their structural integrity [147, 149]. Experiments in in vitro endodontic biofilms have also suggested an effect of EDTA in this regard [150]. In particular, biofilms with a calcified component in their matrix could be targeted by chelators such as EDTA. In theory, such chelators or decalcifying agents could also have a cleansing effect in the root canal by detaching biofilms from the root canal wall. Whether this occurs or not has not been specifically investigated, but could be studied in, for example, flow chambers.

A newer approach in root canal irrigation involves the combined use of NaOCl and a soft chelator in the form of HEDP (1-hydroxyethane 1,1-diphosphonic acid, the chemical designation of etidronic acid). A combined solution containing HEDP (9%) and NaOCl in the concentration of the clinician's choice can be obtained by mixing etidronate powder (Dual Rinse HEDP, Medcem, Weinfelden, Switzerland) into the solution (Fig. 2.44).

Combined NaOCl-HEDP irrigants have to be mixed chair-side and can be used for about 1 h with no relevant loss of any component [151]. Research on extracted teeth has shown that this combination inhibits the formation of a smear layer and accumulated debris during root canal instrumentation [38, 152]. Because of that, bacteria in dentinal tubules become more susceptible to the disinfecting effect of NaOCl [153], even in an abbreviated irrigation protocol when no EDTA is used at all [154]. This becomes especially interesting in conjunction with the anatomical/cleaning file systems mentioned above, such as the XP Endo Finisher or the SAF system. Recent as of yet unpublished research shows that the SAF protocol can be

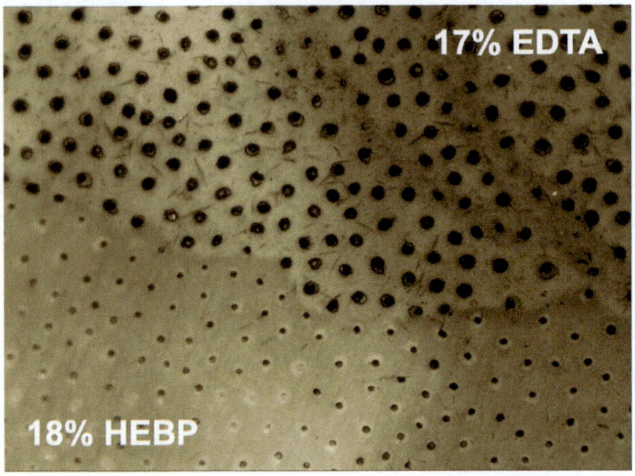

Fig. 2.44 Optical microscopy image showing surface changes of different dentin regions of the same specimen after demineralization with EDTA and HEPB. A well-defined boundary is visible in the interface between the regions etched with EDTA—a strong chelator—and HEBP—a soft chelator. In the region etched by EDTA 17%, the peritubular dentin was destroyed while the original area of intertubular dentin was reduced. In the region etched by the HEPB 18%, both inter- and peritubular dentin areas were preserved

shortened considerably when a HEDP/NaOCl combination is used as the irrigant. However, whether this irrigation concept also detaches biofilms better than a pure NaOCl solution without a chelator remains to be investigated. In experimental biofilms with passive exposure to the NaOCl/HEDP solution, the HEDP had no impact (either positive or negative) on disinfection of biofilm structure [155, 156]. However, HEDP in the main NaOCl irrigant helps to condition the canal walls for subsequent filling procedures [157], in that the dentin is free of a smear layer yet not decalcified [152]. In this context, it should be realized that most dental materials bind to the mineral phase of dentin, and thus continuous "soft" chelation is an easier and probably also better concept than alternating rinses with NaOCl and a strong and noncompatible chelator (EDTA or citric acid) to clean and conditioning the root canal system [158]. This also goes for a core concept in clinical endodontics that has gained little attention: the final seal in the access cavity using composite resins. Newer-generation dentin adhesives, especially those that contain 10-MDP [159], bind directly to calcium, and thus are not expected not to combine well with cavity walls treated by aggressive decalcifying agents such as EDTA or citric acid. However, research on this matter is sparse, as studies have focused on the presence/absence of a smear layer rather than on the decalcification of the dentin itself [160].

2.5 Shaping for Cleaning Irrigation: Clinical Guidelines

Before reaching the minimal canal taper-size enlargement—when the canal space is only partially filled by the irrigant (Fig. 2.45):

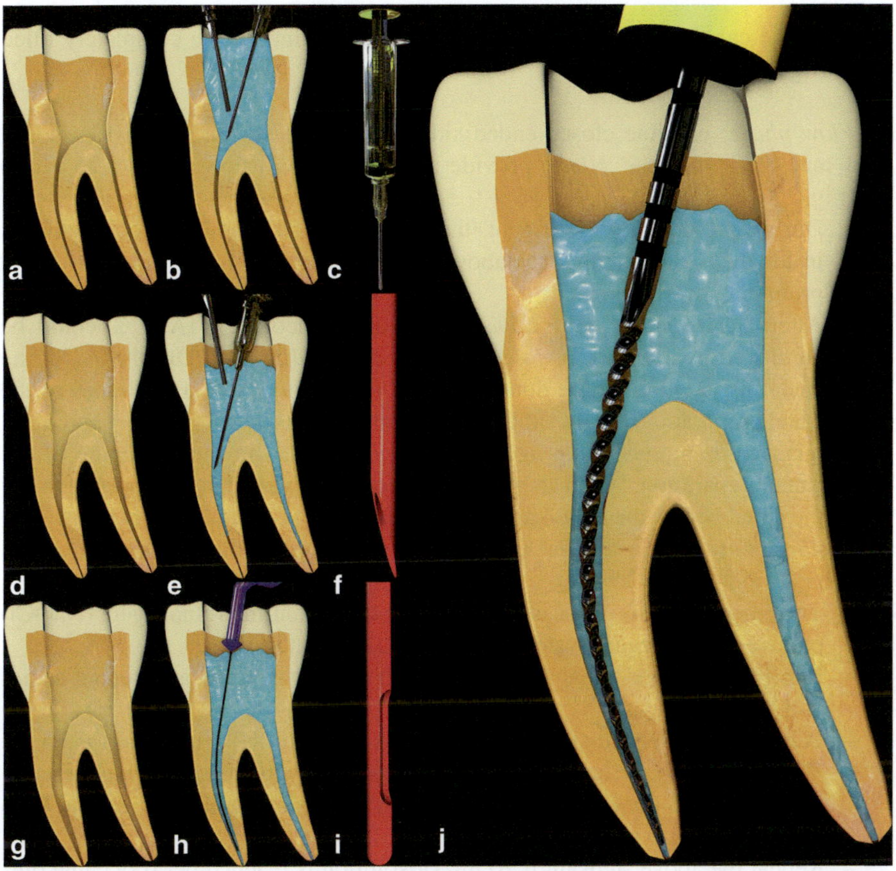

Fig. 2.45 Shaping for Cleaning protocol (preliminary procedures). After (**a**) access preparation and before reaching the final canal enlargement, (**b–f**) irrigation can be performed using larger open-ended needles (~18–20G) adapted to a 5-mL syringe for early disinfection (chemical action) and removal of gross dentinal debris promoted by the high flow rate (physical action). Irrigation must be done on high volumes without binding the needle in the canal. After canal shaping (**g**), the enlarged canal space must be filled with the irrigant using (**h–j**) a fine closed-ended side-vented needle (at least 30G) placed 1 mm short of working length with a high flow rate (~0.25 mL/s)

- Operate the traditional syringe-needle irrigation process using 5-mL syringes with larger open-ended needles (~18–20G)—for an early disinfection during the preflaring phase (chemical action)—and removal of gross dentinal debris promoted by the high flow rate (physical action). This type of ordinary large needles can be used until the end of the cervical third;
- Irrigate on a high-volume scale, but without binding the needle inside the canal. As a suggestion, 1 mL of irrigant after each instrument should be used

After the canal shaping, the enlarged space is assumed to be completely filled with irrigant:

1. *Flow phase*: use fine closed-ended side-vended needles (at least 30G) placed 1 mm short from the WL to provide a relatively high flow rate (~0.25 mL/s) (Fig. 2.46).
   - During the delivery of irrigant, the needle should be moved longitudinally inside the root canal up to the abovementioned point of maximum insertion to promote a flow movement;
   - Alternate irrigation with 2.5% NaOCl and aqueous EDTA 17% could be employed in all cases. In cases of vital pulps with intact PDL, the use of the chelating agent could be done as a final irrigation in the last minutes of the canal preparation. On the other hand, in infected cases and specially in retreatment cases the chelating agent could be used also in the beginning of the canal preparation. When alternate irrigation is employed, it is important to dry the canal before the new irrigant is utilized.
2. *Resting phase*: use of the NaOCl solution as non-agitated intra-visit medication (Fig. 2.47).
   - The purpose of this phase is leaving a fast-acting antimicrobial agent (NaOCl) passively in the canal system during the treatment session;
   - Refill the enlarged canal space with fresh irrigant solution and keep it standstill for 5 min;
   - Place a closed-ended side-vented needle (at least 30G) 1 mm short from the WL and refresh the irrigant moving longitudinally the needle inside the canal for 30 s. Refill the enlarged canal space with fresh irrigant solution and keep it standstill for 5 min;
   - Repeat the above steps until 20 mL of solution is reached per root canal during 20 min.
3. *Agitation phase*: agitate or activate the irrigant with your preferred system should be done with fresh irrigant (use NaOCl and EDTA) (Figs. 2.48 and 2.49).

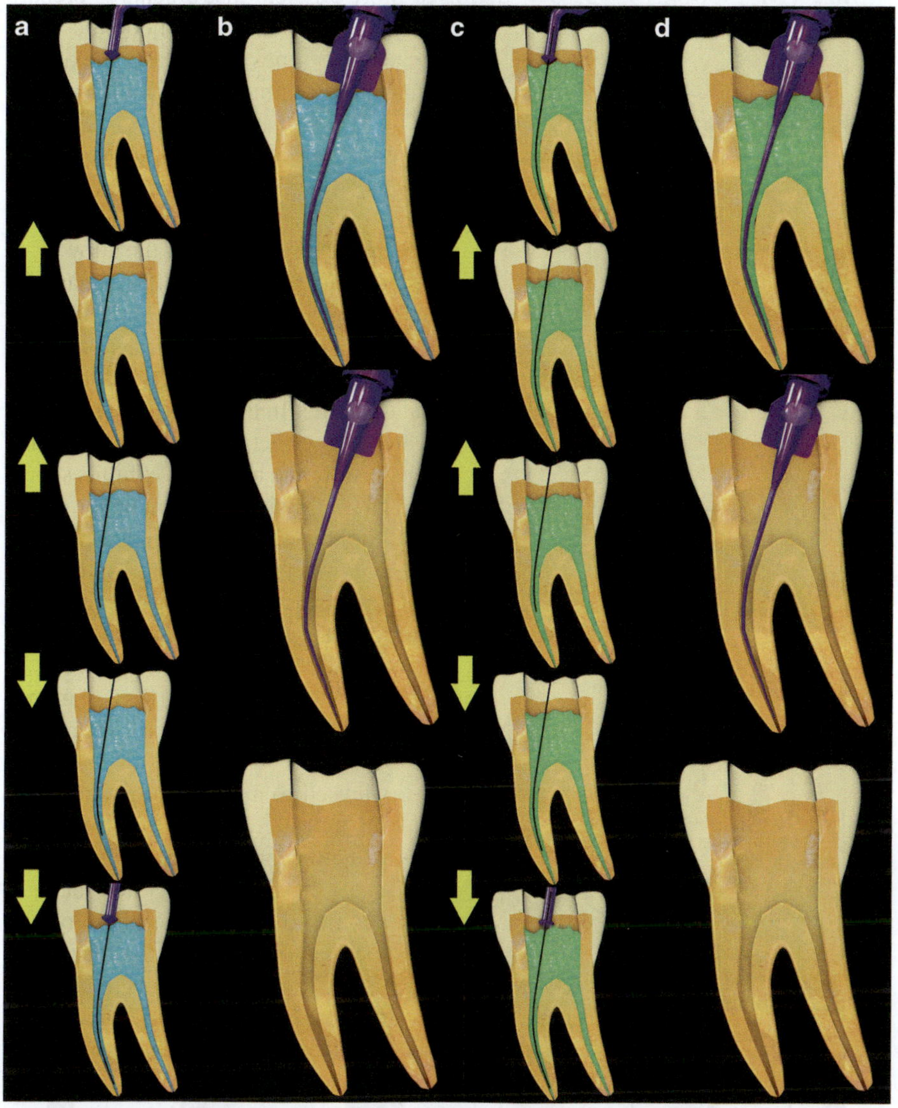

Fig. 2.46 Shaping for Cleaning protocol (Flow Phase). At this phase, the needle should be moved longitudinally inside the root canal while delivering fresh irrigant solution to promote a flow movement (**a** and **c**). It is important to alternate irrigation with (**a**) NaOCl 2.5% and (**c**) aqueous EDTA 17%. (**b** and **d**) When alternate irrigation is employed it is important to dry the canal before the new irrigant is utilized

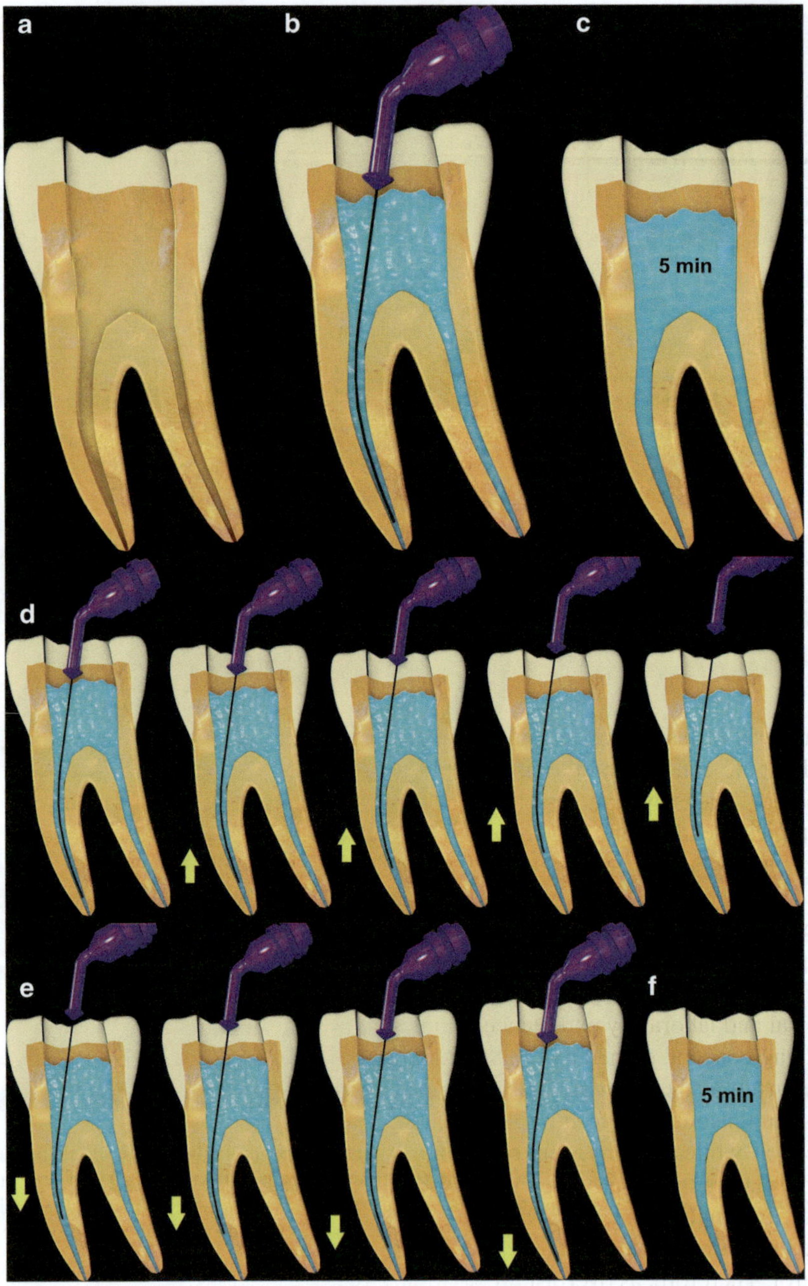

Fig. 2.47 Shaping for Cleaning protocol (Resting Phase). (**a–c**) After drying the root canal, refill the enlarged canal space with fresh irrigant solution and keep it standstill for 5 min. (**d, e**) Then, use the closed-ended side-vented needle 1 mm short from the WL to refresh the irrigant while moving the needle up and down inside the canal for 30 s. (**f**) Finally, refill the canal again with fresh solution and keep it standstill for 5 min. These steps must be repeated until 20 mL of solution is reached per root canal for at least 20 min

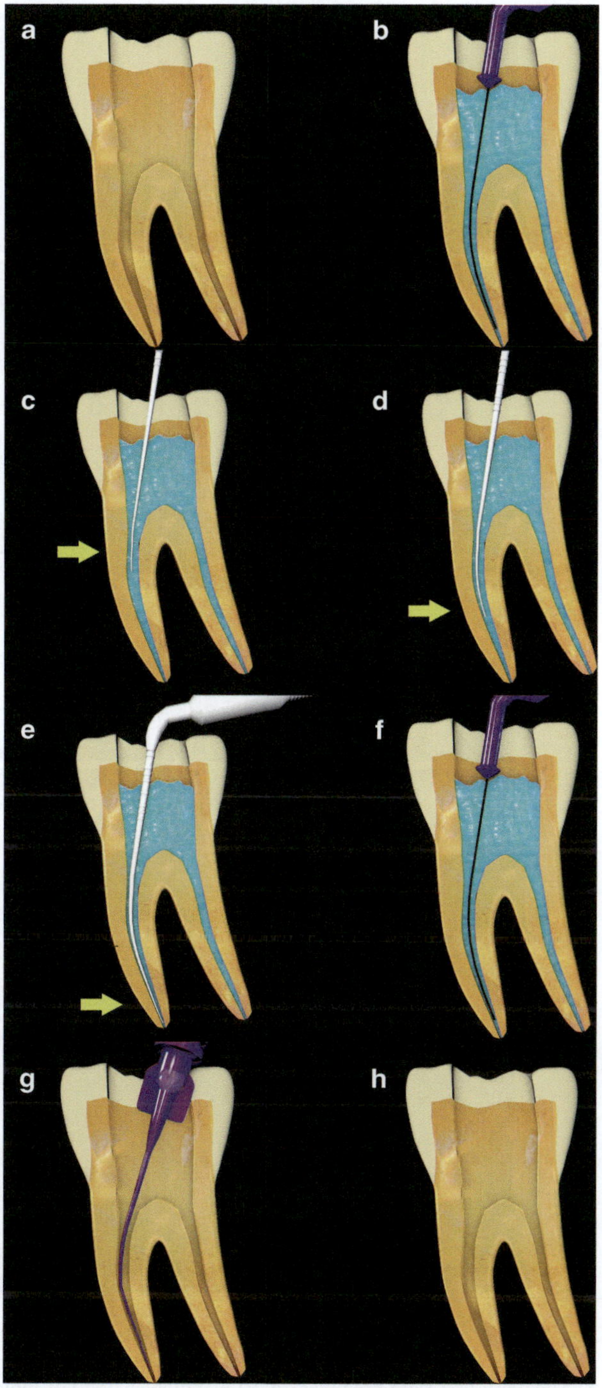

Fig. 2.48 Shaping for Cleaning protocol (Agitation Phase). In this last step, after (**a**) drying the root canal, (**b**) fill it again with fresh irrigant solution and then (**c**–**e**) agitate the solution in all root thirds. Finally, (**f**) irrigate the root canal again, (**g**) dry with paper points and a thin cannula and then (**h**) the root canal system is ready for filling

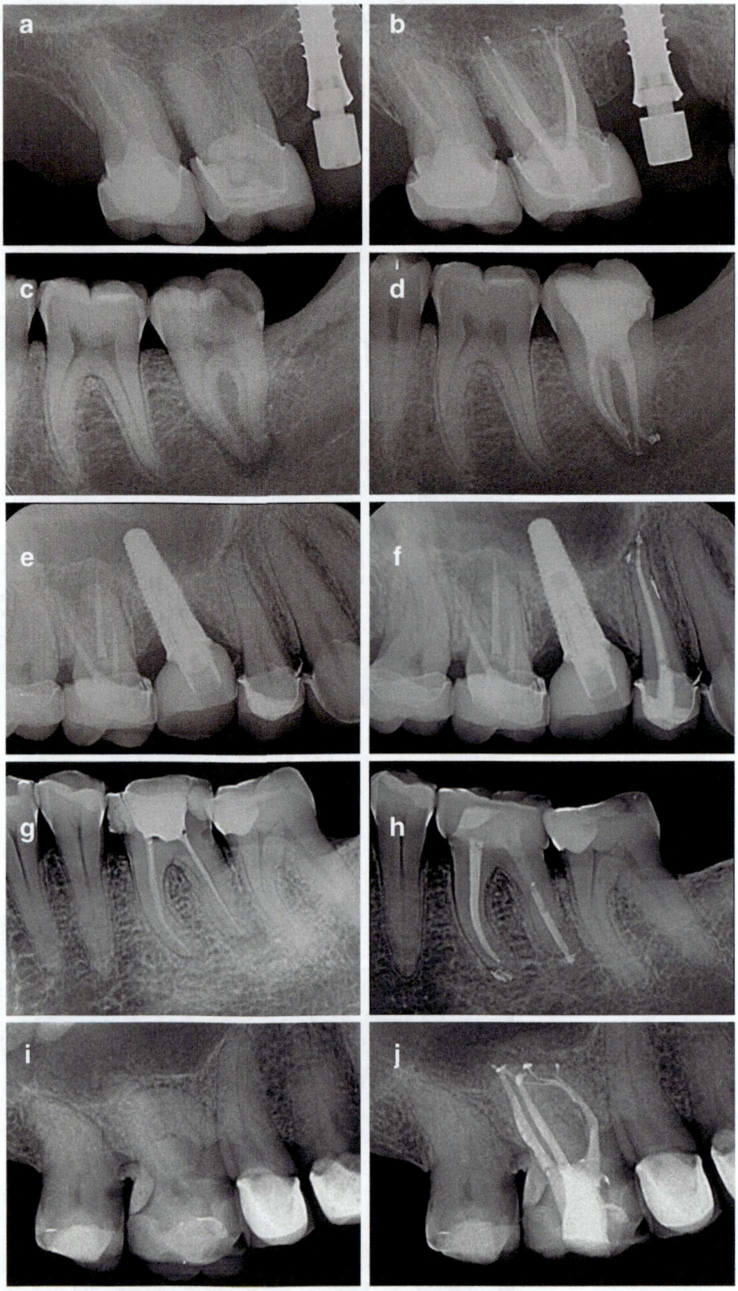

Fig. 2.49 Pre- and postoperative radiographic exams showing clinical cases using the concept of Shaping for Cleaning in a (**a**, **b**) maxillary first left molar. (**c**, **d**) mandibular second left molar. (**e**, **f**) Maxillary first right premolar. (**g**, **h**) mandibular first left molar; and (**i**, **j**) maxillary first right molar. (Courtesy of Dr. Arthur Zuolo, Brazil)

References

1. Sjögren U, Hagglund B, Sundqvist G, Wing K. Factors affecting the long-term results of endodontic treatment. J Endod. 1990;16:498–504.
2. Siqueira JF Jr. Taxonomic changes of bacteria associated with endodontic infections. J Endod. 2003;29:619–23.
3. Siqueira JF Jr, Rôças IN. Clinical implications and microbiology of bacterial persistence after treatment procedures. J Endod. 2008;34:1291–301.e3.
4. Waltimo T, Trope M, Haapasalo M, Orstavik D. Clinical efficacy of treatment procedures in endodontic infection control and one year follow-up of periapical healing. J Endod. 2005;31:863–6.
5. Hatton EH, Skillen WG, Moen OH. Histologic findings in teeth with treated and filled root canals. J Am Dent Assoc. 1928;15:56.
6. Walton RE. Histologic evaluation of different methods of enlarging the pulp canal space. J Endod. 1976;2:304–11.
7. De-Deus G, Belladonna FG, Silva EJ, Marins JR, Souza EM, Perez R, et al. Micro-CT evaluation of non-instrumented canal areas with different enlargements performed by NiTi systems. Braz Dent J. 2015;26:624–9.
8. Peters OA, Boessler C, Paqué F. Root canal preparation with a novel nickel-titanium instrument evaluated with micro-computed tomography: canal surface preparation over time. J Endod. 2010;36:1068–72.
9. Versiani MA, Steier L, De-Deus G, Tassani S, Pécora JD, Sousa-Neto MD. Micro–computed tomography study of oval-shaped canals prepared with the Self-adjusting File, Reciproc, WaveOne, and Protaper Universal systems. J Endod. 2013;39:1060–6.
10. Peters OA, Schönenberger K, Laib A. Effects of four Ni-Ti preparation techniques on root canal geometry assessed by micro computed tomography. Int Endod J. 2001;34:221–30.
11. De-Deus G, Belladonna FG, Cavalcante DM, Simoes-Carvalho M, Silva E, Carvalhal JCA, et al. Contrast-enhanced micro-CT to assess dental pulp tissue debridement in root canals of extracted teeth: a series of cascading experiments towards method validation. Int Endod J. 2020;54:279–93.
12. Senia ES. Canal diameter: the forgotten dimension. Dent Today. 2001;20:58–62.
13. Jou YT, Karabucak B, Levin J, Liu D. Endodontic working width: current concepts and techniques. Dent Clin N Am. 2004;48:323–35.
14. De-Deus G, Barino B, Zamolyi RQ, Souza E, Fonseca A Jr, Fidel S, et al. Suboptimal debridement quality produced by the single-file F2 ProTaper technique in oval-shaped canals. J Endod. 2010;36:1897–900.
15. De-Deus G, Souza EM, Barino B, Maia J, Zamolyi RQ, Reis C, et al. The self-adjusting file optimizes debridement quality in oval-shaped root canals. J Endod. 2011;37:701–5.
16. Varela P, Souza E, de Deus G, Duran-Sindreu F, Mercade M. Effectiveness of complementary irrigation routines in debriding pulp tissue from root canals instrumented with a single reciprocating file. Int Endod J. 2019;52:475–83.
17. Ricucci D, Loghin S, Goncalves LS, Rocas IN, Siqueira JF Jr. Histobacteriologic conditions of the apical root canal system and periapical tissues in teeth associated with sinus tracts. J Endod. 2018;44:405–13.
18. Ricucci D, Loghin S, Siqueira JF Jr. Exuberant biofilm infection in a lateral canal as the cause of short-term endodontic treatment failure: report of a case. J Endod. 2013;39:712–8.
19. Kishen A. Mechanisms and risk factors for fracture predilection in endodontically treated teeth. Endod Topics. 2006;13:57–83.
20. Estrela C, Decurcio DA, Rossi-Fedele G, Silva JA, Guedes OA, Borges AH. Root perforations: a review of diagnosis, prognosis and materials. Braz Oral Res. 2018;32:e73.
21. De-Deus G, Belladonna FG, Simoes-Carvalho M, Cavalcante DM, Ramalho C, Souza EM, et al. Shaping efficiency as a function of time of a new heat-treated instrument. Int Endod J. 2019;52:337–42.

22. Paqué F, Balmer M, Attin T, Peters OA. Preparation of oval-shaped root canals in mandibular molars using nickel-titanium rotary instruments: a micro-computed tomography study. J Endod. 2010;36:703–7.
23. Paqué F, Peters OA. Micro-computed tomography evaluation of the preparation of long oval root canals in mandibular molars with the self-adjusting file. J Endod. 2011;37:517–21.
24. Mickel AK, Chogle S, Liddle J, Jones JJ. The role of apical size determination and enlargement in the reduction of intracanal bacteria. J Endod. 2007;33:21–3.
25. Lacerda MFLS, Marceliano-Alves MF, Perez AR, Provenzano JC, Neves MAS, Pires FR, et al. Cleaning and shaping oval canals with 3 instrumentation systems: a correlative micro-computed tomographic and histologic study. J Endod. 2017;43:1878–84.
26. Lima CO, Barbosa AFA, Ferreira CM, Augusto CM, Sassone LM, Lopes RT, et al. The impact of minimally invasive root canal preparation strategies on the shaping ability of mandibular molars. Int Endod J. 2020;53:1680–8.
27. Rover G, Belladonna FG, Bortoluzzi EA, De-Deus G, Silva E, Teixeira CS. Influence of access cavity design on root canal detection, instrumentation efficacy, and fracture resistance assessed in maxillary molars. J Endod. 2017;43:1657–62.
28. Burleson A, Nusstein J, Reader A, Beck M. The in vivo evaluation of hand/rotary/ultrasound instrumentation in necrotic, human mandibular molars. J Endod. 2007;33:782–7.
29. Vansan LP, Pecora JD, Costa WF, Maia Campos G. Effects of various irrigating solutions on the cleaning of the root canal with ultrasonic instrumentation. Braz Dent J. 1990;1:37–44.
30. Paqué F, Laib A, Gautschi H, Zehnder M. Hard-tissue debris accumulation analysis by high-resolution computed tomography scans. J Endod. 2009;35:1044–7.
31. Robinson JP, Lumley PJ, Claridge E, Cooper PR, Grover LM, Williams RL, et al. An analytical micro-CT methodology for quantifying inorganic dentine debris following internal tooth preparation. J Dent. 2012;40:999–1005.
32. De-Deus G, Roter J, Reis C, Fidel S, Versiani MA, Alves H, et al. Assessing accumulated hard-tissue debris using micro-computed tomography and free software for image processing and analysis. J Endod. 2014;40:271–6.
33. Haapasalo M, Shen Y, Wang Z, Gao Y. Irrigation in endodontics. Br Dent J. 2014;216:299–303.
34. Nair PN, Henry S, Cano V, Vera J. Microbial status of apical root canal system of human mandibular first molars with primary apical periodontitis after "one-visit" endodontic treatment. Oral Surg Oral Med Oral Pathol Oral Radiol Endod. 2005;99:231–52.
35. Portenier I, Haapasalo H, Rye A, Waltimo T, Orstavik D, Haapasalo M. Inactivation of root canal medicaments by dentine, hydroxylapatite and bovine serum albumin. Int Endod J. 2001;34:184–8.
36. Paqué F, Boessler C, Zehnder M. Accumulated hard tissue debris levels in mesial roots of mandibular molars after sequential irrigation steps. Int Endod J. 2011;44:148–53.
37. Paqué F, Rechenberg DK, Zehnder M. Reduction of hard-tissue debris accumulation during rotary root canal instrumentation by etidronic acid in a sodium hypochlorite irrigant. J Endod. 2012;38:692–5.
38. Paqué F, Al-Jadaa A, Kfir A. Hard-tissue debris accumulation created by conventional rotary versus self-adjusting file instrumentation in mesial root canal systems of mandibular molars. Int Endod J. 2012;45:413–8.
39. Siqueira JF Jr, Perez AR, Marceliano-Alves MF, Provenzano JC, Silva SG, Pires FR, et al. What happens to unprepared root canal walls: a correlative analysis using micro-computed tomography and histology/scanning electron microscopy. Int Endod J. 2018;51:501–8.
40. Zehnder M. Root canal irrigants. J Endod. 2006;32:389–98.
41. Berutti E, Castellucci A. Cleaning and shaping the root canal system. In: Castellucci A, editor. Endodontics. Florence: Il Tridente; 2004. p. 396–437.
42. Peters OA, Peters C. Cleaning and shaping of the root canal system. In: Hargreaves KM, Cohen S, editors. Cohen's pathways of the pulp. St. Louis: Mosby; 2011. p. 283–348.
43. Haapasalo M. Current advances in irrigation. Endod Topics. 2013;27:1–2.
44. Papa J, Cain C, Messer HH. Moisture content of vital vs endodontically treated teeth. Endod Dent Traumatol. 1994;10:91–3.

45. Proell F. Über die Eigenschaften des Calxyls und seine Vorzüge vor anderen in der zahnärztlichen Praxis angewandten Medikamenten. Zahnärztl Rdsch. 1949;14:255–9.
46. Behnen MJ, West LA, Liewehr FR, Buxton TB, McPherson JC 3rd. Antimicrobial activity of several calcium hydroxide preparations in root canal dentin. J Endod. 2001;27:765–7.
47. Sjögren U, Figdor D, Spängberg L, Sundqvist G. The antimicrobial effect of calcium hydroxide as a short-term intracanal dressing. Int Endod J. 1991;24:119–25.
48. Hasselgren G, Olsson B, Cvek M. Effects of calcium hydroxide and sodium hypochlorite on the dissolution of necrotic porcine muscle tissue. J Endod. 1988;14:125–7.
49. Zehnder M, Grawehr M, Hasselgren G, Waltimo T. Tissue-dissolution capacity and dentin-disinfecting potential of calcium hydroxide mixed with irrigating solutions. Oral Surg Oral Med Oral Pathol Oral Radiol Endod. 2003;96:608–13.
50. Kvist T, Molander A, Dahlen G, Reit C. Microbiological evaluation of one- and two-visit endodontic treatment of teeth with apical periodontitis: a randomized, clinical trial. J Endod. 2004;30:572–6.
51. Salas H, Vieira GCS, Palomino I, Valero J, Pacheco-Yanes J, Campello AF, et al. Outcome of endodontic treatment with chlorhexidine gluconate as main irrigant: a case series. Aust Endod J. 2020;46:307–14.
52. Naenni N, Thoma K, Zehnder M. Soft tissue dissolution capacity of currently used and potential endodontic irrigants. J Endod. 2004;30:785–7.
53. Zehnder M, Kosicki D, Luder H, Sener B, Waltimo T. Tissue-dissolving capacity and antibacterial effect of buffered and unbuffered hypochlorite solutions. Oral Surg Oral Med Oral Pathol Oral Radiol Endod. 2002;94:756–62.
54. Grigoratos D, Knowles J, Ng YL, Gulabivala K. Effect of exposing dentine to sodium hypochlorite and calcium hydroxide on its flexural strength and elastic modulus. Int Endod J. 2001;34:113–9.
55. Marending M, Stark WJ, Brunner TJ, Fischer J, Zehnder M. Comparative assessment of time-related bioactive glass and calcium hydroxide effects on mechanical properties of human root dentin. Dent Traumatol. 2009;25:126–9.
56. Sim TP, Knowles JC, Ng YL, Shelton J, Gulabivala K. Effect of sodium hypochlorite on mechanical properties of dentine and tooth surface strain. Int Endod J. 2001;34:120–32.
57. Ulin C, Magunacelaya-Barria M, Dahlen G, Kvist T. Immediate clinical and microbiological evaluation of the effectiveness of 0.5% versus 3% sodium hypochlorite in root canal treatment: a quasi-randomized controlled trial. Int Endod J. 2020;53:591–603.
58. Verma N, Sangwan P, Tewari S, Duhan J. Effect of different concentrations of sodium hypochlorite on outcome of primary root canal treatment: a randomized controlled trial. J Endod. 2019;45:357–63.
59. Marending M, Luder HU, Brunner TJ, Knecht S, Stark WJ, Zehnder M. Effect of sodium hypochlorite on human root dentine--mechanical, chemical and structural evaluation. Int Endod J. 2007;40:786–93.
60. Axelsson P, Nystrom B, Lindhe J. The long-term effect of a plaque control program on tooth mortality, caries and periodontal disease in adults. Results after 30 years of maintenance. J Clin Periodontol. 2004;31:749–57.
61. Shen Y, Gao Y, Qian W, Ruse ND, Zhou X, Wu H, et al. Three-dimensional numeric simulation of root canal irrigant flow with different irrigation needles. J Endod. 2010;36:884–9.
62. Thomas AR, Velmurugan N, Smita S, Jothilatha S. Comparative evaluation of canal isthmus debridement efficacy of modified EndoVac technique with different irrigation systems. J Endod. 2014;40:1676–80.
63. van der Sluis LWM, Verhaagen B, Macedo R, Versluis M. The role of irrigation in endodontics. In: Olivi G, De Moor R, DiVito E, editors. Lasers in endodontics: scientific background and clinical applications. 1st ed. Cham: Springer; 2016. p. 298.
64. Boutsioukis C, Van der Sluis L. Syringe irrigation: blending endodontics and fluid dynamics. In: Bettina B, editor. Endodontic irrigation: chemical disinfection of the root canal system. Cham: Springer; 2015. p. 45–64.
65. Grossman LI. Irrigation of root canals. J Am Dent Assoc. 1943;30:1915–7.

66. Psimma Z, Boutsioukis C, Kastrinakis E, Vasiliadis L. Effect of needle insertion depth and root canal curvature on irrigant extrusion ex vivo. J Endod. 2013;39:521–4.
67. Psimma Z, Boutsioukis C, Vasiliadis L, Kastrinakis E. A new method for real-time quantification of irrigant extrusion during root canal irrigation ex vivo. Int Endod J. 2013;46:619–31.
68. Ram Z. Effectiveness of root canal irrigation. Oral Surg Oral Med Oral Pathol. 1977;44:306–12.
69. Kahn FH, Rosenberg PA, Gliksberg J. An in vitro evaluation of the irrigating characteristics of ultrasonic and subsonic handpieces and irrigating needles and probes. J Endod. 1995;21:277–80.
70. Saini M, Kumari M, Taneja S. Comparative evaluation of the efficacy of three different irrigation devices in removal of debris from root canal at two different levels: an in vitro study. J Conserv Dent. 2013;16:509–13.
71. Perez R, Neves AA, Belladonna FG, Silva EJ, Souza EM, Fidel S, et al. Impact of the needle insertion depth on the removal of hard-tissue debris. Int Endod J. 2016;50:560–8.
72. Boutsioukis C, Kastrinakis E, Lambrianidis T, Verhaagen B, Versluis M, van der Sluis LW. Formation and removal of apical vapor lock during syringe irrigation: a combined experimental and computational fluid dynamics approach. Int Endod J. 2014;47:191–201.
73. Boutsioukis C, Lambrianidis T, Kastrinakis E, Bekiaroglou P. Measurement of pressure and flow rates during irrigation of a root canal ex vivo with three endodontic needles. Int Endod J. 2007;40:504–13.
74. Šnjarić D, Čarija Z, Braut A, Halaji A, Kovačević M, Kuiš D. Irrigation of human prepared root canal—ex vivo based computational fluid dynamics analysis. Croat Med J. 2012;23:470–9.
75. Fernandez Rivas D, Verhaagen B, Seddon JR, Zijlstra AG, Jiang LM, van der Sluis LW, et al. Localized removal of layers of metal, polymer, or biomaterial by ultrasound cavitation bubbles. Biomicrofluidics. 2012;6:34114.
76. van der Sluis LW, Versluis M, Wu MK, Wesselink PR. Passive ultrasonic irrigation of the root canal: a review of the literature. Int Endod J. 2007;40:415–26.
77. Shankar PN, Deshpande MD. Fluid mechanics in the driven cavity. Annu Rev Fluid Mech. 2000;32:93–136.
78. Tay FR, Gu LS, Schoeffel GJ, Wimmer C, Susin L, Zhang K, et al. Effect of vapor lock on root canal debridement by using a side-vented needle for positive-pressure irrigant delivery. J Endod. 2010;36:745–50.
79. Agarwal A, Deore RB, Rudagi K, Nanda Z, Baig MO, Fareez MA. Evaluation of apical vapor lock formation and comparative evaluation of its elimination using three different techniques: an in vitro study. J Contemp Dent Pract. 2017;18:790–4.
80. Vera J, Arias A, Romero M. Effect of maintaining apical patency on irrigant penetration into the apical third of root canals when using passive ultrasonic irrigation: an in vivo study. J Endod. 2011;37:1276–8.
81. Vera J, Arias A, Romero M. Dynamic movement of intracanal gas bubbles during cleaning and shaping procedures: the effect of maintaining apical patency on their presence in the middle and cervical thirds of human root canals-an in vivo study. J Endod. 2012;38: 200–3.
82. Vera J, Hernandez EM, Romero M, Arias A, van der Sluis LW. Effect of maintaining apical patency on irrigant penetration into the apical two millimeters of large root canals: an in vivo study. J Endod. 2012;38:1340–3.
83. Berbert A, Bramante CM. Endodontia prática. São Paulo: Sarvier; 1980.
84. Gutmann JL, Zehnder M, Levermann VM. Historical perspectives on the roots of the apical negative pressure irrigation technique in endodontics. J Hist Dent. 2014;62:32–40.
85. Abarajithan M, Dham S, Velmurugan N, Valerian-Albuquerque D, Ballal S, Senthilkumar H. Comparison of Endovac irrigation system with conventional irrigation for removal of intracanal smear layer: an in vitro study. Oral Surg Oral Med Oral Pathol Oral Radiol Endod. 2011;112:407–11.
86. Buldur B, Kapdan A. Comparison of the EndoVac system and conventional needle irrigation on removal of the smear layer in primary molar root canals. Niger J Clin Pract. 2017;20:1168–74.

87. Buldur B, Kapdan A. Comparison of the antimicrobial efficacy of the EndoVac system and conventional needle irrigation in primary molar root canals. J Clin Pediatr Dent. 2017;41:284–8.
88. de Miranda RG, Gusman HD, Colombo AP. Antimicrobial efficacy of the EndoVac system plus PDT against intracanal Candida albicans: an ex vivo study. Braz Oral Res. 2015;29:S1806–83242015000100308.
89. Nielsen B, Craig Baumgartner J. Comparison of the EndoVac system to needle irrigation of root canals. J Endod. 2007;33:611–5.
90. Parente JM, Loushine RJ, Susin L, Gu L, Looney SW, Weller RN, et al. Root canal debridement using manual dynamic agitation or the EndoVac for final irrigation in a closed system and an open system. Int Endod J. 2010;43:1001–12.
91. Mitchell RP, Yang SE, Baumgartner JC. Comparison of apical extrusion of NaOCl using the EndoVac or needle irrigation of root canals. J Endod. 2010;36:338–41.
92. Howard RK, Kirkpatrick TC, Rutledge RE, Yaccino JM. Comparison of debris removal with three different irrigation techniques. J Endod. 2011;37:1301–5.
93. Schoeffel GJ. The EndoVac method of endodontic irrigation, part 2—efficacy. Dent Today. 2008;27:82, 4, 6–7.
94. Silva CC, Ferreira VMD, De-Deus G, Herrera DR, Prado MD, Silva E. Effect of intermediate flush using different devices to prevent chemical smear layer formation. Braz Dent J. 2017;28:447–52.
95. Silva EJNL, Carvalho CR, Belladonna FG, Prado MC, Lopes RT, De-Deus G, et al. Micro-CT evaluation of different final irrigation protocols on the removal of hard-tissue debris from isthmus-containing mesial root of mandibular molars. Clin Oral Investig. 2019;23:681–7.
96. Siu C, Baumgartner JC. Comparison of the debridement efficacy of the EndoVac irrigation system and conventional needle root canal irrigation in vivo. J Endod. 2010;36:1782–5.
97. Venumbaka NR, Baskaran P, Mungara J, Chenchugopal M, Elangovan A, Vijayakumar P. Comparative evaluation of Endovac and conventional irrigating syringe on apical extrusion in primary molars. An in vitro study. J Clin Pediatr Dent. 2018;42:355–60.
98. Velmurugan N, Sooriaprakas C, Jain P. Apical extrusion of irrigants in immature permanent teeth by using EndoVac and needle irrigation: an in vitro study. J Dent (Tehran). 2014;11:433–9.
99. Kungwani ML, Prasad KP, Khiyani TS. Comparison of the cleaning efficacy of EndoVac with conventional irrigation needles in debris removal from root canal. An in-vivo study. J Conserv Dent. 2014;17:374–8.
100. Căpută PE, Retsas A, Kuijk L, Chavez de Paz LE, Boutsioukis C. Ultrasonic irrigant activation during root canal treatment: a systematic review. J Endod. 2019;45:31–44. e13.
101. Dioguardi M, Gioia GD, Illuzzi G, Laneve E, Cocco A, Troiano G. Endodontic irrigants: different methods to improve efficacy and related problems. Eur J Dent. 2018;12:459–66.
102. Plotino G, Cortese T, Grande NM, Leonardi DP, Di Giorgio G, Testarelli L, et al. New technologies to improve root canal disinfection. Braz Dent J. 2016;27:3–8.
103. Silva E, Rover G, Belladonna FG, Herrera DR, De-Deus G, da Silva Fidalgo TK. Effectiveness of passive ultrasonic irrigation on periapical healing and root canal disinfection: a systematic review. Br Dent J. 2019;227:228–34.
104. Rius L, Arias A, Aranguren JM, Romero M, de Gregorio C. Analysis of the smear layer generated by different activation systems: an in vitro study. Clin Oral Investig. 2021;25:45–51.
105. Urban K, Donnermeyer D, Schäfer E, Bürklein S. Canal cleanliness using different irrigation activation systems: a SEM evaluation. Clin Oral Investig. 2017;21:2681–7.
106. Ma JZ, Shen Y, Al-Ashaw AJ, Khaleel HY, Yang Y, Wang ZJ, et al. Micro-computed tomography evaluation of the removal of calcium hydroxide medicament from C-shaped root canals of mandibular second molars. Int Endod J. 2015;48:333–41.
107. Neuhaus KW, Liebi M, Stauffacher S, Eick S, Lussi A. Antibacterial efficacy of a new sonic irrigation device for root canal disinfection. J Endod. 2016;42:1799–803.
108. Richman MJ. The use of ultrasonic in root canal therapy and root resection. J Dent Med. 1957;12:8–12.

109. Weller RN, Brady JM, Bernier WE. Efficacy of ultrasonic cleaning. J Endod. 1980;6:740–3.
110. Gu LS, Kim JR, Ling J, Choi KK, Pashley DH, Tay FR. Review of contemporary irrigant agitation techniques and devices. J Endod. 2009;35:791–804.
111. Blank-Goncalves LM, Nabeshima CK, Martins GH, Machado ME. Qualitative analysis of the removal of the smear layer in the apical third of curved roots: conventional irrigation versus activation systems. J Endod. 2011;37:1268–71.
112. Lee SJ, Wu MK, Wesselink PR. The effectiveness of syringe irrigation and ultrasonics to remove debris from simulated irregularities within prepared root canal walls. Int Endod J. 2004;37:672–8.
113. Metzler RS, Montgomery S. Effectiveness of ultrasonics and calcium hydroxide for the debridement of human mandibular molars. J Endod. 1989;15:373–8.
114. Al-Jadaa A, Paqué F, Attin T, Zehnder M. Necrotic pulp tissue dissolution by passive ultrasonic irrigation in simulated accessory canals: impact of canal location and angulation. Int Endod J. 2009;42:59–65.
115. de Gregorio C, Estevez R, Cisneros R, Paranjpe A, Cohenca N. Efficacy of different irrigation and activation systems on the penetration of sodium hypochlorite into simulated lateral canals and up to working length: an in vitro study. J Endod. 2010;36:1216–21.
116. Nagendrababu V, Jayaraman J, Suresh A, Kalyanasundaram S, Neelakantan P. Effectiveness of ultrasonically activated irrigation on root canal disinfection: a systematic review of in vitro studies. Clin Oral Investig. 2018;22:655–70.
117. Kosarieh E, Bolhari B, Sanjari Pirayvatlou S, Kharazifard MJ, Sattari Khavas S, Jafarnia S, et al. Effect of Er:YAG laser irradiation using SWEEPS and PIPS technique on dye penetration depth after root canal preparation. Photodiagn Photodyn Ther. 2020;33:102136.
118. Bronnec F, Bouillaguet S, Machtou P. Ex vivo assessment of irrigant penetration and renewal during the final irrigation regimen. Int Endod J. 2010;43:663–72.
119. Gao Y, Haapasalo M, Shen Y, Wu H, Li B, Ruse ND, et al. Development and validation of a three-dimensional computational fluid dynamics model of root canal irrigation. J Endod. 2009;35:1282–7.
120. Machtou P. Investigations sur l'irrigation en endodontie [Thèse de doctorat en sciences odontologiques]. Paris: Université Paris; 1980.
121. Andrabi SM, Kumar A, Mishra SK, Tewari RK, Alam S, Siddiqui S. Effect of manual dynamic activation on smear layer removal efficacy of ethylenediaminetetraacetic acid and SmearClear: an in vitro scanning electron microscopic study. Aust Endod J. 2013;39:131–6.
122. Çapar ID, Aydinbelge HA. Surface change of root canal dentin after the use of irrigation activation protocols: electron microscopy and an energy-dispersive X-ray microanalysis. Microsc Res Tech. 2013;76:893–6.
123. Saber Sel D, Hashem AA. Efficacy of different final irrigation activation techniques on smear layer removal. J Endod. 2011;37:1272–5.
124. Boutsioukis C, Psimma Z, van der Sluis LW. Factors affecting irrigant extrusion during root canal irrigation: a systematic review. Int Endod J. 2013;46:599–618.
125. Desai P, Himel V. Comparative safety of various intracanal irrigation systems. J Endod. 2009;35:545–9.
126. Wu MK, Wesselink PR. A primary observation on the preparation and obturation of oval canals. Int Endod J. 2001;34:137–41.
127. Hof R, Perevalov V, Eltanani M, Zary R, Metzger Z. The self-adjusting file (SAF). Part 2: mechanical analysis. J Endod. 2010;36:691–6.
128. Metzger Z. The self-adjusting file (SAF) system: an evidence-based update. J Conserv Dent. 2014;17:401–19.
129. Metzger Z, Teperovich E, Zary R, Cohen R, Hof R. The self-adjusting file (SAF). Part 1: respecting the root canal anatomy - a new concept of endodontic files and its implementation. J Endod. 2010;36:679–90.
130. Adiguzel O, Yigit-Ozer S, Kaya S, Uysal I, Ganidagli-Ayaz S, Akkus Z. Effectiveness of ethylenediaminetetraacetic acid (EDTA) and MTAD on debris and smear layer removal using a self-adjusting file. Oral Surg Oral Med Oral Pathol Oral Radiol Endod. 2011;112:803–8.

131. Metzger Z, Teperovich E, Cohen R, Zary R, Paqué F, Hülsmann M. The self-adjusting file (SAF). Part 3: removal of debris and smear layer—a scanning electron microscope study. J Endod. 2010;36:697–702.
132. Lin J, Shen Y, Haapasalo M. A comparative study of biofilm removal with hand, rotary nickel-titanium, and self-adjusting file instrumentation using a novel in vitro biofilm model. J Endod. 2013;39:658–63.
133. Siqueira JF Jr, Alves FR, Almeida BM, de Oliveira JC, Roças IN. Ability of chemomechanical preparation with either rotary instruments or self-adjusting file to disinfect oval-shaped root canals. J Endod. 2010;36:1860–5.
134. De-Deus G, Accorsi-Mendonca T, de Carvalho e Silva L, Leite CA, da Silva D, Moreira EJ. Self-adjusting file cleaning-shaping-irrigation system improves root-filling bond strength. J Endod. 2013;39:254–7.
135. Abramovitz I, Relles-Bonar S, Baransi B, Kfir A. The effectiveness of a self-adjusting file to remove residual gutta-percha after retreatment with rotary files. Int Endod J. 2012;45:386–92.
136. Solomonov M, Paqué F, Kaya S, Adiguzel O, Kfir A, Yigit-Ozer S. Self-adjusting files in retreatment: a high-resolution micro-computed tomography study. J Endod. 2012;38: 1283–7.
137. Voet KC, Wu MK, Wesselink PR, Shemesh H. Removal of gutta-percha from root canals using the self-adjusting file. J Endod. 2012;38:1004–6.
138. Siqueira JF Jr, Alves FR, Versiani MA, Rôças IN, Almeida BM, Neves MA, et al. Correlative bacteriologic and micro-computed tomographic analysis of mandibular molar mesial canals prepared by self-adjusting file, reciproc, and twisted file systems. J Endod. 2013;39:1044–50.
139. Costerton JW, Geesey GG, Cheng KJ. How bacteria stick. Sci Am. 1978;238:86–95.
140. Costerton JW, Lewandowski Z, Caldwell DE, Korber DR, Lappin-Scott HM. Microbial biofilms. Annu Rev Microbiol. 1995;49:711–45.
141. Nair PN, Luder HU. [Root canal and periapical flora: a light and electron microscopy study]. Schweiz Monatsschr Zahnmed. 1985;95:992–1003.
142. Zobell CE. The effect of solid surfaces upon bacterial activity. J Bacteriol. 1943;46:39–56.
143. Schaudinn C, Carr G, Gorur A, Jaramillo D, Costerton JW, Webster P. Imaging of endodontic biofilms by combined microscopy (FISH/cLSM—SEM). J Microsc. 2009;235:124–7.
144. Flemming HC, Wingender J. The biofilm matrix. Nat Rev Microbiol. 2010;8:623–33.
145. Karygianni L, Ren Z, Koo H, Thurnheer T. Biofilm matrixome: extracellular components in structured microbial communities. Trends Microbiol. 2020;28:668–81.
146. Oppenheimer-Shaanan Y, Sibony-Nevo O, Bloom-Ackermann Z, Suissa R, Steinberg N, Kartvelishvily E, et al. Spatio-temporal assembly of functional mineral scaffolds within microbial biofilms. NPJ Biofilms Microbiomes. 2016;2:15031.
147. Busanello FH, Petridis X, So MVR, Dijkstra RJB, Sharma PK, van der Sluis LWM. Chemical biofilm removal capacity of endodontic irrigants as a function of biofilm structure: optical coherence tomography, confocal microscopy and viscoelasticity determination as integrated assessment tools. Int Endod J. 2019;52:461–74.
148. Tawakoli PN, Ragnarsson KT, Rechenberg DK, Mohn D, Zehnder M. Effect of endodontic irrigants on biofilm matrix polysaccharides. Int Endod J. 2017;50:153–60.
149. Banin E, Brady KM, Greenberg EP. Chelator-induced dispersal and killing of *Pseudomonas aeruginosa* cells in a biofilm. Appl Environ Microbiol. 2006;72:2064–9.
150. Chavez de Paz LE, Bergenholtz G, Svensater G. The effects of antimicrobials on endodontic biofilm bacteria. J Endod. 2010;36:70–7.
151. Zollinger A, Mohn D, Zeltner M, Zehnder M. Short-term storage stability of NaOCl solutions when combined with dual rinse HEDP. Int Endod J. 2018;51:691–6.
152. Lottanti S, Gautschi H, Sener B, Zehnder M. Effects of ethylenediaminetetraacetic, etidronic and peracetic acid irrigation on human root dentine and the smear layer. Int Endod J. 2009;42:335–43.
153. Morago A, Ordinola-Zapata R, Ferrer-Luque CM, Baca P, Ruiz-Linares M, Arias-Moliz MT. Influence of smear layer on the antimicrobial activity of a sodium hypochlorite/etidronic acid irrigating solution in infected dentin. J Endod. 2016;42:1647–50.

154. Giardino L, Del Fabbro M, Morra M, Pereira T, Bombarda de Andrade F, Savadori P, et al. Dual rinse((R)) HEDP increases the surface tension of NaOCl but may increase its dentin disinfection efficacy. Odontology. 2019;107:521–9.
155. Arias-Moliz MT, Ordinola-Zapata R, Baca P, Ruiz-Linares M, Ferrer-Luque CM. Antimicrobial activity of a sodium hypochlorite/etidronic acid irrigant solution. J Endod. 2014;40:1999–2002.
156. Arias-Moliz MT, Ordinola-Zapata R, Baca P, Ruiz-Linares M, Garcia Garcia E, Hungaro Duarte MA, et al. Antimicrobial activity of chlorhexidine, peracetic acid and sodium hypochlorite/etidronate irrigant solutions against *Enterococcus faecalis* biofilms. Int Endod J. 2015;48:1188–93.
157. Neelakantan P, Varughese AA, Sharma S, Subbarao CV, Zehnder M, De-Deus G. Continuous chelation irrigation improves the adhesion of epoxy resin-based root canal sealer to root dentine. Int Endod J. 2012;45:1097–102.
158. De-Deus G, Namen F, Galan J Jr, Zehnder M. Soft chelating irrigation protocol optimizes bonding quality of resilon/epiphany root fillings. J Endod. 2008;34:703–5.
159. Carrilho E, Cardoso M, Marques Ferreira M, Marto CM, Paula A, Coelho AS. 10-MDP based dental adhesives: adhesive interface characterization and adhesive stability—a systematic review. Materials (Basel). 2019;12:790.
160. De-Deus G, Reis C, Paciornik S. Critical appraisal of published smear layer-removal studies: methodological issues. Oral Surg Oral Med Oral Pathol Oral Radiol Endod. 2011;112:531–43.

The Glide Path Matter

3

Gustavo De Deus, Emmanuel J. N. L. Silva, Erick Souza, Marco A. Versiani, and Mario Zuolo

3.1 Introduction

Historically, nickel-titanium (NiTi) rotary instruments are marked by concerns regarding a somehow unpredictable risk of fracture. There is a significant accumulated body of applied and scientific knowledge on the sequence of physical processes that result in the fracture of a NiTi instrument driven under continuous rotary kinematics. Although studies have reported fracture rates of NiTi rotary instruments from 2 to 26% [1–5], the main difference between rotary and reciprocating movement is clear, as studies that evaluated reciprocating instruments have always shown a low separation rate [6–8]. There are two main causes of instrument fracture: cyclic fatigue and torsional failure. The former occurs as a consequence of the repeated use of the instrument under flexion (Fig. 3.1a), while the torsional fracture is a result of the continuous screwing of the instrument within a narrow-reduced canal space (Fig. 3.1b). Essentially, what happens in the torsional failure is that the tip of the instrument locks in the root canal while the rest of the body continues to rotate until the fracture occurs. The rotary instrument is repeatedly engaged to the dentin in order to cut it during the

G. De Deus (✉)
Fluminense Federal University, Niterói, Brazil
e-mail: endogus@gmail.com

E. J. N. L. Silva
Fluminense Federal University, Grande Rio University, Rio de Janeiro State University, Niterói, Brazil

E. Souza
Federal University of Maranhão, São Luis, Brazil

M. A. Versiani
Dental Specialty Center, Brazilian Military Police, Minas Gerais, Brazil

M. Zuolo
Dental School of APCD – FAOA, São Paulo, Brazil

G. De Deus et al. (eds.), *Shaping for Cleaning the Root Canals*,
https://doi.org/10.1007/978-3-030-84617-6_3

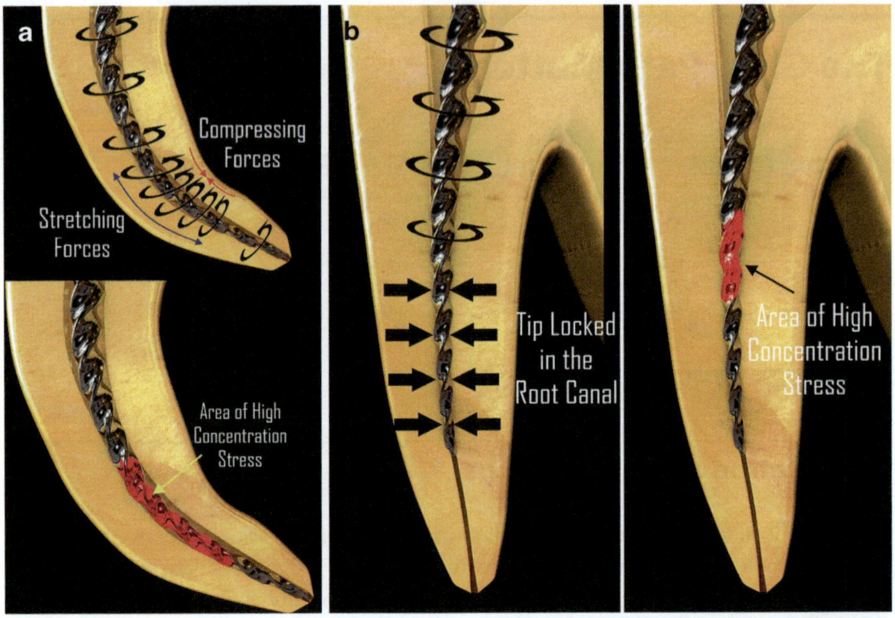

Fig. 3.1 (**a**) Cyclic fatigue occurs as a consequence of the repeated use of the instrument under flexion, while (**b**) torsional stress results from the continuous screwing of the instrument within a narrow-reduced canal space

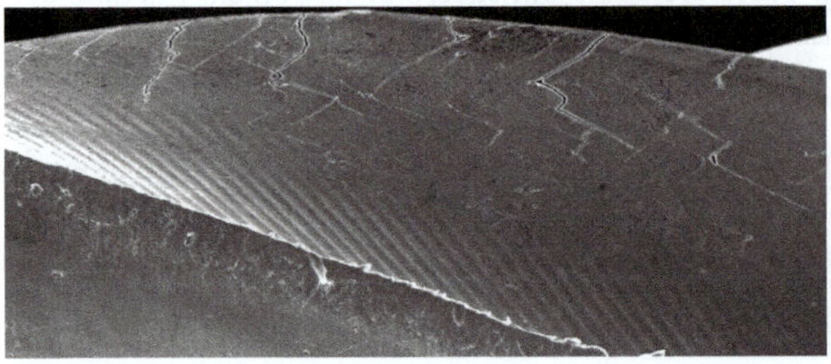

Fig. 3.2 Scanning electron microscopy of a rotary NiTi instrument showing several microstructural damages on its surface after being clinically used to prepare the root canals of a mandibular molar. (Courtesy of Prof. Victor Talarico Leal Vieira)

shaping procedure while forces start and increase as the instrument moves toward the apex. During this process, the instrument is progressively submitted to physical contact with the dentinal walls, which may lead to microstructural surface damages (Fig. 3.2) that accumulate very fast due to the continuous rotary movement. Then, its tip may bind into the canal lumen creating more stress, ending up in torsional failure (Fig. 3.3). In summary, the high torque levels lead the instrument to exceed its elastic limit and the torsional fracture takes place. As it is well documented in the literature, this represents the major cause of separation and deformation of NiTi rotary instruments [3, 9] (Fig. 3.4).

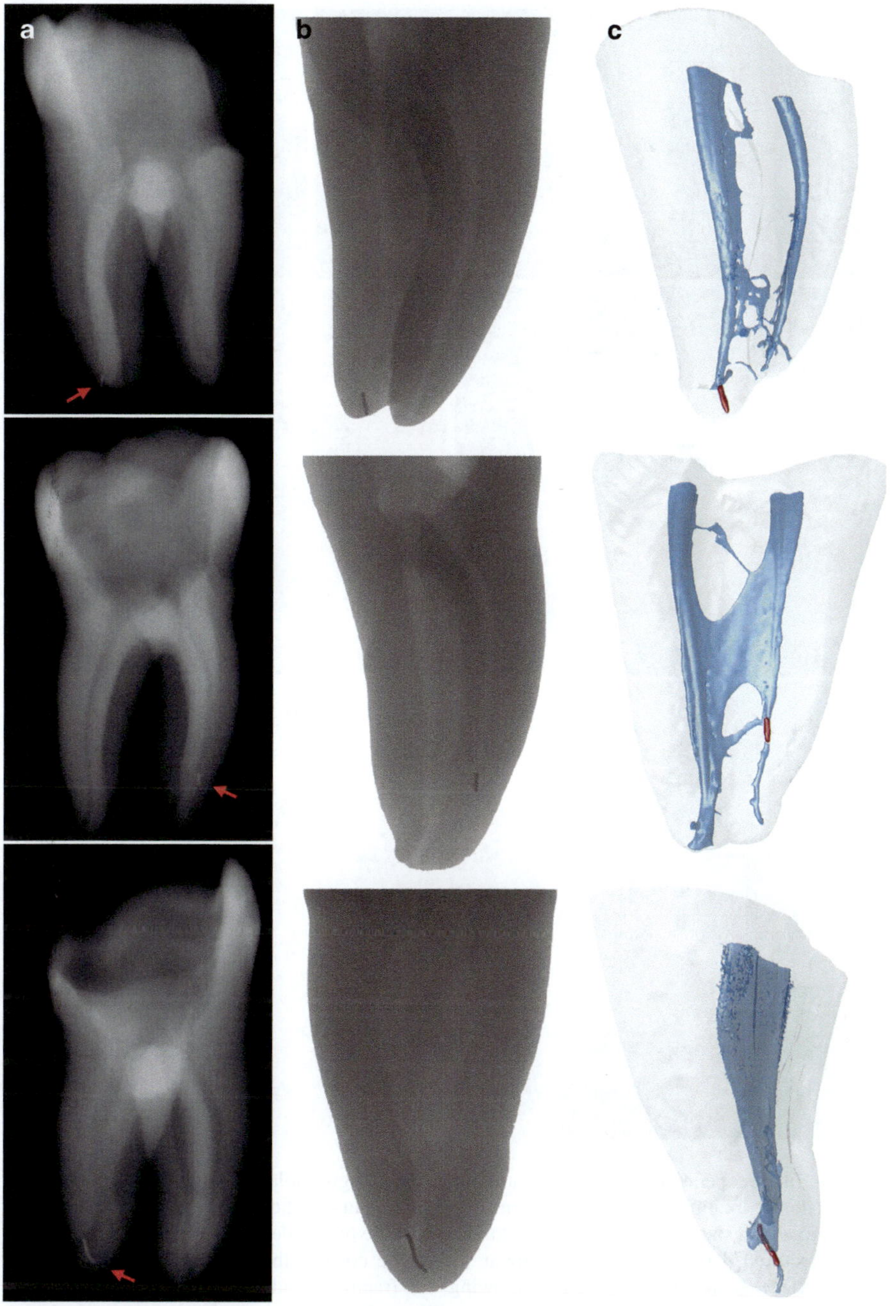

Fig. 3.3 (**a**) Radiographic images of 3 mandibular molar teeth with fractured NiTi pathfinder instruments within the root canal system (red arrows). (**b**) Micro-CT projection images highlighting the position of the fragments. (**c**) Representative 3D models depicting the root canals (in blue) and the fractured instruments (in red). These are typical cases in which the main cause of instrument separation was the accumulated torsional stress

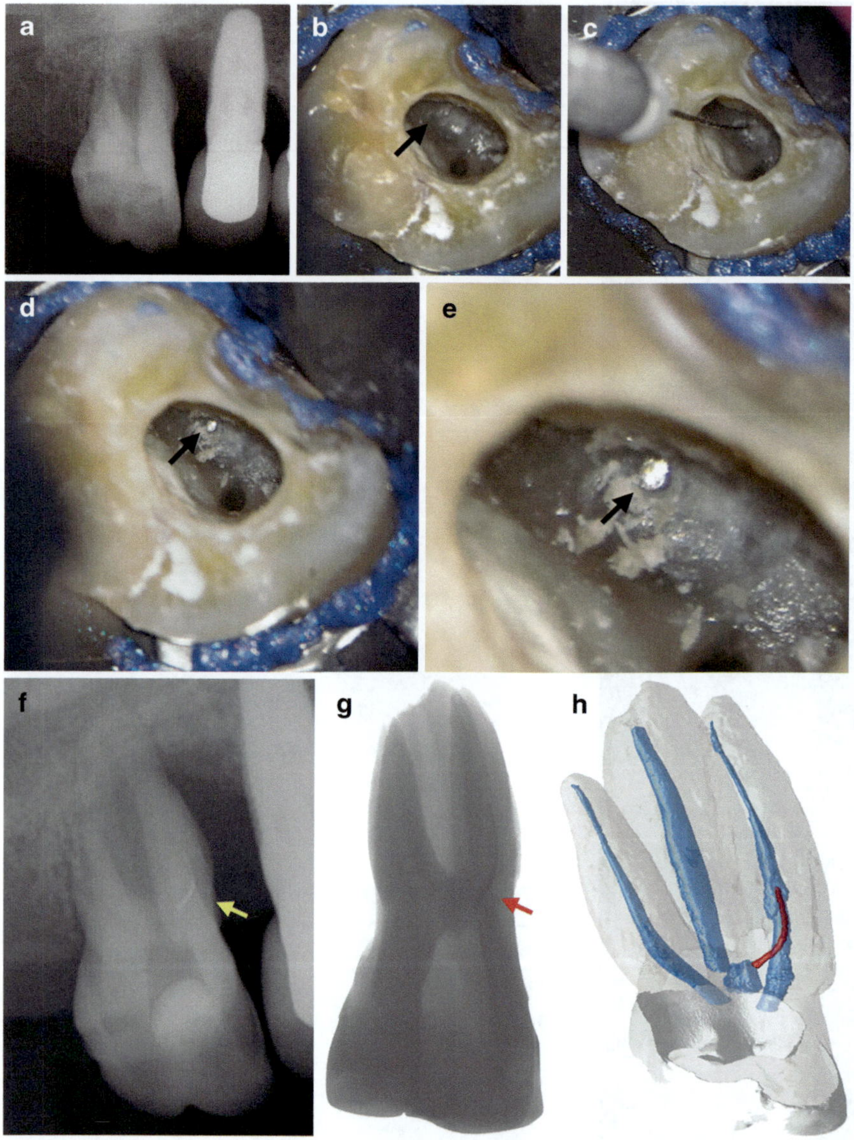

Fig. 3.4 (**a**) Preoperative radiograph of a maxillary first right molar with narrow canals referred for endodontic treatment. (**b**) Localization of the MB2 canal orifice (black arrow). (**c**) Scouting procedure with a size 08 C-Pilot file prior to the use of the pathfinder NiTi instrument. (**d**, **e**) View of the fractured pathfinder NiTi instrument within the coronal third of the MB2 canal (black arrow). (**f**) Transoperative radiograph showing the fractured pathfinder NiTi instrument in a severely curved MB2 canal (yellow arrow). (**g**) Micro-CT projection image acquired after tooth extraction highlighting the level and length of the broken fragment (red arrow). The extraction was done because changes in treatment planning. (**h**–**j**) Different views of a micro-CT 3D model of the extracted tooth depicting the root canals (in blue) and the fragment of the instrument (in red). The instrument separation possibly occurred due to the interplay of two factors: (1) the screwing of the instrument within a narrow-reduced canal space at the coronal third and (2) the tip of the instrument was lost in finding the natural canal path at the beginning of the middle third (black arrows in **j**)

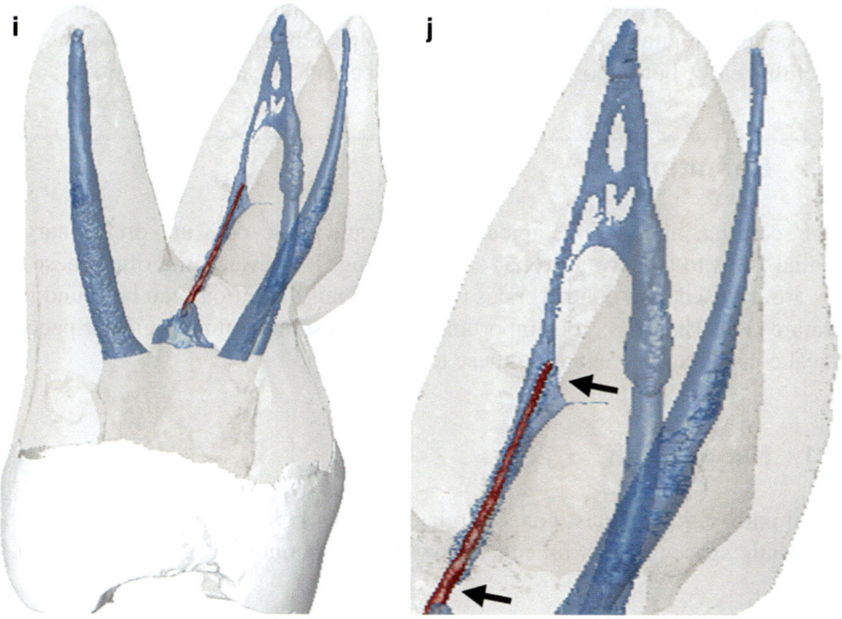

Fig. 3.4 (continued)

One of the proposals to minimize the fracture rate of rotary instruments was made in the early 2000s when John West [10] coined the glide path concept. As a matter of fact, at that time, experienced clinicians were already aware that a pre-enlargement of the root canal space with manual files was a basic requirement for the safe usage of the engine-driven NiTi rotary instruments. However, it is fair to say that West [10] moved things forward when introducing the term "glide path." He organized the overall idea of pre-instrumentation with manual files into a logical rationale on what, how, when and why the safety of rotary canal preparation is dependent on the quality of this early preparation procedure. This way, West [10] streamlined the overall glide path idea as "the secret to rotary safety" because the procedure is able to reduce instrument fracture caused by torsional stress. Consequently, as time went by, glide path became a mandatory step in the preparation of the root canal system with rotary NiTi instruments due to the improvements in safety and efficiency.

The problem takes place when, at the same time as being mandatory for engine-based shaping, the glide path represents a highly technically demanding transoperative maneuver that can often be challenging, laborious, and time-consuming, requiring the utmost patience and diligence even from masterful endodontic clinicians. Therefore, this represents an interesting problematic paradoxical situation: while one problem is controlled (risk of instrument fracture), another serious one is created, as the glide path often demands clinical experience and skills. As a consequence, the effective use of rotary-driven NiTi instruments requires a considerable long learning curve until proper competence is achieved.

The aim of the present chapter is to clarify the nomenclature and definitions of the procedures related to the glide path and to present and discuss different protocols of this early, but important stage of the mechanical canal preparation.

3.2 Definitions

Canal scouting, negotiation, apical patency, and glide path are preliminary but essential steps to achieve a proper canal shaping. However, quite often these concepts are misused, and controversies regarding their definitions can be found in the literature [11]. Therefore, it is important to discuss some terminological aspects and clinical considerations regarding these terms.

3.2.1 Natural Path

Natural path is the simplest concept related to this topic and it means the existing hollow pulp space that instruments follow during shaping procedures (Fig. 3.5).

3.2.2 Canal Scouting

Canal scouting precedes the establishment of the apical patency. It refers to the initial canal negotiation/exploration with passive, small and flexible files attempting to progress toward the apex up to the working length. It is worth noting that, under the framework of endodontics, “exploration” and “scouting” are synonyms of “negotiation.”

Canal scouting is a passive penetration that smooths out the irregularities on the canal walls but without the intention of cutting dentin. As a general rule, small-sized and more rigid instruments are suitable for narrow canals, while precurved instruments are more effective to overcome abrupt canal curvatures [12–14]. The point is to balance the small sizes with the adequate rigidity of the instruments to overcome the natural resistance and thus explore the natural canal path while advancing toward the apex.

Canal scouting allows the operator to understand and become acquainted with not only the internal anatomy of the tooth, but also to verify the level of resistance in order to advance the file toward the apex [11]. This procedure is done by using thin stainless steel hand K-files, such as sizes 06, 08 or 10, in a watch-winding movement with gentle apical pressure (Fig. 3.6a–i). This allows the clinician to obtain as much information as possible on the internal anatomy of the tooth including the overall configuration, length, width and the presence of calcification and/or curvatures [11] (Figs. 3.7 and 3.8). By preemptively identifying these anatomical factors, clinicians can obtain a guiding overview for planning the sequential steps of the treatment before effectively starting the mechanical preparation [15]. This information along with that obtained by radiographic or CBCT images allow the

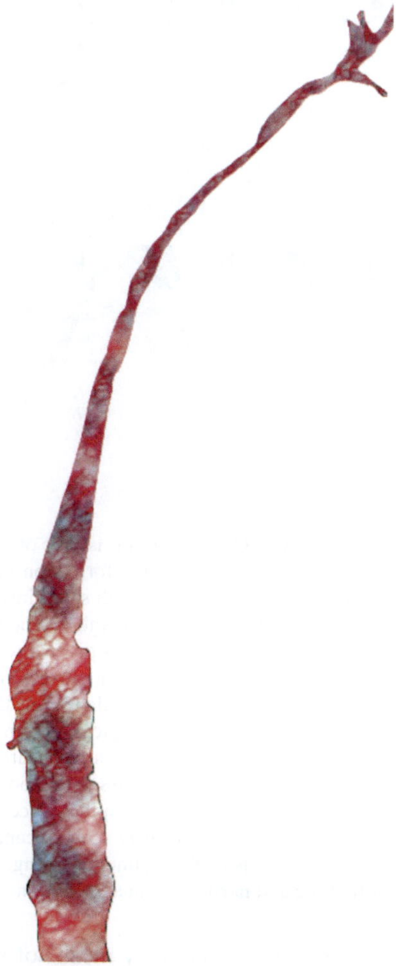

Fig. 3.5 Natural path is the existing pulp space that instruments follow during shaping procedures. Preliminary steps before root canal preparation, such as scouting, patency and glide path may be more complicated or not depending if the natural path is narrow or not

professional to create a true-to-life visualization of the three-dimensional status of the original root canal. The better the 3D map of the root canal conditions mentally created by the clinician, the smoother the canal shaping will flow.

3.2.3 Apical Patency

In his classic study from 1974, Schilder [16] discussed in detail the mechanical preparation of root canals and addressed the apical patency concept. However, it was not until almost a decade later that the modern concept of apical patency was formalized by Buchanan [17]. Today, apical patency is described in the *Glossary of Endodontic Terms* published by the American Association of Endodontists [18] as a

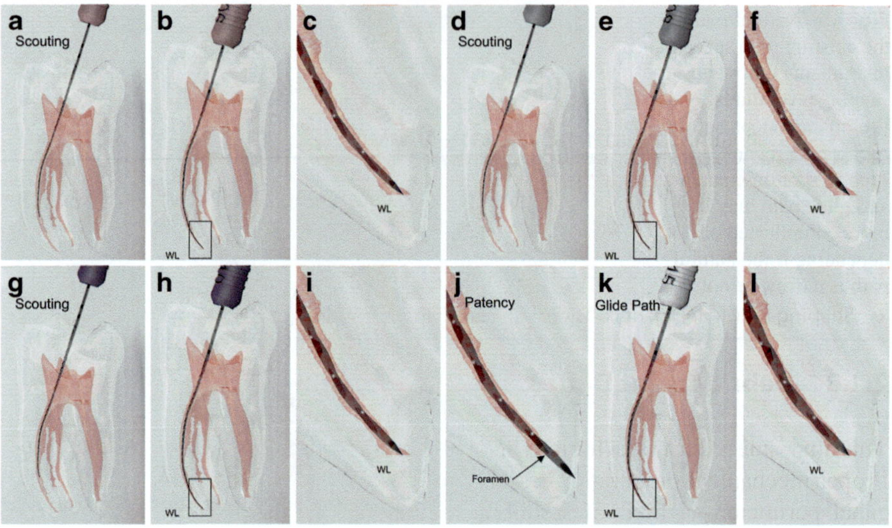

Fig. 3.6 (**a–i**) Canal scouting is part of the glide path procedure and refers to an early step in which the clinician gathers information and insights on the root canal anatomy through tactile sensitivity while advancing with small instruments toward the apex. It consists in a passive penetration of the instrument to smooth out the irregularities on the canal walls without the intention of cutting the dentinal tissue. This procedure is done by using thin stainless steel hand K-files sizes 06, 08, or 10 in a watch-winding movement with gentle apical pressure in order to verify the level of resistance and advance the file toward the apex. (**j**) Patency is the last stage of the micro glide path procedure in which the apical portion of the canal is maintained free of debris by recapitulation with a small file passing passively through the apical foramen. It refers to the ability to pass a small K-file beyond the confines of the root length ensuring the clinician has full access to the main apical foramen during the shaping procedures. (**k, l**) The glide path per se consists in a small enlargement of the previously scouted canal space. It aims to create a smooth canal path to minimize the incidence of instrument binding, controlling the torsional stress to reduce the incidence of fracture and iatrogenic canal deviation

preparation technique by means of which the "apical portion of the canal is maintained free of debris by recapitulation with a small file through the apical foramen" (Figs. 3.9 and 3.10). In other words, apical patency refers to the ability to pass a small K-file beyond the confines of the root length (Fig. 3.6j), ensuring the clinician has full access to the main apical foramen during the shaping procedures (Fig. 3.11), once soft tissue and dentinal debris may accumulate during canal shaping causing undesirable apical blockage and loss of working length [19]. In the workflow of the glide path procedure, the establishment of the apical patency is completed by the electronic determination of the canal terminus (Fig. 3.12).

At this moment, although it may be considered as basic knowledge, it is timely to clarify the difference between working length and canal terminus. The latter is the endpoint of the root canal, the virtual vertex of the major anatomical foramen. It is the anatomical landmark where the reading of the electronic apex locator (EAL)

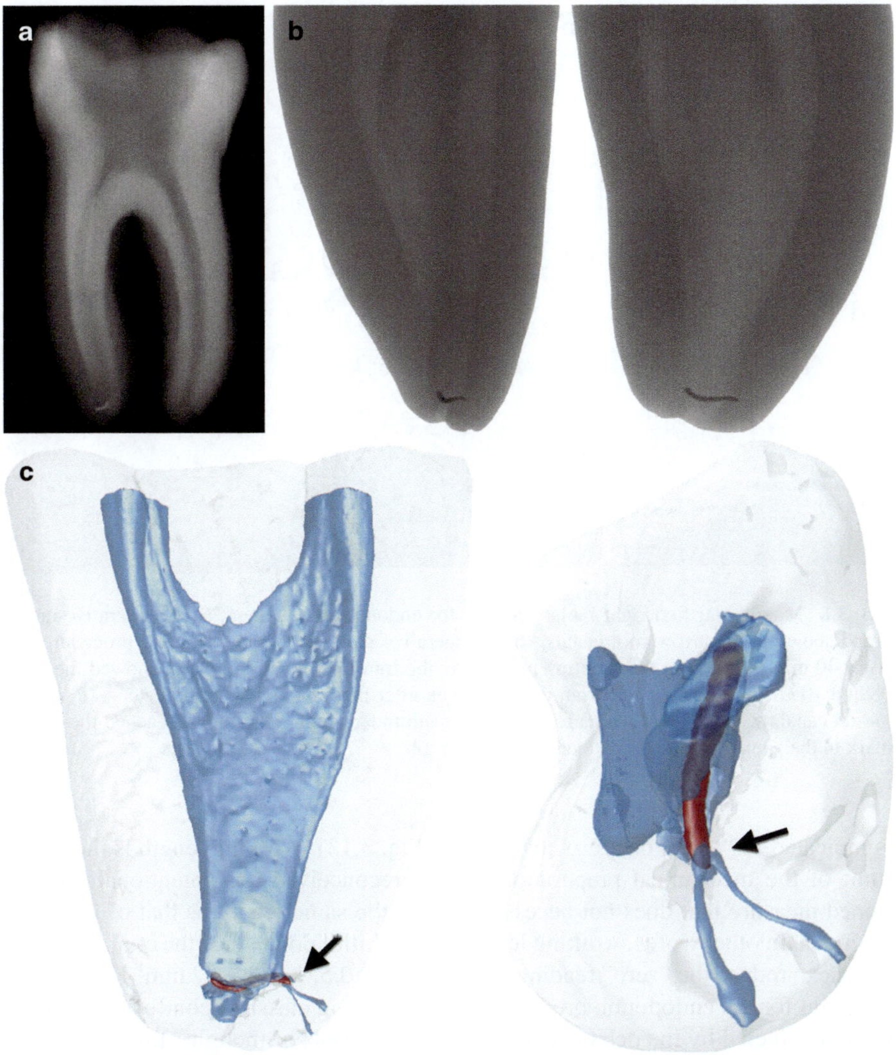

Fig. 3.7 Canal configuration, canal length, canal width, calcifications, curvatures, and bifurcations are core challenges for achieving apical patency. (**a**) Radiographic image of a mandibular molar with a pathfinding instrument fractured at the apical third. (**b**) Micro-CT projection images showing different views of the mandibular molar in (**a**). (**c**) Different views of the micro-CT 3D model of the mandibular molar in (**a**) in which it is possible to observe the intricate canal anatomy at the apical third. In fact, the close view of the apex shows a bifurcation in which the pathfinder instrument got itself unable to follow the natural canal pathway, ending up in its fracture

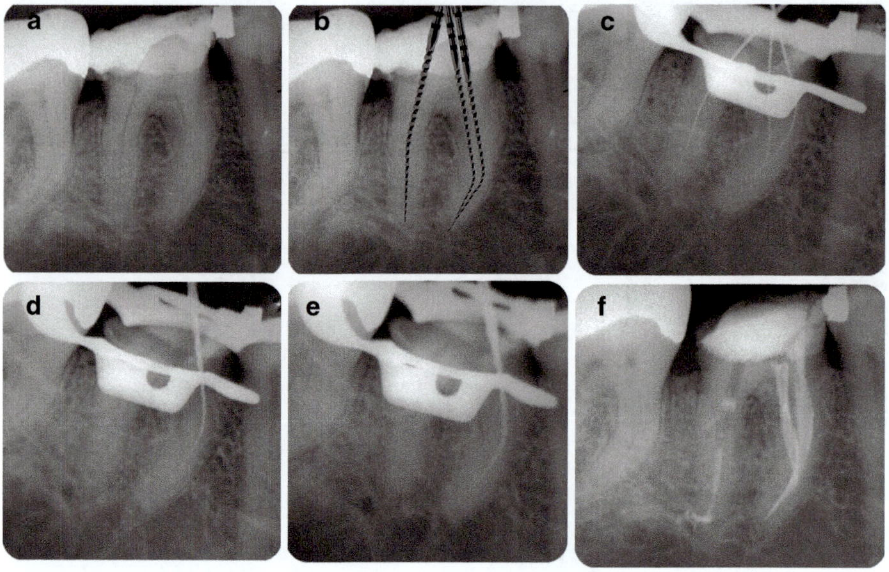

Fig. 3.8 Mandibular first right molar referred for endodontic treatment. (**a**) Preoperative radiograph showing its narrow root canals. (**b**) Preoperative planning for the scouting procedure. (**c**) After 40 min performing the scouting procedure, the transoperative radiograph showed the sizes 08 and 10 C-Pilot files still far from the apex even after meticulous negotiation steps. (**d**, **e**) The mesial canals were scouted with a reciprocating pathfinder instrument until it reached the "zero" mark in the apex locator. (**f**) Postoperative radiograph

is indicated as "apex" or "zero" by default (Fig. 3.13). Working length is the apical limit of the mechanical preparation and a preconceived and intentionally determined measure that does not necessarily have the same length as that of the canal terminus. In other words, working length is an arbitral point since the clinicians may choose to reduce the "zero" reading in the EAL by 0.5, 1 or even 2 mm. The optimal endpoint for the endodontic procedures is an ongoing classical controversy in endodontics, fueled by the debate among different schools of thought. Taken into consideration that the "zero" reading indicated by the EALs is the only accurate measure from the canal length [20, 21], we do not believe that the dispute between 0.5 and 1 mm over the optimal endpoint of root canal treatment is of clinical relevance. In simple terms, we think that using the "zero" reading indicated by the EALs is a practical and convenient clinical strategy that streamlines the earliest sequence of root canal treatment: negotiation, canal patency confirmation, and working length determination—which, in our group, is considered as being at the canal terminus. This means that, at this particular point, we follow most of the North American dental schools, which advocate extending the shaping procedures up to the canal terminus. This clinical approach started off with Schilder in his classical paper [16] in which he stated that the apex, as seen on the radiographic film, is the unique reference point for the clinician. However, nowadays, it is well established that the

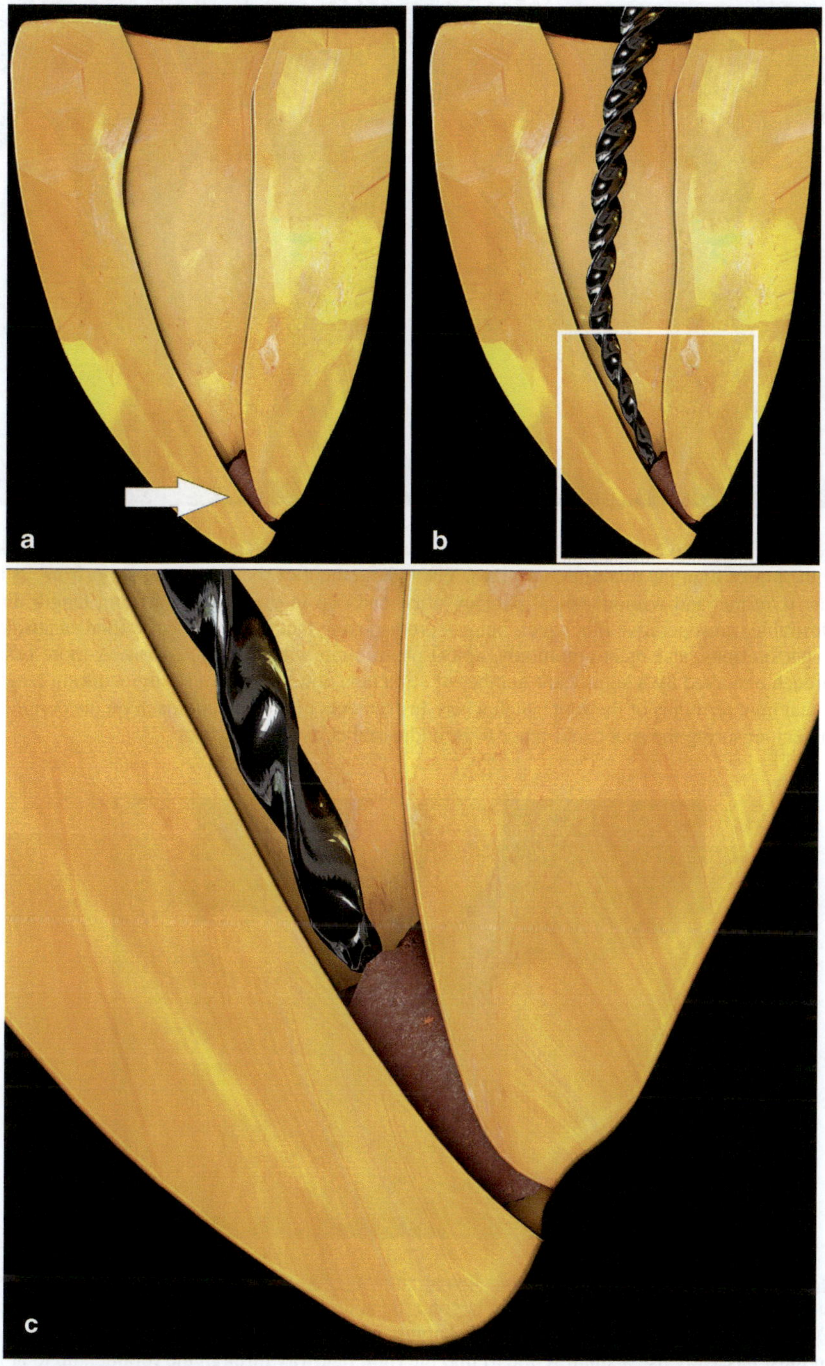

Fig. 3.9 Illustrative images showing the presence of debris created at the apical canal (arrow in **a**) by hand or mechanical preparation. (**b, c**) The presence of accumulated debris hinders the performance of the shaping for cleaning procedures at this level as such apical blockage may be unable to be bypassed by the clinician

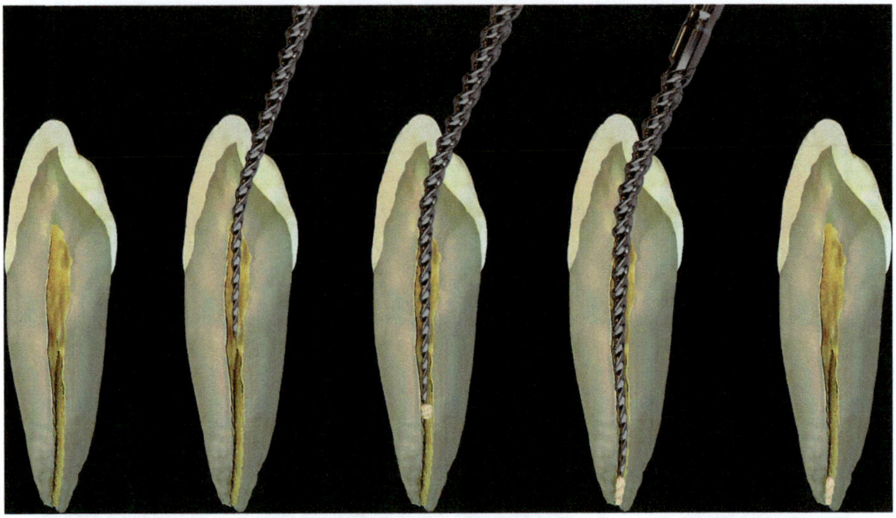

Fig. 3.10 Illustrative images showing the sequential steps of shaping procedures with working length shorter than the anatomic terminus. The enlargement of the root canal short from its anatomic terminus and without apical patency often ends up in the loss of working length due to undesirable transoperative blockages, being a predisposing factor to unclean/unfilled canals, ledging, perforations, and most commonly, apical obstruction with dentinal debris. A more reliable approach endorsed by a significant number of clinicians nowadays is to set the working length at the anatomic terminus of the root canal, where instruments may often encroach on the periodontal ligament, ensuring the root canal space to be addressed at its full extension

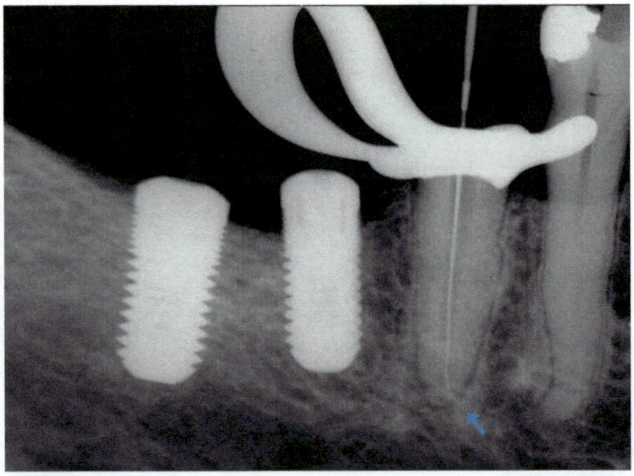

Fig. 3.11 Transoperative radiographic image showing the patency file (small tip-sized instrument) being passively extended slightly beyond the apical foramen (blue arrow), a maneuver that must be continuously repeated throughout shaping procedures. To perform this properly, the clinician must passively use a small K-file to find the right pathway through the foramen up to at least 1 mm longer than the working length

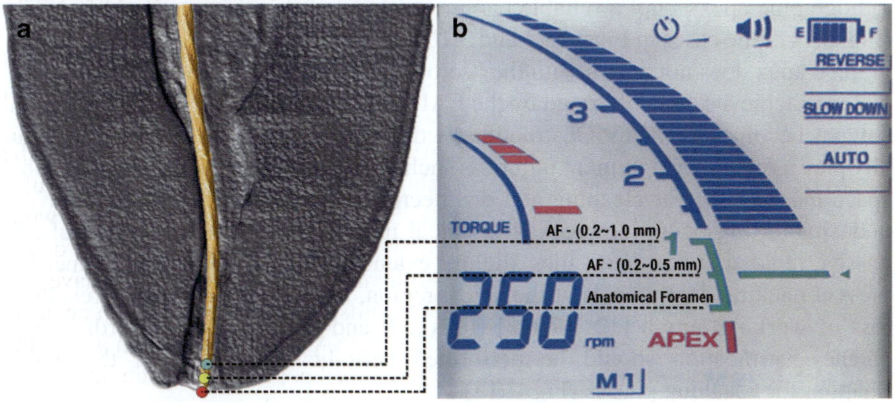

Fig. 3.12 (**a**) Longitudinal micro-CT cross section of the apical third of a single-rooted teeth with the tip of a stainless steel instrument (in yellow) positioned at the anatomical foramen. (**b**) LCD display screen of an electronic apex locator showing its reading marks and their corresponding anatomical landmarks at the canal terminus. (Courtesy of Dr. Marco Simões, Rio de Janeiro, Brazil)

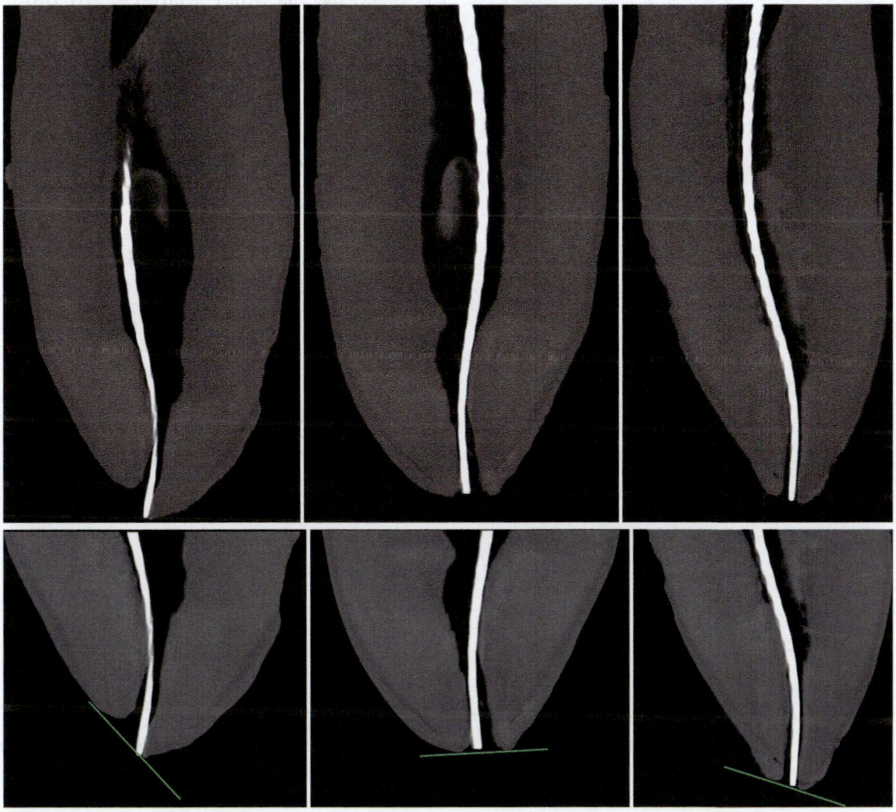

Fig. 3.13 Longitudinal micro-CT cross sections of the apical third of single-rooted teeth showing the tip of a stainless steel endodontic file positioned at the "apex" or "zero" reading mark of the electronic apex locator. (Courtesy of Dr. Marco Simões, Rio de Janeiro, Brazil)

radiographic apex is not a reliable parameter to determine the true canal terminus (Fig. 3.14). The cases in Figs. 3.15 and 3.16 illustrate a situation in which the radiographic apex does not match with the "zero" mark indicated by the EAL.

Once achieved and confirmed by the EAL reading, the maintenance of the apical patency becomes the focus. Obstructions, ledges, zips, and canal transportation usually play a role in the treatment failure as such incidents may leave parts of the canal space inaccessible for cleaning and disinfection procedures (Fig. 3.17). To avoid undesirable transoperative blockages, apical patency is kept by systematical and passive reuse of small hand files slightly extended beyond the main foramen, to prevent packing dentin chips at the apical region, a problem that usually results in loss of working length [12, 17, 22] (Figs. 3.9 and 3.10). In other words, apical patency verification should be performed periodically throughout the whole Shaping for Cleaning phases (Fig. 3.18).

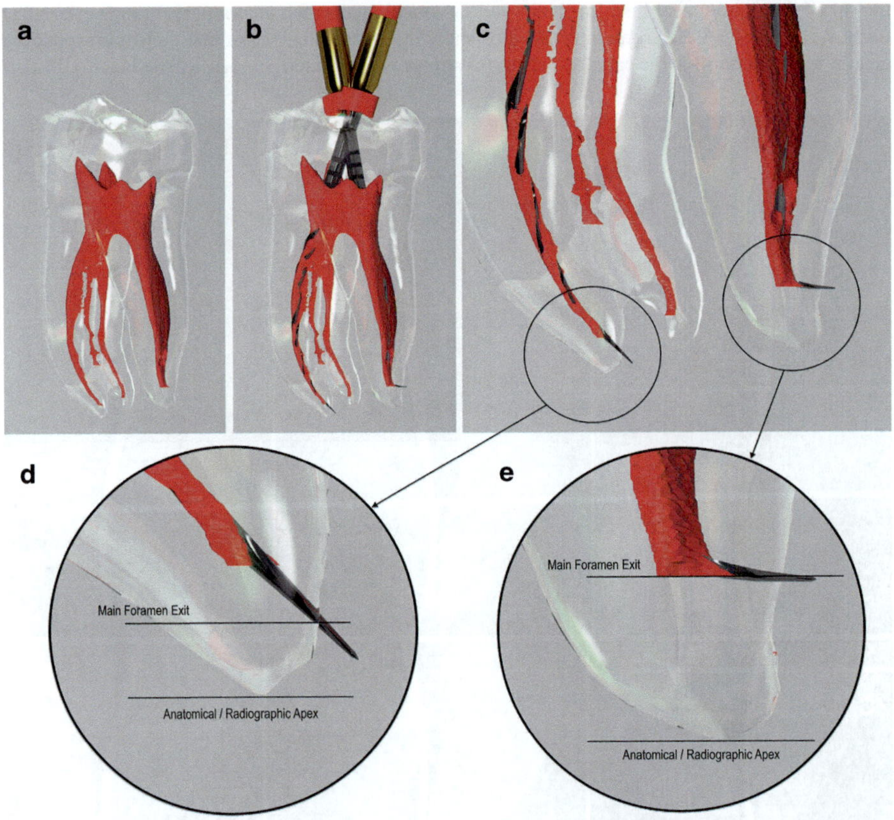

Fig. 3.14 (**a**) 3D model of a real mandibular first molar acquired using a micro-CT imaging system and reconstructed with dedicated software. (**b**) Simulation of patency procedure with rotary instruments using advanced computational tools. (**c–e**) Detailed images of the apical third of the mesial and distal roots showing that anatomical/radiographic apex is not a reliable parameter to determine the true canal terminus considering that in most teeth apical foramen is located at the lateral aspect of the root

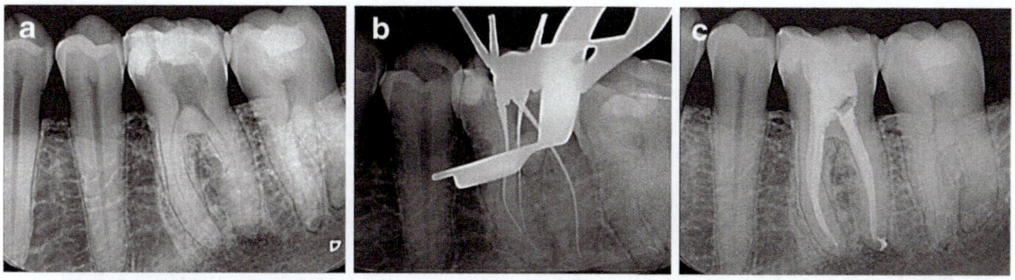

Fig. 3.15 (**a**) Preoperative radiograph of a mandibular first left molar with apical periodontitis referred for root canal treatment. (**b**) Scouting procedure was performed to the working length with sizes 10 and 15 K-files in the mesial and distal canals, respectively, determined by the electronic apex locator at the "zero" reading mark. Note that there is no coincidence at the working length determined by the apex locator ("zero" reading) and the radiographic apex. (**c**) Postoperative radiograph

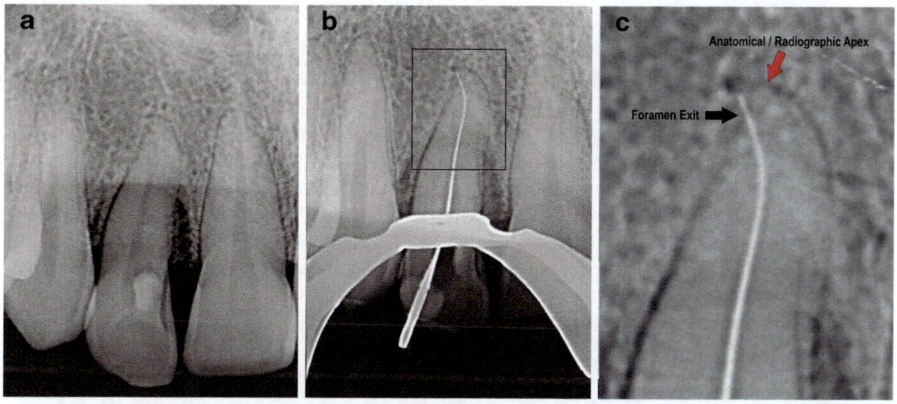

Fig. 3.16 Clinical case illustrating the classical situation of an eccentric foramen position. (**a**) Preoperative radiograph of a maxillary right lateral incisor referred for root canal treatment. (**b**) Working length determination with an electronic apex locator set at the "zero" reading mark. (**c**) Magnification of the area squared in (**b**) showing that the anatomical/radiographic apex does not coincide with the position of the major foramen exit, the anatomical landmark determined by the apex locator

Patency also improves irrigation by significantly reducing gas bubbles at the apical area, overcoming the adverse effects of the vapor-look phenomenon [23]. Moreover, it provides a direct route for drainage, allowing the exudates to outflow toward the canal space. Considering that inflammatory exudates often accumulate in the periapical tissues, a patent foramen is an important physical-local factor to provide relief to the patient. Evidence from clinical studies has demonstrated that apical patency yields a low degree of postoperative pain [23–26].

Considering the aforementioned elements, it is reasonable to say that, without the conquest and maintenance of the apical patency, the treatment outcome is, at least to some extent, compromised. This statement is supported by the study of Ng et al. [27] that found 1.54- and 1.97-fold reduction in the treatment and retreatment success outcome, respectively, when canal patency could not be established.

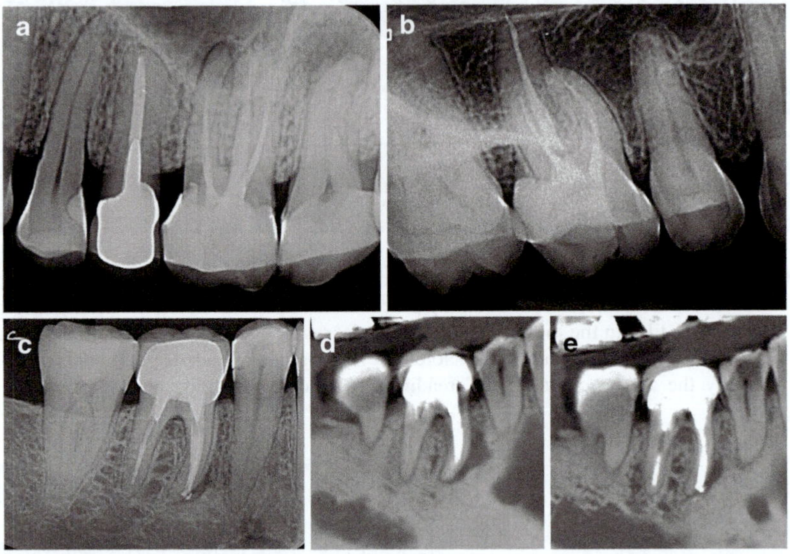

Fig. 3.17 Clinical cases showing (**a**, **b**) suboptimal mechanical shaping and (**c**–**e**) procedural erros in the root canal treatment of molars. (**a**) Maxillary first left molar with deviation and inadequate apical preparation limit in the mesibuccal root. (**b**) Maxillary first right molar with incomplete canal shaping and apical periodontitis observed in preoperative radiograph image. (**c**–**e**) Mandibular right first molar with canal deviation, perforation at the apical third and extensive bone loss at the level of the defect observed in the (**c**) radiograph, (**d**) parasagittal and (**e**) axial tomographic images

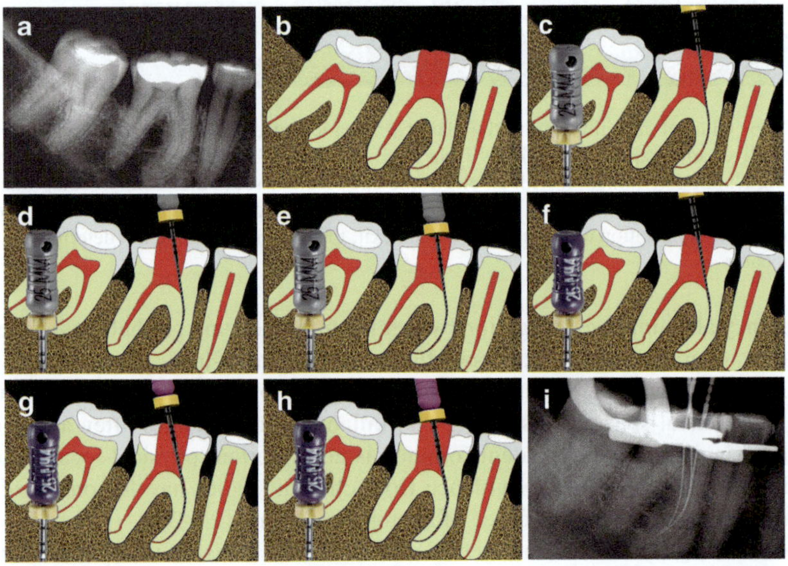

Fig. 3.18 (**a**) Preoperative radiograph of a mandibular first left molar with apical periodontitis referred for root canal treatment. (**b**–**h**) Illustrative images showing the sequential steps of the canal scouting procedure. It starts by moving a small stainless steel K-file (usually sizes 08 or 10) in short amplitude vertical strokes toward the anatomic terminus of the canal. (**i**) Postoperative radiograph showing the scouting files at the anatomic terminus

3.2.4 Glide Path

In aeronautics, glide path (or glide slope) alludes to the final approach path in the landing. It refers to an imaginary line at an optimal angle that travels from the final approach of the runway upwards to the aircraft that is about to land (Fig. 3.19). When an aircraft is correctly on the glide slope, the aircraft will land at the correct touchdown point and at the optimal speed. In endodontics, it is commonplace for the glide path to be a mandatory step; however, its precise definition has not been straightforwardly established. Its traditional definition was coined by West [10, 28] as a "smooth radicular tunnel from canal orifice to physiologic terminus." Ideally, the glide path must confirm the existence of sufficient and smooth available space in the canal lumen, and that the root canal microenvironment is ready for the next enlargement step using NiTi mechanical instruments (Fig. 3.20). In fact, the glide path has been conceptualized in different ways leading to ongoing controversies fueled by misinformation and the natural difficulty to discuss the topic per se. Aside from the lack of consensual definition in the literature, what does seem to be agreed on is that the glide path is essentially achieved when a thin file can go from the canal entrance up to the apex in a repeatable, smooth and predictable manner. In general, its minimum size should be equivalent to a "super loose" ISO size 10 hand file [29, 30] or a loose ISO size 15 K-file (Fig. 3.21) to minimize the incidence of instrument binding, to control the torsional stress of the instrument, and to reduce the incidence of fracture and/or iatrogenic canal deviations (Fig. 3.22).

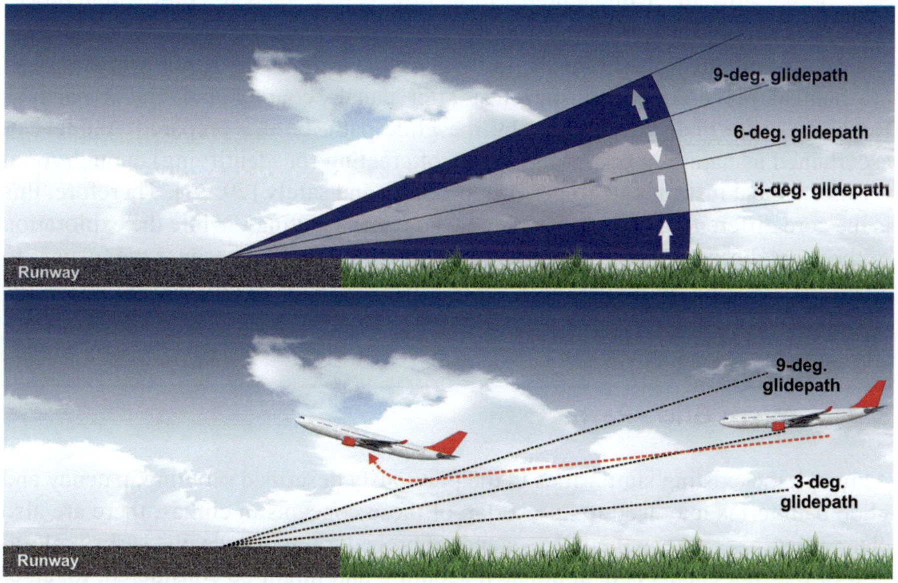

Fig. 3.19 Twists in the glide path of an aircraft. (Top) Polarity reversals on an instrument landing system glideslope occur near the 6° "false" glideslope (blue shading) and above the 9° false glideslope. (Bottom) Reversals cause the autopilot to pitch the aircraft away from the desired 3° glideslope. (Adapted from https://aviationweek.com/twists-glidepath)

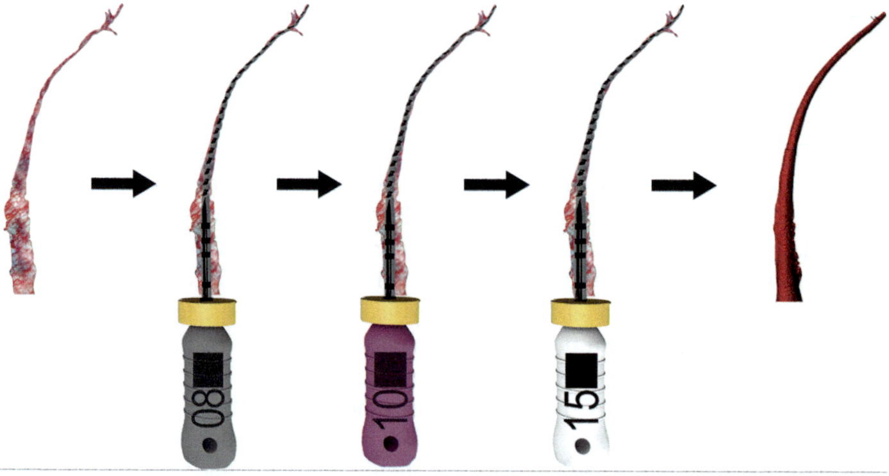

Fig. 3.20 Sequential illustrative images of the preliminary canal enlargement procedures in a simulated canal from scouting with small tip-sized files (sizes 08 and 10) up to glide path procedure with a size 15 K-file aiming to change the irregular anatomy of the canal lumen into a smooth path

In simple terms, the glide path can be seen as a matter of the canal size (Fig. 3.23). This is indeed a point of note because the canal size is a result of the original anatomy, or the active mechanical preparation, usually described as a preshaping procedure. According to West [29], it is likely that as many as 50% of canals are already essentially smooth-walled tunnels. In these cases, a glide path is not necessary and mechanical preparation can start just after canal scouting and apical patency. Regardless, the main role played by the glide path, be it a prepared "tunnel" or ascertained as naturally occurring, is that of creating (or identifying) enough room for mechanical instruments to perform properly and safely [29, 31]. Therefore, this is the core difference between glide path and canal scouting—while the exploration of the canal during scouting procedures is essentially passive because the focus is to reach the apex, the glide path procedure effectively cuts dentin and promotes the enlargement of the canal space (Fig. 3.24).

3.3 Micro Glide Path

Although the existing similarities in the previously described scouting, patency and glide path terms may lead to an overlap of these concepts in clinics, there are also clear differences among them. In a standard procedural sequence, the early exploration of the root canals is denominated scouting and might be considered, together with the apical patency maneuver, as a glide path to the glide path instruments. Following this, it is important to locate the main apical foramen and keep it unobstructed, a procedural step known as apical patency. Establishing and maintaining a

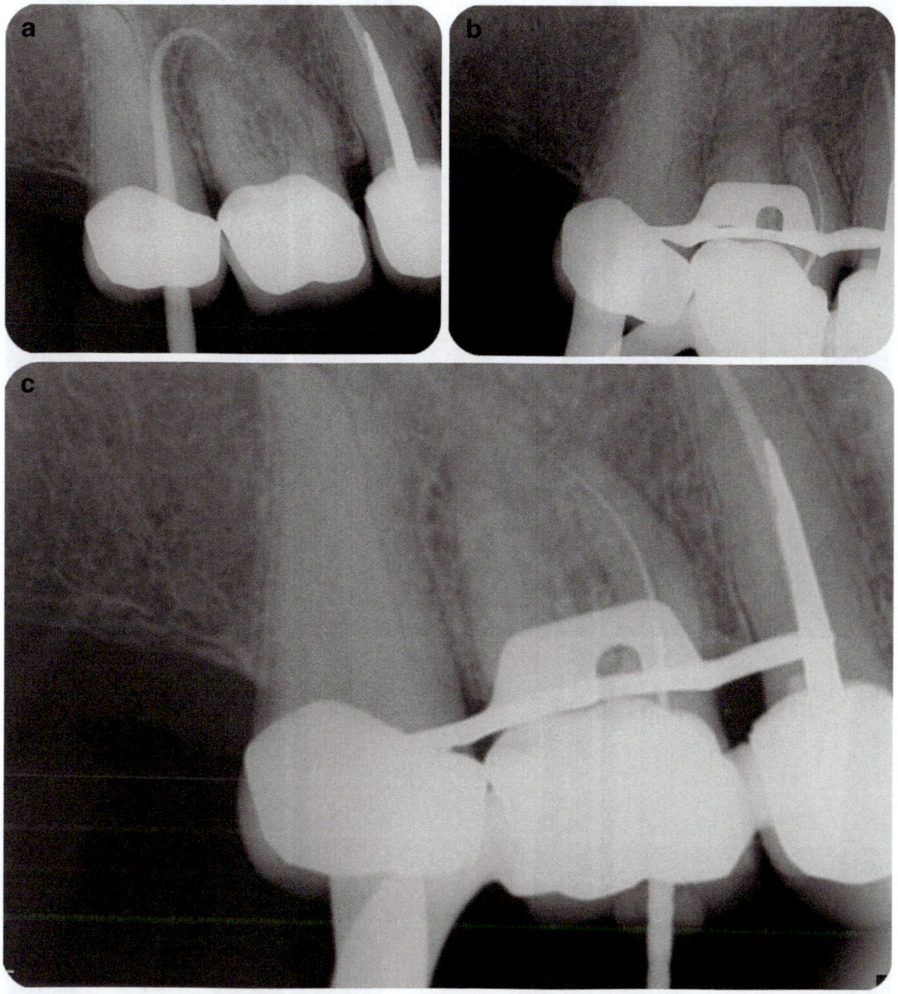

Fig. 3.21 (**a**) Preoperative radiograph of a maxillary first right molar with apical periodontitis and fistula referred for root canal treatment. (**b**) Canal scouting with a size 10 K-file at the anatomical terminus of the canal determined by an apex locator. (**c**) A super loose size 15 K-file positioned at the canal terminus indicating the glide path procedure is completed

patent root canal is an important goal of the mechanical preparation [32]. Didactically, canal scouting and apical patency can be referred to as a micro glide path, following the rationale introduced by van der Vyver [33]. The anatomical variability, particularly at the apical third, may make scouting and patency procedures challenging and time-consuming. Actually, the ability to gain canal patency is often considered a benchmark of the clinician's skills. However, it is important to bear in mind that this canal path should not be mechanically altered or fabricated; instead, it should be made always maintaining the original anatomy. One major issue of the

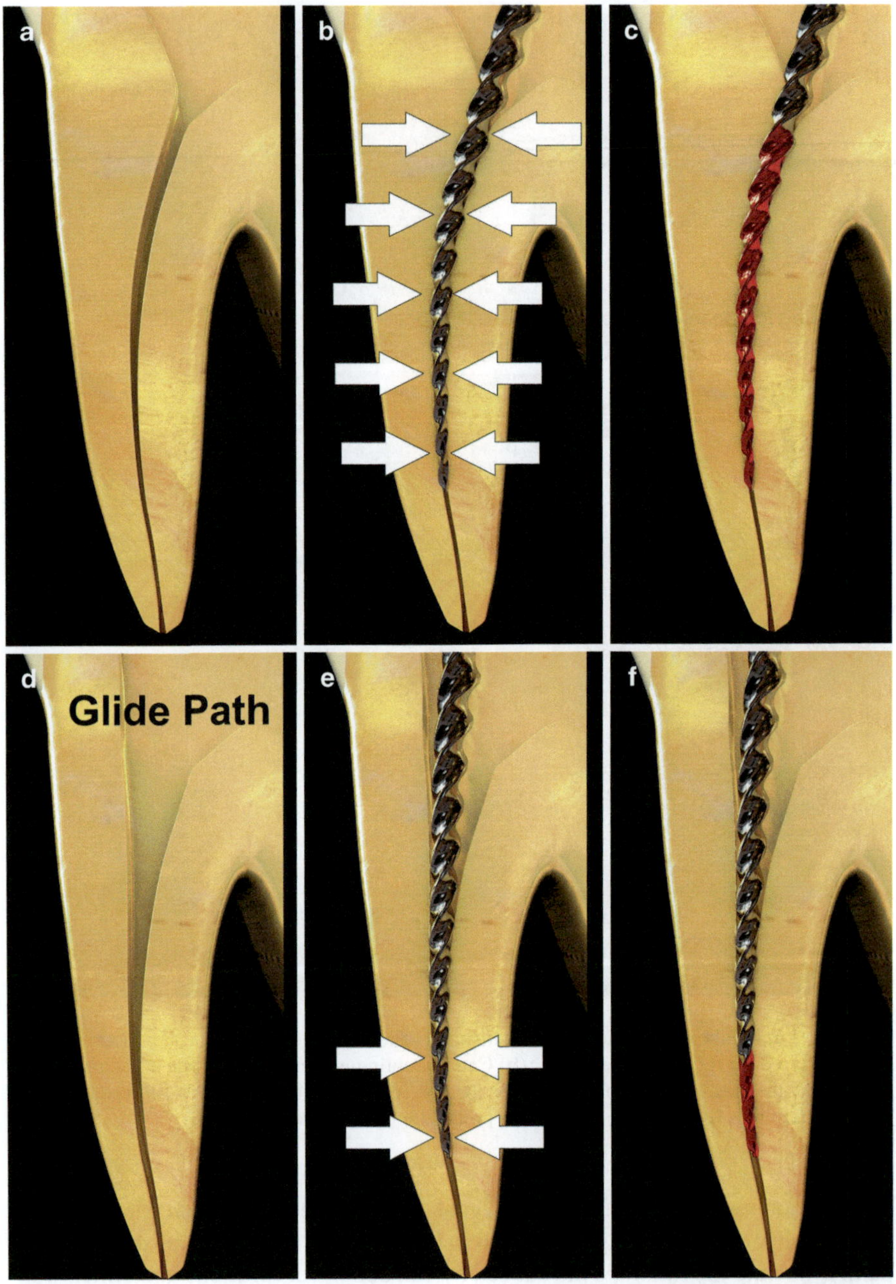

Fig. 3.22 Illustrative images showing the torsional stress (red areas) over the shaping instrument (**a–c**) before and (**d–f**) after glide path procedure in a narrow root canal. Glide path procedure is achieved when a thin file can go from the canal orifice up to the apex in a repeatable, smooth and predictable manner minimizing the incidence of instrument binding, the torsional stress and, consequently, the incidence of fracture

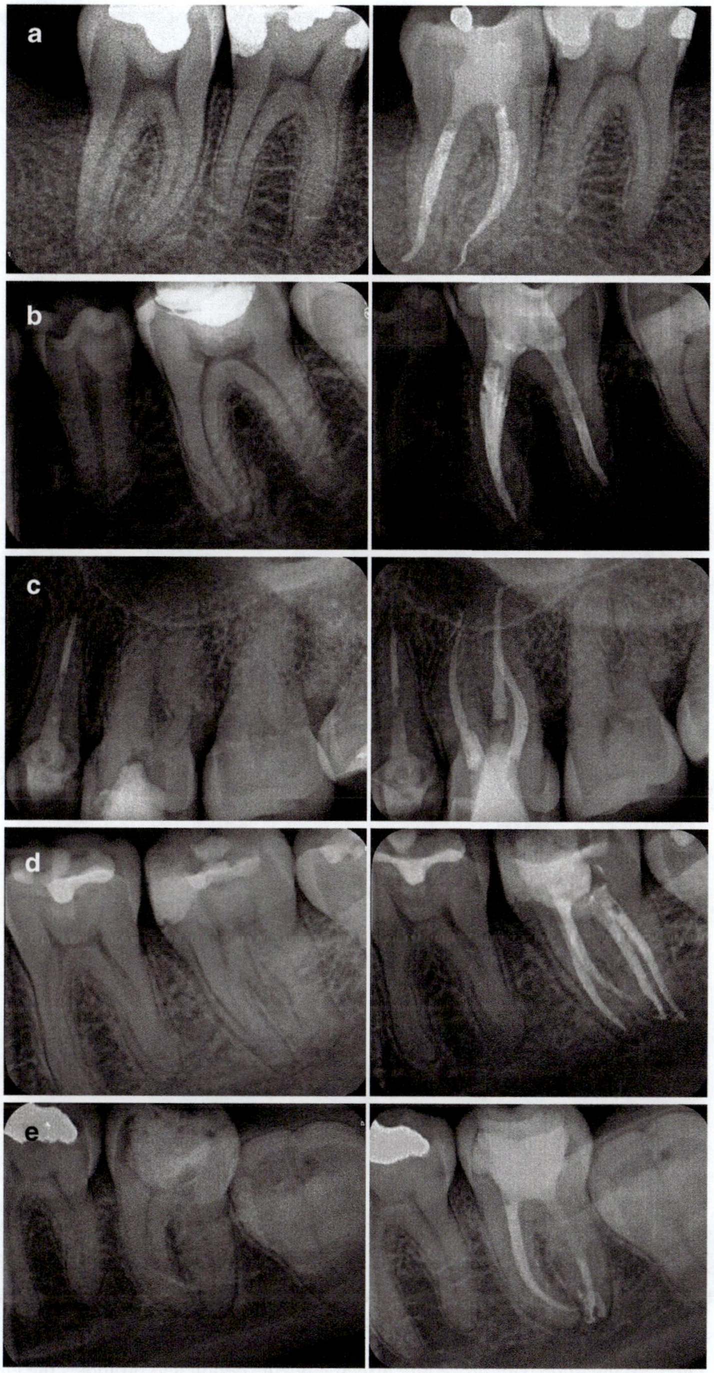

Fig. 3.23 Clinical cases illustrating situations in which (**a**, **b**) a natural glide path is present and (**c**–**e**) teeth that require to perform micro and macro glide path procedures to predictably shape the root canals

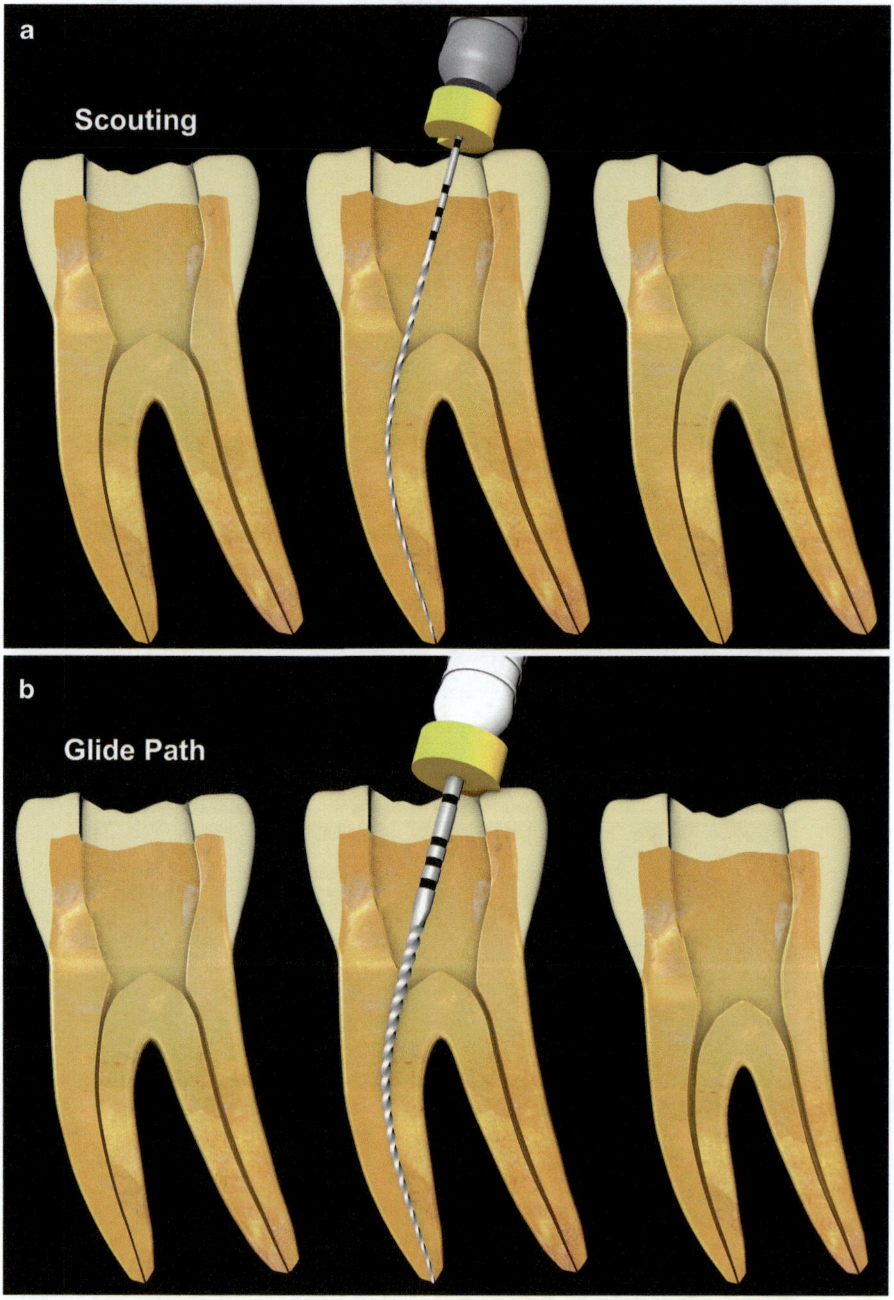

Fig. 3.24 (**a**) The root canal scouting procedure is essentially passive because the focus is to reach the apex, while (**b**) the glide path procedure effectively cuts dentin and promotes the enlargement of the canal space

micro glide path technique is the fact that it is usually performed with hand instruments and may take a considerable amount of time. In addition, it is heavily reliant upon the proper technique mastery of the clinician and, consequently, may lead to poor results [34]. Once verified that the micro glide path is completed (by means of inserting a file size 08 or 10 to the working length, pulling back 5 mm and pushing it back again without any interferences) this reproducible canal path can now be expanded by cutting the dentin tissue with other instruments (the glide path procedure) to create a smoother "tunnel" throughout the main root canal, providing safety for large-tapered rotary or reciprocating instruments to be used [29, 35]. The glide path (reproducible smooth canal "tunnel") is usually completed when the canal reaches approximately the same size or one size larger than the tip of the first instrument to be used in sequence. In summary, the micro glide path (scouting and apical patency) and the glide path represent the initial steps prior to the Shaping for Cleaning procedures (Table 3.1 and Fig. 3.25).

3.3.1 Guidelines for Canal Scouting

As a rule of thumb, stainless steel K-files or special instruments such as C+ (Dentsply Sirona, Switzerland) or C-pilot (VDW, Germany) files are used to routinely scout the root canals (Fig. 3.26). Often, the diameter of the initial scouting instrument is

Table 3.1 Glide path procedures

Micro glide path	Scouting	Refers to the early steps of the shaping procedures, where clinicians can gather information and insights on the root canal anatomy through tactile sensitivity while advancing with small scouting instruments—usually sizes 08 or 10—toward the apex
	Patency	Preparation technique by means of which the apical portion of the canal is maintained free of debris by recapitulation with a small file through the apical foramen
Glide path	Enlargement of the scouted canal space	To create a smooth "tunnel" to minimize the incidence of instrument binding, controlling the torsional stress to reduce the incidence of fracture and iatrogenic canal deviations

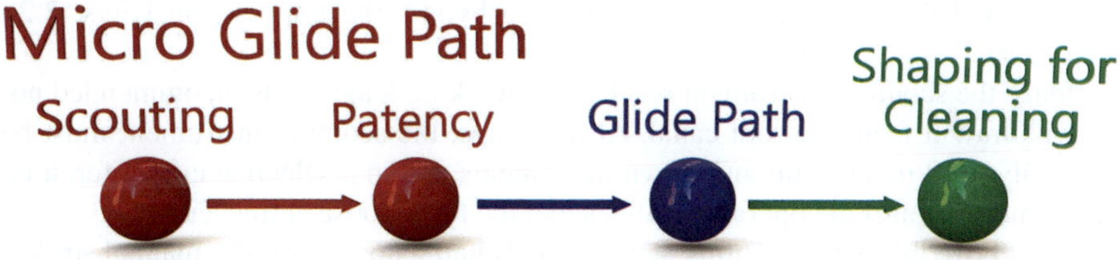

Fig. 3.25 Micro glide path (scouting and apical patency) and the glide path represents the initial steps prior to the shaping for cleaning procedures

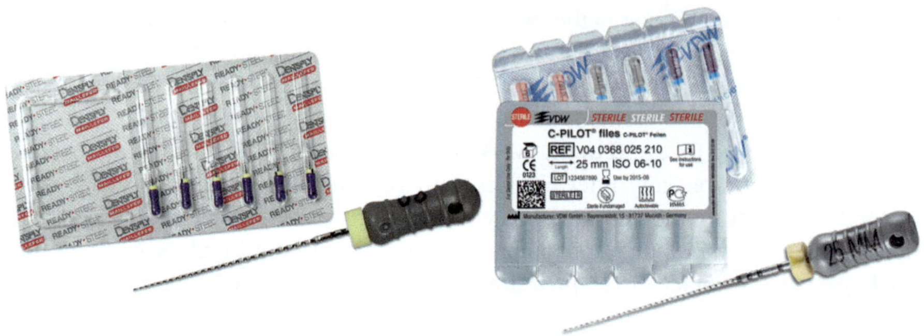

Fig. 3.26 C+ (Dentsply Sirona, Switzerland) (on the left) and C-Pilot (VDW, Germany) (on the right) endodontic files

larger than the canal lumen itself and thus, some difficulty may be experienced by the clinician at this initial step. In such cases, 21 mm-length instruments are suggested to be used, as this length presents great buckling resistance, facilitating the scouting procedure. The same rationale applies to the C+ or C-pilot, two instruments specifically designed for canal scouting with features that improve the buckling resistance and stiffness of their shafts, allowing more vertical pressure to be applied during the negotiation of the original canal path. Moreover, such instruments provide the operator with exceptional tactile feedback.

The canal scouting starts by moving a small stainless steel K-file, usually sizes 08 or 10, in short amplitude vertical strokes toward the provisional working length determined on the preoperative radiograph (Fig. 3.27). Firstly, scouting instruments are used to explore the coronal third of the root canal with a watch-winding motion and careful short amplitude vertical strokes. The file is removed and the irrigant solution renewed. In difficult anatomies, it may be necessary to preflare the coronal two-thirds of the canal as long as this facilitates the instrument movement toward the apex. Coronal preflaring also improves the tactile sensitivity of the operator during the scouting procedures [36]. After gaining the coronal two thirds of the canal, the scouting instrument is used to negotiate the apical third, the most delicate part of the procedure. It is worth mentioning that, in clinical routine, the tip of the scouting file should never be forced apically, but be passively introduced. In case of difficulty in progressing the file up to working length, remove it from the canal, clean the flutes, bend its last 2 mm, and try again. Now, it is possible to explore and find out the correct position to bypass the impediment (Figs. 3.28 and 3.29).

Once the scouting instrument reaches the working length, it is recommended not to withdraw it from the root canal. At this stage, the scouting instrument must be carefully used in short up-and-down movements and in a selective circumferential filing motion, until the operator realizes that the file is loose at this length. As stated by West [10], this early scouting step demands half a dozen or more manual strokes or whatever it takes to get the file loose at this position.

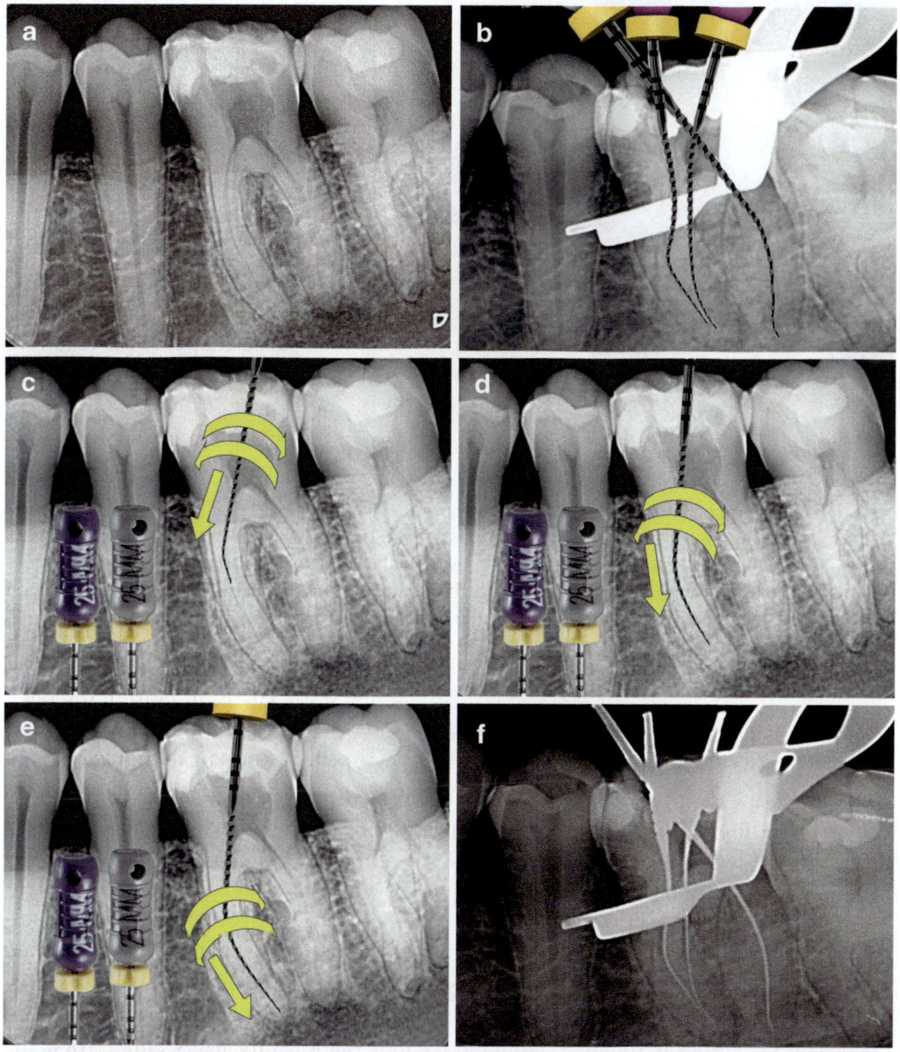

Fig. 3.27 Illustrative sequence showing the dynamic of the scouting procedure. (**a**) Preoperative periapical radiograph of a mandibular left first molar referred for root canal treatment. (**b**) Preoperative planning of the scouting procedure. (**c**) Firstly, scouting instruments—small stainless steel K-files, usually sizes 08 or 10—are used at the coronal third with a watch-winding motion and careful short amplitude vertical strokes. (**d**, **e**) The files advance in short amplitude vertical strokes toward the provisional working length determined on the preoperative radiograph. (**f**) Radiographic image showing the end of the scouting procedure determined when apical patency is achieved

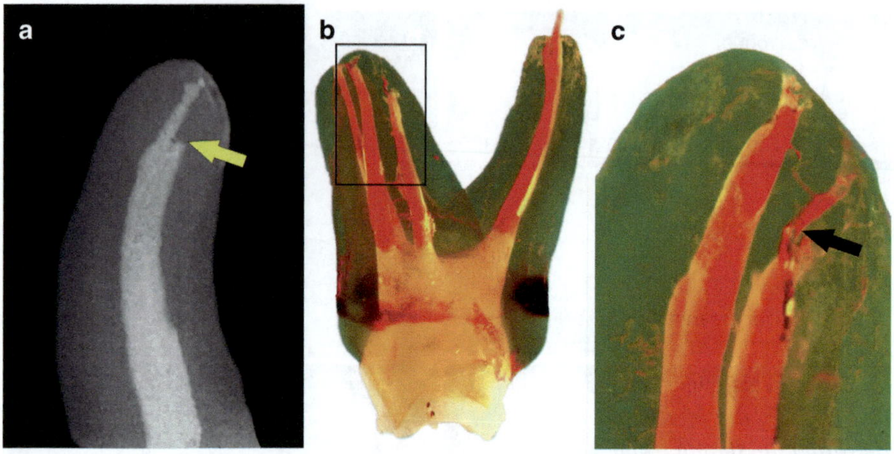

Fig. 3.28 The negotiation of the apical third is the most challenging step of the scouting procedure. (**a**) Radiographic image of the mesiobuccal root of an extracted maxillary first molar after shaping and filling procedures in which it is possible to observe that instruments were unable to reach and completely prepare the last 2 mm of the apical canal (yellow arrow). (**b**) Extracted tooth of (**a**) after clearing (diaphanization) technique that rendered it transparent. (**c**) High magnification of the mesiobuccal root showing a size 06 K-file unable to scout the last apical 2 mm of the canal. (Courtesy of Dr. Holm Reuver, Germany)

Even when scouting is easily performed, sometimes it may not be quite smooth or reproducible. This is the case when the scouting file can slide back to the working length without major interferences, but even so it may find obstacles on its way back. Accordingly, the scouting procedure must be considered finished only when the scouting file is able to travel 4–5 mm short of the working length up to the apical foramen using only light finger pressure.

3.3.2 Guidelines for Establishing the Apical Patency

Once canal scouting is finished, apical patency is the missing step required to complete the micro glide path procedure. To accomplish this task, the apical 2 mm of the root canal must be scouted and the main exit (major foramen) successfully located. Afterwards, the patency file must be passively extended slightly beyond the apical foramen, a maneuver that must be continuously repeated throughout shaping procedures. To perform this properly, the clinician must passively use a small K-file to find the right pathway through the foramen up to at least 1 mm longer than the working length (Fig. 3.30). Taking into consideration the vast blood supply and immune capabilities of the periradicular tissues, inserting such a small-tip-sized instrument in this area is a safe procedure from both biological and mechanical standpoints. In summary, it is only possible to achieve apical patency as a consequence of meticulous negotiation steps [33].

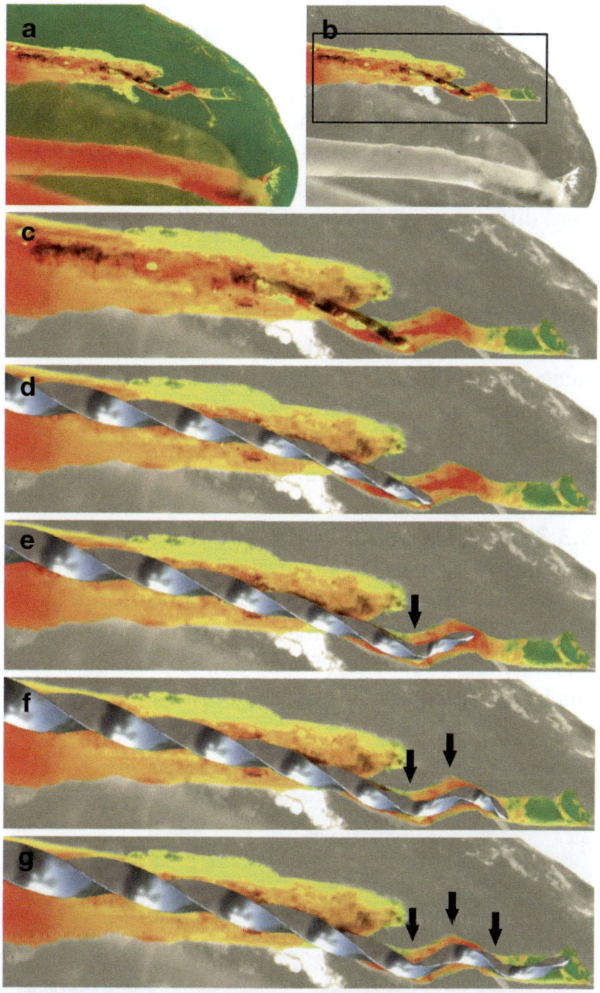

Fig. 3.29 (**a**, **b**) Mesiobuccal root of a maxillary molar after clearing technique as described in Fig. 3.28. (**c**) High magnification of the squared image in (**b**) depicting the tortuosity of the apical canal third and the level in which the file stopped. (**d**) Computational virtual modeling of the real file showed in (**c**). (**e**–**g**) Simulation of the apical canal scouting using the virtual instrument in (**d**) bypassing the first curvature (**e**), the second curvature (**f**) and the third curvature (**g**) to reach the major foramen (apical patency). In clinics, it is unlikely that this apical tortuosity could be properly scout even using small-tipped instruments. (Courtesy of Dr. Holm Reuver, Germany)

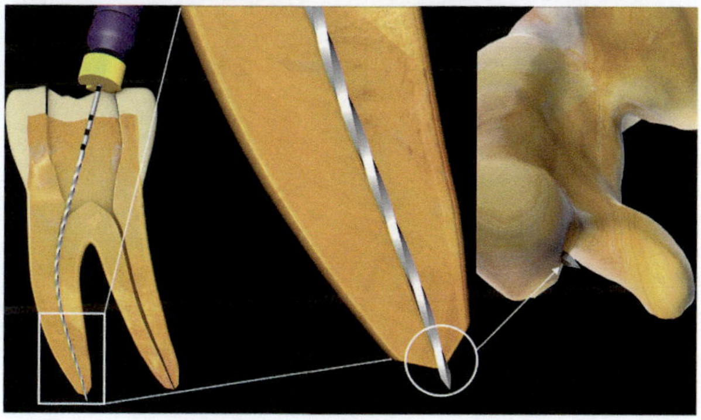

Fig. 3.30 Illustrative images showing that patency must be achieved using a small K-file that extends passively and slightly beyond the apical foramen, a maneuver that must be continuously repeated throughout shaping procedures

3.3.3 Challenges in Scouting and Patency Procedures

A reliable micro glide path procedure is the initial step to prevent iatrogenic mishaps, such as instrument fracture, allowing the canal anatomy to remain as close as possible to its original shape, during the subsequent mechanical canal shaping [37]. According to the level of negotiation, root canals can be didactically classified into easy, difficult or non-negotiable, as follows:

3.3.3.1 Easily Negotiable Root Canals

Easily negotiable root canals are those in which the working length can be reached with minimal efforts by the clinician, even during the scouting procedure. In this category, canals are typically wide and straight, or with minimal curvature, allowing even large-tapered instruments to reach the working length without major difficulties (Fig. 3.31). In some cases, canal scouting can be effortlessly performed only after some dentinal removal attained by the preflaring procedure.

3.3.3.2 Root Canals with Difficult Negotiation

In some root canals, scouting procedures using small-sized instruments such as 06 or 08 may be hard or even impossible to perform. In others, although canal scouting can be adequately performed with those instruments, a reliable glide path using instruments sizes 10 or 15 may not be possible. These are typical canal types that can be classified as challenging or difficult to negotiate.

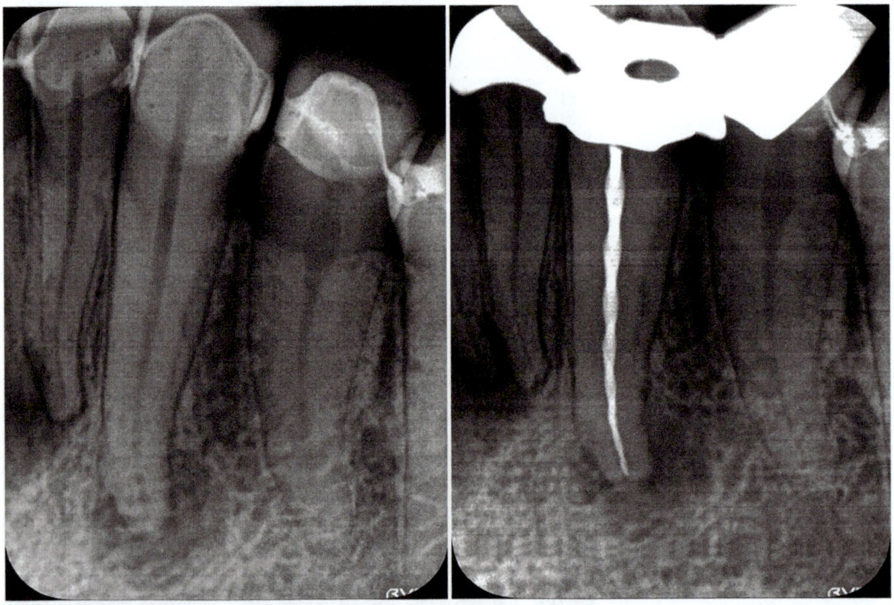

Fig. 3.31 Clinical case illustrating a wide and straight root canal easy to negotiate. The reciprocating instrument was driven to the working length without the need of a previous scouting or glide path procedures

Routine challenges in achieving the apical patency are usually related to three main factors: (1) physiologically formed blockages within the root canal, such as the deposition of cementum [22] or as a host response to wall-off the bacterial ingress; (2) intricate root canal anatomy in the last 1–2 mm of the canal (Fig. 3.32); and (3) iatrogenically created blockages that may hamper the location of the main foramen and thus the establishment of apical patency. Regarding the latter, the loss of the working length due to undesirable transoperative blockages is a relatively common adverse event, especially among less experienced clinicians. Apical blockage is usually caused by the accumulation of dentinal debris or an iatrogenic ledge created by intentional engagement of the instrument.

Preventing working length loss due to the previously mentioned reasons demands careful and more zealous approach in the following points: (1) systematically rechecking the apical patency by passing the tip of the file at least 1 mm beyond the foramen; and (2) employing diligent and generous irrigations between each instrument used. In the quest to regain apical patency, it is mandatory to be careful when trying to advance beyond the blockage point as the instrument should not be forced in the conviction that it would be able to unblock the canal pathway. Actually, in forcing the instrument, there is a real risk of proceeding in the wrong way by creating a "false canal". Once the last apical millimeters of the canal are blocked, regaining the apical patency demands a calm approach because it can be a laborious, time-consuming and unexpected transoperative event that may compromise the treatment outcome. The dentist needs to rely on attentive and slow-moving canal renegotiation with small, precurved scouting K-file fueled by copious syringe-needle and ultrasonic irrigation (Fig. 3.33).

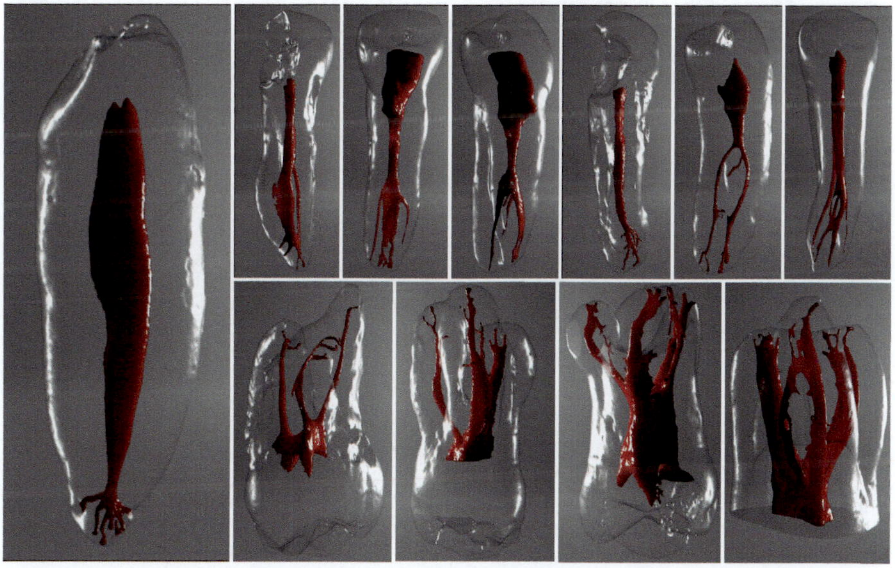

Fig. 3.32 Micro-CT 3D models of different real teeth illustrating challenges in achieving the apical patency caused by the intricate canal anatomy at the apical third

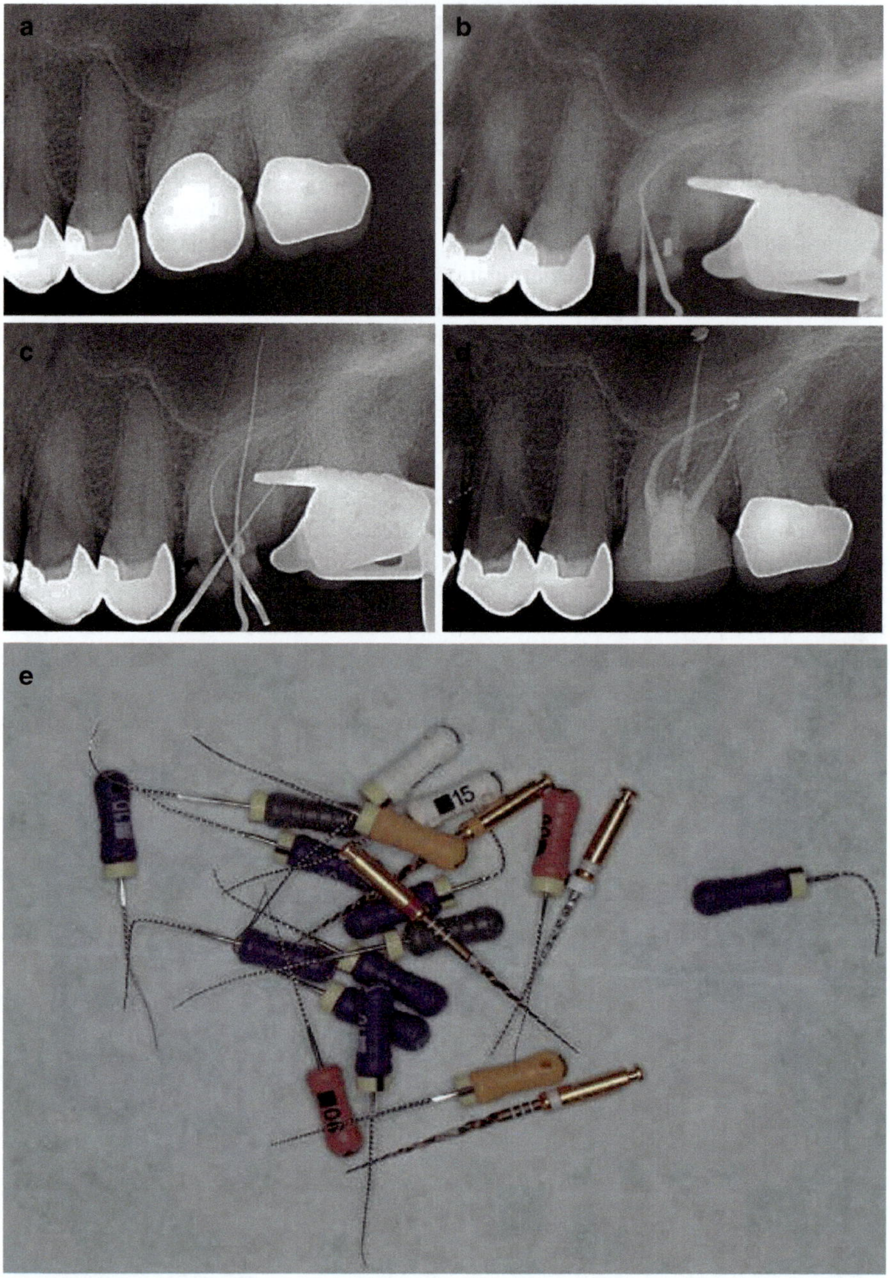

Fig. 3.33 Root canal treatment of a maxillary first left molar showing the difficulty in performing glide path with manual and rotary instruments. (**a**) Preoperative radiograph. (**b**) Glide path performed with hand stainless steel files. (**c**) Glide path with hand files on the MB1 and MB2 canals. (**d**) Postoperative radiograph. (**e**) Distorted instruments used during the glide path procedure. (Courtesy of Dr. Leandro Gomila, Spain)

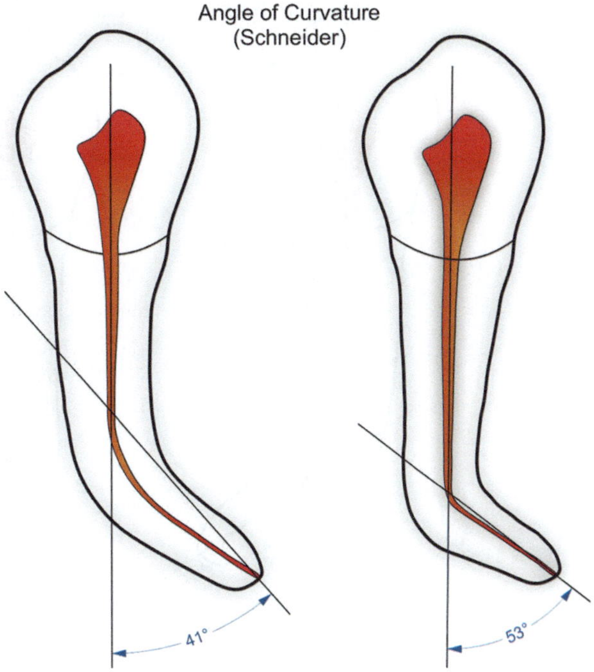

Fig. 3.34 Schneider method. Curvature is calculated based on the angle that is obtained by two straight lines. The first is parallel to the long axis of the root canal, and the second passes through the apical foramen until intersecting with the first line at the point in which the curvature starts. The formed angle (α) is named according to the degree of root canal curvature into straight (5°), moderate (10–20°) or severe (>25°)

It is important to note that the interplay between the original pulp space and the degree of curvature should be taken into account in order to classify the difficulty degree of glide path preparation. In large canals, even the most challenging curvature can be handled effortlessly. On the other hand, curved narrow canals are much more difficult to treat. In addition, although most teeth present root curvature in only one direction, some may display double or multiplanar curvatures, which is another factor that may hamper the treatment.

In the literature, the degree of canal curvature has been addressed by Schneider's method [38] (Fig. 3.34), although Pruett [39] proposed the radius as a more appropriate way to describe the canal curvature of human teeth (Fig. 3.35). In this book, we will consider the interplay between the original anatomy and the radius of curvature of the root canal when classifying clinical cases according to its difficulty to negotiate, as follows:

– *Canals with difficult coronal negotiation*. In several cases, the coronal third of the root canal may present some resistance to negotiation. A typical example is the second canal of the mesiobuccal root of maxillary molars, the so-called MB2 [40–42]. The MB2 orifice is usually covered by a dentin shelf that creates an abrupt curvature at the first 2–3 mm of the canal to the distal direction (Fig. 3.36) [43]. For this reason, if the canal is scouted with rigid manual stainless steel files, its tip is guided by the dentin shelf that covers the canal orifice toward the mesial wall (Fig. 3.37). At this point, a small ledge or irregularity may be created, thus

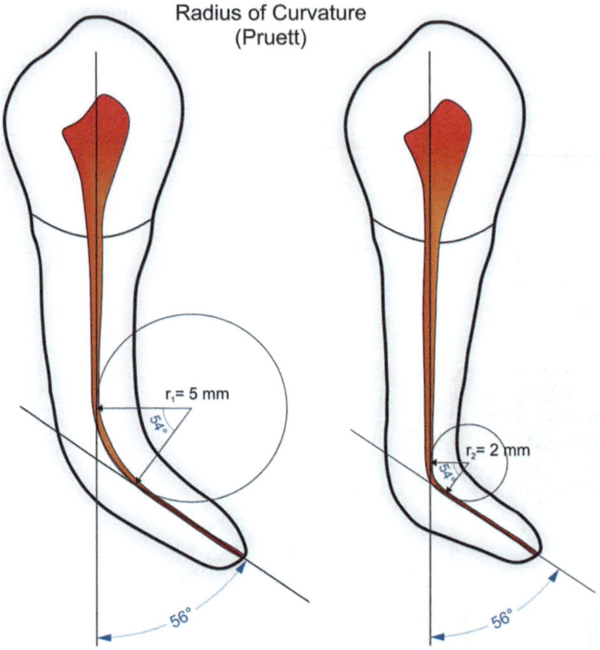

Fig. 3.35 Pruett method. The effect of the radius of curvature as an independent variable should be considered in studies evaluating root canal instrumentation since two root canals measured at the same angle in degrees by the Schneider's method could have different radii or abruptness of curvature. To determine the radius of curvature, two lines perpendicular to the lines along the long axes of the coronal and apical portions of the root canal space are drawn. Then, a circle is drawn touching the points wherein the canal deviates from the straight lines and either begin or end the curved portion of the root canal space. The arc lies on a circle whose size is specified by its radius, and the circle's radius is taken to be the radius of curvature of the canal in that local area. The circle's radius is the radius of the curved portion of the root canal space and defines how abruptly the canal curves

impairing the proper scouting at the coronal third. Therefore, the early removal of the dentin shelf with either low-speed burs or ultrasonic tips is the key for obtaining straight-line access to the canal pathway.

- *Narrow canals with continuous curvature and radius higher than 2–3 mm.* Scouting narrow curved canals is also a great challenge [44]. In narrow canals with continuous curvatures, the pathway toward the apex is usually not smooth when using manual K-file size 10 with gentle watch-winding movements. Thus, clinicians should pay special attention to avoid the creation of iatrogenic mishaps. Accidents such as ledges and perforations, mainly at the apical third, can occur during the scouting of this type of canal and this may compromise the treatment outcome [45] (Fig. 3.17). Typically, K-type files have reduced resistance to buckling, which frequently creates difficulties in the scouting of narrow, curved canals [44].
- *Canals with abrupt apical curvature and radius lower than 2–3 mm.* In this class of root canals, clinicians must never force stainless steel manual files toward the

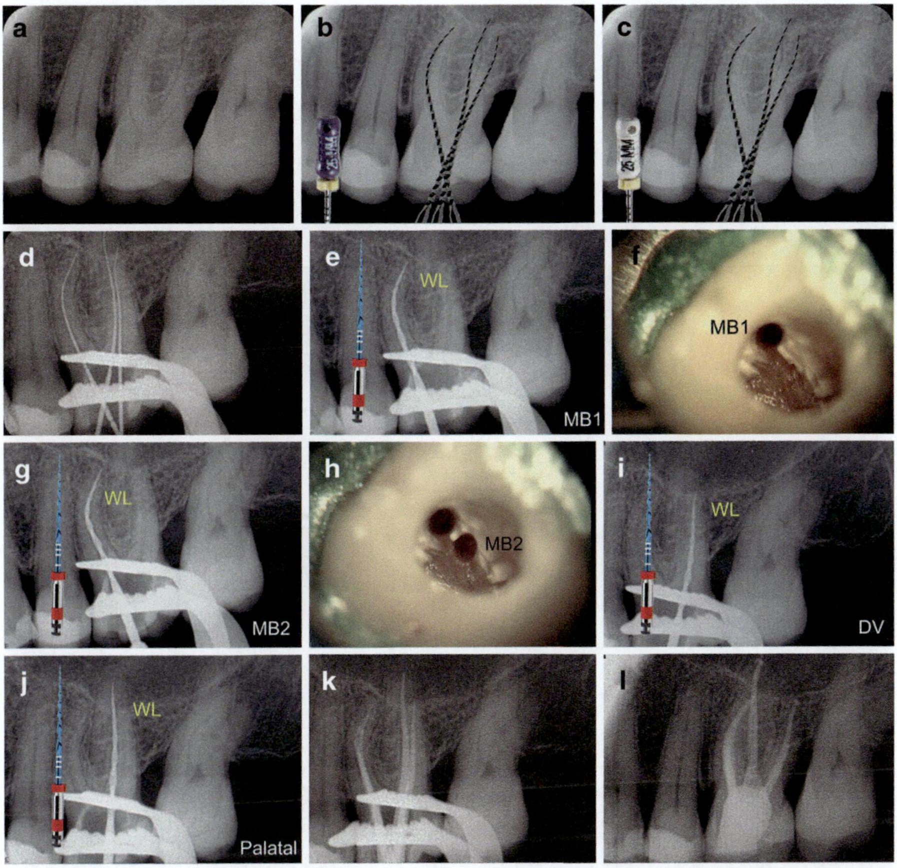

Fig. 3.36 The orifice of the second canal of the mesiobuccal root of maxillary molars (MB2) is usually covered by a dentin shelf that creates an abrupt curvature at the first 2–3 mm of the canal in a distal direction. This clinical case shows (**a**) a maxillary first left molar referred for root canal treatment in which (**b**) canal scouting was performed with a size 10 K-file, followed by (**c**, **d**) glide path with a size 15 K-file to the working length. Canals were scouted with manual stainless steel files and their tips were guided toward the mesial wall by the dentin shelf that covered the canal orifices. After preliminary procedures, canal shaping of (**e**, **f**) MB1, (**g**, **h**) MB2, (**i**) distobuccal and (**j**) palatal canals were done with a Reciproc Blue R25 instrument. (**k**, **l**) Then, filling procedures were done by single-cone technique using an epoxy-based canal sealer

apex because even small alterations of the original anatomy may create serious difficulties in completing the scouting procedure or even render it impossible. Precurving the instrument tip is a well-known practice that is successfully used to overcome the scouting challenges in such canals. Therefore, in these cases, the 1–3 mm of the file tip must be precurved with a sharp bend (60–90°) before scouting. The challenge, however, is to reach the apical third with this instrument without losing its prebending. For that, a slight coronal preflaring to the point where the canal curves is often helpful. The goal is to remove the surrounding dentin that narrows the canal lumen, thus creating enough space for the pre-bent

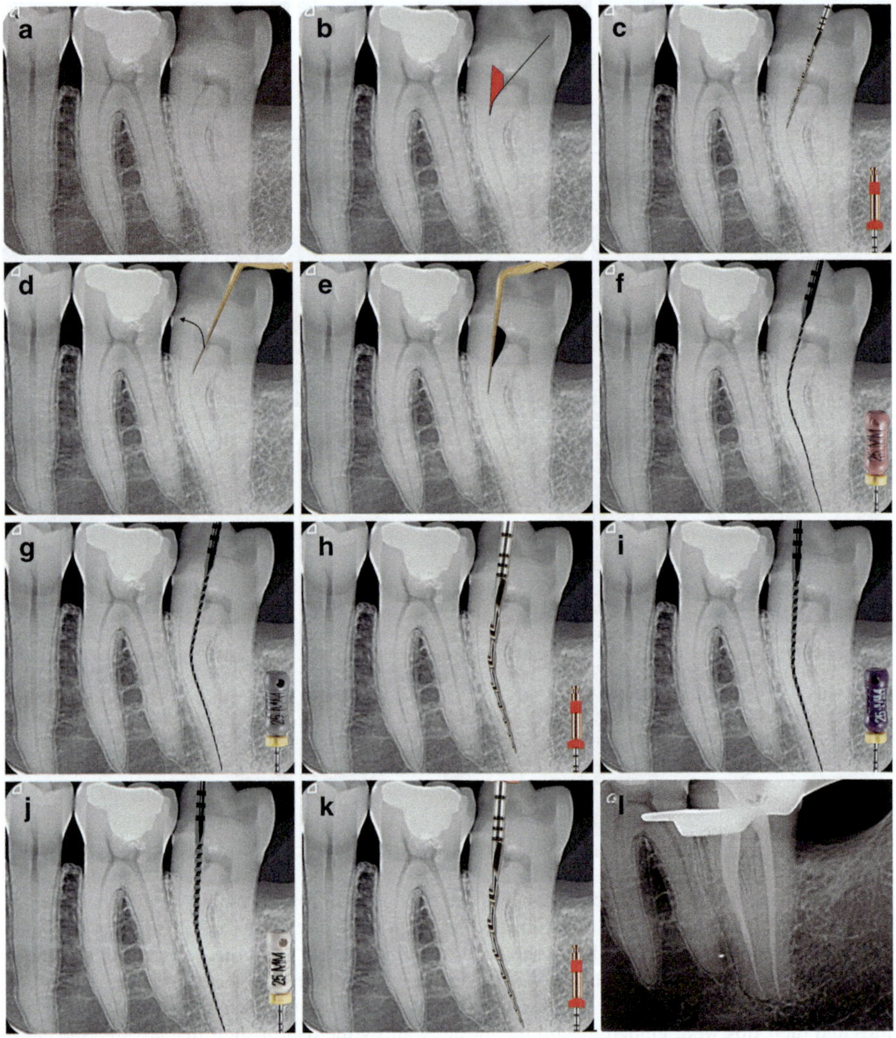

Fig. 3.37 The mesial orifice of mandibular molars is usually covered by a dentin shelf that creates an abrupt curvature at the first 2–3 mm of the canal in a distal direction. This clinical case shows a (**a**) mandibular second left molar referred for root canal treatment. (**b**) At the preoperative radiograph it is possible to observe the dentin shelf covering the mesial canals orifices (in red). A line was drawn digitally to demonstrate that the direction of the instrument's tip will be guided toward the distal aspect of the crown. (**c**) Root canal was first explored with a reciprocating instrument, followed by (**d**, **e**) the removal of the dentin shelf (in black) using an ultrasonic tip. Then, (**f**, **g**) canal scouting was performed with sizes 06 and 08 K-files, followed by (**h**) a Reciproc R25 instrument up to the apical third but without reaching the working length. (**i**, **j**) Glide path was performed with sizes 10 and 15 K-files at the working length and (**k**) final enlargement was finished after the Reciproc R25 instrument reached the apical foramen. (**l**) Radiograph showing the final stage of filling procedure

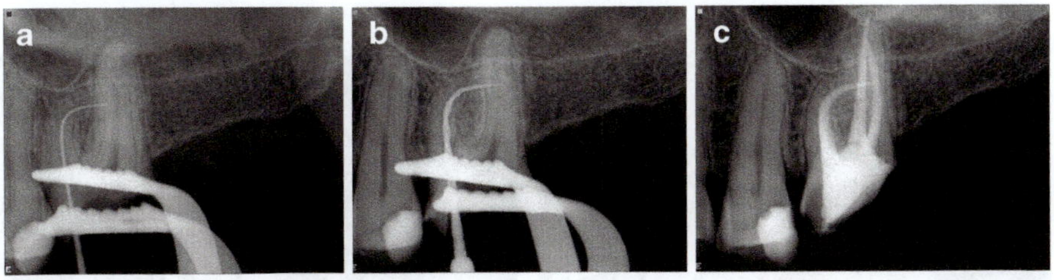

Fig. 3.38 Preflaring procedure enables the clinician to guide the bent tip of the instruments in different positions and inclinations to explore the correct direction of the apical curvature. This clinical case shows a maxillary first left molar with (**a**) the glide path file and (**b**) the Reciproc R25 instrument positioned at the working length of a mesial canal having a 90° curvature. (**c**) Postoperative radiograph. (Courtesy of Dr. José Eduardo de Mello Júnior)

file to reach the apex. Under this circumstance, it is recommended to reduce the vertical scouting movement length to 1 mm to prevent the risk of creating ledges and blockages. Furthermore, frequent and thorough irrigation with sodium hypochlorite and chelating agents, such as EDTA 17%, is strongly recommended to lubricate the canal walls for the scouting instrument and avoid accumulation of debris in the apical area, which would create additional challenges for achieving apical patency. The previous enlargement created by this preflaring procedure will enable the clinician to guide the bent tip of the instruments in different positions and inclinations to explore the correct direction of the apical curvature and, ultimately, succeed in scouting the whole canal length (Fig. 3.38). The general recommendation is to initiate the procedure with a K-file size 06 or 08 using gentle quarter-turn movements. After reaching the working length, the instrument must not be withdrawn from the canal because it may be difficult to put it back in the same position again. So, with the instrument at the working length, the operator must perform watch-winding movements with minimal apico-coronal strokes; these slight movements will aid in achieving the canal patency, overcoming the abrupt apical canal curvature. A clinical tip to identify the direction of the apical curvature is to use the marker on the silicone stop.

3.3.3.3 Non-negotiable Apical Canal Anatomies

Despite technological advancements and continuous developments in alloys and instrument kinematics, some extremely challenging canals cannot be scouted up to the apex due to anatomical complexities [46] (Figs. 3.39 and 3.40). Non-negotiable canals refer to some anatomies that, even after several attempts, are not possible to be fully explore. Although more than 20% of root canals can be non-patent, they may not be doomed to failure once the endodontic treatment outcome depends on several other factors [47] (Figs. 3.41 and 3.42). Such non-patent canals may require more intensive care on the chemical component of the treatment, which implies copious irrigation to improve the overall cleaning condition. This means optimizing the removal of organic and inorganic contents by delivering irrigants where instruments are unable to mechanically act. Another important factor to consider in canal

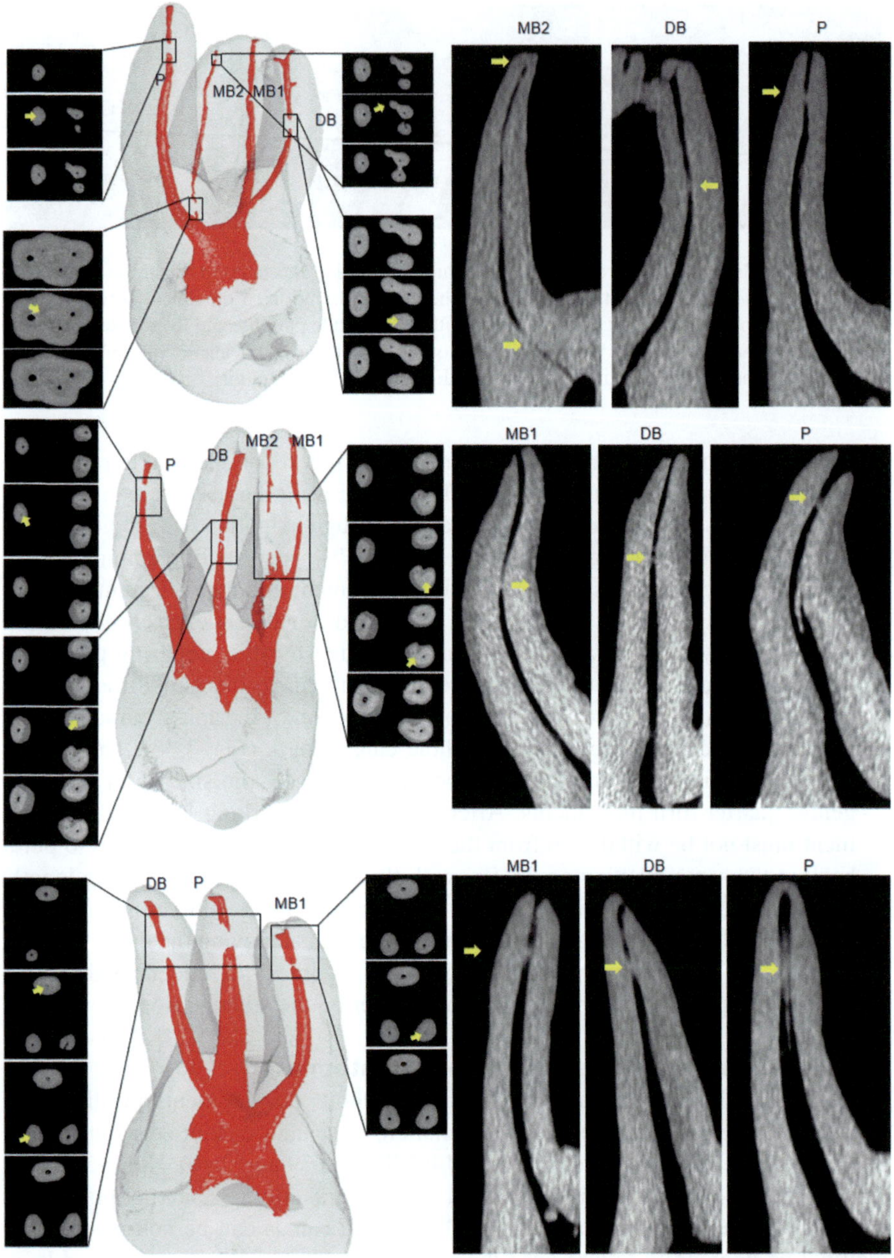

Fig. 3.39 Although the continuous technological advancements in alloys and instrument kinematics, some canals cannot be scouted up to the apex because of anatomical complexities. These illustrative images show 3D models and cross-sectional images of three maxillary first molars having calcifications (yellow arrows) in the mesiobuccal, distobuccal and palatal canals (black squares). The presence of calcifications can be also observed in axial and sagittal cross sections at different levels of the roots. (Courtesy of Dr. Ali Keles, Turkey)

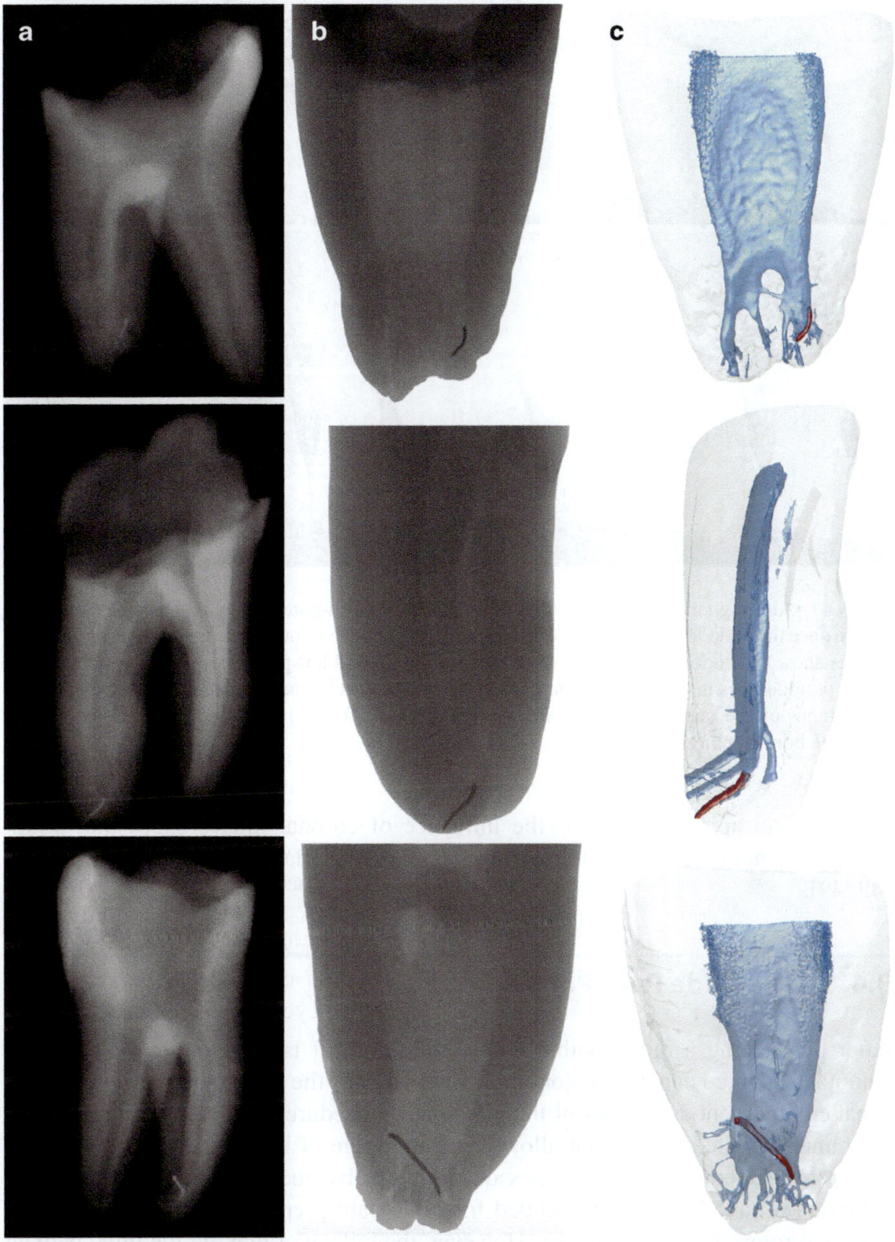

Fig. 3.40 (**a**) Radiographic images of 3 mandibular molar teeth with fractured NiTi pathfinder instruments at their apical thirds. (**b**) Micro-CT projection images in different views highlighting the fragment of the instruments. (**c**) 3D models of the mandibular molars in (**a**) depicting the root canals (in blue) and the fractured instruments (in red) to demonstrate typical cases in which the main cause of fracture was the high complexity of the canal anatomy at the apical third

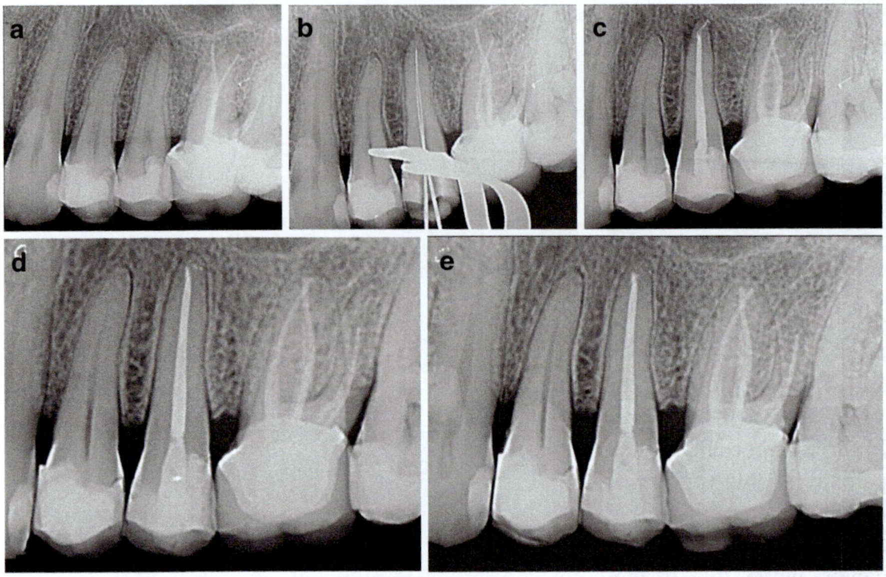

Fig. 3.41 Although more than 20% of root canals can be non-patent, they may not be doomed to failure once the endodontic treatment outcome depends on several other factors. (**a**–**e**) Radiographic images show the endodontic treatment of a maxillary second left premolar having a preoperative apical periodontitis in which apical patency was not achieved by using small hand files. Follow-up radiographs of the maxillary second left premolar taken after (**d**) one and (**e**) and 2 years show complete bone healing

scouting and apical patency is the influence of coronal interferences that might change the incidence angle of the instruments' cutting blades on the root canal walls [48, 49].

3.4 The Glide Path Per Se

After performing a reproducible micro glide path, it is necessary to enlarge the smoothed scouted canal to major sizes, which means the glide path per se [33]. The canal enlargement as a result of the glide path procedure must create a smooth and biomimetic-walled tunnel that allows the safe usage of large-tapered NiTi engine-driven instruments toward the apex during the subsequent canal shaping. Several approaches have been recommended for glide path preparation, such as specially designed rotary NiTi instruments. However, the fallacy of making the glide path an easy procedure represents the main appeal of the NiTi pathfinder instruments, a topic addressed later in this chapter. It is important to point out that in all glide path protocols, the previous establishment of working length and irrigation after each instrument are recommended to avoid debris accumulation.

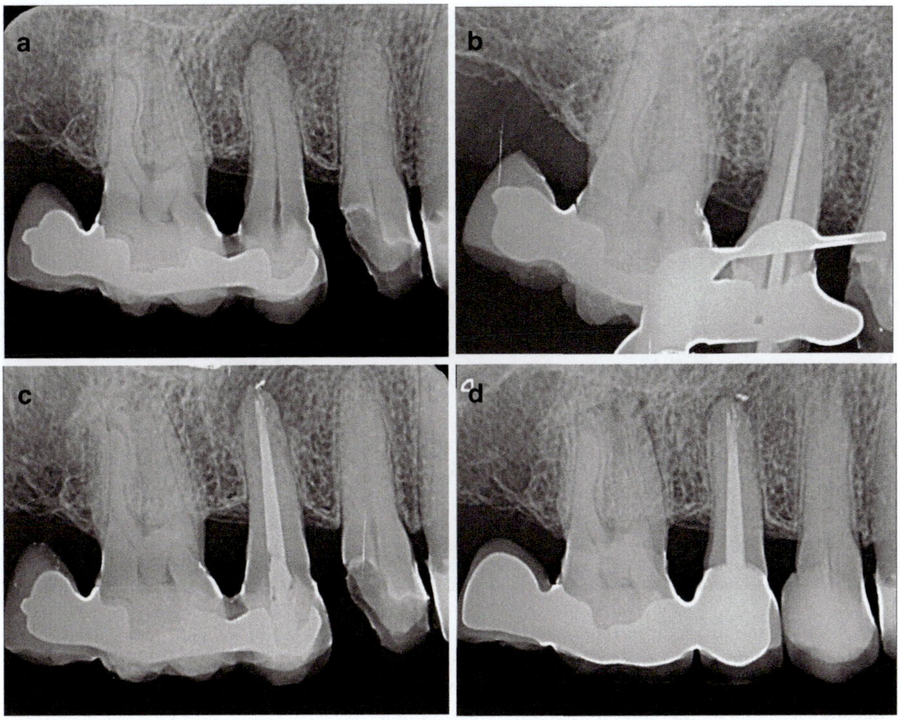

Fig. 3.42 Radiographic images show the endodontic treatment of (**a–c**) a maxillary second right premolar having a preoperative apical periodontitis in which apical patency was not achieved by using small hand files. (**d**) Follow-up radiograph after 36 months shows complete bone healing

3.4.1 Manual Glide Path Preparation

Hand files are used for the scouting procedures using either watch-winding or quarter-turn/pull movement applied with a gentle slight apical pressure. The file progress toward the apex is a result of systematic but careful repetition of these movements, until the instrument reaches the canal terminus and conquers the foraminal patency [44]. During the micro glide path, the canal is slightly enlarged, and the dentinal walls are smoothed by removing irregularities. Afterwards, a sequence of increased file sizes (usually K-file sizes 08 and 10) creates a pathway for the shaping instruments. Throughout the glide path procedure, files should be used up to the main apical foramen and canal patency constantly rechecked. The glide path is considered to be concluded when either a K-file size 10 is super loose or a K-file size 15 is loose in the canal. This means that the last file of the sequence must easily achieve the apical foramen and, when pulled backward for 4–5 mm and introduced again with a light finger pressure, it can reach the working length without any interference [50]. Normally, a size 15 K-file does not easily reach the apical foramen in a canal scouted with a size 10 K-file, which is quite understandable considering the corresponding percentage of increase in its tip diameter. This was

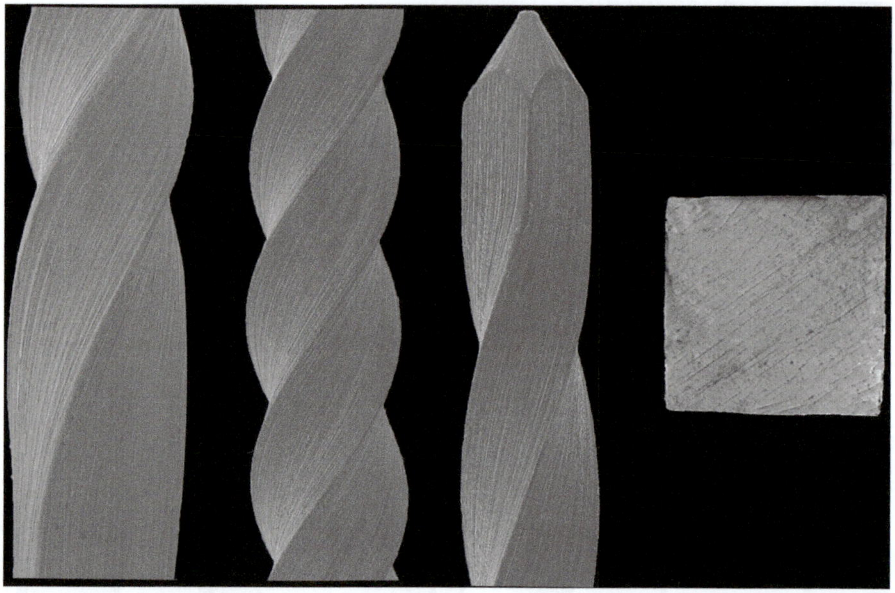

Fig. 3.43 Scanning electron microscopic images of the KCC file (VDW, Germany) showing its intermediary region, helical shaft, the conical and circular tip, and squared cross section present in the sizes 06, 08, 10, 12.5, 15, 17.5, 20, and 25 instruments. KCC instruments ISO sizes 30 to 140 (not shown in this image) have a triangular cross section

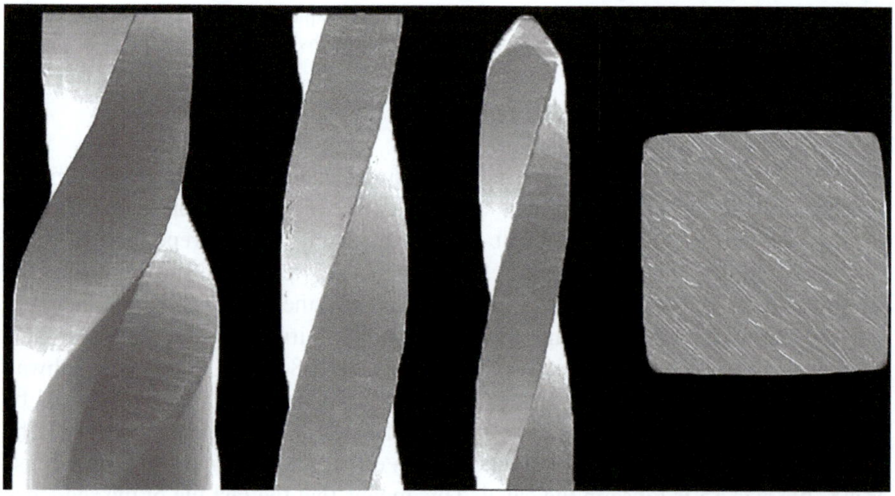

Fig. 3.44 Scanning electron microscopic images of the C+ instrument (Dentsply Maillefer, Switzerland) showing its intermediary region, helical shaft, the conical and circular tip, and squared cross section

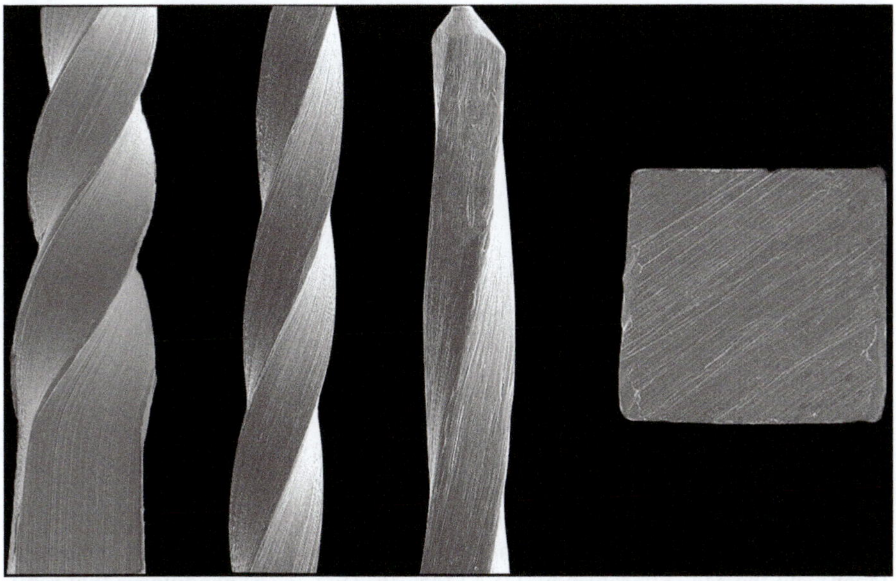

Fig. 3.45 Scanning electron microscopic images of the C-Pilot (VDW, Germany) instrument showing its intermediary region, helical shaft, the conical and circular tip, and squared cross section

the reason why West [10] advised that the size 15 K-file is one of the most dangerous instruments that can be used for glide path procedures because several iatrogenic errors have been associated with its usage.

On the market there are several available brands of stainless steel K-files, but some of them were specially designed for glide path, including the constant tapered (0.02 mm/mm) KCC file (VDW, Germany) sizes 06, 08, 10, 12.5, 15, 17.5, [50] (Fig. 3.43); the C+ files (Dentsply Maillefer, Switzerland) sizes 06, 08, 10, and 15 (Fig. 3.44), designed mainly for calcified root canals, with a taper of 0.04 mm/mm in the first 4 mm from the tip and 0.02 mm/mm along the rest of the helical shaft; the C-Pilot file sizes 06, 08, 10, 12.5, and 15 (VDW, Germany) (Fig. 3.45), designed for severely curved or calcified root canals, and tapered 0.02 mm/mm along the entire shaft [44]; and the Hi-5 file sizes 06, 08, 10, and 15 (Miltex, Inc., York, USA), designed with helical ground flutes and a pentagonal cross section, also recommended for narrowed or calcified root canals.

3.4.2 Glide Path Using Hand Files in Dedicated Oscillatory Pneumatic Contra-Angles

Glide path procedures can also be performed using manual files mounted in specific oscillatory handpieces that have a special chuck that strongly locks the cable of regular stainless steel or NiTi hand files. This way, the hand files can be activated

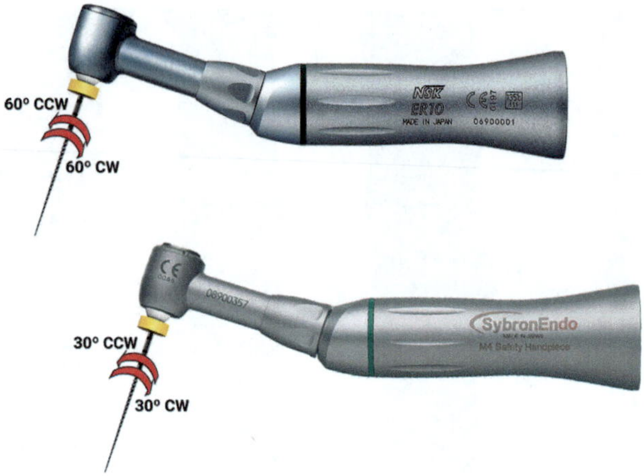

Fig. 3.46 TEP ER10 (NSK Nakanishi, Japan) and M4 (SybronEndo, USA) oscillatory handpieces. These handpieces have a special chuck that locks the cable of regular stainless steel or NiTi hand files and allow them to oscillate in specific angles

by either electric or pneumatic engines, applying a vertical 1–3 mm up-and-down movement [51]. Examples of these handpieces are the TEP ER10 (NSK Nakanishi, Japan) and the M4 (SybronEndo, USA) [45, 46] (Fig. 3.46) handpieces that replicate the oscillatory movement [51, 52] by constant angles of 30°/30° (M4) or 45°/45° (TEP E16R). The TEP E16R is a 16:1 reduction handpiece that can be used with a speed rotation of 625 rpm [53], while the M4 (18:1 reduction) can be driven at 900 rpm [51] (Fig. 3.46). The final result of the mechanical glide path with oscillatory handpieces is similar to the manual approach, but with two main advantages: (1) a low risk of instrument separation; and (2) reduced preparation time. Despite the lack of formal evidence, the use of hand files adapted to oscillatory handpieces is a safe and efficient way to perform the enlargement required to complete the glide path procedure. Considering the accumulated knowledge on reciprocating movement available nowadays, it is possible to assume that such features result from the symmetrical small oscillatory angles performed by these handpieces. In simple terms, hand files operating in small forward and reverse angles hardly reach their plastic limit of resistance to fracture. Besides, the use of the intermediate-sized files such as 12.5 and 17 sizes can provide a more gradual and smoother canal enlargement than the traditional ISO sequence of K-file sizes 10 and 15 (Fig. 3.47).

3.4.3 Rotary NiTi Glide Path Preparation

Glide path procedures using NiTi engine-driven rotary instruments, the so-called pathfinders, have been associated with lower canal deviation, apical transportation, and less preparation time compared to manual preparation [54–56]. In addition, rotary instruments can promote less extrusion of debris than manual preparation with a linear movement to the apical direction [57]. However, it is important to underline that, before the use of rotary instruments for glide path preparation, it is

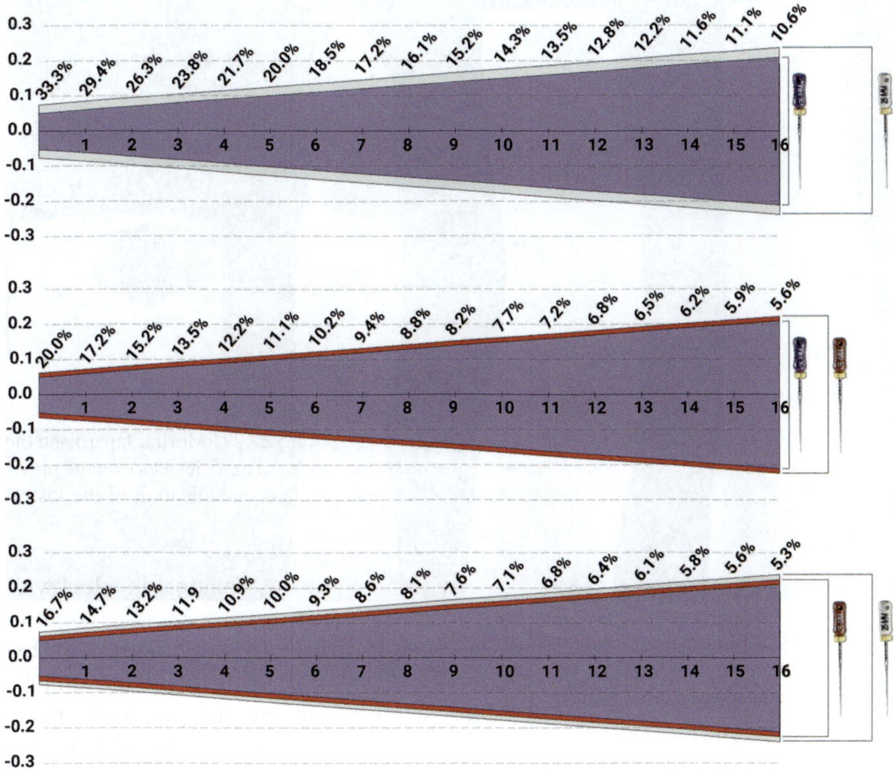

Fig. 3.47 Graphic representation of the differences in the transition of instruments used to perform the glide path and the percentage increase required in each millimeter for this transition. Note that the use of the intermediate-sized files such as the K-file size 12.5 between the K-files sizes 10 and 15 (middle and bottom graphics) can provide a more gradual and smoother canal enlargement than the traditional ISO sequence of K-files sizes 10 and 15 (top graphic)

mandatory to complete the canal scouting and apical patency procedures—the micro glide path—which means that engine-driven pathfinder NiTi instruments are indicated only for the glide path per se [33, 58, 59]. Nowadays, there are some pathfinder systems available on the market, including the following:

3.4.3.1 PathFile

PathFile (Dentsply Maillefer, Switzerland) was the first system specifically designed to perform the glide path with rotary instruments. This system is composed of three constant tapered (0.02 mm/mm) NiTi instruments manufactured with a conventional NiTi alloy (Fig. 3.48) to be used sequentially: PathFile 1 (purple; tip size 13), PathFile 2 (white; tip size 16), and PathFile 3 (yellow; tip size 19). The instruments are operated at 300 rpm and 3 N·cm torque in short and smooth in-and-out movements (3–5 s) until they reach the working length [59]. A preliminary manual scouting with a size 10 K-file is recommended before using this system.

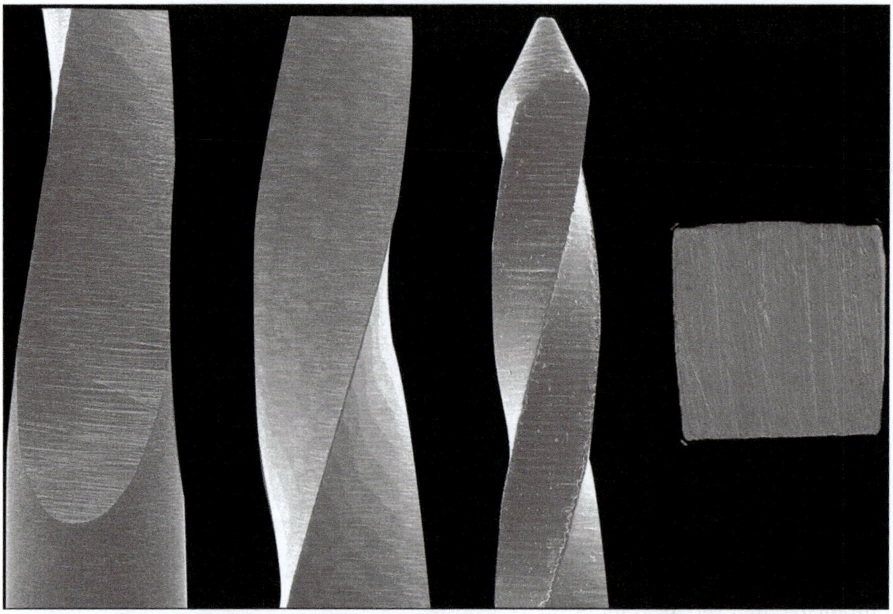

Fig. 3.48 Scanning electron microscopic images of the PathFile rotary glide path instrument (Dentsply Maillefer, Switzerland) showing its intermediary region, helical shaft, the conical and circular tip, and squared cross section

3.4.3.2 ScoutRaCe

ScoutRaCe (FKG Dentaire, Switzerland) rotary instruments have a 0.02 taper and ISO tip sizes of 10 (purple), 15 (white), and 20 (yellow) (Fig. 3.49). They are used in sequence after exploring the canal up to the working length with a K-file size 06 or 08 [54].

3.4.3.3 ProGlider

ProGlider instrument (Dentsply Sirona, Switzerland) is manufactured with heat-treated NiTi M-Wire alloy, which enhances its flexibility and flexural strength [60] (Fig. 3.50). This instrument has a progressive taper (0.02 at tip level up to 0.085) aiming to create an additional enlargement at the coronal and middle portions of the root canal to facilitate the use of subsequent large-tapered rotary instruments [60, 61]. The manufacturer recommends using the ProGlider at 300 rpm and 5 N·cm torque [62] after scouting the root canal with at least a K-file size 10.

3.4.3.4 The Critical Role of Micro Glide Path for Rotary Pathfinder Instruments

As previously described, pathfinder instruments were specifically developed to mechanize the glide path procedure. Compared to manual preparation, evidence points out that pathfinders would be able to significantly reduce the transoperative time, the postoperative pain and the incidence of flare-ups [50, 53, 57], as well as to achieve more centered preparations [54]. Yet, oddly enough, until 2016, there was no

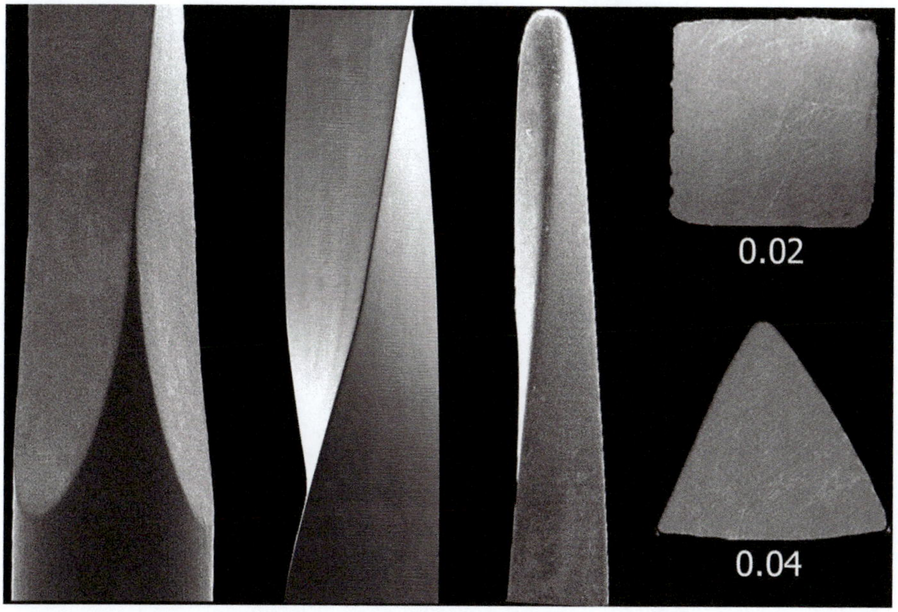

Fig. 3.49 Scanning electron microscopic images of the ScoutRaCe rotary glide path instrument (FKG Dentaire, Switzerland) showing its intermediary region, helical shaft, the conical and circular tip, and squared cross-section. The RaCe system also has a similar instrument but with different taper (0.04) and a triangular cross section design

study analyzing the two main critical aspects of such instruments: efficiency and safety, where efficiency refers to their ability to scout the canal and reach the apex, and safety to their fracture rate. Taken together, efficiency and safety are the most important outcomes that can reflect the real performance of a given pathfinder instrument and should be considered as default parameters in research studies on this topic.

In 2016, De-Deus and colleagues [46] tested these parameters for the first time, comparing the performance and safety of four pathfinder instruments available in the market: ScoutRace 10/0.02 (FKG Dentaire, Switzerland), MTwo 10/0.04 (VDW, Germany), ProGlider 16/0.02 (Dentsply Maillefer, Switzerland) and ProDesign 25/0.01 (Easy Equipamentos Odontológicas, Brazil). The experimental design included moderately curved molars (120 upper and 120 lower molars) with typical anatomy and was focused on the ability of these instruments to perform the mechanical glide path by reaching the apical foramen. The results were quite surprising since the overall efficiency of the instruments in getting the apex was only 53.75%. Even worse was their safety considering that the fracture rate ranged from 3 to 12%, with an average of 6.5%. ScoutRace 10/0.02 showed the best overall performance, the ProDesign 25/0.01 instrument had the least efficiency in reaching the apex, and the ProGlider had the highest fracture rate (Fig. 3.51). The conclusions were discouraging as they indicate that glide path procedures using engine-driven pathfinder instruments were unpredictable in terms of safety and efficiency. It is worth noting that the pathfinders were intentionally not used as recommended by the manufacturers which

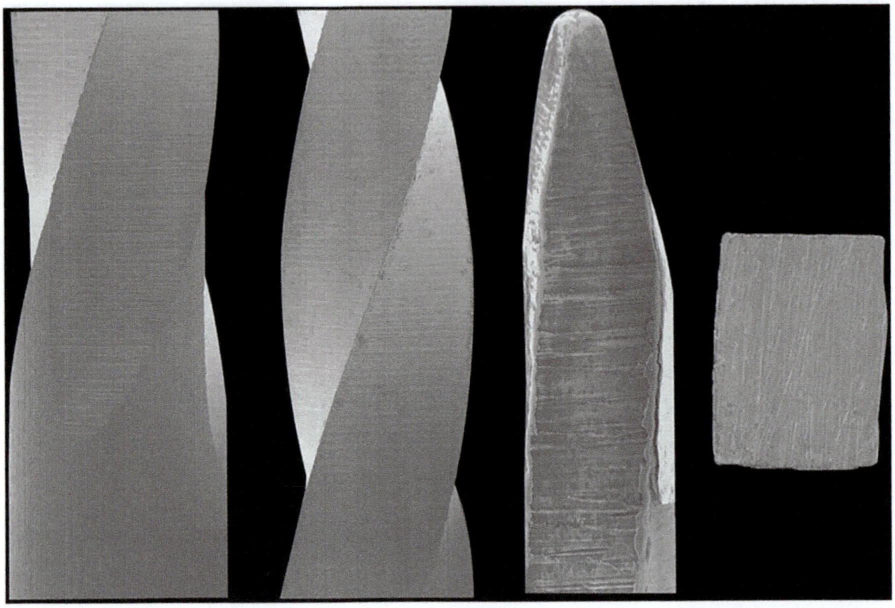

Fig. 3.50 Scanning electron microscopic images of the ProGlider rotary glide path instrument (Dentsply Sirona, Switzerland) showing its intermediary region, helical shaft, the conical and circular tip, and squared cross section

Fig. 3.51 Graphic representation of the results obtained in the study of De-Deus et al. [46] for ProDesign, Mtwo, Scout Race and ProGlider instruments. (**a**) Percentage means efficiency to reach the working length and (**b**) safety represented by the percentage of instrument fracture

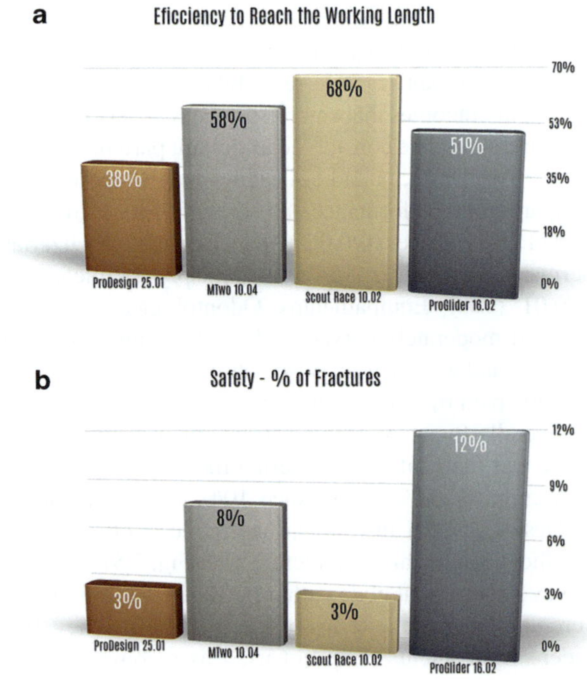

includes a previous scouting of the root canals to their full extension with a size 10 K-file, i.e., a reliable micro glide path must be confirmed before using the engine-driven pathfinder instruments. This means that current engine-driven pathfinder instruments are recommended only for the glide path per se but CANNOT BE USED for canal scouting, which is the most challenging step of the glide path procedure. Taking this into consideration, authors [46] deliberately ignored the manufacturers' recommendations in order to evaluate the real ability of those instruments in performing the complete mechanical canal negotiation. In another study [63] with a similar design to that of De-Deus et al. [46], Jaiswal and collaborators compared the performance and safety of the MTwo 10/0.04 (VDW, Germany), ProGlider 16/0.02 (Dentsply Maillefer, Switzerland) and OneG 14/0.03 (Micro-Mega AS, France) rotary pathfinders. However, at this time authors performed the micro glide path with K-file sizes 08 and 10 before using the pathfinders. Interestingly, results were quite similar to those obtained by De-Deus et al. [46], with the MTwo, OneG and ProGlider instruments reaching the working length in only 53%, 63% and 86% of the root canals, respectively. In addition, the fracture rate ranged from 6% (ProGlider) to 26% (Mtwo and OneG) (Fig. 3.52). Interestingly enough, these results indirectly pointed out that getting a loose size 10 K-file may not be sufficient to provide safety standards for using pathfinder instruments.

Taken together, these results clearly speak to the technical challenges involved in the micro glide path procedures. Moreover, they bear witness to the fact that the rotary-driven pathfinders are far away from achieving the so-called full mechanical canal negotiation in an efficient and safe way.

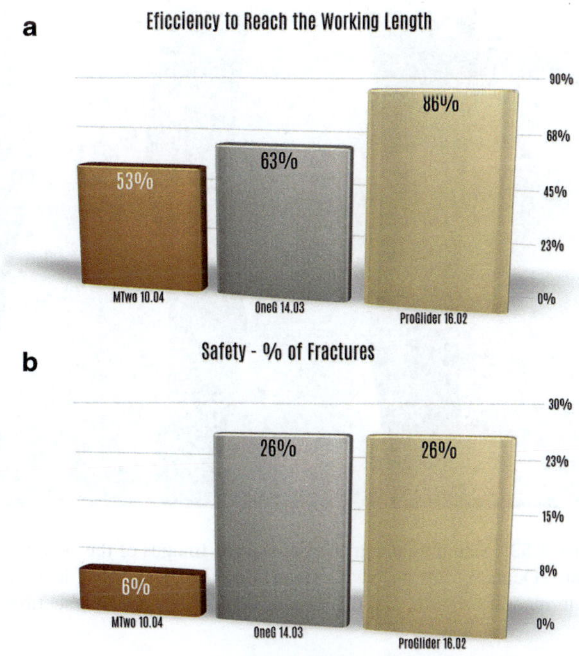

Fig. 3.52 Graphic representation of the results obtained by Mtwo, OneG and ProGlider instruments in the study of Jaiswal et al. [63]. (**a**) Percentage means efficiency to reach the working length and (**b**) safety represented by the percentage of instrument fracture

3.4.4 Reciprocating NiTi Glide Path Preparation

Instead of a continuous rotary motion, there are pathfinder instruments specifically designed to be driven under asymmetric reciprocating movement. The rationale behind this proposal is the well-known ability of reciprocating instruments to scout the canal and progress toward the apex with a better controlled risk of fracture [63]. Currently, there are two available reciprocating pathfinders on the market:

3.4.4.1 WaveOne Gold Glider

WaveOne Gold Glider (Dentsply Sirona, Switzerland) is made of a thermo-mechanically treated alloy termed "Gold" by the manufacturer (Fig. 3.53). This

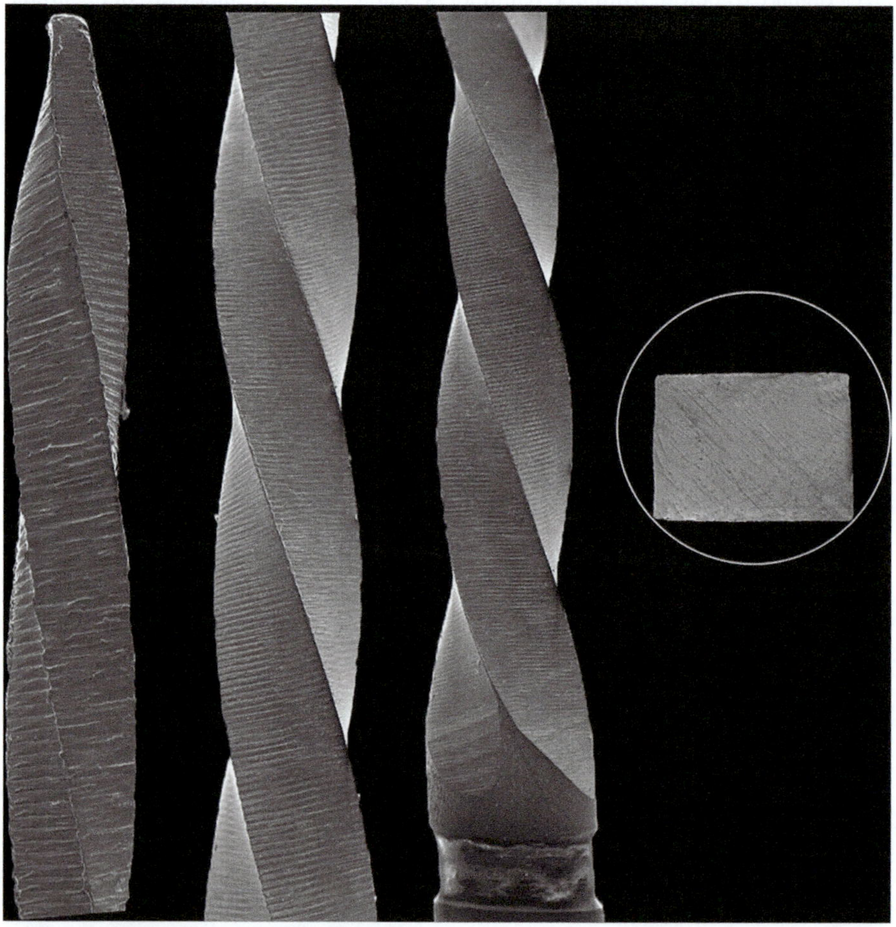

Fig. 3.53 Scanning electron microscopic images of the WaveOne Gold Glider reciprocating glide path (Dentsply Sirona, Switzerland) instrument showing its conical and circular tip, helical shaft, intermediary region, and the parallelogram-shaped cross section

instrument has a 0.15 mm tip diameter and a 2% taper that progressively increases up to 6% at D16, with a parallelogram-shaped cross section with two cutting edges [64]. It is driven under reciprocating motion in a dedicated motor following the preset program "WaveOne All" (350 rpm, 170° counterclockwise and 50° clockwise). A preliminary scouting with a size 10 K-file is recommended before its use.

3.4.4.2 R-Pilot

R-Pilot (VDW, Germany) is manufactured from M-Wire NiTi alloy and has a 0.125 mm tip diameter with 4% constant taper and an S-shaped cross section [64] (Fig. 3.54). This instrument is driven under reciprocating movement (150° counter-clockwise and 30° clockwise) in a dedicated motor following the preset program

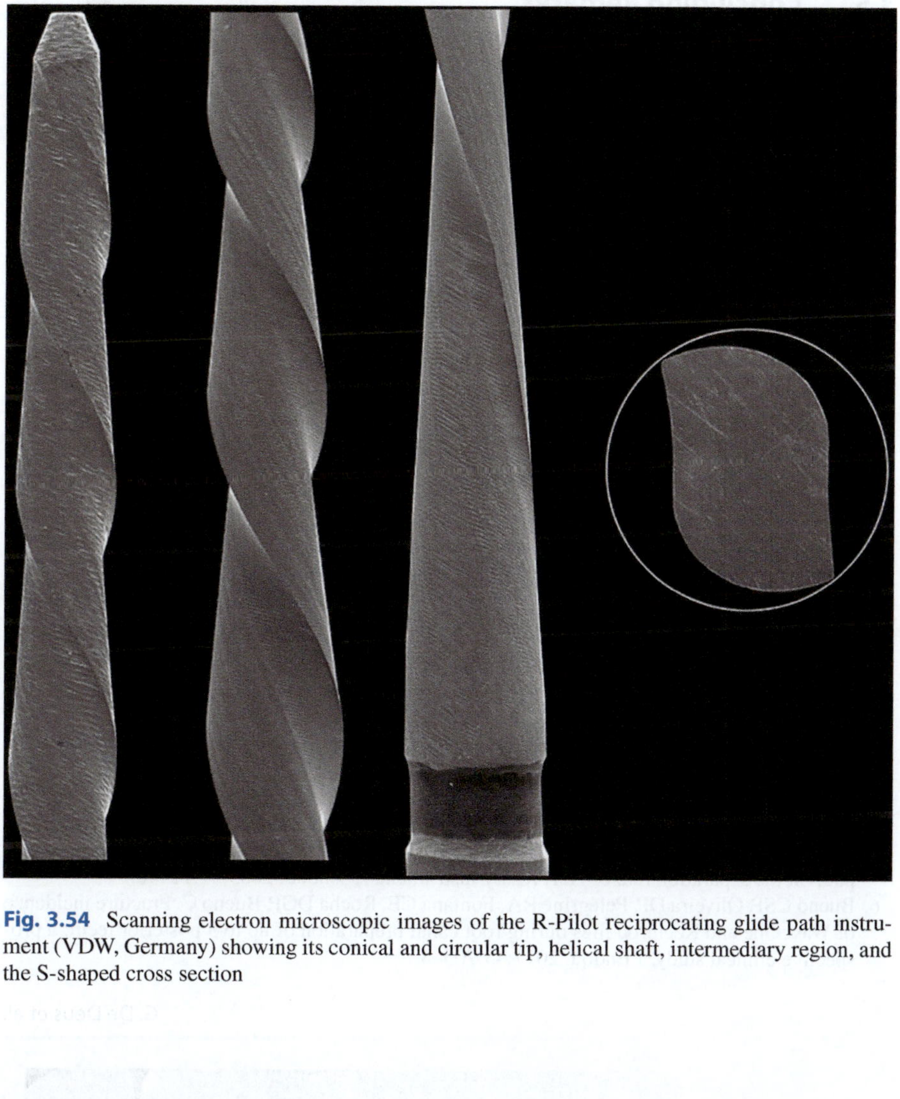

Fig. 3.54 Scanning electron microscopic images of the R-Pilot reciprocating glide path instrument (VDW, Germany) showing its conical and circular tip, helical shaft, intermediary region, and the S-shaped cross section

"Reciproc ALL" mode at 300 rpm. Following three pecking motions, the instrument is withdrawn to be cleaned and the canal irrigated. This procedure is repeated until the established working length is achieved. A preliminary scouting with a size 08 K-file is recommended before using this instrument.

It should be noted that the same critical aspect discussed in the use of rotary pathfinders applies to the R-Pilot and WaveOne Glider instruments, since previous canal scouting is still required. Yet, at least some progress can be observed as the R-Pilot manufacturer specifies canal scouting up to the ISO file size 08, instead of sizes 10 or 15, as recommended for most rotary pathfinders. Although several studies have tested the mechanical properties of R-Pilot and WaveOne Glider instruments, to date, however, there is a lack of laboratorial and clinical studies evaluating their performance (safety and ability to reach the apex).

3.5 Concluding Remarks

The glide path procedure is generally accepted as a challenging transoperative procedure that sometimes is laborious and time-consuming, requiring patience and diligence even from masterful clinicians. However, the role that the glide path plays for the further enlargement of the root canal space with the engine-driven shaping instruments is also irrefutable. Thus, the glide path represents an essential skill for all endodontic practitioners that must be trained to improve their skills to perform this procedure in a safe and predictable way whenever necessary. Although some rotary pathfinder instruments have been made available in the market over the last decade, evidence in terms of safety and efficiency in reaching the apex does not support their ability in replacing manual instrument maneuvers. On the other hand, reciprocating movement seems to be a promising approach for performing the glide path procedure, despite the lack of evidence so far. Canal scouting, apical patency and glide path per se are considered the initial steps that allow the Shaping for Cleaning strategy.

References

1. Inan U, Gonulol N. Deformation and fracture of Mtwo rotary nickel-titanium instruments after clinical use. J Endod. 2009;35:1396–9.
2. Peng B, Shen Y, Cheung GS, Xia TJ. Defects in ProTaper S1 instruments after clinical use: longitudinal examination. Int Endod J. 2005;38:550–7.
3. Sattapan B, Nervo GJ, Palamara JE, Messer HH. Defects in rotary nickel-titanium files after clinical use. J Endod. 2000;26:161–5.
4. Shen Y, Coil JM, Haapasalo M. Defects in nickel-titanium instruments after clinical use. Part 3: a 4-year retrospective study from an undergraduate clinic. J Endod. 2009;35:193–6.
5. Patiño PV, Biedma BM, Liebana CR, Cantatore G, Bahillo JG. The influence of a manual glide path on the separation rate of NiTi rotary instruments. J Endod. 2005;31:114–6.
6. Bueno CSP, Oliveira DP, Pelegrine RA, Fontana CE, Rocha DGP, Bueno C. Fracture incidence of WaveOne and Reciproc files during root canal preparation of up to 3 posterior teeth: a prospective clinical study. J Endod. 2017;43:705–8.

7. Caballero-Flores H, Nabeshima CK, Binotto E, Machado MEL. Fracture incidence of instruments from a single-file reciprocating system by students in an endodontic graduate programme: a cross-sectional retrospective study. Int Endod J. 2019;52:13–8.
8. Cunha RS, Junaid A, Ensinas P, Nudera W, Bueno CE. Assessment of the separation incidence of reciprocating WaveOne files: a prospective clinical study. J Endod. 2014;40:922–4.
9. Yared G, Kulkarni GK. Accuracy of the TCM Endo III torque-control motor for nickel-titanium rotary instruments. J Endod. 2004;30:644–5.
10. West J. Endodontic update 2006. J Esthet Restor Dent. 2006;18:280–300.
11. Plotino G, Nagendrababu V, Bukiet F, Grande NM, Veettil SK, De-Deus G, et al. Influence of negotiation, glide path, and preflaring procedures on root canal shaping-terminology, basic concepts, and a systematic review. J Endod. 2020;46:707–29.
12. Buchanan LS. Management of the curved root canal. J Calif Dent Assoc. 1989;17:18–25, 7.
13. Kiefner P, Connert T, ElAyouti A, Weiger R. Treatment of calcified root canals in elderly people: a clinical study about the accessibility, the time needed and the outcome with a three-year follow-up. Gerodontology. 2017;34:164–70.
14. Nehammer CF, Stock CJ. Preparation and filling of the root canal. Br Dent J. 1985;158:285–91.
15. Ruddle CJ. Finishing the apical one third. Endodontic considerations. Dent Today. 2002;21:66–70, 2–3.
16. Schilder H. Cleaning and shaping the root canal. Dent Clin N Am. 1974;18:269–96.
17. Buchanan LS. Working length and apical patency: the control factors. Endod Rep. 1987:16–20.
18. AAE. Glossary of endodontics terms. 9th ed. Chicago: American Association of Endodontists; 2016.
19. Tsesis I, Amdor B, Tamse A, Kfir A. The effect of maintaining apical patency on canal transportation. Int Endod J. 2008;41:431–5.
20. Higa RA, Adorno CG, Ebrahim AK, Suda H. Distance from file tip to the major apical foramen in relation to the numeric meter reading on the display of three different electronic apex locators. Int Endod J. 2009;42:1065–70.
21. Stoll R, Urban-Klein B, Roggendorf MJ, Jablonski-Momeni A, Strauch K, Frankenberger R. Effectiveness of four electronic apex locators to determine distance from the apical foramen. Int Endod J. 2010;43:808–17.
22. Cailleteau JG, Mullaney TP. Prevalence of teaching apical patency and various instrumentation and obturation techniques in United States dental schools. J Endod. 1997;23:394–6.
23. Vera J, Arias A, Romero M. Effect of maintaining apical patency on irrigant penetration into the apical third of root canals when using passive ultrasonic irrigation: an in vivo study. J Endod. 2011;37:1276–8.
24. Souza RA. The importance of apical patency and cleaning of the apical foramen on root canal preparation. Braz Dent J. 2006;17:6–9.
25. Vera J, Arias A, Romero M. Dynamic movement of intracanal gas bubbles during cleaning and shaping procedures: the effect of maintaining apical patency on their presence in the middle and cervical thirds of human root canals-an in vivo study. J Endod. 2012;38:200–3.
26. Yaylali IE, Kurnaz S, Tunca YM. Maintaining apical patency does not increase postoperative pain in molars with necrotic pulp and apical periodontitis: a randomized controlled trial. J Endod. 2018;44:335–40.
27. Ng YL, Mann V, Gulabivala K. A prospective study of the factors affecting outcomes of non-surgical root canal treatment: part 1: periapical health. Int Endod J. 2011;44:583–609.
28. West J. Finishing: the essence of exceptional endodontics. Dent Today. 2001;20:36–41.
29. West JD. The endodontic glidepath: "secret to rotary safety". Dent Today. 2010;29:86, 8, 90–3.
30. Yared G. Canal preparation using only one Ni-Ti rotary instrument: preliminary observations. Int Endod J. 2008;41:339–44.
31. Ruddle CJ, Machtou P, West JD. Endodontic canal preparation: innovations in glide path management and shaping canals. Dent Today. 2014;33:118–23.
32. Peters OA. Current challenges and concepts in the preparation of root canal systems: a review. J Endod. 2004;30:559–67.
33. Van der Vyver PJ. Creating a glide path for rotary NiTi instruments: part one. Int Dent. 2011;13:6–10.

34. Ungerechts C, Bårdsen A, Fristad I. Instrument fracture in root canals—where, why, when and what? A study from a student clinic. Int Endod J. 2014;47:183–90.
35. Berutti E, Paolino DS, Chiandussi G, Alovisi M, Cantatore G, Castellucci A, et al. Root canal anatomy preservation of WaveOne reciprocating files with or without glide path. J Endod. 2012;38:101–4.
36. Stabholz A, Rotstein I, Torabinejad M. Effect of preflaring on tactile detection of the apical constriction. J Endod. 1995;21:92–4.
37. Gunes B, Yesildal Yeter K. Effects of different glide path files on apical debris extrusion in curved root canals. J Endod. 2018;44:1191–4.
38. Schneider SW. A comparison of canal preparations in straight and curved root canals. Oral Surg Oral Med Oral Pathol. 1971;32:271–5.
39. Pruett JP, Clement DJ, Carnes DL Jr. Cyclic fatigue testing of nickel-titanium endodontic instruments. J Endod. 1997;23:77–85.
40. Hasan M, Raza Khan F. Determination of frequency of the second mesiobuccal canal in the permanent maxillary first molar teeth with magnification loupes (× 3.5). Int J Biomed Sci. 2014;10:201–7.
41. Somma F, Leoni D, Plotino G, Grande NM, Plasschaert A. Root canal morphology of the mesiobuccal root of maxillary first molars: a micro-computed tomographic analysis. Int Endod J. 2009;42:165–74.
42. Sujith R, Dhananjaya K, Chaurasia VR, Kasigari D, Veerabhadrappa AC, Naik S. Microscope magnification and ultrasonic precision guidance for location and negotiation of second mesiobuccal canal: an in vivo study. J Int Soc Prev Community Dent. 2014;4:S209–12.
43. Plotino G, Grande NM, Pecci R, Bedini R, Pameijer CH, Somma F. Three-dimensional imaging using microcomputed tomography for studying tooth macromorphology. J Am Dent Assoc. 2006;137:1555–61.
44. Lopes HP, Elias CN, Mangelli M, Lopes WS, Amaral G, Souza LC, et al. Buckling resistance of pathfinding endodontic instruments. J Endod. 2012;38:402–4.
45. Jafarzadeh H, Abbott PV. Ledge formation: review of a great challenge in endodontics. J Endod. 2007;33:1155–62.
46. De-Deus G, Belladonna FG, Souza EM, Alves Vde O, Silva EJ, Rodrigues E, et al. Scouting ability of 4 pathfinding instruments in moderately curved molar canals. J Endod. 2016;42:1540–4.
47. Allen JS. Apical patency and its effect on endodontic outcomes. Maryland: University of the Health Sciences; 2012.
48. Alovisi M, Pasqualini D, Musso E, Bobbio E, Giuliano C, Mancino D, et al. Influence of contracted endodontic access on root canal geometry: an in vitro study. J Endod. 2018;44:614–20.
49. Pedullà E, La Rosa GRM, Virgillito C, Rapisarda E, Kim HC, Generali L. Cyclic fatigue resistance of nickel-titanium rotary instruments according to the angle of file access and radius of root canal. J Endod. 2020;46:431–6.
50. Vorster M, van der Vyver PJ, Paleker F. Influence of glide path preparation on the canal shaping times of WaveOne Gold in curved mandibular molar canals. J Endod. 2018;44:853–5.
51. Cassim I, Van der Vyver PJ. An in vitro comparison of different techniques for glide path preparation. Saudi Dent J. 2015;70:452–6.
52. Nahmias Y, Cassim I, Glassman G. "Own the canal": the importance of a reproducible glide path. Oral Health J. 2013;5:74–82.
53. Hartmann MS, Fontanella VR, Vanni JR, Fornari VJ, Barletta FB. CT evaluation of apical canal transportation associated with stainless steel hand files, oscillatory technique and pro taper rotary system. Braz Dent J. 2011;22:288–93.
54. Ajuz NC, Armada L, Goncalves LS, Debelian G, Siqueira JF Jr. Glide path preparation in S-shaped canals with rotary pathfinding nickel-titanium instruments. J Endod. 2013;39:534–7.
55. Alovisi M, Cemenasco A, Mancini L, Paolino D, Scotti N, Bianchi CC, et al. Micro-CT evaluation of several glide path techniques and ProTaper Next shaping outcomes in maxillary first molar curved canals. Int Endod J. 2017;50:387–97.
56. Hartmann RC, Peters OA, de Figueiredo JAP, Rossi-Fedele G. Association of manual or engine-driven glide path preparation with canal centring and apical transportation: a systematic review. Int Endod J. 2018;51:1239–52.

57. Pasqualini D, Mollo L, Scotti N, Cantatore G, Castellucci A, Migliaretti G, et al. Postoperative pain after manual and mechanical glide path: a randomized clinical trial. J Endod. 2012;38:32–6.
58. Passi S, Kaler N, Passi N. What is a glide path? Saint Int Dent J. 2016;2:32–7.
59. Zanette F, Grazziotin-Soares R, Flores ME, Camargo Fontanella VR, Gavini G, Barletta FB. Apical root canal transportation and remaining dentin thickness associated with ProTaper Universal with and without PathFile. J Endod. 2014;40:688–93.
60. Gavini G, Santos MD, Caldeira CL, Machado MEL, Freire LG, Iglecias EF, et al. Nickel-titanium instruments in endodontics: a concise review of the state of the art. Braz Oral Res. 2018;32:e67.
61. Berutti E, Alovisi M, Pastorelli MA, Chiandussi G, Scotti N, Pasqualini D. Energy consumption of ProTaper Next X1 after glide path with PathFiles and ProGlider. J Endod. 2014;40:2015–8.
62. Zheng L, Ji X, Li C, Zuo L, Wei X. Comparison of glide paths created with K-files, PathFiles, and the ProGlider file, and their effects on subsequent WaveOne preparation in curved canals. BMC Oral Health. 2018;18:152.
63. Jaiswal NU, Mantri SP, Paul B, Dube K, Singh V, Bhatnagar N. Comparative evaluation of the effectiveness and fracture rate of three pathfinding nickel-titanium rotary instruments, Mtwo, OneG, and ProGlider, in mechanically negotiating moderately curved molar canals to the full working length. J Conserv Dent. 2019;22:260–5.
64. Özyürek T, Uslu G, Gündoğar M, Yılmaz K, Grande NM, Plotino G. Comparison of cyclic fatigue resistance and bending properties of two reciprocating nickel-titanium glide path files. Int Endod J. 2018;51:1047–52.

NiTi Rotary Systems: From Revolution to the "More of the Same" Phenomenon

4

Emmanuel J. N. L. Silva, Erick Souza, Gustavo De Deus, Marco A. Versiani, and Mario Zuolo

4.1 Nickel-Titanium Alloy: History and Properties

In the literature, no one has summarized the impact of the introduction of nickel-titanium (NiTi) rotary instruments in endodontics better than Buchanan [1]. According to him,

> Nickel titanium rotary shaping files fundamentally changed everything in endodontics; conceptually, procedurally and economically as well. NiTi rotary files made root canal therapy more accessible and kinder of fun for dentists, and dental companies were loved for making files that cost four times more than SS hand files but delivered a ten times improvement.

In summary, the introduction of NiTi alloy to produce instruments for shaping the root canal moved endodontics to the next level.

Improvements on the NiTi metallurgical technology allowed the development of a variety of new instruments with innovative designs, mainly on the tip and blade geometry, which ended up in an overall improved efficiency [2–8]. The intrinsic characteristics of the NiTi alloy enabled the development of instruments that were prone to better control the occurrence of ordinary iatrogenic mishaps such as

E. J. N. L. Silva (✉)
Fluminense Federal University, Grande Rio University, Rio de Janeiro State University, Niterói, Brazil
e-mail: nogueiraemmanuel@hotmail.com

E. Souza
Federal University of Maranhão, São Luis, Brazil

G. De Deus
Fluminense Federal University, Niterói, Brazil

M. A. Versiani
Dental Specialty Center, Brazilian Military Police, Minas Gerais, Brazil

M. Zuolo
Dental School of APCD – FAOA, São Paulo, Brazil

G. De Deus et al. (eds.), *Shaping for Cleaning the Root Canals*,
https://doi.org/10.1007/978-3-030-84617-6_4

deviation and perforation [3, 9, 10]. In fact, it is fair to say that shaping outcomes with NiTi rotary instruments are more predictable and the canal enlargement procedure is more pleasant and simpler for dentists when compared to the manual preparation with stainless steel files [4].

The NiTi alloy was developed in the United States by William Buehler in 1963 and was firstly named NiTiNOL, an acronym for nickel (Ni), titanium (Ti), and Naval Ordnance Laboratory (NOL) [11]. In dentistry, Andreasen and Morrow [12] initially applied the NiTiNOL in orthodontics due to its low modulus of elasticity, shape memory effect and super flexibility. In 1975, Civjan and colleagues [13] published a manuscript containing suggestions for its use in different dental specialties, including endodontics. The authors concluded that the low modulus of elasticity of the NiTi alloy would allow the production of more efficient instruments to prepare curved canals. The first study using prototypes made from NiTi orthodontic wires for root canal preparation concluded that they had 2–3 times more elastic flexibility in bending and superior resistance to torsional fracture compared to similar instruments manufactured in stainless steel alloy [14].

The NiTi alloys used in the production of endodontic instruments have almost equiatomic ratios of nickel and titanium elements [14] and contain three microstructural phases named austenite, martensite, and R-phase. The respective amount of each one of these phases will determine the mechanical properties of the alloy [3, 8, 15, 16]. The transformation of austenite into martensite (also called classic martensitic transformation) is caused by the ability of the alloy to modify its atomic arrangement. The alteration of its crystalline microstructure and transformation characteristics directly influence the mechanical properties of the alloy. Martensite, the low-temperature phase, is relatively soft and ductile. In this phase, the alloy can be easily deformed and possesses the shape memory effect [3, 8, 16]. In contrast, austenite, the high-temperature phase, is relatively stiff and hard, and exhibits superelasticity [8, 16]. The phase composition of the NiTi alloy is dependent on the ambient temperature and whether the alloy is cooled or heated to a specific temperature (Fig. 4.1). If the temperature is above the austenite finish temperature (A_f), the NiTi alloy is in the austenitic state, displaying a body-centered cubic structure. If the temperature is below the martensite finish temperature (M_f), the NiTi is in the martensitic state, because of a classic linear thermal contraction that initiates at the M_i and becomes linear until the M_f, the point at which the alloy reaches 100% of monoclinic martensite phase [3, 8, 16]. Reheating this martensite phase will eventually reverse the process and yield an austenite form.

Among the main properties of the NiTi alloys used to manufacture endodontic instruments are the shape memory effect and superelasticity [3, 8, 16]. When the NiTi wire is submitted to external stress, the austenite form is reconverted to the martensite (stress-induced martensite) form (Fig. 4.2). This form is not stable at room temperature, so an immediate transformation to the austenitic phase occurs once the stress is released, which is known as superelasticity. In other words, superelasticity is characterized by the ability of the alloy to recover its original shape merely by the removal of the tension applied, even after large strains, without the need for heating (Figs. 4.3 and 4.4) [16, 17]. This stress-induced change without a

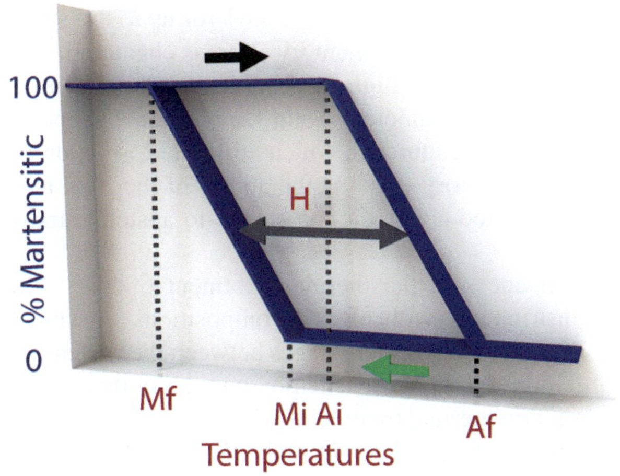

Fig. 4.1 Temperature hysteresis diagram of nickel-titanium (NiTi) alloy showing the martensite start temperature (M_i), the martensite finish temperature (M_f), the austenite start temperature (A_i), and the austenite finish temperature (A_f). If temperature is above the austenite finish temperature (A_f), the NiTi alloy is in the austenitic state, displaying a body-centered cubic structure. On the other hand, if temperature is below the martensite finish temperature (M_f), the NiTi is in the martensitic state, considering the classical linear thermal contraction that initiates at the M_i and becomes linear until the M_f, the point at which the alloy reaches 100% of monoclinic martensite phase

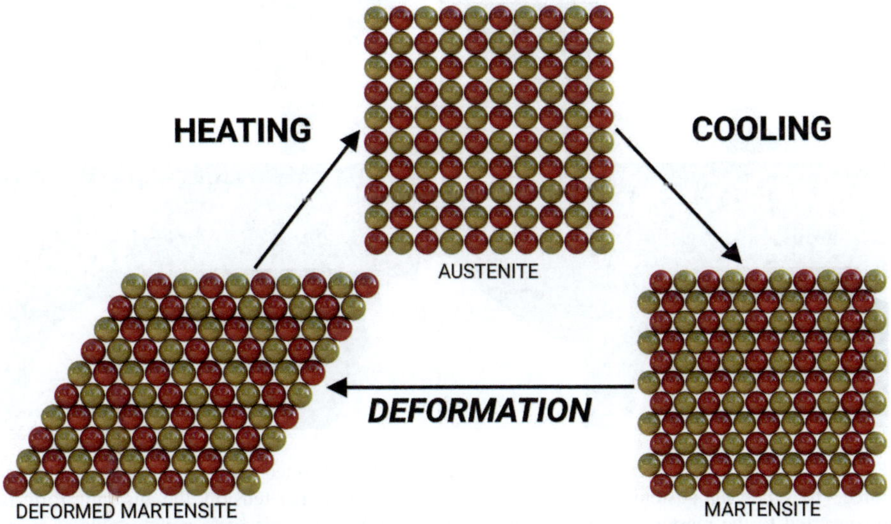

Fig. 4.2 Schematic illustration of shape memory alloy (SMA) phase transformation between austenite and martensite of NiTi. The transformation of the austenite phase into martensite results from cooling the NiTi alloy. The deformation of the alloy in a martensite phase results in a deformed martensite crystal structure, which returns to the austenite phase at high temperature. The shape memory effect is a direct consequence of this reversible transition between austenite and martensite phases

permanent deformation is possible in NiTi alloys for up to 8% strain, as opposed to 1% in stainless steel [6]. The shape memory effect is characterized as a property by means of which, after relatively high deformations at temperatures below the full formation of martensite, instruments regain their original shape and size through subsequent heating at temperatures in which austenite formation occurs (Fig. 4.5). In other words, shape memory effect is the ability of the NiTi alloy to recover its original shape when heated above the martensite-to-austenite transformation temperature (Fig. 4.6).

Technological advances in the thermal treatment of NiTi alloys allowed the development of instruments with altered compositions in which the crystalline structure of the alloy is in intermediate stages between the austenitic and martensitic phases, with substantial stable martensite phase under body temperature [3, 8, 18]. Examples of proprietary thermal treatments of NiTi alloys developed by some companies are the M-wire (Dentsply Tulsa Dental, USA), R-phase (SybronEndo, USA), CM-wire (DS Dental, USA), EDM (Coltène/Whaledent AG, Switzerland), Gold and Blue treatments (Dentsply Tulsa Dental, USA), T-wire (MicroMega, France),

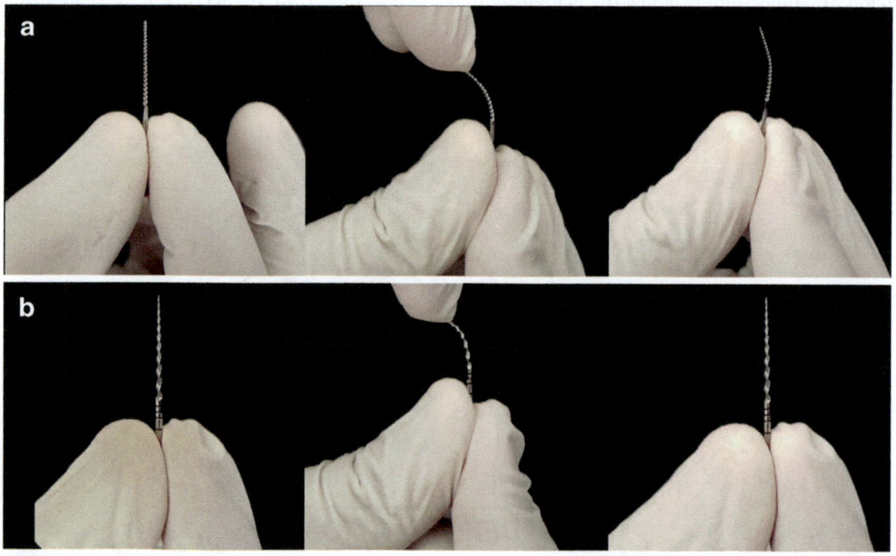

Fig. 4.3 (**a**) Stainless steel instrument being plastically deformed after application of tension force. (**b**) When the austenitic NiTi wire is submitted to a similar tension, the austenite form is reconverted to the martensite (stress-induced martensite) form. This form is not stable at room temperature, so an immediate transformation to the austenitic phase occurs once the stress is released meaning that NiTi austenitic instruments can recover to their original shape after applying forces

and MaxWire (FKG Dentaire, Switzerland). While M-wire and R-phase instruments maintain an austenitic state, CM-Wire, Gold and Blue heat-treated instruments are composed of substantial amounts of martensite. According to the manufacturer (FKG Dentaire, Switzerland), MaxWire is in the martensitic state at room temperature and changes to the austenitic state at intracanal temperature, recovering the shape of the instrument.

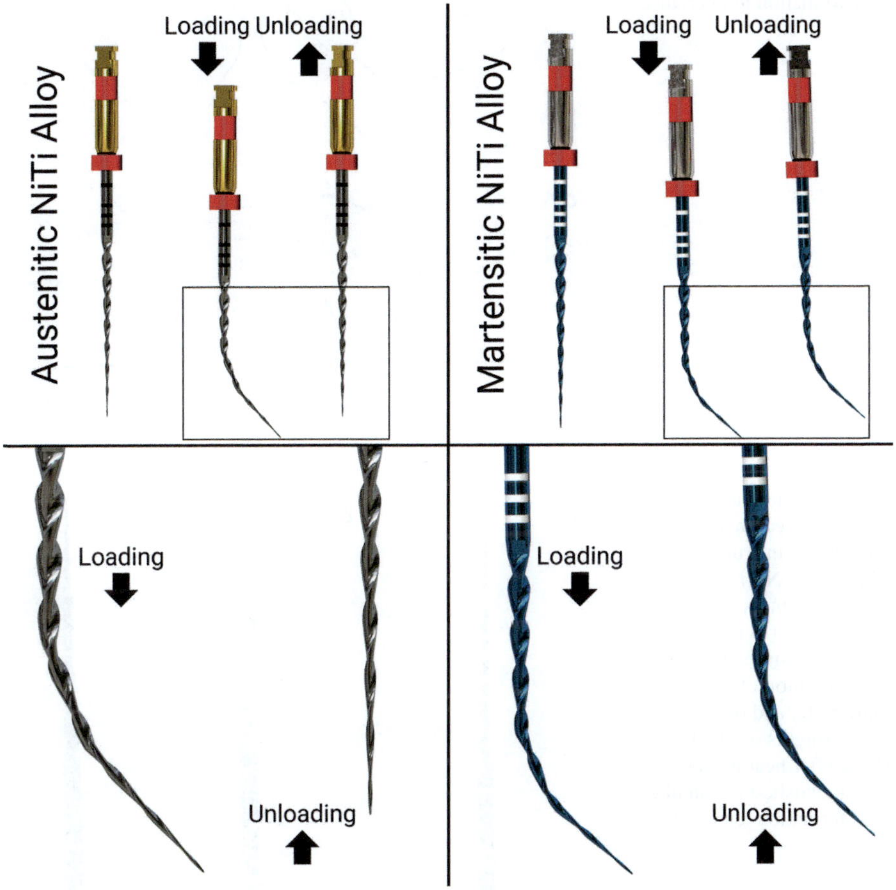

Fig. 4.4 Different behavior of NiTi austenitic alloy (which possesses superelastic properties) and NiTi martensitic alloys (which possess shape memory properties) endodontic instruments during and after application of tension forces. While the instrument made of austenitic NiTi alloy (on the left) recover to its original shape by removing the tension applied, the martensitic NiTi alloy instrument (on the right) has apparent deformation at temperatures below the full formation of martensite

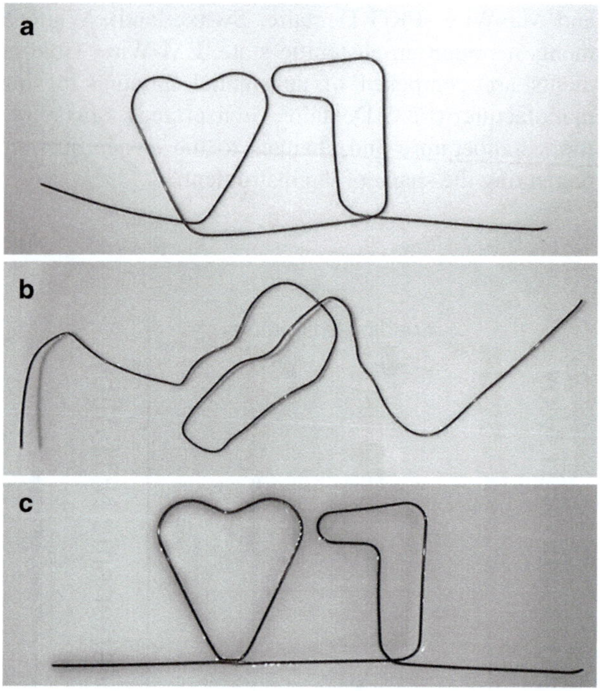

Fig. 4.5 The shape memory effect. (**a**) Martensitic NiTi alloy wire in its original shape. (**b**) This same wire is deformed at a temperature below the full formation of martensite and (**c**) recover to its original shape after being heated above the martensite-to-austenite transformation temperature

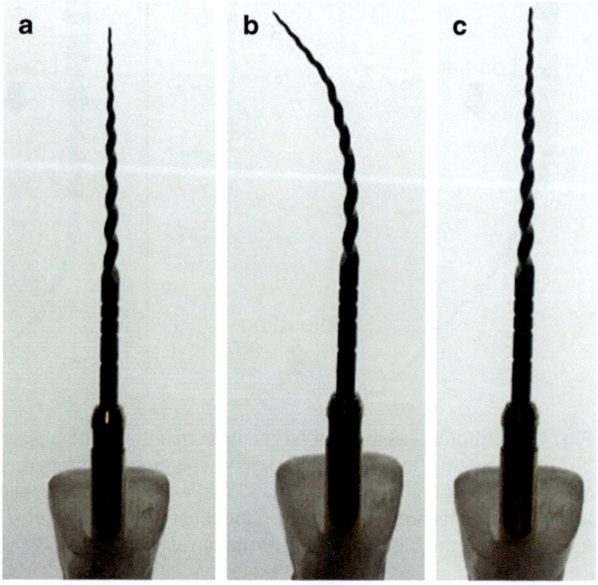

Fig. 4.6 The shape memory effect in an endodontic instrument. (**a**) Martensitic NiTi instrument in its original shape being (**b**) deformed at a temperature below the full formation of martensite, and (**c**) recovering its original shape after heating above the martensite-to-austenite transformation temperature

4.2 NiTi Alloys and Specific Features

4.2.1 Austenitic NiTi Alloy

4.2.1.1 Conventional NiTi Alloy

As previously stated, conventional NiTi instruments have near-equiatomic proportions of nickel and titanium elements, and have superelasticity as their main property. These instruments have their austenite finish temperature below body temperature and, therefore, are mainly constituted of the austenite phase. This phase is relatively stiff and hard [7, 8] and the use of these instruments might produce an in situ elastic deformation that follows a linear stress function. If the stress increases, the superelasticity deformation appears so that the strain remains constant until the NiTi mass has entirely shifted to the martensitic phase. Continuing activation beyond that point will result in typical martensitic deformation. But, if the load is relieved before the plastic deformation limit, the deformation is reversible. Because of the superelasticity, the manufacturing process of these instruments involves the traditional grinding method, which may result in defects, such as microcracks, debris and milling grooves on their surfaces, especially at the cutting edges (Fig. 4.7). Logical reasoning dictates that such defects may negatively impact on the fatigue resistance, corrosion and cutting efficiency.

4.2.1.2 Electropolishing Treatment

Additional metallurgical treatments on the NiTi alloys, such as the electropolishing and some heat treatments, were developed in order to improve the clinical performance of endodontic instruments. Electropolishing is a surface finishing process

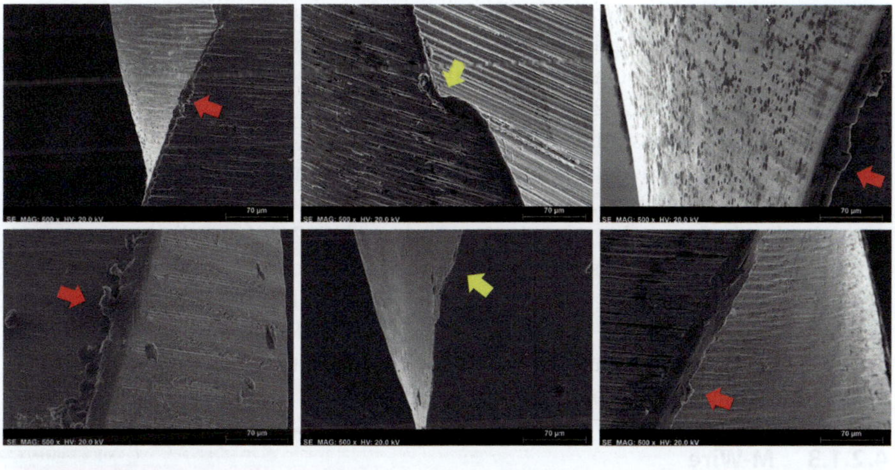

Fig. 4.7 Scanning electron microscopy of endodontic instruments made by the grinding method which it is possible to observe distinct machining marks resulting from the manufacturing process. Red arrows show barbs at the cutting edge of some instruments, while yellow arrows depict cutting edge discontinuity

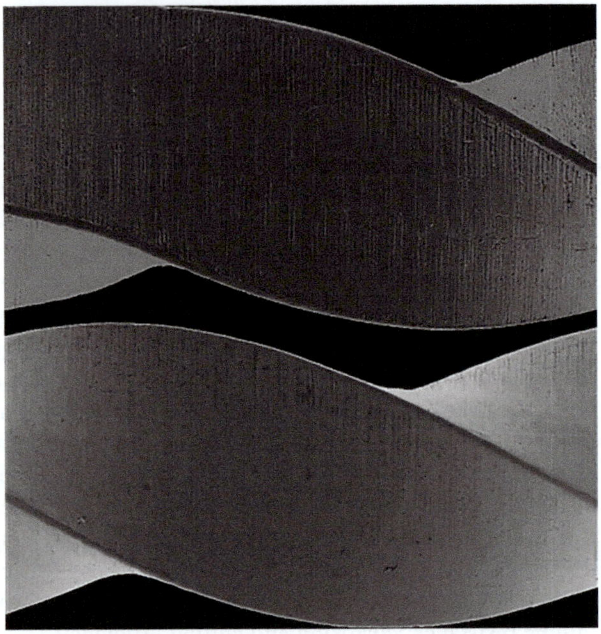

Fig. 4.8 Scanning electron microscopy of the same rotary NiTi instrument before (on top) and after (below) electropolishing procedure, demonstrating the improvement of the surface finishing

that electrolytically remove components from metal parts in a highly ionic solution using an external source of electrical current. In this process, a very thin layer of the material on the instruments' surfaces is removed, resulting in the reduction of micro asperities that characterize metal surfaces. This process can be used to remove surface irregularities, cracks, and residual stress caused by the grinding process during manufacturing. The electropolishing of NiTi mechanized instruments not only improves their metallic surface, leading to a smoother surface with increased gloss, but also makes it more rigid [19–21] (Fig. 4.8). This process might also result in an improved corrosion resistance without affecting the superelasticity and cutting efficiency of instruments [22, 23].

However, although studies have demonstrated that electropolishing treatment might improve the cyclic fatigue resistance of NiTi instruments [21–23] by reducing microcracks, surface debris, and milling grooves [19, 20], this method is unable to avoid the development of structural microfractures [19, 24]. According to these studies, microcracks of non-polished instruments are nucleated and run along the machining grooves in conventional NiTi instruments, while in electropolished instruments a fine, irregular, zigzag crack pattern can be observed [19, 24]. This means that more cycles are needed to increase the severity of the defects in electropolished instruments when compared to non-polished counterparts.

4.2.1.3 M-Wire

In 2007, a new NiTi alloy known as M-Wire was introduced by Dentsply Tulsa Dental. This alloy was developed using a proprietary thermomechanical manufacturing procedure applied before the instruments are machined, which renders an improved flexibility and cyclic fatigue resistance when compared to conventional NiTi alloys [15, 25, 26]. The austenite finish temperature of M-Wire was found to be around 43–50 °C [27, 28] and, consequently, high above the A_f of conventional NiTi, indicating that M-Wire is not completely composed of austenite under body temperature. In this condition, metallurgical studies reported that M-Wire alloy contains three crystalline phases: small amounts of deformed and micro-twinned martensite, R-phase, and austenite [27–29].

4.2.1.4 R-Phase

The NiTi R-phase alloy, also called pre-martensitic, was developed by the Sybron Endo company in 2008 from a series of distinct thermal treatments (heating and cooling) that allowed the formation and maintenance of this specific crystallographic phase. The R-phase alloy is characterized as an intermediate crystalline phase that occurs along a very narrow temperature range on the heating or cooling curve between martensitic and austenitic forms. Similar to the martensite and austenite phases, the intermediate R-phase also has specific temperatures for its formation, represented as R_i for the beginning of phase formation, and R_f for the end [5–8]. This additional phase change in the crystal structure of the alloy results in lower resistance to elastic deformation (high flexibility and low rigidity), increasing its resistance to cyclic fatigue, but reducing its torsional resistance [15] when compared to conventional alloys [15, 30].

The Twisted File (TF) and K3XF, both manufactured by Sybron Endo, are the main examples of R-Phase instruments. The manufacturing process of TF includes three new methods: the R-phase heat treatment, the twisting of the metal wire (produced by means of plastic deformation followed by heat-treating the metal into recrystallization), and a special surface conditioning process, performed with an oxidation bath, which increases the hardness of the instrument without changing its flexibility. Through the twisting of the metal wire, a greater integrity of the crystal lattice structure of the metal is ensured, as the core of the structure is never sectioned, nor are there any cross-sectional striations (which facilitate fracture propagation) machined into the instrument. In other words, the grooves of the twisted instrument face the direction opposite to that of crack propagation, which is not the case with machined instruments. Defects in the TF are in the long axis while in conventional machining instruments they are perpendicular to it (Fig. 4.9). In contrast to TF, K3XF instruments, a new generation of the K3 system, are manufactured by the traditional grinding process with a post-machining R-phase treatment.

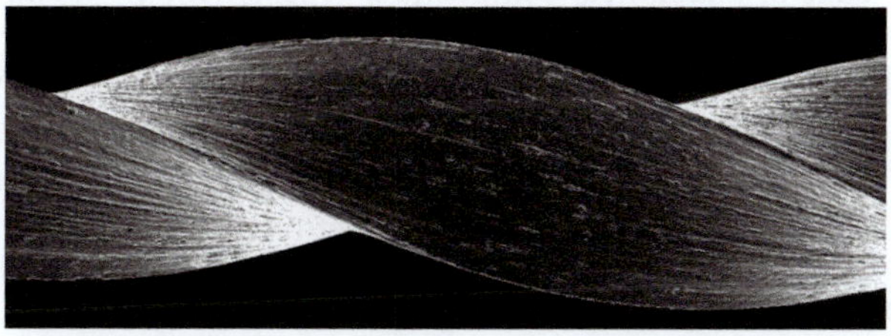

Fig. 4.9 Scanning electron microscopy of the Twisted File Adaptive NiTi instrument showing some defects on its active part

4.2.2 Martensitic NiTi Alloy

When the alloy is subject to a heat treatment the M_f is raised, allowing instruments to have the martensite as the main phase at room temperature [2, 5–8]. The martensitic phase of NiTi alloy has greater elasticity than its austenitic phase, reaching large percentages of deformation with relatively low stress. NiTi instruments made of martensitic alloy are soft, ductile and more resistant to cyclic fatigue. Even under great deformation, these instruments can return to their original state because of the shape memory effect [2, 5–8]. Similarly to the shape memory effect, reorientation of the martensitic microstructure allows stress deformations up to 8%. Thus, after being used for root canal preparation, instruments do not show high increase in their internal stress or plastic deformation, returning to their original state when heated [2, 5–8].

From a practical point of view, instruments made of this thermomechanically treated alloy have increased fatigue resistance and flexibility when compared to conventional NiTi instruments [31–37]. Therefore, martensitic instruments are recommended to be used in severely curved canals (Fig. 4.10), once they are supposed to provide a better maintenance of the original canal path [9, 38–40]. However, Arslan et al. [38] reported no difference in the centering ability of ProTaper Gold, Reciproc and ProTaper Universal in the preparation of severely curved mesial roots of mandibular molars. Similar results were found by Duque et al. [41] comparing root canal preparation of mandibular molars with ProTaper Universal and ProTaper Gold. Another study from Bürklein et al. [42] demonstrated that corresponding instruments manufactured with M-Wire, Gold or Blue alloys maintained the original canal curvature without significant differences among them and no instrument fracture. Similar results were observed by Belladonna et al. [43], who reported similar shaping ability of the original M-Wire Reciproc with Reciproc Blue instruments in the preparation of curved canals of mandibular molars. It is important to emphasize that some of these studies [42, 43] used instruments in reciprocating motion, a movement that will be discussed in Chap. 5. However, taken together, these results show that conventional NiTi and M-Wire instruments have enough flexibility to maintain the canal curvature in most of the cases, and that more flexible alloys, such as Gold and Blue instruments, would be better indicated in severely curved canals. Moreover, the possibility of bending the martensitic instruments would also help in the preparation of difficult cases. For instance, in case of patients with restricted mouth opening, martensitic instruments can be pre-bent, providing access to the canal entrance (Figs. 4.11 and 4.12). In addition, the possibility of pre-bending the instrument may allow the regaining of the original canal pathway in the presence of ledge or anatomical complexities (Figs. 4.13, 4.14, and 4.15).

The major limitation of these instruments is that the martensitic crystalline phase has a low transition temperature, so it requires less energy for deformation. This means that plastic deformation and unwinding of these instruments can be experienced more often (Fig. 4.16). Under torsion, martensitic thermally treated instruments have a high angular deflection, so they can sustain great rotation before fracture; however, the torque needed to deform and fracture these instruments is

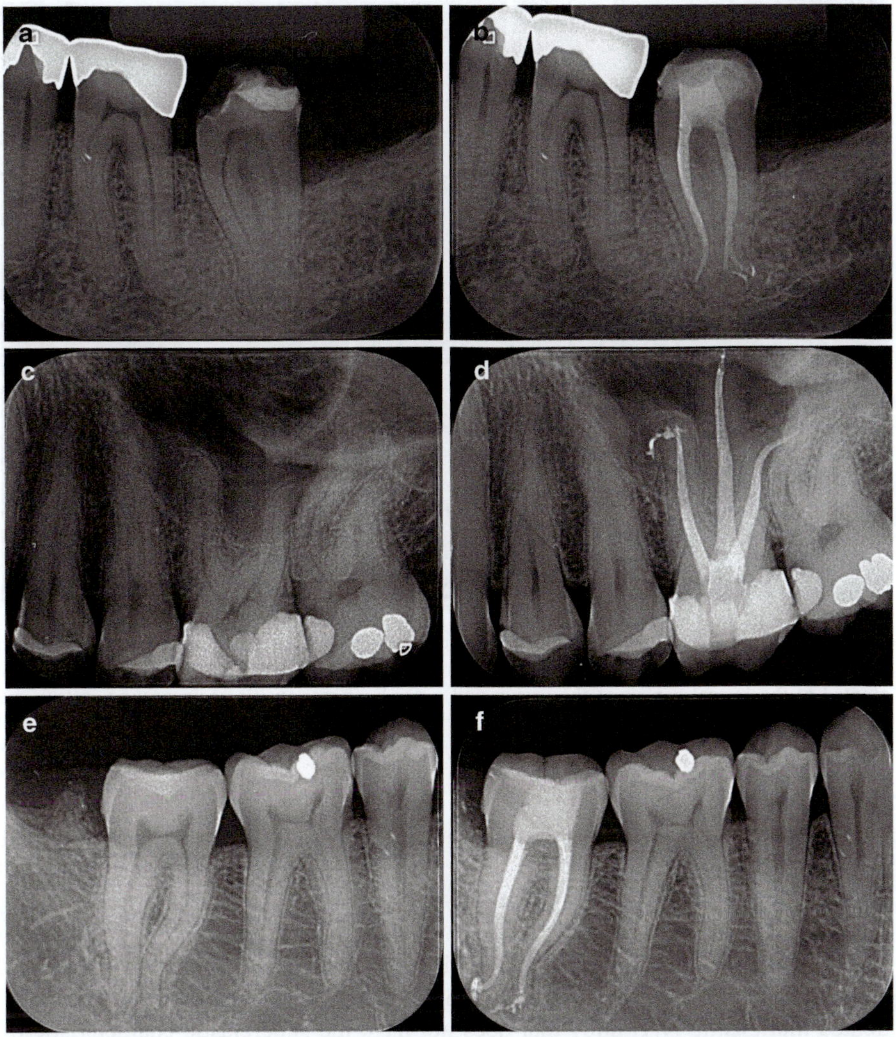

Fig. 4.10 Clinical cases showing the preparation of curved canals of (**a**, **b**) a mandibular second left molar, (**c**, **d**) a maxillary first left molar, and (**e**, **f**) a mandibular second right molar, with martensitic NiTi alloy instruments. (Courtesy of Dr. Iracema Ehrhardt, Brazil)

lower than austenitic intruments [34–37, 44]. Furthermore, extremely flexible alloys may compromise the ability of a given instrument to advance toward the apex. For this reason, in the clinical setting, the overall perception is of difficulty in preparing narrow root canals, with an enhanced risk of instrument distortion and fracture. In contrast, austenitic instruments show high torque values at fracture under torsion and thus they can be more efficient for shaping straight or slightly curved narrow canals, as well as in retreatment cases. Therefore, depending on the case, it is

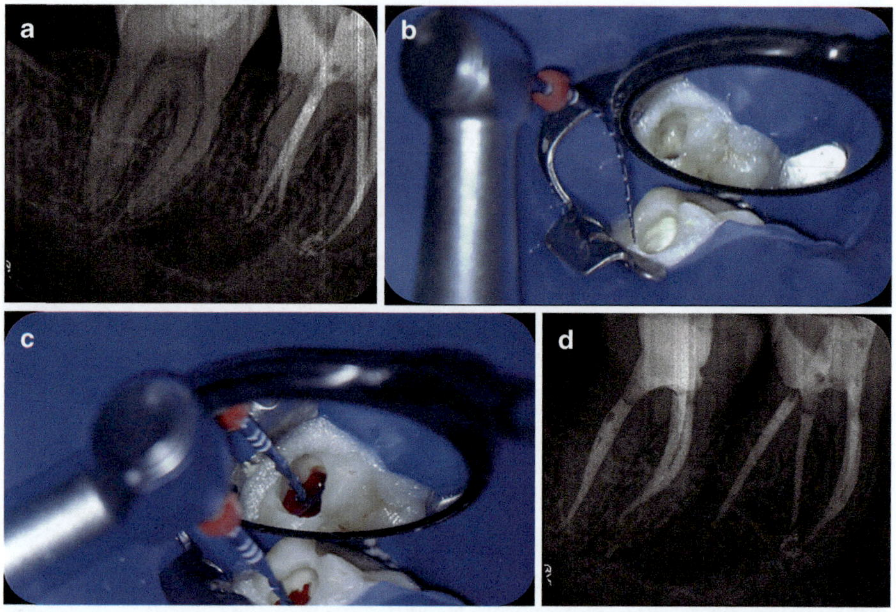

Fig. 4.11 Alternative use of a martensitic instrument. (**a**) Patient with limited mouth opening demanding root canal treatment in a mandibular second right molar. (**b**) Access preparation was granted at the buccal aspect of the crown and a pre-bent martensitic reciprocating instrument (Reciproc Blue R25) was used (**c**) to prepare the root canals and allow (**d**) their filling

important to find a balance between the mechanical properties of flexibility and resistance to torsion.

4.2.2.1 CM-Wire

In 2010, instruments manufactured in CM-Wire (controlled memory) thermal treatment technology were introduced by DS Dental (USA). The CM-Wire is a heat-treated martensitic NiTi alloy that does not have the superelastic characteristic of the austenite phase, which means a lack of rebound effect after unloading, and the original shape of the instrument is restored after heat application or autoclaving sterilization. This happens because the variation in its chemical composition, through the reorientation of the martensite crystalline phase, allows the alloy deformation as a function of the stress to which the instrument is submitted [5, 6]. According to the manufacturer, the use of instruments made of CM-Wire alloy reduces the occurrence of errors during canal shaping because of their high flexibility, provided by their controlled memory effect, preventing the instrument to return to its original geometry during unloading. Besides, this feature allows instruments to be bent before insertion into the root canal. They also have superior resistance to cyclic fatigue, but with an increased tendency to plastic deformations during use, which might be considered as their major drawback.

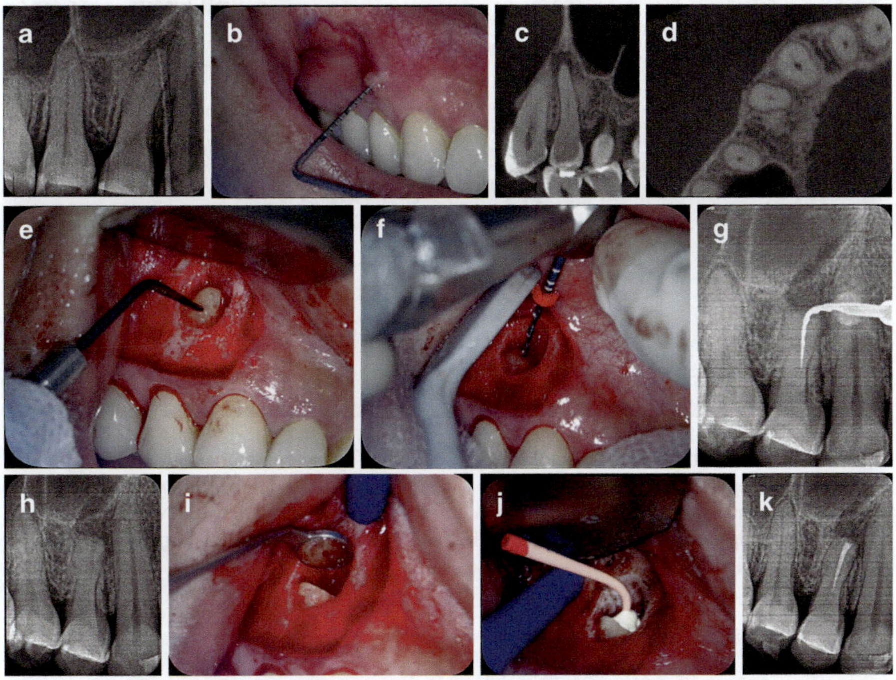

Fig. 4.12 Alternative use of a martensitic instrument. (**a**) Radiograph of a maxillary right first premolar with a partially calcified root canal system displaying apical lesion and (**b**) fistula. (**c, d**) CBCT examination revealed the presence of a single and patent canal only at the middle and apical thirds. (**e**) Considering the mesiodistal constriction of the tooth at the CEJ level, an apical surgery was performed and (**f, g**) a martensic pre-bent instrument (Reciproc Blue R25) was used for retro-preparation, after which (**h–k**) the prepared canal was filled with a single-cone technique using an epoxy-resin based sealer

4.2.2.2 Electrical Discharge Machining

Electrical discharge machining (EDM) technology is a noncontact thermal erosion process that consists of sparks produced by high energy and high-frequency electric discharges between the metal workpiece and an electrode. This leads to melting and evaporation of small portions of the workpiece material, resulting in a finished product of the desired geometry [45]. Rotary NiTi instruments produced using this technique have sharp cutting edges, built-in abrasive properties, variable changing profiles, and a progressive flexibility [44, 45]. In endodontics, HyFlex EDM (Coltène/Whaledent, Switzerland) and NeoNiti (Neolix SAS, France) are instruments that undergo this type of alloy treatment [46–48] (Fig. 4.17).

4.2.2.3 Gold and Blue Wires

Heat-treated instruments have been developed with proprietary heating and cooling treatments, which result in a deposition of extra layers of titanium oxide at their surfaces. Differences in the thickness of these layers are responsible for changing the color of the instrument and, currently, the most common variations are blue

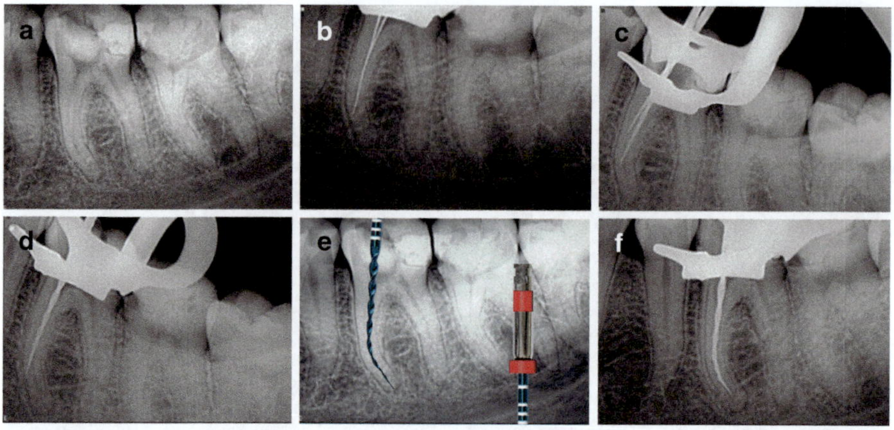

Fig. 4.13 (**a**) Mandibular first left molar with a moderate apical curvature of the mesial root. (**b**) During canal preparation a ledge was formed with stainless steel hand instruments and (**c**, **d**) austenitic instruments were not able to overcome it. (**e**, **f**) A pre-bent martensitic NiTi reciprocating instrument (Reciproc Blue R25) allowed to find and follow the original canal path. (Courtesy of Dr. Evaldo Rodrigues, Brazil)

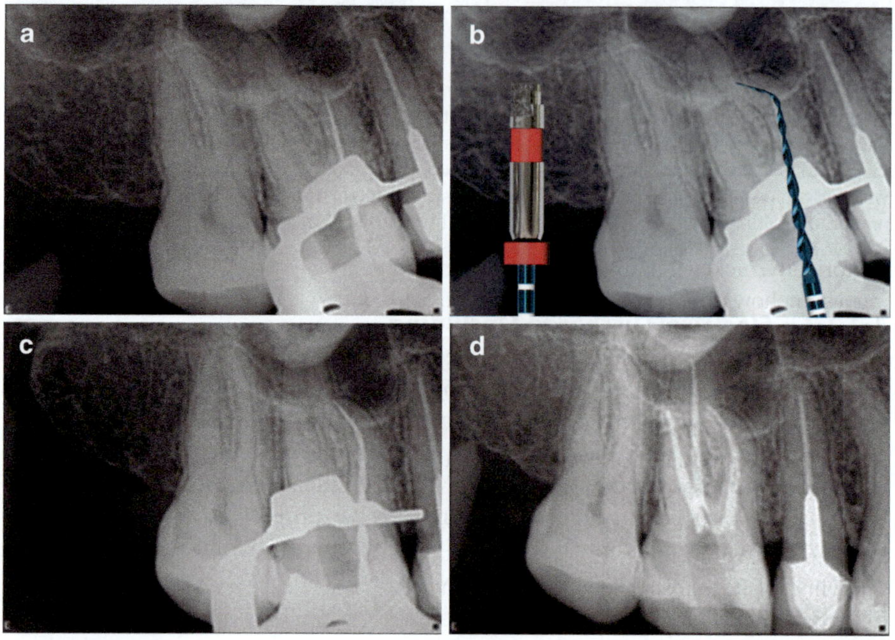

Fig. 4.14 (**a**) Radiography of a maxillary first right molar showing an austenitic NiTi instrument positioned at a ledge created by the previous preparation. (**b**) The tip of a martensitic NiTi instrument (Reciproc Blue R25) was bent, (**c**) allowing its passage through the ledge and (**d**) filling of the original canal. (Courtesy of Dr. Evaldo Rodrigues, Brazil)

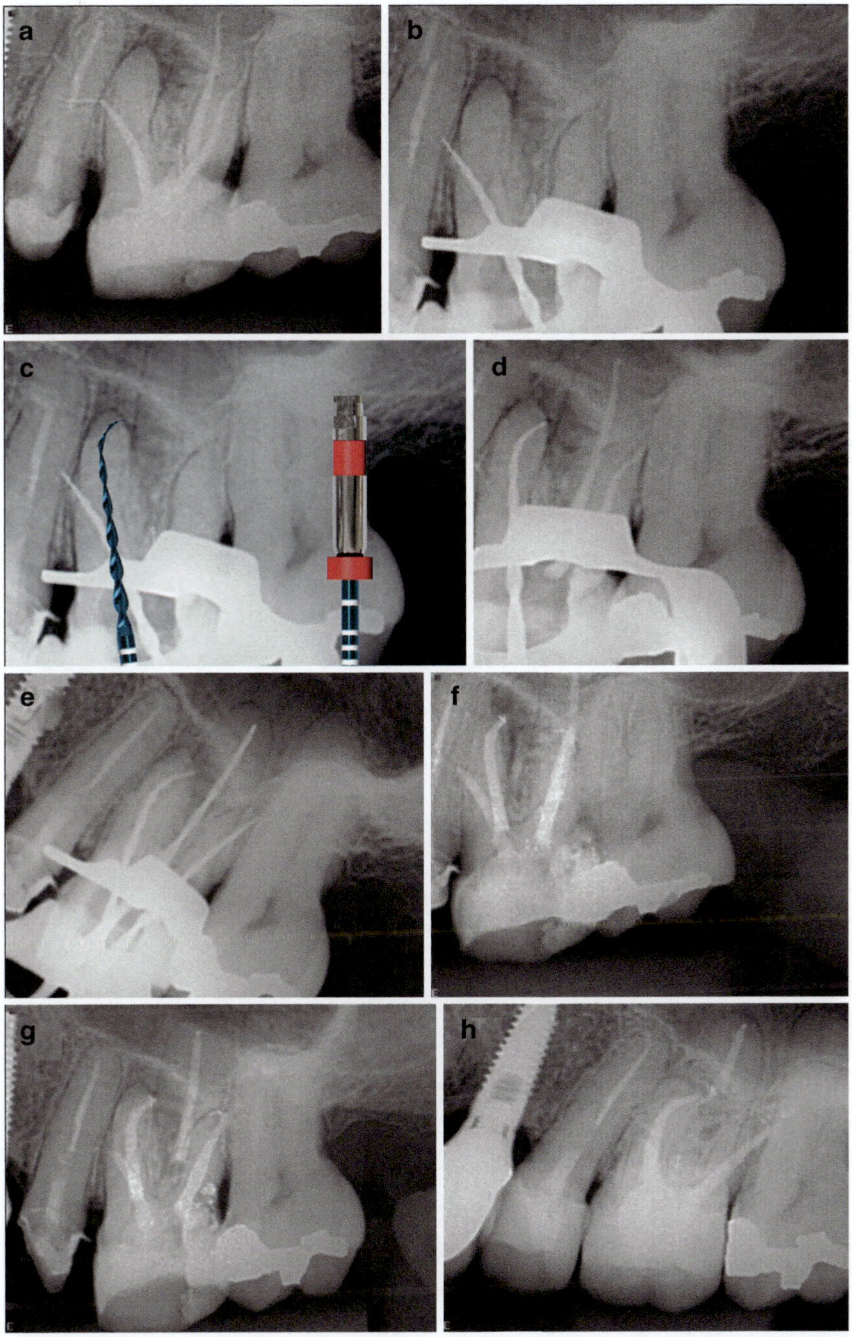

Fig. 4.15 (**a**, **b**) Radiographic images of a maxillary first left molar with root canal deviation and perforation at the middle third of the mesiobuccal root. (**c**, **d**) A pre-bent martensitic NiTi instrument was used to overcome the deviation and (**e**, **f**) further prepared the original canal path and sealed perforation with MTA HP Repair (Angelus, Brazil). (**g**, **h**) 6-month and 1-year radiographic follow-ups showing favorable treatment outcome. (Courtesy of Dr. Evaldo Rodrigues, Brazil)

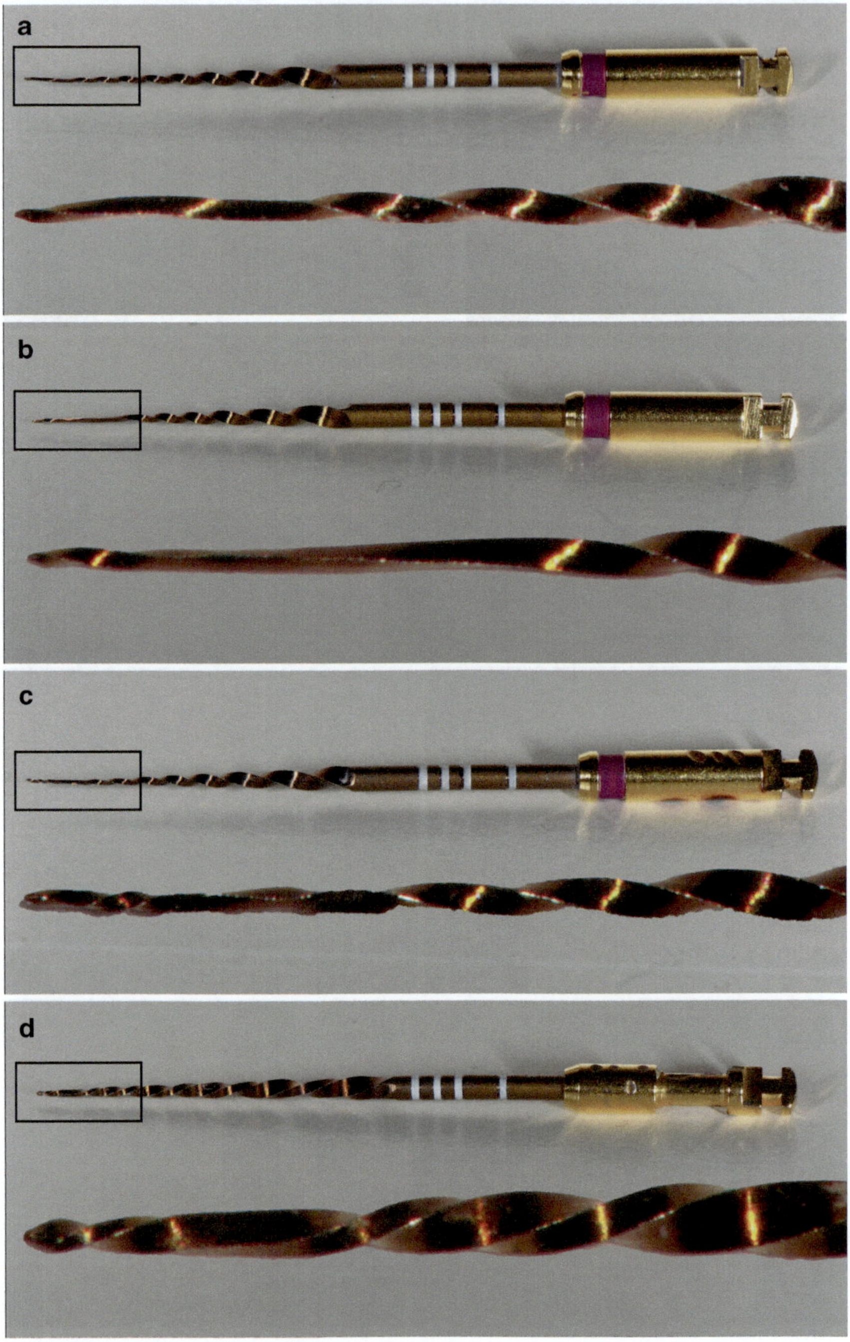

Fig. 4.16 Images showing deformation on the tip of the (**a–c**) ProTaper Gold and (**d**) WaveOne Gold martensitic instruments. The martensitic crystalline phase of NiTi alloy has a low transition temperature and requires less energy for deformation, so that plastic deformation and unwinding of these types of instruments can be observed more often. (Courtesy of Dr. Jorge Martins, Portugal)

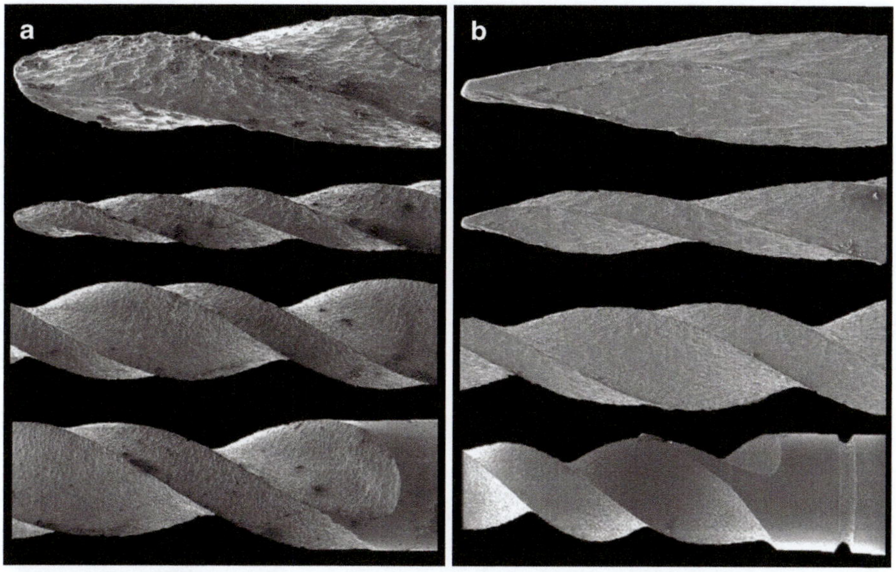

Fig. 4.17 Scanning electron microscopy of electrical discharge machining instruments. (**a**) NeoNiTi instruments (Neolix SAS, France). (**b**) HyFlex EDM instruments (Coltène/Whaledent, Switzerland)

and gold. In general, Blue heat-treated instruments show austenite formation at 38.5 °C, which is close to the body temperature. These instruments have large amounts of stabilized NiTi martensite crystalline phase compared to the M-Wire alloy, which makes them softer and more ductile. In gold-colored instruments, austenite is formed at temperatures close to 50 °C, which indicates that martensite and R-Phase are predominant during clinical use. Regarding the mechanical properties, both Blue and Gold heat-treated instruments have greater flexibility and resistance to fatigue than instruments made with M-Wire or conventional NiTi alloy. ProTaper Gold (Dentsply, Switzerland), WaveOne Gold (Dentsply, Switzerland) and Reciproc Blue (VDW, Germany) are examples of this type of instrument.

4.2.3 MaxWire

MaxWire alloy (Martensite-Austenite-electropolish-fileX), introduced by FKG Dentaire (Switzerland), allowed the development of the first endodontic instruments that combine shape memory effect and superelasticity properties for clinical application. Thermomechanical treatment of the alloy results in the presence of martensite at room temperature (static state), with M_i around 20 °C, and the austenitic phase during clinical use (dynamic state), where A_i is observed at 35 °C [2, 6, 8]. Hence, these instruments have the shape memory effect when inserted into the canal (martensite state to austenite state), while exhibit superelasticity during canal preparation. Studies on these instruments reported great resistance to cyclic fatigue and low resistance to torsion [36, 37] (Fig. 4.18).

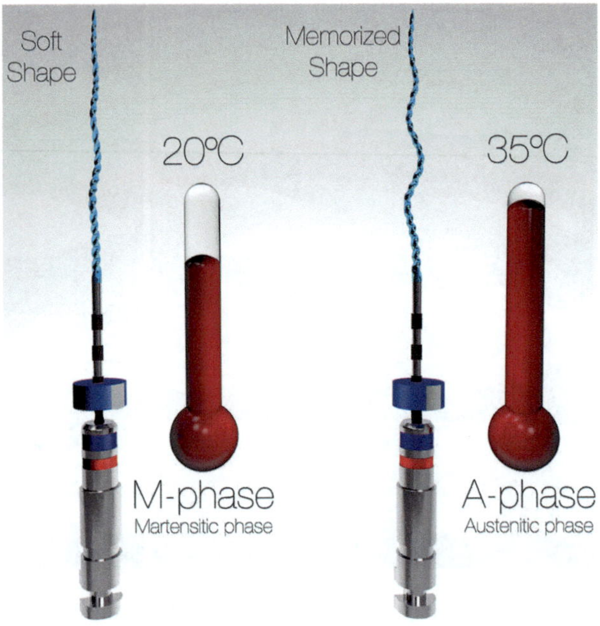

Fig. 4.18 XP-endo Shaper instrument (FKG, Switzerland). Thermomechanical treatment of the MaxWire alloy results in the presence of martensite at room temperature (static state), with M_i around 20 °C (on the left), and the austenitic phase during clinical use (dynamic state), where A_i is observed at 35 °C (on the right)

4.3 The Genealogical Tree of NiTi Systems

Root canal preparation instruments can be classified according to multiple criteria, such as introduction date, geometry (active part, cross-sectional design, tip, taper, helical angle, etc.), NiTi alloy, manufacturing process, and activation kinematics (Fig. 4.19). However, a more comprehensive classification divide the instruments into generations (Fig. 4.20), according to the evolution of their components and designs, as properly described by Haapasalo and Shen [3] (Table 4.1).

4.3.1 The Patriarchs (First Generation)

In 1990, John McSpadden and Ben Johnson developed the first nickel-titanium rotary instruments for the mechanized preparation of root canals. However, it was only in 1992, at the IFEA congress in Paris, that it has been officially launched on the market. This marked a new era in the preparation of root canals. The first generation of NiTi rotary instruments was characterized by instruments having passive cutting radial lands, constant taper, and a neutral or negative attack angle. The main deficiency of the systems in this generation was the number of instruments required to achieve the complete canal preparation, and the rather complex required protocols. A representative clinical study also demonstrated an elevated number of accidents and errors when using these instrument [49]. In that study, the type and frequency of defects of the NiTi Quantec Series 2000 were evaluated after routine

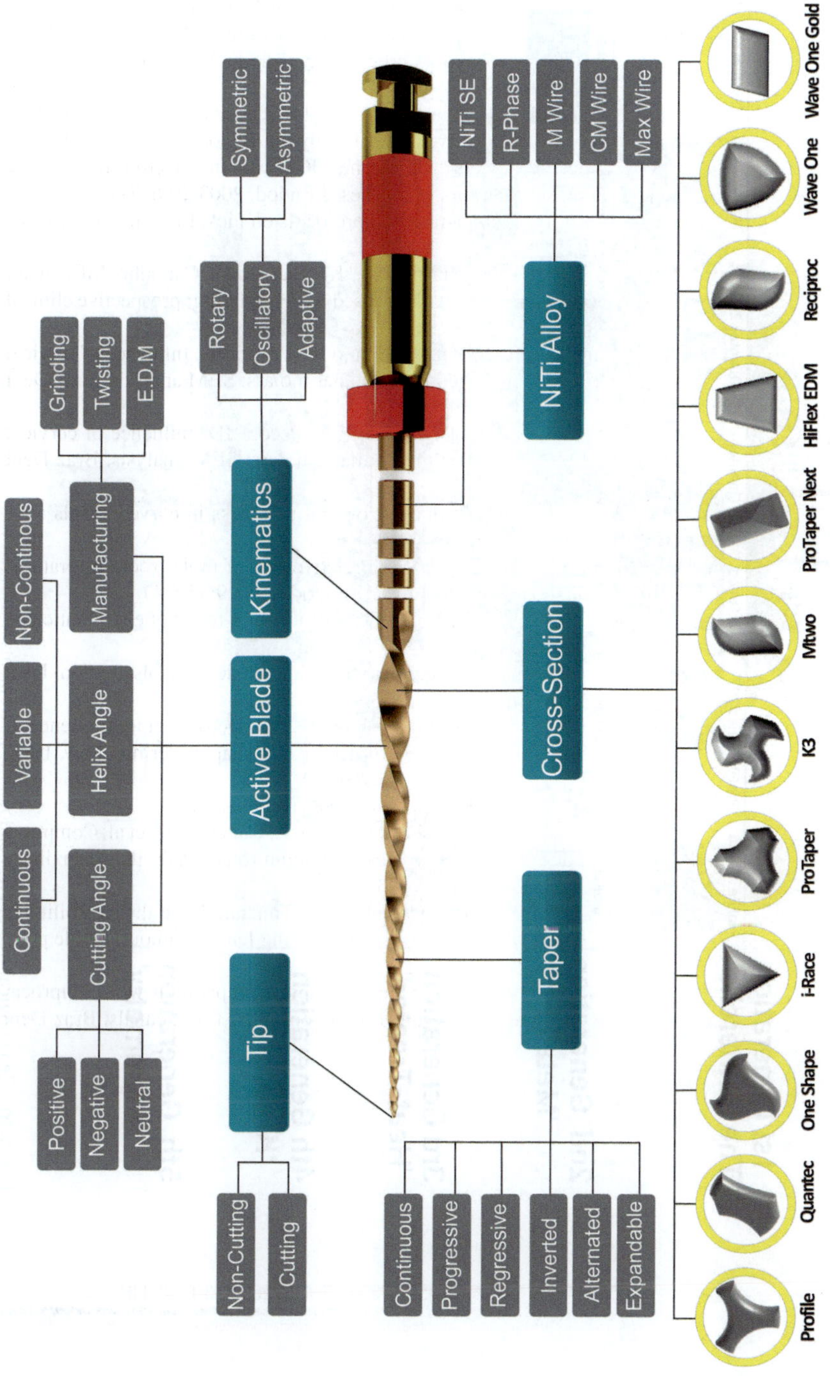

Fig. 4.19 Summary of the geometric and kinematic features of the most known NiTi rotary and reciprocating endodontic instruments

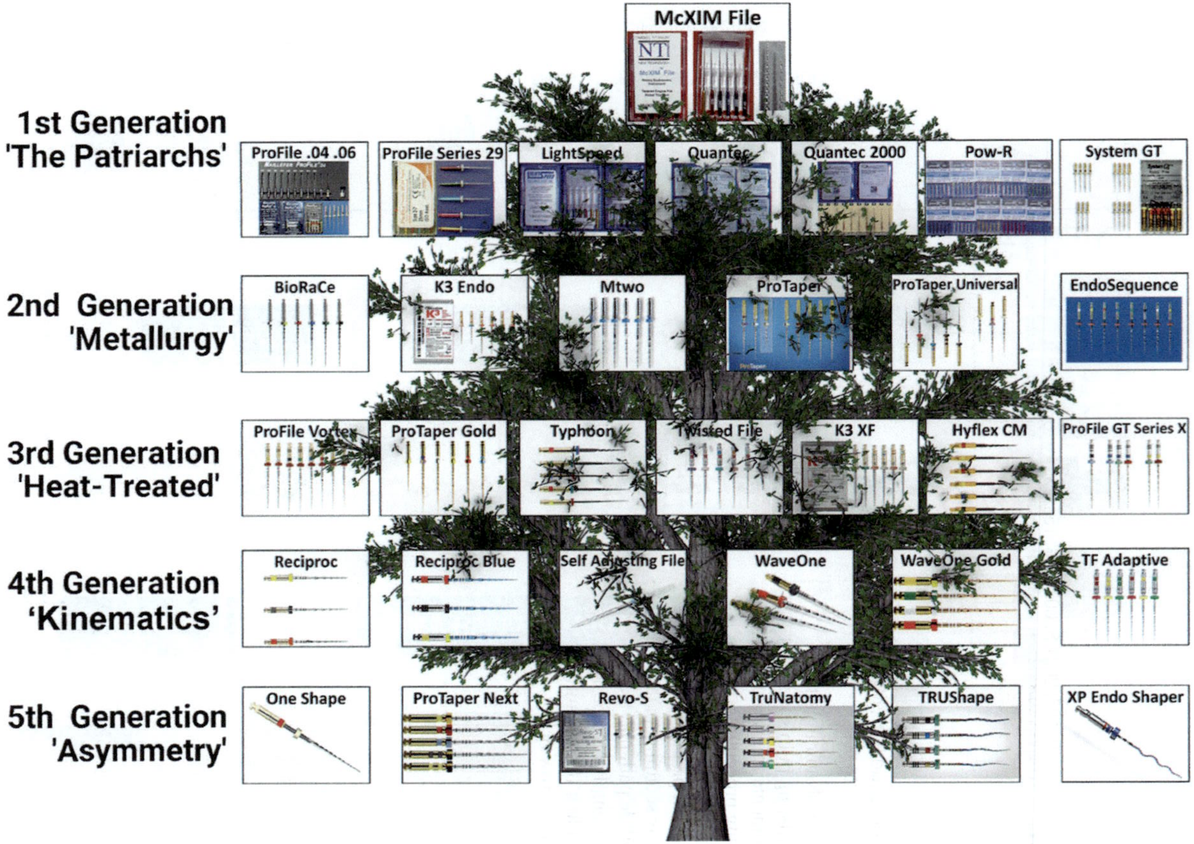

Fig. 4.20 Genealogical tree of NiTi endodontic instruments illustrated with some commercial systems launched in each generation

Table 4.1 Different generations of NiTi rotary and reciprocating instruments

Generation	Examples
First generation "The Patriarchs"	McXim File (NT Company) GT system (Dentsply) LightSpeed (LightSpeed Technology) Pow-R (Moyco) ProFile (Dentsply) ProFile Series 29 (Dentsply) Quantec (Tycom) Quantec 2000 (Tycom) Rapid Body Shaper (Moyco)
Second generation Improving metallurgical properties	BioRaCe (FKG) EndoSequence (Brasseler) K3 (Sybron) Mtwo (VDW) ProTaper Universal (Dentsply)
Third generation Heat treatment is good!	HyFlex CM (Coltène) K3XF (Sybron Endo) ProFile GT Series X (Dentsply) ProFile Vortex (Dentsply) ProFile Vortex Blue (Dentsply) ProTaper Gold (Dentsply) Twisted File (Sybron) Typhoon (Clinician's Choice)
Fourth generation No! Kinematic is better!	Reciproc (VDW) Reciproc Blue (VDW) WaveOne (Dentsply) WaveOne Gold (Dentsply) Twisted File Adaptive (Sybron Endo)
Fifth generation The asymmetrical revolution	OneShape (MicroMega) ProTaper Next (Dentsply) Revo-S (MicroMega) Rotary Files (VDW) TruNatomy (Dentsply) TruShape (Dentsply) XP-endo Shaper (FKG)

Adapted from Haapasalo and Shen [3]

clinical use. The results demonstrated that almost 50% of the instruments showed some visible defect. In fact, 21% of the instruments were fractured and 28% had defects without fracture. In another clinical study, Al-Fouzan [50] used ProFile instruments in 419 mandibular and maxillary molars and found 19 instruments with visible signs of plastic deformation (4.5% of the cases) and 21 fractured during treatment (5% of the cases). This high fracture rate, especially when compared to manual instrumentation, may be related to the quality of the manufacturing process of instruments of this first generation, along with the lack of knowledge of clinicians regarding the best ways to prevent accidents.

4.3.2 Improving Metallurgical Properties (Second Generation)

From the end of the 1990s, manufacturers were concerned in developing safer and more efficient instruments through the treatment of their metallic surface (electropolishing and ion implantation) along with changes in their helical angles, tapers and cutting edges. Instruments of this generation have active cutting edges with a great cutting efficiency, and most of them do not have radial lands. These improvements led to a smaller number of instruments required to achieve complete canal preparation.

Studies demonstrated the higher efficiency in the preparation of root canals and a lower fracture rate when compared to the previous generation [51–54]. Wolcott et al. [53] evaluated the separation incidence of the ProTaper Universal rotary system in 4,652 treated root canals and observed an overall fracture rate of 2.4% with no significant difference over the first four uses. Ehrhardt and colleagues [51] evaluated the incidence of separation of Mtwo instruments during the preparation of mandibular and maxillary molars and premolars with previous coronal preflaring, and showed a separation rate of 1.98%. Similar results were observed by Wu et al. [54], who demonstrated an overall instrument separation incidence of 2.6%. This almost ten-fold reduction of fracture rate compared to the first generation is certainly related to improvements in the quality of the manufacturing process, as well as a better understanding of influential factors responsible for instrument fracture, coupled with an increased knowledge of the proper way to use them. These results, however, are not supported by other studies in which the fracture rate was as high as those of the first generation [55, 56]. Inan et al. [55] evaluated 593 Mtwo rotary instruments after clinical use and demonstrated a fracture rate of 16.02% and that 25.8% had some type of deformation, mostly in instruments sizes 10/0.04 and 15/0.05. These results were in line with Ehrhardt et al. [51], who found that all fractures occurred on 10/0.04 (90.01%) and 15/0.05 (9.09%) instruments. Patiño et al. [56] also found a fracture rate of 26% when rotary NiTi instruments were used without previous glide path preparation, compared to 12% when glide path was performed.

It is clear that the improvements brought by advancements in the manufacturing process and mastery of operators of this second generation of rotary instruments had a positive impact on their performance. Nonetheless, fractures were still a major concern, and preliminary clinical procedures were recommended in order to avoid them, such as glide path and coronal preflaring, which proved to reduce fracture occurrence. When faced with complex anatomical features, instruments of this generation generally require careful inspection in order to identify any sustained distortions and, eventually, to be discarded. Furthermore, despite requiring a fewer number of instruments to complete the preparation procedures, compared to the previous generation, a considerable number are still required to ensure overall safety.

4.3.3 Heat Treatment Is the Pathway to Follow! (Third Generation)

This generation is characterized by the evolution of the metallurgy of the instruments, mainly regarding the heat treatment of the NiTi alloy and the manufacturing methods to improve its mechanical properties. Heat treatment is one of the fundamental approaches to adjust the crystalline transition phase of a metal alloy and, consequently, to improve its resistance to fatigue. In 2007, new thermomechanical procedures began to be used by the manufacturers of endodontic instruments, and each company developed and patented a different method. Following the implementation of these technologies, the instruments became safer, with a good performance in shaping ability, especially in the preparation of anatomical challenges such as curved root canals, while few clinical studies reported low fracture rates [6, 57]. The same precautions reported for the previous generations are also recommended to use these instruments in a clinical setup; however, most of these systems have a lower number of instruments to complete the canal shaping compared to previous generations.

4.3.4 No! Kinematic Is Better (Fourth Generation)

To the metallurgical improvements of the previous generation, a change in the kinematics was added, ranging from continuous rotary to asymmetric (reciprocating) oscillatory motion. The reciprocating motion relieves stress on the instrument by a special counterclockwise motion rotation to cut dentin and a short clockwise rotation to relieve the instrument. In comparison to continuous rotation, these movements extend the NiTi instrument lifespan by increasing its resistance to fatigue. Similar motion is provided by the Optimum Torque Reverse (OTR) function present in the dedicated TriAuto ZX2 cordless motor (J Morita, Japan). Under this motion, instruments are activated under continuous clockwise rotation when minimal load resistance is met. Once the given torque values for an instrument are exceeded (trigger torque), it automatically reverses rotation to the counterclockwise direction for 90° and switches back to the cutting direction for 180°; this cycle repeats itself until the torque becomes less than the set value. The reciprocating movement will be further address in Chap. 5.

4.3.5 The Asymmetrical Proposition (Fifth Generation)

This is the most recent group of NiTi instruments, which also show new metallographic treatments and major changes in the geometric configuration of the active blades, allowing eccentric or asymmetric rotation (the axis of rotation is off-center). The ProTaper Next system (Dentsply Sirona, USA), with its asymmetrical rectangular cross section, is an instrument in which the axis of rotation is off-centered. The TruNatomy system (Dentsply Sirona, USA) and the XP-endo Shaper (FKG,

Switzerland) are other systems with asymmetrical motion. The XP-endo Shaper instrument expands beyond the size of its core at temperatures equal to or greater than 35 °C (temperature-dependent morphology) due to a change in the crystalline phase of the alloy, as previously explained. Overall, instruments with an off-centered axis of rotation claim an improved shaping ability by promoting a greater contact between the surface of the instrument and the canal walls. However, most studies have failed to demonstrate a significant shaping improvement compared with conventional NiTi instruments [58, 59].

4.4 Clinical Recommendations for Safe Use

The safe use of a rotary NiTi instrument for root canal preparation must involve maximum benefits while minimizing the risk of accidents, especially those related to instrument fracture. Regarding the latter, nowadays there is a significant accumulated clinical and scientific knowledge about the physical events involved in that process. It is well known that instruments fracture due to cyclic fatigue, that is the repeated use of the instrument under flexion, and torsional failure, a result of the continuous screwing of an instrument in a narrow space within the root canal. Essentially, what happens during torsional failure is that the tip of the instrument gets locked within the root canal while the bulk continues to rotate until fracture occurs. During the penetration of a rotary instrument toward the apical canal, different forces are triggered and tend to increase as the it moves further. These forces result from a combination of the excessive contact of the instrument with the root canal walls and the continuous rotary motion. If the instrument locks within the canal walls and continues to rotate at high torque, it will inevitably reach its elastic resistance limit and the torsional fracture will occur. To avoid both types of fractures, some clinical procedures are recommended.

Firstly, it is important that prior to any clinical use of a new NiTi system, the professional accomplished an adequate laboratory training to get proficiency with that system. Thus, previous training in resin blocks and extracted teeth is mandatory. It is also important that clinicians know the design, the mechanical behavior, and the NiTi alloy of the instrument. Technically speaking, the only way to provide a minimal control of instrument fracture is to create a reliable and reproducible glide path, as well as, a proper coronal preflaring inasmuch as the instrument is naturally submitted to a low mechanical load. Nevertheless, coronal preflaring demands attention to avoid an exaggerated removal of dental structures, which might impact on the long-term outcome of the treatment by reducing the resistance strength of the teeth.

Another important recommendation is to use the manufacturers' settings in a dedicated torque-controlled motor. This approach keeps the instrument usually below its elastic limit, since changing it on its own might result in unexpected failure as the operator is often unaware of the required torque and rotation speed values for each endodontic instrument that may prevent its fracture. Thus, endodontic instruments must be used with the lowest possible rotation speed, as long as it does not hamper its cutting ability. Generally, manufacturers provide the recommended torque and speed values for each instrument, and adhering to their instructions is a good way to avoid complications. Regarding the proper number of uses, there is still no consensus and even the manufacturers and independent research fail to provide conclusive answers. Therefore, manufacturers recommend the single-use approach, given that fracture rate naturally increases with the reuse of instruments.

As a rule, rotary instruments should be used by applying gentle pressure, with in-and-out motions and short vertical amplitude movements (1–3 mm toward the apical direction) intercalated with complete withdraws from the canal. Greater advances of the instrument to the apical direction increase the contact area and resistance when cutting the dentinal walls, which may cause total or partial immobilization of its tip, inducing a load higher than its torsional fracture resistance limit. In addition, following every withdrawal, the instruments should be cleaned prior to reinsert them into the canal, as dentin scraps in the helical shaft may decrease the cutting efficiency and increase the chance of the instrument to be locked and fractured within the canal walls.

In curved canals, stay for as short a time as possible with the instrument rotating inside the curvature and also consider single use or at least early replacement. The usage time is cumulative, therefore the shorter the time the instrument rotates at the same position, the greater will be its fatigue life span. Thus, in curved canals, always keep the instrument in a constant forward and backward movements to the apical direction. This procedure aims to avoid the concentration of tensions in specific areas of the instrument.

4.5 Rotary NiTi Systems: "The MORE of the SAME" Phenomenon

Even after all the aforementioned developments, NiTi rotary instruments still present non-negligible limitations, which have always been a matter of concern for both clinicians and the scientific community. Their main limitations can be summarized as the unpredictable fracture rate, the difficulty in enlarging the canal space while progressing toward the apex, and the ability to mechanically debride the whole surface area of the canal walls. In other words, the efficiency of rotary systems demands a lot of work and energy to achieve their goal. An efficient instrument must have a high cutting ability to enlarge the canal space into its final taper-size with less time, torque and/or pressure. As McSpadden [60] highlighted so well: "*The less pressure, torque and time required, the more likely file failure can be prevented*". As a further drawback, the high cost of implementing their use on a daily clinical routine is still a relevant factor, especially when considering the single-use approach. The great complexity of most rotary systems (large instrument sequence and great variability of instruments' design) is also an important disadvantage that cannot be overlooked, as it directly impacts on the learning curve of techniques and protocols, as well as, on the clinical workflow.

Beyond these issues, over the last decade, the mechanical canal shaping has been marked by a further aspect that deserves our attention: the massive increase in the number of NiTi rotary systems. With a digital search, it is possible to realize that hundreds of rotary systems produced by several companies worldwide are currently available on the market. However, which would render a myriad of possibilities is indeed a rich substrate for reflection:

What's the problem of having hundreds of available NiTi rotary systems on the market?

The answer is neither easy nor straightforward. For a better understanding, it is necessary to unfold what stimulates the systematic launching of new NiTi rotary systems. The origin of such a phenomenon has a twofold basis: the overall limitations of the current technology for mechanical preparation of the root canal system, and the goal of providing dentists with more choices than ever by bringing endodontics into a fast-paced era of endless new products.

Actually, this scenario stands for what is usually called the "MORE of the SAME" phenomenon, which features a choice overload created by speed-rules advertisement-based environments. "MORE of the SAME" is a relatively well-known phenomenon typical of the capitalist narrative and, from one side, its origin is explained by (1) the popular wisdom that the more choices the people have, the better off they are; and (2) that getting good results is only possible when an array of choices is at hand. Moreover, the "MORE of the SAME" phenomenon is boosted by the fact that when people have no or very reduced possibilities of choice, life is almost unbearable [61]. However, the point is that some choices are good and beneficial, but these do not necessarily mean that an overload of choices is really better. Barry Schwartz [61], in his amazing book *The Paradox of Choice* was accurate: "In particular, increased choice among goods and services may contribute little or nothing to the kind of freedom that really counts. Indeed, it may impair freedom by taking time and energy we'd be better off devoting to other matters." In other words, there is an undeniable personal cost of having an overkill of choices. As the professional no longer knows what NiTi system they should invest their time, energy and money in, a critical and persistent problem is created by a no small amount of self-doubt and anxiety to find the best pathway [61]. In general, each new NiTi system raises the overall expectation that almost always leads to disappointment due to the lack of real innovation or advantages, which is demonstrated as time goes by.

The other side that inflames such scenario is based on the fact that it is easier to develop and launch "new innovative" products since the "MORE of the SAME" almost always comprise three aspects:

1. None or little real innovation;
2. Easy penetration by marketing and advertising methods;
3. None or poor scientific background.

It is worth mentioning that the easy penetration into the market is promoted by an industry of skilled marketers and advertisers who make the new products difficult or even impossible to ignore, as well as, our natural tendency to look around at what others are doing and mistakenly use them as reference for comparison.

At a glance, it seems that, by creating a huge array of options for canal shaping, manufacturers undoubtedly did a favor to dentists by offering rotary NiTi systems with instruments in several sizes, tapers, alloy types, and sequences. With regard to the latter, in general, NiTi system protocols are often complex, requiring several instruments and procedural stages, which unsurprisingly lead to a steep learning curve until achieving shaping competence with the need of considerable chairside time. Taken together, these factors are components that favor poor results and the habitual occurrence of inadequacy or iatrogeny. Besides, these different possibilities of shaping forge an apparently scientific approach based on the idea that "there is a suitable instrument for every root canal anatomy." However, within the "MORE of the SAME" scenario, overall, the rotary NiTi systems have not only similar advantages, but also limitations. Peters et al. [62] described the beginning of this scenario as early as 2010: "Similarly to the development of composite resins in restorative dentistry, the development of new files is a fast and market-driven process. With new instruments becoming available, the clinician may find it difficult to pick the file and technique most suitable for an individual case." As a consequence of the increased number of choices, another critical question emerges:

How can we trust in a recently launched NiTi rotary system?

This question is valid once almost all new systems are launched basically without any scientific evidence. When independent studies start to build up a body of evidence after 2 to 4 years, most of the time the system is unsurprisingly withdrawn from the market, or has already been replaced by an "updated" and "better" version of itself. Actually, the entire "MORE of the SAME" strategy depends on short life cycles in which the products are removed from the market before they are improved and their lack of innovation is called out by independent studies. Thus, the mainstream created by this new short-life market cycle clearly has significant critical aspects to be considered by the clinician with each new rotary NiTi system launched on the market:

- What is the instrument's fracture rate?
- Does its shaping ability outperform my current system?
- Is the new system able to improve my final results in difficult cases?
- Does it carry real technological innovations to justify the price?
- Does the new system show better handling properties to make my daily workflow easier?

Ideally, in the framework of a biomedical area like endodontics, scientific evidence should be the right tool to help narrow the choices and thus facilitate the decision-making process for the clinicians. Moreover, in the search for reliable information, dentists would have to go beyond advertisements and look toward disinterested unbiased sources, such as certified consumer reports and sound scientific evidence, but unfortunately most give substantial weight to anecdotal evidence, the inventor's name and, more than anything else, information that comes easily from advertising. As a general and current rule, dentists are getting more and more recommendations and "education" from salespeople, internet tools, and social media. In fact, it is virtually impossible to provide a scientific basis for new systems since the fast-pace in which they are developed and launched is much greater than the articulation capacity of international research groups committed to test them. Overall, it is fair to say that the "MORE of the SAME" mainstream distorts the evidence-based decision-making process by the chronic lack of scientific background and also by offering easy advertising routes to information. In summary, all that remains to guide the endodontist in the decision is his/her personal critical thinking ability plus clinical experience.

In brief, the "MORE of the SAME" phenomenon has become a major problem as it does not contribute to raise the bar in endodontics as a specialty of the biomedical field. Thus, there is a clear necessity to move the endodontic community to pressure the manufacturers toward a more scientific-based narrative, not only to provide products that incorporate real innovations, but also to offer independent and unbiased scientific evidence to support their use.

References

1. Buchanan S. New additions to the NiTi rotary file market: What to bring in and what to leave out. Dental Tribune U.S. Edition. 2011;6:19–20.
2. Gavini G, Santos MD, Caldeira CL, Machado MEL, Freire LG, Iglecias EF, et al. Nickel-titanium instruments in endodontics: a concise review of the state of the art. Braz Oral Res. 2018;32:e67.
3. Haapasalo M, Shen Y. Evolution of nickel-titanium instruments: from past to future. Endod Topics. 2013;29:3–17.
4. Peters OA. Current challenges and concepts in the preparation of root canal systems: a review. J Endod. 2004;30:559–67.
5. Shen Y, Coil JM, Zhou H, Zheng Y, Haapasalo M. HyFlex nickel-titanium rotary instruments after clinical use: metallurgical properties. Int Endod J. 2013;46:720–9.
6. Shen Y, Zhou HM, Zheng YF, Peng B, Haapasalo M. Current challenges and concepts of the thermomechanical treatment of nickel-titanium instruments. J Endod. 2013;39:163–72.
7. Zhou H, Peng B, Zheng YF. An overview of the mechanical properties of nickel-titanium endodontic instruments. Endod Topics. 2013;29:42–54.
8. Zupanc J, Vahdat-Pajouh N, Schafer E. New thermomechanically treated NiTi alloys—a review. Int Endod J. 2018;51:1088–103.
9. Sousa-Neto MD, Silva-Sousa YC, Mazzi-Chaves JF, Carvalho KKT, Barbosa AFS, Versiani MA, et al. Root canal preparation using micro-computed tomography analysis: a literature review. Braz Oral Res. 2018;32:e66.
10. Del Fabbro M, Afrashtehfar KI, Corbella S, El-Kabbaney A, Perondi I, Taschieri S. In vivo and in vitro effectiveness of rotary nickel-titanium vs manual stainless steel instruments for root canal therapy: systematic review and meta-analysis. J Evid Based Dent Pract. 2018;18:59–69.
11. Buehler W, Gilfrich J, Wiley RC. Effects of low-temperature phase changes on the mechanical properties of alloys near composition TiNi. Int J Appl Phys. 1963;34:1475–7.

12. Andreasen GF, Morrow RE. Laboratory and clinical analyses of nitinol wire. Am J Orthod. 1978;73:142–51.
13. Civjan S, Huget EF, DeSimon LB. Potential applications of certain nickel-titanium (nitinol) alloys. J Dent Res. 1975;54:89–96.
14. Walia HM, Brantley WA, Gerstein H. An initial investigation of the bending and torsional properties of nitinol root canal files. J Endod. 1988;14:346–51.
15. Lopes HP, Gambarra-Soares T, Elias CN, Siqueira JF Jr, Inojosa IF, Lopes WS, et al. Comparison of the mechanical properties of rotary instruments made of conventional nickel-titanium wire, M-wire, or nickel-titanium alloy in R-phase. J Endod. 2013;39:516–20.
16. Ōtsuka K, Wayman CM. Shape memory materials. Cambridge: Cambridge University Press; 1998.
17. Otsuka K, Ren X. Physical metallurgy of Ti-Ni based shape memory alloys. Prog Mater Sci. 2005;50:511–678.
18. Thompson SA. An overview of nickel-titanium alloys used in dentistry. Int Endod J. 2000;33:297–310.
19. Anderson M, Price J, Parashos P. Fracture resistance of electropolished rotary nickel–titanium endodontic instruments. J Endod. 2007;33:1212–6.
20. Lopes HP, Elias CN, Vieira MV, Vieira VT, de Souza LC, Dos Santos AL. Influence of surface roughness on the fatigue life of nickel-titanium rotary endodontic instruments. J Endod. 2016;42:965–8.
21. Lopes HP, Elias CN, Vieira VT, Moreira EJ, Marques RV, de Oliveira JC, et al. Effects of electropolishing surface treatment on the cyclic fatigue resistance of BioRace nickel-titanium rotary instruments. J Endod. 2010;36:1653–7.
22. Bui TB, Mitchell JC, Baumgartner JC. Effect of electropolishing ProFile nickel-titanium rotary instruments on cyclic fatigue resistance, torsional resistance, and cutting efficiency. J Endod. 2008;34:190–3.
23. Praisarnti C, Chang JW, Cheung GS. Electropolishing enhances the resistance of nickel-titanium rotary files to corrosion-fatigue failure in hypochlorite. J Endod. 2010;36:1354–7.
24. Shen Y, Winestock E, Cheung GS, Haapasalo M. Defects in nickel-titanium instruments after clinical use. Part 4: an electropolished instrument. J Endod. 2009;35:197–201.
25. Arias A, Perez-Higueras JJ, de la Macorra JC. Influence of clinical usage of GT and GTX files on cyclic fatigue resistance. Int Endod J. 2014;47:257–63.
26. Çapar ID, Kaval ME, Ertas H, Sen BH. Comparison of the cyclic fatigue resistance of 5 different rotary pathfinding instruments made of conventional nickel-titanium wire, M-wire, and controlled memory wire. J Endod. 2015;41:535–8.
27. Alapati SB, Brantley WA, Iijima M, Clark WA, Kovarik L, Buie C, et al. Metallurgical characterization of a new nickel-titanium wire for rotary endodontic instruments. J Endod. 2009;35:1589–93.
28. Ye J, Gao Y. Metallurgical characterization of M-wire nickel-titanium shape memory alloy used for endodontic rotary instruments during low-cycle fatigue. J Endod. 2012;38:105–7.
29. Pirani C, Paolucci A, Ruggeri O, Bossu M, Polimeni A, Gatto MR, et al. Wear and metallographic analysis of WaveOne and Reciproc NiTi instruments before and after three uses in root canals. Scanning. 2014;36:517–25.
30. Perez-Higueras JJ, Arias A, de la Macorra JC. Cyclic fatigue resistance of K3, K3XF, and twisted file nickel-titanium files under continuous rotation or reciprocating motion. J Endod. 2013;39:1585–8.
31. Braga LC, Faria Silva AC, Buono VT, de Azevedo Bahia MG. Impact of heat treatments on the fatigue resistance of different rotary nickel-titanium instruments. J Endod. 2014;40:1494–7.
32. De-Deus G, Silva EJ, Vieira VT, Belladonna FG, Elias CN, Plotino G, et al. Blue thermomechanical treatment optimizes fatigue resistance and flexibility of the Reciproc files. J Endod. 2017;43:462–6.
33. Plotino G, Testarelli L, Al-Sudani D, Pongione G, Grande NM, Gambarini G. Fatigue resistance of rotary instruments manufactured using different nickel-titanium alloys: a comparative study. Odontology. 2014;102:31–5.

34. Silva E, Vieira VTL, Belladonna FG, Zuolo AS, Antunes HDS, Cavalcante DM, et al. Cyclic and torsional fatigue resistance of XP-endo Shaper and TRUShape instruments. J Endod. 2018;44:168–72.
35. Silva EJNL, Giraldes JFN, de Lima CO, Vieira VTL, Elias CN, Antunes HS. Influence of heat treatment on torsional resistance and surface roughness of nickel-titanium instruments. Int Endod J. 2019;52:1645–51.
36. Silva EJNL, Hecksher F, Antunes HDS, De-Deus G, Elias CN, Vieira VTL. Torsional fatigue resistance of blue-treated reciprocating instruments. J Endod. 2018;44:1038–41.
37. Silva EJNL, Vieira VTL, Hecksher F, Dos Santos Oliveira MRS, Dos Santos Antunes H, Moreira EJL. Cyclic fatigue using severely curved canals and torsional resistance of thermally treated reciprocating instruments. Clin Oral Investig. 2018;22:2633–8.
38. Arslan H, Yildiz ED, Gunduz HA, Sumbullu M, Bayrakdar IS, Karatas E, et al. Comparative study of ProTaper Gold, Reciproc, and ProTaper Universal for root canal preparation in severely curved root canals. J Conserv Dent. 2017;20:222–4.
39. Bürklein S, Hinschitza K, Dammaschke T, Schäfer E. Shaping ability and cleaning effectiveness of two single-file systems in severely curved root canals of extracted teeth: Reciproc and WaveOne versus Mtwo and ProTaper. Int Endod J. 2012;45:449–61.
40. Plotino G, Ahmed HM, Grande NM, Cohen S, Bukiet F. Current assessment of reciprocation in endodontic preparation: a comprehensive review—part II: properties and effectiveness. J Endod. 2015;41:1939–50.
41. Duque JA, Vivan RR, Cavenago BC, Amoroso-Silva PA, Bernardes RA, Vasconcelos BC, et al. Influence of NiTi alloy on the root canal shaping capabilities of the ProTaper Universal and ProTaper Gold rotary instrument systems. J Appl Oral Sci. 2017;25:27–33.
42. Bürklein S, Flüch S, Schäfer E. Shaping ability of reciprocating single-file systems in severely curved canals: WaveOne and Reciproc versus WaveOne Gold and Reciproc blue. Odontology. 2019;107:96–102.
43. Belladonna FG, Carvalho MS, Cavalcante DM, Fernandes JT, de Carvalho Maciel AC, Oliveira HE, et al. Micro-computed tomography shaping ability assessment of the new blue thermal treated reciproc instrument. J Endod. 2018;44:1146–50.
44. Pedullá E, Lo Savio F, Boninelli S, Plotino G, Grande NM, La Rosa G, et al. Torsional and cyclic fatigue resistance of a new nickel-titanium instrument manufactured by electrical discharge machining. J Endod. 2016;42:156–9.
45. Pirani C, Iacono F, Generali L, Sassatelli P, Nucci C, Lusvarghi L, et al. HyFlex EDM: superficial features, metallurgical analysis and fatigue resistance of innovative electro discharge machined NiTi rotary instruments. Int Endod J. 2016;49:483–93.
46. Gündoğar M, Özyürek T. Cyclic fatigue resistance of OneShape, HyFlex EDM, WaveOne Gold, and Reciproc Blue nickel-titanium instruments. J Endod. 2017;43:1192–6.
47. Nabavizadeh MR, Sedigh-Shams M, Abdolrasoulnia S. Cyclic fatigue life of two single file engine-driven systems in simulated curved canals. Iran Endod J. 2018;13:61–5.
48. Rubio J, Zarzosa JI, Pallares A. A comparative study of cyclic fatigue of 10 different types of endodontic instruments: an in vitro study. Acta Stomatol Croat. 2019;53:28–36.
49. Sattapan B, Nervo GJ, Palamara JE, Messer HH. Defects in rotary nickel-titanium files after clinical use. J Endod. 2000;26:161–5.
50. Al-Fouzan KS. Incidence of rotary ProFile instrument fracture and the potential for bypassing in vivo. Int Endod J. 2003;36:864–7.
51. Ehrhardt IC, Zuolo ML, Cunha RS, De Martin AS, Kherlakian D, Carvalho MC, et al. Assessment of the separation incidence of mtwo files used with preflaring: prospective clinical study. J Endod. 2012;38:1078–81.
52. Wang NN, Ge JY, Xie SJ, Chen G, Zhu M. Analysis of Mtwo rotary instrument separation during endodontic therapy: a retrospective clinical study. Cell Biochem Biophys. 2014;70:1091–5.
53. Wolcott S, Wolcott J, Ishley D, Kennedy W, Johnson S, Minnich S, et al. Separation incidence of protaper rotary instruments: a large cohort clinical evaluation. J Endod. 2006;32:1139–41.
54. Wu J, Lei G, Yan M, Yu Y, Yu J, Zhang G. Instrument separation analysis of multi-used ProTaper Universal rotary system during root canal therapy. J Endod. 2011;37:758–63.

55. Inan U, Gonulol N. Deformation and fracture of Mtwo rotary nickel-titanium instruments after clinical use. J Endod. 2009;35:1396–9.
56. Patiño PV, Biedma BM, Liebana CR, Cantatore G, Bahillo JG. The influence of a manual glide path on the separation rate of NiTi rotary instruments. J Endod. 2005;31:114–6.
57. Gambarini G, Piasecki L, Di Nardo D, Miccoli G, Di Giorgio G, Carneiro E, et al. Incidence of deformation and fracture of twisted file adaptive instruments after repeated clinical use. J Oral Maxillofac Res. 2016;7:e5.
58. Lacerda M, Marceliano-Alves MF, Perez AR, Provenzano JC, Neves MAS, Pires FR, et al. Cleaning and shaping oval canals with 3 instrumentation systems: a correlative micro-computed tomographic and histologic study. J Endod. 2017;43:1878–84.
59. Versiani MA, Carvalho KKT, Mazzi-Chaves JF, Sousa-Neto MD. Micro-computed tomographic evaluation of the shaping ability of XP-endo Shaper, iRaCe, and EdgeFile systems in long oval-shaped canals. J Endod. 2018;44:489–95.
60. McSpadden JT. Mastering endodontic instrumentation. Ramsey: Arbor Books, Inc.; 2007.
61. Schwartz B. The paradox of choice: why more is less. 1st ed. New York: Ecco; 2004.
62. Peters OA, Paqué F. Current developments in rotary root canal instrument technology and clinical use: a review. Quintessence International. 2010;41:479–88.

Reciprocating Movement: Mastering the Mechanical Preparation

5

Gustavo De Deus, Emmanuel J. N. L. Silva, Erick Souza, Marco A. Versiani, Ghassan Yared, Hans-Willi Herrmann, and Mario Zuolo

5.1 Reciprocating Steel Instruments: The First Beginning!

Automated mechanical preparation of the root canals was an early clinician's desire at the beginning of the twentieth century, when pioneers tried to develop mechanical instruments [1]. Over the years, several different mechanized root canal preparation systems were launched in the market. The first commercially available endodontic motor introduced in 1925 and named Endocursor (W&H, Burmoos, Austria) allowed the use of conventional K or Reamer stainless-steel (SS) files with a complete 360° rotating motion combined with vertical strokes [1]. The main problem with SS instruments is their intrinsic stiffness that does not allow them to be

G. De Deus (✉)
Fluminense Federal University, Niterói, Brazil
e-mail: endogus@gmail.com

E. J. N. L. Silva
Fluminense Federal University, Grande Rio University, Rio de Janeiro State University, Niterói, Brazil

E. Souza
Federal University of Maranhão, São Luis, Brazil

M. A. Versiani
Dental Specialty Center, Brazilian Military Police, Minas Gerais, Brazil

G. Yared
Private Practice, Beirut, Lebanon

H.-W. Herrmann
Private Practice Limited to Endodontics, Bad Kreuznach, Germany

M. Zuolo
Dental School of APCD – FAOA, São Paulo, Brazil

G. De Deus et al. (eds.), *Shaping for Cleaning the Root Canals*,
https://doi.org/10.1007/978-3-030-84617-6_5

continuously rotated up to the working length without procedural errors [2, 3]. In fact, continuous rotation associated with SS instruments could never be safely implemented and, for this reason, reciprocating kinematics using equal angles in both directions was further successfully introduced. This type of symmetric reciprocation, also termed complete oscillating reciprocation (Figs. 5.1a, b and 5.2), resembles the classic watch-winding movement using manual SS files [4].

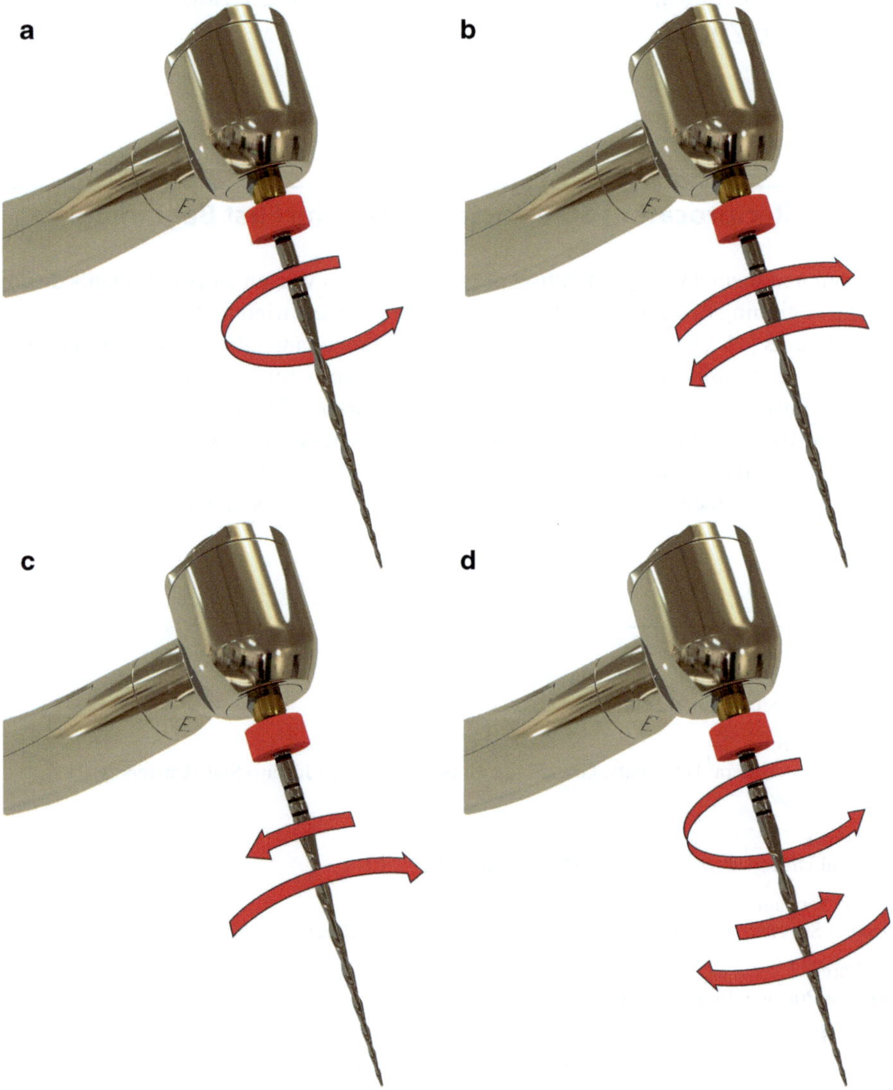

Fig. 5.1 Representation of different activation movements of NiTi instruments for root canal preparation. (**a**) Rotary movement. (**b**) Symmetric reciprocation. (**c**) Asymmetric reciprocation. (**d**) Combined movement—rotary and asymmetric reciprocation

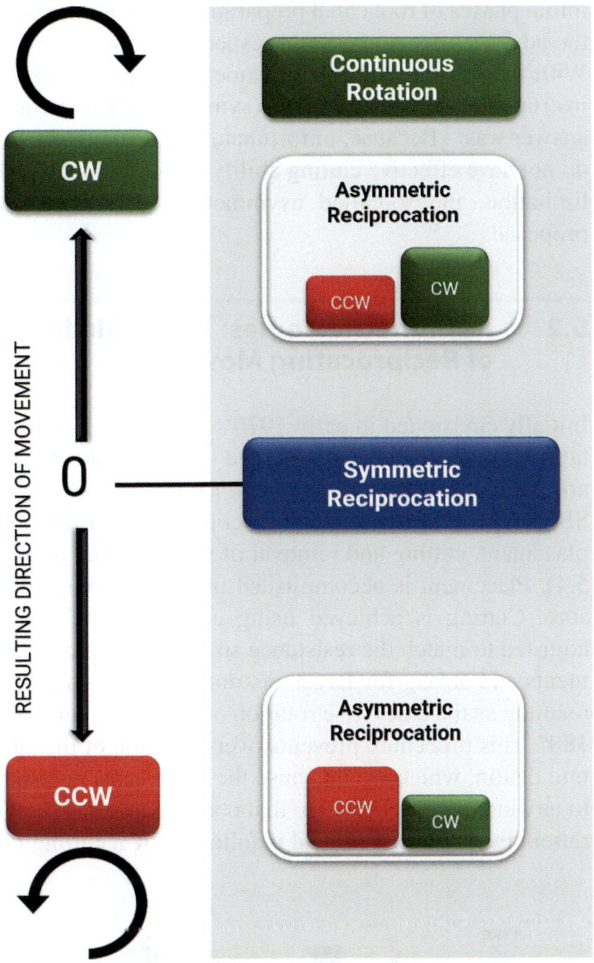

Fig. 5.2 Representative chart of different activation movements of NiTi instruments. The resulting direction of the movement can be clockwise (CW) or counterclockwise (CCW). Symmetric reciprocation, also termed as complete oscillating reciprocation, refers to identical CW and CCW angulations. Asymmetric reciprocation uses different CW and CCW angulations. In such a way, a rotational effect is observed after some cycles of this unequal reciprocation movement. Endodontic motors nowadays can perform continuous rotation movement, but also symmetric and/or asymmetric reciprocating movements. (Adapted from Gambarini et al. [4])

In the 1960s, different reciprocating handpieces were manufactured including the *Giromatic* (MicroMega, France), designed to reciprocate at 90°, and similar handpieces such as the *Intra-Endo 3 LD* (KaVo, Germany), which works with an alternating 80° rotational movement, and *Dynatrak* (Dentsply-DeTrey, Germany). Usually, these motors work at higher speeds (between 3,000 and 6,000 oscilations/min) for greater efficiency. In the last decades, other handpieces for use with SS manual files in reciprocating motion were launched for root canal preparation, including the *M4 Safety Handpiece* (30°) (SybronEndo/Kerr, USA), the *Endo-Gripper* (45°) (Moyco/Union Broach, USA) and the *NSKTEP-E10R* (90°) (Nakanishi Inc., Japan). Although there are several dedicated symmetric reciprocating handpieces on the market, the overall results regarding their shaping ability are similar to those for conventional preparation with manual files [5, 6]; however, a higher incidence of iatrogenic errors was observed [7–11], limiting their use to the initial phases of root canal preparation such as the glide path procedure, to minimize the adverse effects of SS files especially when using larger and stiffer instruments. With the advent of NiTi instruments, a question has arisen: "Why not use NiTi instruments in an oscillatory (symmetrical) movement to improve safety?". The answer was: "Because, unfortunately, in symmetrical movement, these instruments do not have effective cutting ability to properly shape the root canal." In face of this limitation, the so-called asymmetric oscilating movement (reciprocating) was proposed.

5.2 Asymmetric Angles: The Rebirth of Reciprocating Movement

Initially envisioned in early 1970's and after 12 years of trial-and-error experimentation, Roane et al. [12] published one of the most creative and important scientific articles regarding a new approach for the preparation of curved canals with manual SS files: the "balanced force" concept in which instrumentation is refined into placement, cutting and removal of the file using only rotary motions (Figs. 5.3 and 5.4). Placement is accomplished using clockwise rotation and light, inward pressure. Cutting is achieved using counterclockwise rotation and inward pressure adjusted to match the resistance strength of the file, i.e., very light for small instruments and strong for larger instruments. The balanced force concept is similar to reaming as the clockwise rotation of the instrument must be limited to no more than 180°. This procedure prevents over-insertion of the apical portion of the instrument into dentin, which would cause the tip to cease turning and allow the rotating force to unwind the file coronal to that point, increasing the likelihood of instrument separation. Each placement load is followed by a cutting motion with counterclockwise

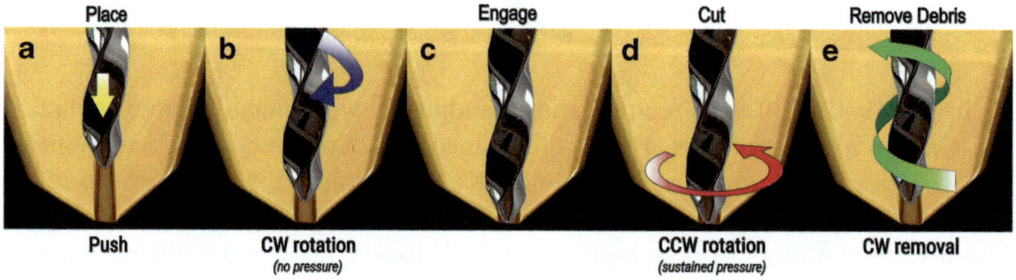

Fig. 5.3 Balanced Force Technique (**a**) Pressureless insertion of the instrument into the root canal space. (**b**) Rotate the file in a 90° clockwise direction by applying light apical pressure, which seats the file with a slight screwing-in motion. (**c**) Engage the file in the dentinal canal walls. (**d**) Turn the file in between 180° and 270° counterclockwise (depending on its cross-section) as it is held in place with enough inward pressure (sustained pressure). At this moment, the shear strength of the dentin is exceeded and a "stripping" action occurs when it is common to hear a slight "click" sound. (**e**) Turn the file completely in the clockwise direction to load the debris into its flutes and withdraw it from the root canal space. (Adapted from Pierre Machtou; unpublished personal communication)

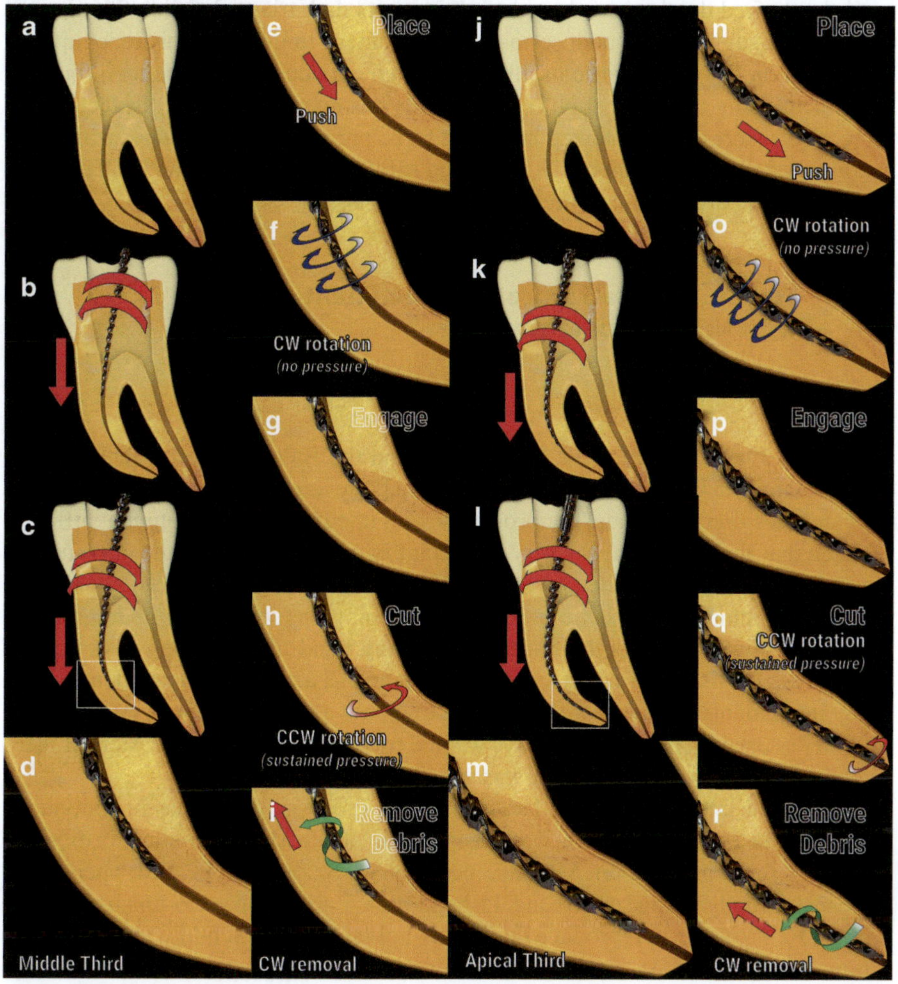

Fig. 5.4 In 1985, Roane et al. [12] advocated an original preparation method for curved root canals which allowed the same quality of the enlarging procedure obtained for straight canals, while avoiding ledge formation, transportation of the foramen or perforation, the so-called Balanced Force Technique. This schematic illustration shows the step-by-step use of this technique to enlarge the middle (**a**–**i**) and the apical (**j**–**r**) thirds of a curved mesial canal of a mandibular molar. Briefly, the hand file must be inserted into the root canal without pressure (**a**–**d**, **j**–**m**). Then, rotate it 90° in a clockwise direction by applying light pressure until it engages the canal walls (**e**–**g**, **n**–**p**). The file must be then rotated 180–270° counterclockwise at the same position with enough inward pressure (**h**, **q**) and, finally, removed from the canal space by turning it fully clockwise to remove debris (**i**, **r**)

rotation of 120° or greater (depending on the cross-sectional shape of the instrument) in order to finish the canal enlargement to the file's dimensions, free the instrument and allow its deeper placement when the next clockwise rotation is applied. Clockwise placement and counterclockwise cutting rotations are repeated until the desired depth or working length is reached. A triangular file with a modified tip was suggested as a close-to-ideal instrument to use with this technique. It was based on this asymmetric oscillatory movement concept that the reciprocating movement using mechanical NiTi instruments has arisen (Fig. 5.1c).In fact, it can be read as a sort of automatized balanced force pressureless technique, which is a rationale often used to support its increased safety, performance, and shorter learning curve compared to rotary preparation (Fig. 5.2).

5.2.1 The Story of Reciprocating Movement with NiTi Instruments

Ghassan Yared

It all started with the article of James Roane on the Balanced Force Technique in 1985. Roane showed that it was possible to shape severely curved canals with large SS hand files used in manual reciprocation with unequal angles. From that article, I realized that reciprocation was very important in order to maintain the curvature of a canal. That was toward the end of the 1980s. I kept this crucial information in the back of my mind. At the same time, I was teaching endodontics to undergraduate students; I always noticed their struggle in using hand files to shape a root canal. They struggled like I did when I was a student and as a newly graduate dentist. Too many instruments and steps were required to obtain a tapered shape. I was teaching Schilder's serial preparation. I always wanted to make the procedure easier for them (and myself) but I could not. That was my other ongoing struggle.

Toward the end of the 1990s, I started testing ProTaper prototypes in continuous rotation. The ProTaper system was designed to obtain shapes similar to those of Schilder's serial preparation. My sequence was S1, S2, F1, and F2 after opening up the canal initially with sizes 10 and 15 hand files. I always liked to finish my cases with an F2 ProTaper to reproduce the results I obtained with Schilder's serial preparation. At the same time, my research was focused on endodontic motors. ATR Italy, a manufacturer of dental motors, sent me an endodontic motor, the ATR (Automatic Torque Reduction) Tecnika (ATR, Italy), to test for continuous rotation. I noticed that the motor had a reciprocating feature (Figs. 5.5 and 5.6). The light bulb in the back of my brain lit up instantly: I had the concept of Roane, a motor that works in reciprocation and rotary NiTi instruments with a good cutting ability. I thought if Roane was able to prepare severely curved canals with large and rigid SS hand files used in manual reciprocation, I should be able to obtain even better results with engine-driven flexible NiTi instruments. I did a few tests with the ProTaper prototypes in curved canals in resin blocks. The instruments were used with the reciprocation feature of the ATR motor in the same sequence as described above. I changed the reciprocation parameters a few times and then I discovered that these instruments worked well in reciprocation with unequal angles to prepare the artificial canals. I was very excited. With the end in mind, i.e., an F2 ProTaper instrument at length, I tried to use this instrument alone for the canal preparation. After many trials and errors, the

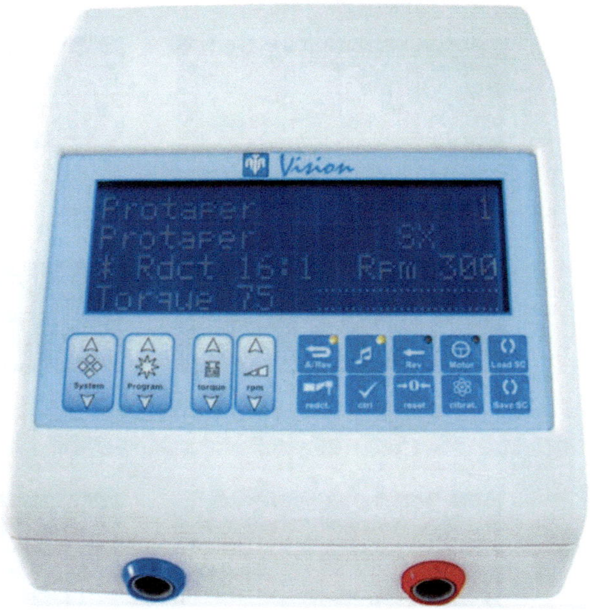

Fig. 5.5 ATR (Automatic Torque Reduction) Tecnika electric motor (ATR, Italy) adjusted for reciprocating motion with ProTaper F2 instrument

instrument driven by reciprocation with the ATR and my motivation driven by the need to simplify the endodontic procedure for my students (and myself), I discovered that I could prepare a curved canal in a resin block with only the F2 ProTaper instrument. That was in the summer of 1999 just before I moved from Lebanon to Canada. I knew that I had in my hands a concept with great potential.

I continued my tests in Toronto, Canada, on hundreds of artificial canals and hundreds of extracted teeth. I did the first video clip of the preparation of an artificial curved canal with an F2 ProTaper used in unequal reciprocation with the ATR motor in 2000, at the University of Toronto. I continued those tests until 2001. I was still at that time in my practice in Toronto using the rotary ProTaper system. I had a large stock of those instruments worth several thousand dollars. I contacted Tulsa Dentsply and asked to exchange all of my SX, S1, F1, and F3 ProTaper instruments for F2 ProTaper instruments. I still remember the shock of the salespeople at Dentsply: What is wrong with this guy? Why is he exchanging all of the instruments for only F2 instruments? No one knew what was happening. I switched my technique of preparation then, in 2001, from continuous rotation to unequal reciprocation using only one NiTi (F2) instrument. I have not used continuous rotation since then. After several years of clinical experience, I had confirmation that single-file reciprocation was very safe and efficient. I published an article about this novel concept in 2008 in the *International Endodontic Journal*. This approach using a ProTaper F2 in reciprocating movement was based on a series of experiments conducted in Toronto designed to estimate the maximal rotational angle before plastic deformation, the elastic limit of the instrument (Fig. 5.7) [13]. A forward angle of 144° (attack angle) followed by a reverse rotation of 72° (relief angle) was thus

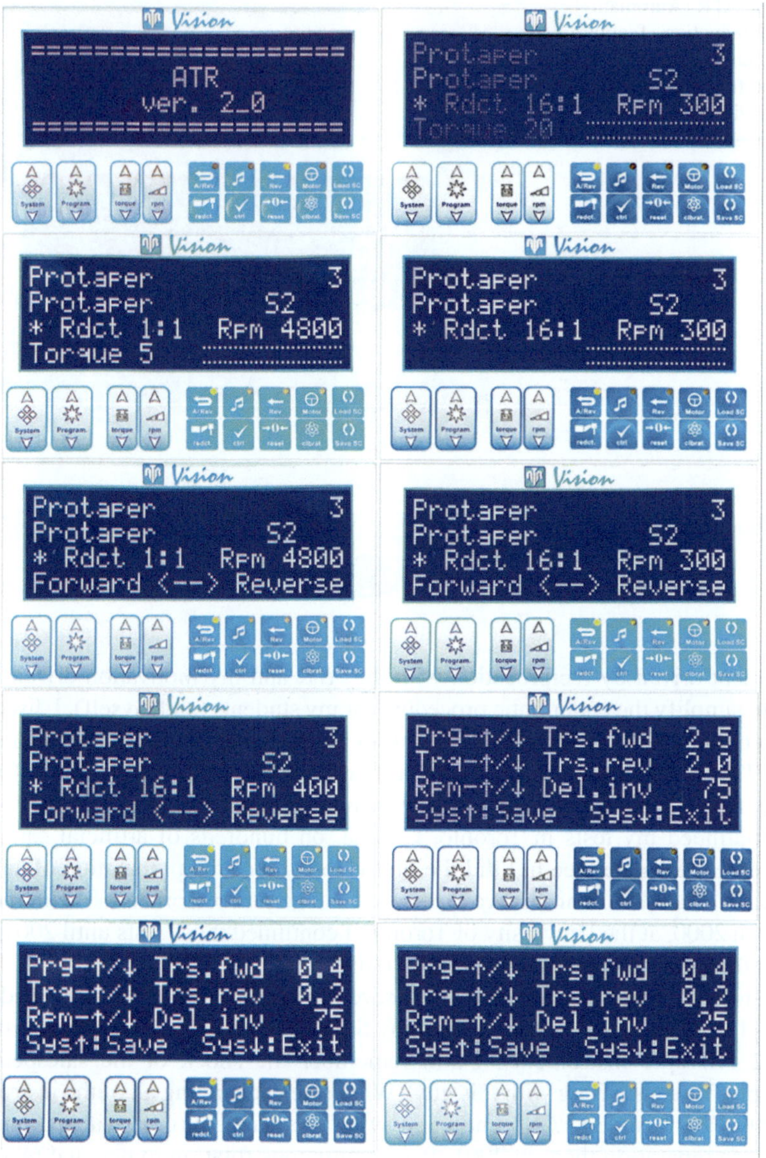

Fig. 5.6 Adjusting the ATR motor for reciprocating motion with ProTaper F2 instrument according to Dr. Ghassan Yared. (1) Find a preset that you would never use. For e.g., "PF Or. Shaper #1". (2) Decrease the torque to 5, using the "torque" down button. (3) Press the "redct." button to change the reduction to 1:1. (4) Press the "ctrl" (the check mark) and the "torque" increase buttons at the same time. "Forward-Reverse" will appear on the screen. (5) Press the "redct." button to change the reduction back to 16:1. (6) Press the "rpm" up button to increase the RPM to 400. (7) Press the "ctrl" button (the check mark) and the music note button directly above it, at the same time. (8) Use the "Program" down button to decrease the "trs. fwd" to 0.4. (9) Use the "torque" down button to decrease the "trs. rev" to 0.2. (10) Use the "rpm" down button to decrease the "del. inv" to 25. (11) Hit the "system" up button to save the settings. After these steps your ATR motor is ready to operate under asymmetric reciprocation motion

Torsional Fatigue Profile of the F2 ProTaper Instrument

Deflection Angle	Cycles to Fracture
360°	3.5
270°	6.9
252°	9.7
216°	29.8
180°	66.6
162°	302.5
144°	397.5
126°	712.5
108°	4029.3
90°	42941.9

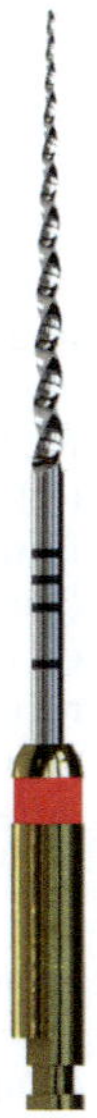

Fig. 5.7 Table on the torsional fatigue profile of the ProTaper Universal F2 instrument showing the negative correlation between the deflection angle and the number of cycles needed to fracture i.e., the lower the deflection angle, the safer the movement. (Adapted from Thompson [13])

achieved, which renders a difference of 72° between the reciprocating movements; as a result, a complete 360° revolution cycle is achieved after five complete reciprocating cycles, producing the so-called rotational effect (Fig. 5.8). A contact was established with VDW and Dentsply, and modern single-file reciprocation with unequal angles was born in 2010 under the names WaveOne and Reciproc. Hundreds of articles from international researchers and mainly from the authors of this textbook have confirmed the efficiency and safety of the Reciproc system.

5.3 Reciprocating Systems

In the years that followed the first publication [14] in which Ghassan Yared proposed the use of the NiTi ProTaper F2 instrument in reciprocating movement, two commercial systems based on the same kinematics were launched in the market: Reciproc (VDW, Germany) and WaveOne (Dentsply Maillefer, Switzerland). Both systems were developed based on the concept of preparing root canals with a single instrument using asymmetric oscillatory movements, in order to mitigate the drawbacks of rotary systems (e.g., taper lock, fatigue fracture, threading-in). WaveOne and Reciproc feature a constant taper from D0 to D3 and a variable regressive taper to D16. Due to commercial reasons, they are machined with left-leaning flutes, which means that the cutting direction for both is counterclockwise. This exclusive feature creates a linked dependency between these instruments and the engine drive (motor). The practical result is that both WaveOne and Reciproc instruments need to be driven by dedicated motors to allow cutting in a counterclockwise direction. For both instruments, different angles in the cutting and non-cutting directions always render a difference of 120° between movements. As a result, a complete

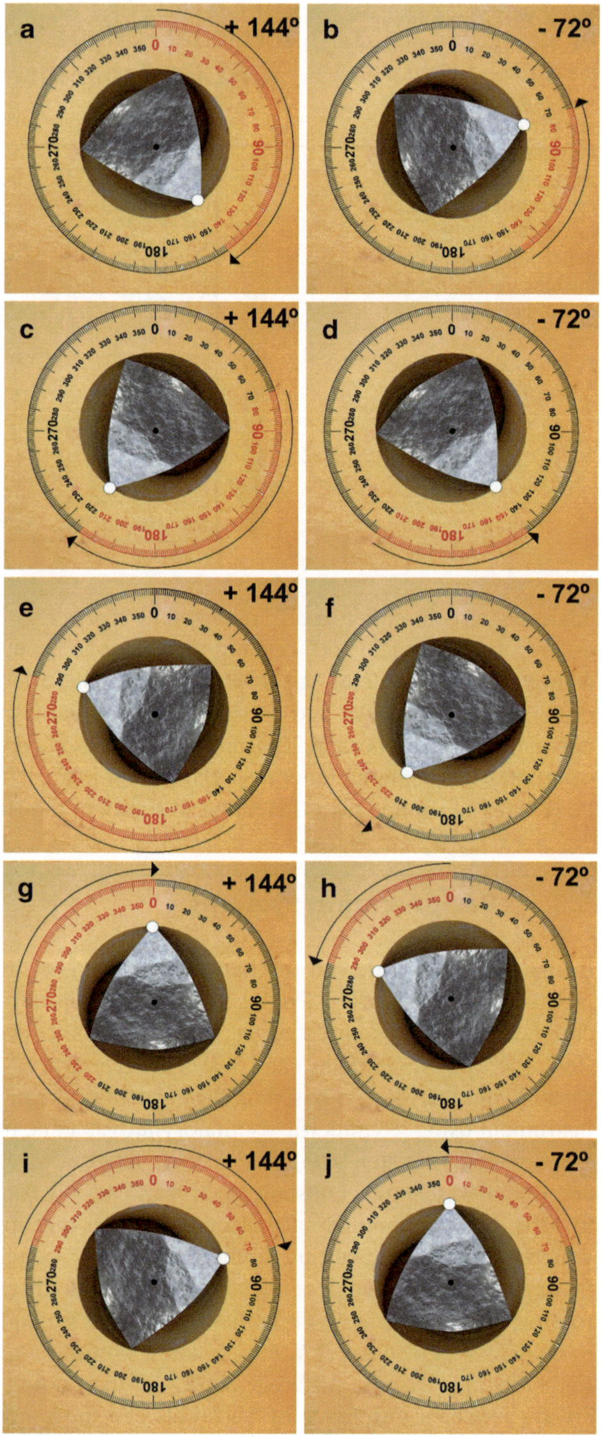

Fig. 5.8 Schematic illustration demonstrating the reciprocating movement configured in the software of the ATR (Automatic Torque Reduction) Tecnika electric motor (ATR, Italy) for the ProTaper F2 reciprocation technique. (**a, c, e, g, i**) The forward angle is 144° (attack angle) followed by (**b, d, f, h, j**) a reverse rotation of 72° (relief angle), which renders a difference of 72° between the reciprocating movements; as a result, a complete 360° revolution cycle is achieved after five complete reciprocating cycles, producing the so-called rotational effect

360° revolution cycle occurs after three complete reciprocating cycles, also producing the previously described rotational effect, which is one of the pillars responsible for the optimal overall performance of asymmetric reciprocating systems. Reciproc employs 150°/30° with an average speed of 300 rpm (Fig. 5.9a and b), while WaveOne uses 170°/50° with an average speed of 350 rpm (Fig. 5.9c and d), and these parameters are within the torsional elastic limit of each instrument.

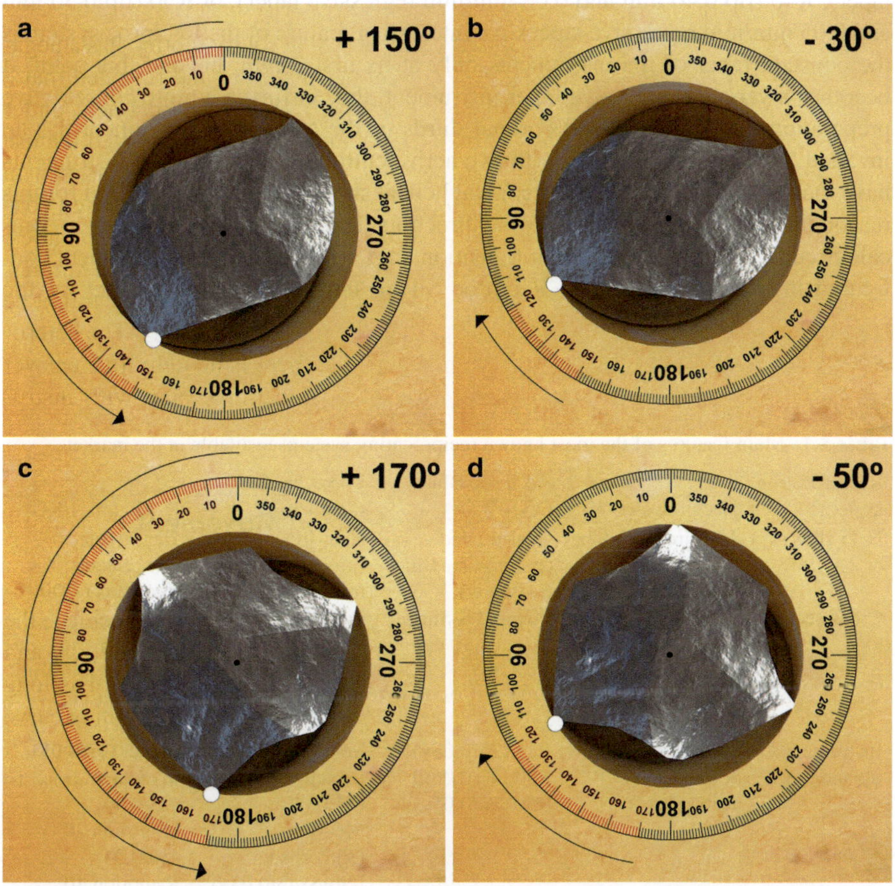

Fig. 5.9 Schematic illustrations demonstrating (**a, b**) the reciprocating movement configured in the software of the VDW electric motor for the Reciproc instrument (RECIPROC ALL program) and (**c, d**) in the Dentsply electric motor for the WaveOne instrument (WAVE ONE ALL program). The Reciproc movement initially works with a (**a**) 150° counterclockwise to cut dentin followed by (**b**) a clockwise 30° (relief movement), while the WaveOne starts with (**c**) 170° counterclockwise to cut dentin followed by (**d**) a clockwise 50° (relief movement). For both settings, after each cycle of counterclockwise and clockwise movements, a 120° difference is achieved which corresponds to the effective cutting forward advancement. This difference of 120° means that a complete rotation of 360° occurs after three cycles. Although the applied kinematics is reciprocating, at high speed, the phenomenon known as "rotational effect" can be observed, which means that the resultant of the movements allows the complete rotation of the instrument

5.3.1 Reciproc M-Wire

The Reciproc system is a set of reciprocating instruments machined from an M-Wire patented heat-treated NiTi alloy (Table 5.1). The M-Wire alloy presents greater resistance to cyclic fatigue and greater flexibility than traditional NiTi alloys [15]. The manufacturer of Reciproc suggests the use of one of the three available instruments depending on the canal size: R25 (tip 0.25 mm and 0.08 mm/mm regressive taper), R40 (tip 0.40 mm and 0.06 mm/mm regressive taper), or R50 (tip 0.50 mm and 0.05 mm/mm regressive taper). An interesting feature of the Reciproc system is the constant taper of the instruments only at its first 3 mm; beyond this point, it becomes a variable regressive-taper instrument, thus ensuring a more conservative preparation of the middle and coronal thirds of the canal. The instrument has an inverted S-shape cross-section with two active cutting edges. Reciproc instruments have their spirals arranged on the conical helical shaft from left to right, and for this reason they cut in a counterclockwise direction. The tip of the instruments is conical, circular, and truncated with a transition angle (Fig. 5.10). The movement configured in the software of the Reciproc Silver and Gold electric motors for the

Table 5.1 Main features of the most known reciprocating systems available in the market

Reciprocating systems	Reciproc (VDW)	Reciproc Blue (VDW)	WaveOne Gold (Dentsply)	R-Motion (FKG)
NiTi alloy	M-Wire	Heat-treated (proprietary Blue treatment)	Heat-treated (proprietary Gold treatment)	Heat-treated (proprietary treatment)
Cross-section	Inverted S-Shape	Inverted S-Shape	Parallelogram-shape with 1 or 2 cutting edges	Rounded triangular cross-section with sharp cutting edges
Instruments' tip and taper	R25 (25/0.08v) R40 (40/0.06v) R50 (50/0.05v)	R25 (25/0.08v) R40 (40/0.06v) R50 (50/0.05v)	Small (20/0.07v) Primary (25/0.07v) Medium (35/0.06v) Large (45/0.05v)	Glider (15/0.03) R-motion 25 (25/0.06) R-motion 30 (30/0.04) R-motion 40 (40/0.04) R-motion 50 (50/0.04)
Available lengths	21, 25, and 31 mm	21, 25, and 31 mm	21, 25, and 31 mm	21, 25, and 31 mm
Kinematics (activation)	"RECIPROC ALL" setting. Rotation angle of 150° counterclockwise and 30° clockwise	"RECIPROC ALL" setting. Rotation angle of 150° counterclockwise and 30° clockwise	"WAVEONE ALL" setting. Rotation angle of 170° counterclockwise and 50° clockwise	"WAVEONE ALL" setting. Rotation angle of 170° counterclockwise and 50° clockwise

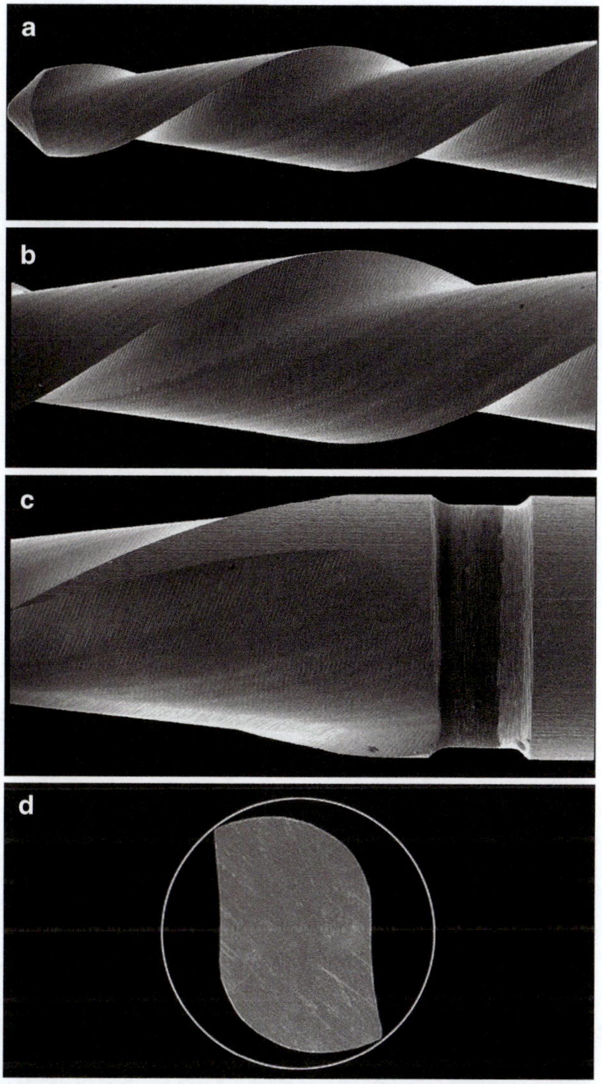

Fig. 5.10 Scanning electron microscopic images of the Reciproc M-Wire instrument design showing its (**a**) conic, circular and truncated tip with a transition angle, (**b**) the helical shaft, (**c**) the intermediary region, and (**d**) the inverted S-shaped cross-section

Reciproc system (RECIPROC ALL program) works with a 150° counterclockwise to cut dentin followed by a clockwise 30°, where the instrument is relieved of its cutting function. Thus, after each cycle of counterclockwise and clockwise movements, a 120° difference is created which corresponds to the effective cutting forward advancement. With this difference of 120° in the reciprocating movement, a complete rotation of 360° occurs after three cycles. Although the applied kinematics is reciprocating, at high speed, the phenomenon known as "rotational effect" can be observed, which means that the resultant of the movements allows the complete rotation of the instrument (Fig. 5.11).

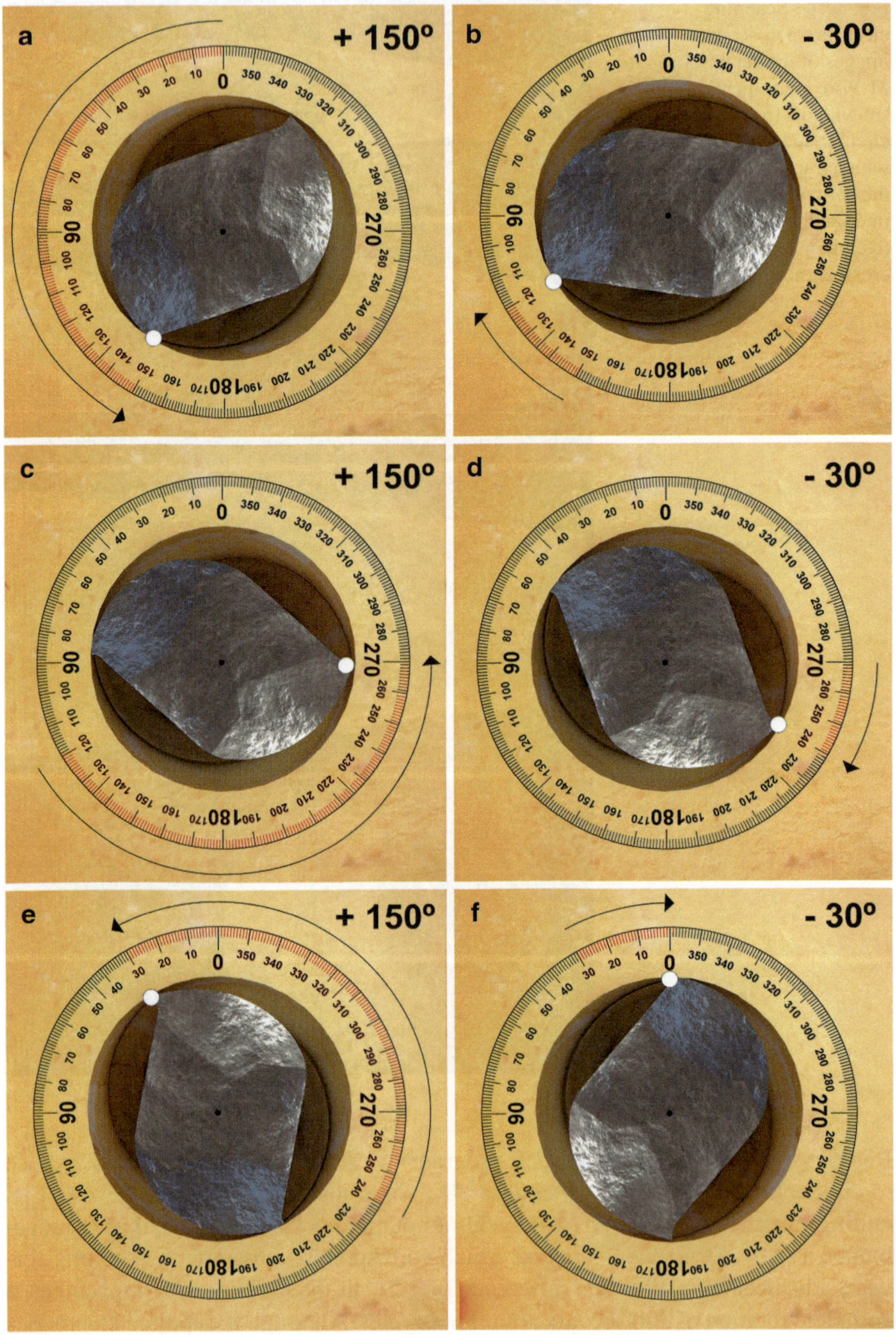

Fig. 5.11 Schematic illustrations demonstrating the complete rotational effect (360°) of the reciprocating movement with a Reciproc instrument adapted to a dedicated electric motor set at RECIPROC ALL motion, after three cycles of (**a, c, e**) 150° counterclockwise cutoff for the dentin followed by (**b, d, f**) a clockwise 30° movement

5.3.1.1 Manufacturer Guidelines (Fig. 5.12)

- Create a straight-line access to the root canal;
- Fill the access cavity with the irrigating agent;
- Insert the Reciproc instrument into the root canal and activate the motor when inside the canal;
- Move the instrument in a slow in- and-out-motion (pecking motion). The amplitude of the movements must not exceed 3 mm. Light apical pressure should be applied. The instrument will advance in the canal in the apical direction. An in- and out-movement is equal to one peck. Remove the instrument after three pecks;
- Clean the instrument blades to remove cutting debris;
- Irrigate the root canal;
- Check with a manual instrument size 10 if the canal is free at approximately 3 mm beyond the previously prepared canal;
- Continue to use the Reciproc instrument as described above until it reaches 2/3 of the estimated canal length. Determine root canal length and continue with Reciproc until it reaches the working length.

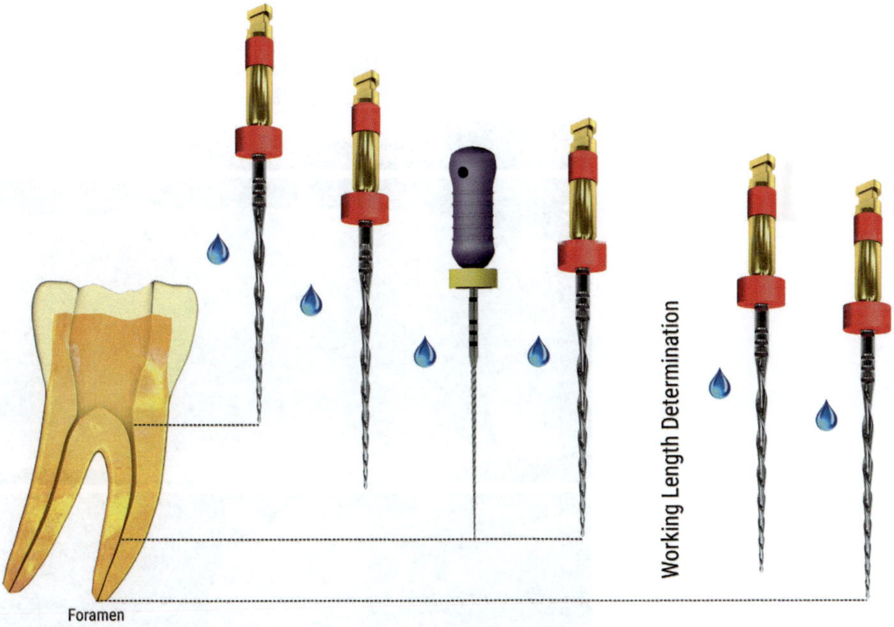

Fig. 5.12 Schematic illustration of the step-by-step manufacturer guidelines recommended for the use of the Reciproc M-Wire. Reciproc M-Wire is used at the entrance of the canal followed by a manual file to explore the canal up to two-thirds of the root length. After working length determination, the Reciproc instrument is progressively driven up to the working length

5.3.2 Reciproc Blue

The heat treatment of NiTi alloys has been successfully used to improve the mechanical properties of endodontic instruments. This thermomechanical processing optimizes the microstructural behavior and phase transformation of NiTi alloys, directly influencing the mechanical properties of NiTi instruments [16, 17]. The Reciproc Blue system is similar in design to the original Reciproc M-wire system (Table 5.1), but with the benefit of being manufactured using a thermally treated NiTi alloy that exhibits greater flexibility and resistance to cyclic fatigue than the original Reciproc. In this way, Reciproc Blue instruments can be used with increased safety in anatomically challenging teeth, such as in cases of sharp curvatures and narrow canals.

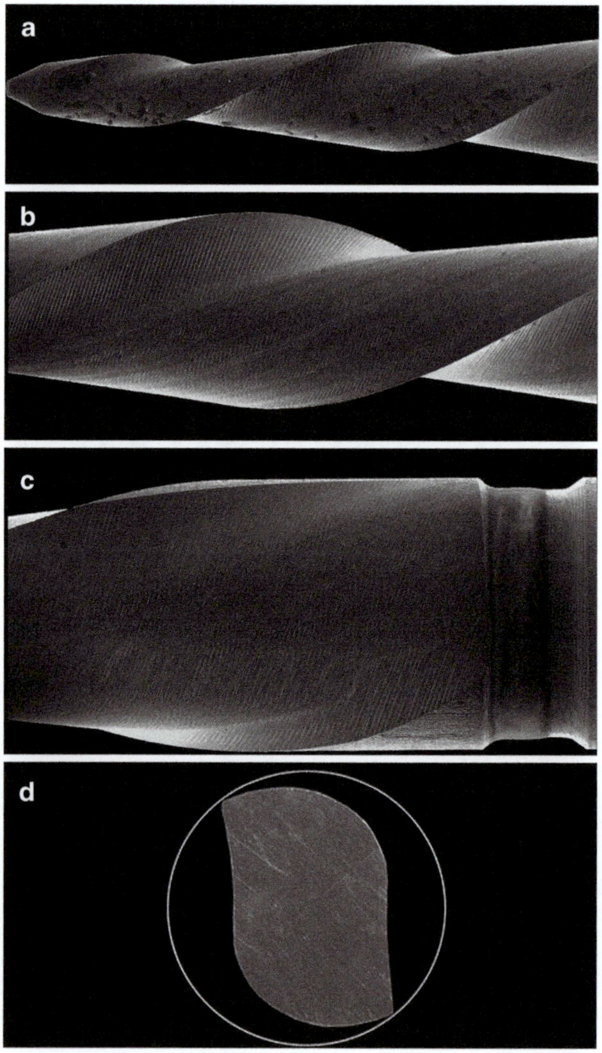

Fig. 5.13 Scanning electron microscopic images of the Reciproc Blue instrument design showing its (**a**) conic, circular, and truncated tip with a transition curve, (**b**) the helical shaft, (**c**) the intermediary region, and (**d**) its inverted S-shaped cross-section

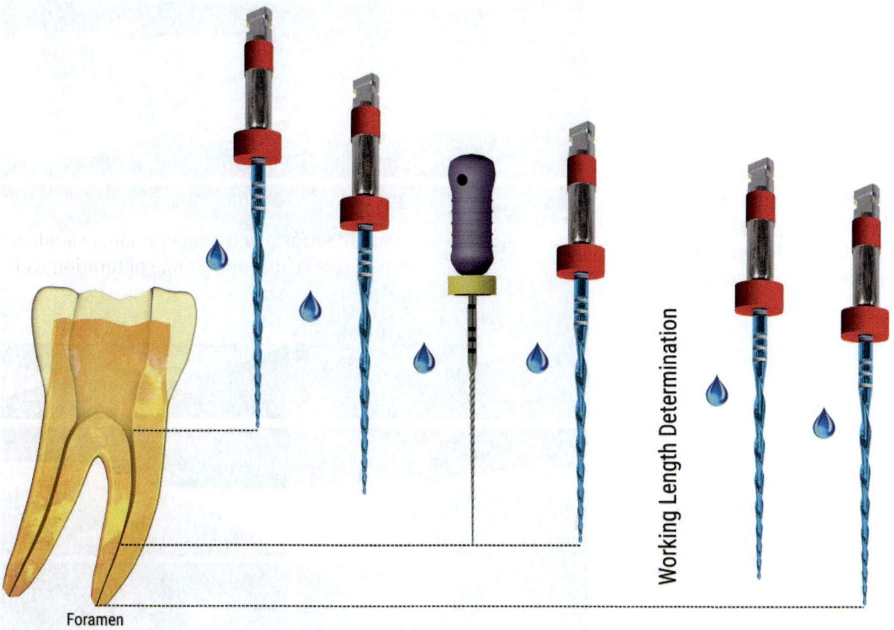

Fig. 5.14 Schematic illustration of the step-by-step manufacturer guidelines recommended for the use of the Reciproc Blue. Reciproc Blue is used at the entrance of the canal followed by a manual file exploring the canal up to two-thirds of the root length. After working length determination, the Reciproc Blue instrument is progressively driven up to the working length

Overall, Reciproc Blue instruments are similar but not identical to Reciproc M-Wire instruments. The tip size, cross-section and regressive taper are equal, but the tip geometry of Reciproc Blue instruments differs from that of the original Reciproc as it has a circular truncated conical shape with a transition curve and both ends are inactive (Fig. 5.13). According to the manufacturer recommendations, Reciproc Blue is used in the same manner as Reciproc M-wire (Fig. 5.14).

5.3.3 WaveOne Gold

The WaveOne Gold system (Dentsply Maillefer, Ballaigues, Switzerland) is an updated version of the original WaveOne system which, according to the manufacturer, kept the simplicity with additional benefits as it is built from a NiTi alloy treated with repeated heating and cooling cycles (Table 5.1). This treatment promotes an improvement in instrument's resistance and flexibility, allowing its use in different anatomical challenges. In addition, WaveOne Gold instruments have a parallelogram-shaped cross-section with one or two cutting edges, varying according to the location along the instrument, thus minimizing the "screw-in" effect and reducing the instrument's torque within the root canal walls. WaveOne Gold instruments are available in four sizes: small (tip 0.20 mm and 0.07 mm/mm regressive taper), primary (tip 0.25 mm and 0.07 mm/mm regressive taper), medium (tip

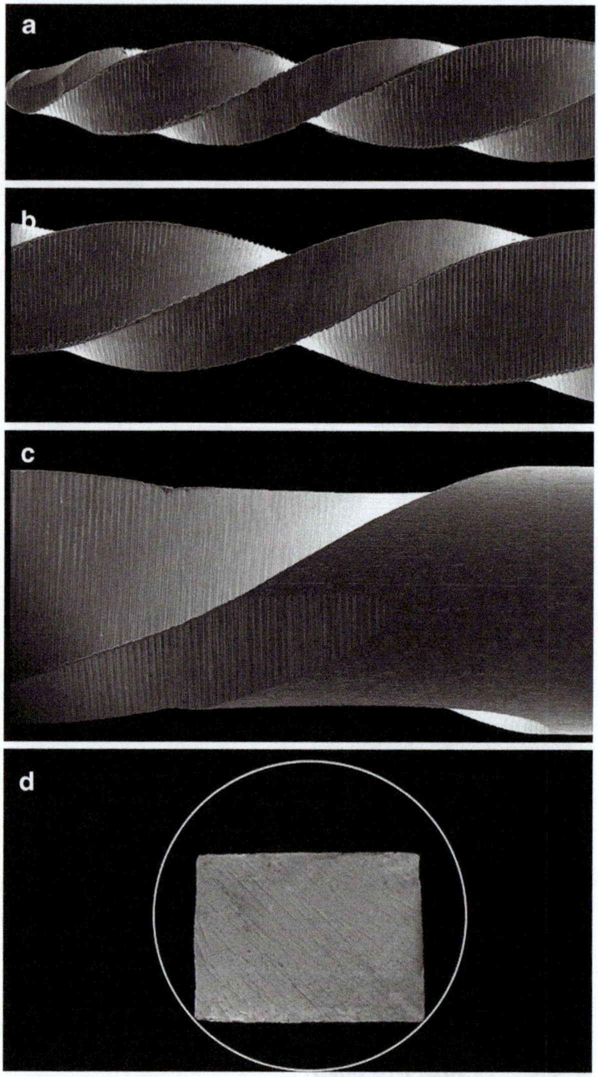

Fig. 5.15 Scanning electron microscopic images of the WaveOne Gold instrument design showing its (**a**) conic, circular and truncated tip with a transition curve, (**b**) the helical shaft, (**c**) the intermediary region, and (**d**) its parallelogram-shaped cross-section

0.35 mm and 0.06 mm/mm regressive taper) and large (tip 0.45 mm and 0.05 mm/mm regressive taper). The tip is inactive and the taper is constant only in the first 3 mm from the tip (Fig. 5.15). Beyond this point, the taper is regressive, thus ensuring a more conservative preparation of the middle and coronal thirds of the canals. The side cutting rods are oriented to cut in a counterclockwise direction. The kinematics configured in the WaveOne system software (X-Smart Plus) initially work with a counterclockwise cut of 170°, followed by a clockwise movement of 50° by relieving the instrument (WAVEONE ALL). Thus, in each cycle, the instrument achieves an effective advance of 120°, requiring three cycles to complete a full rotation (Fig. 5.16).

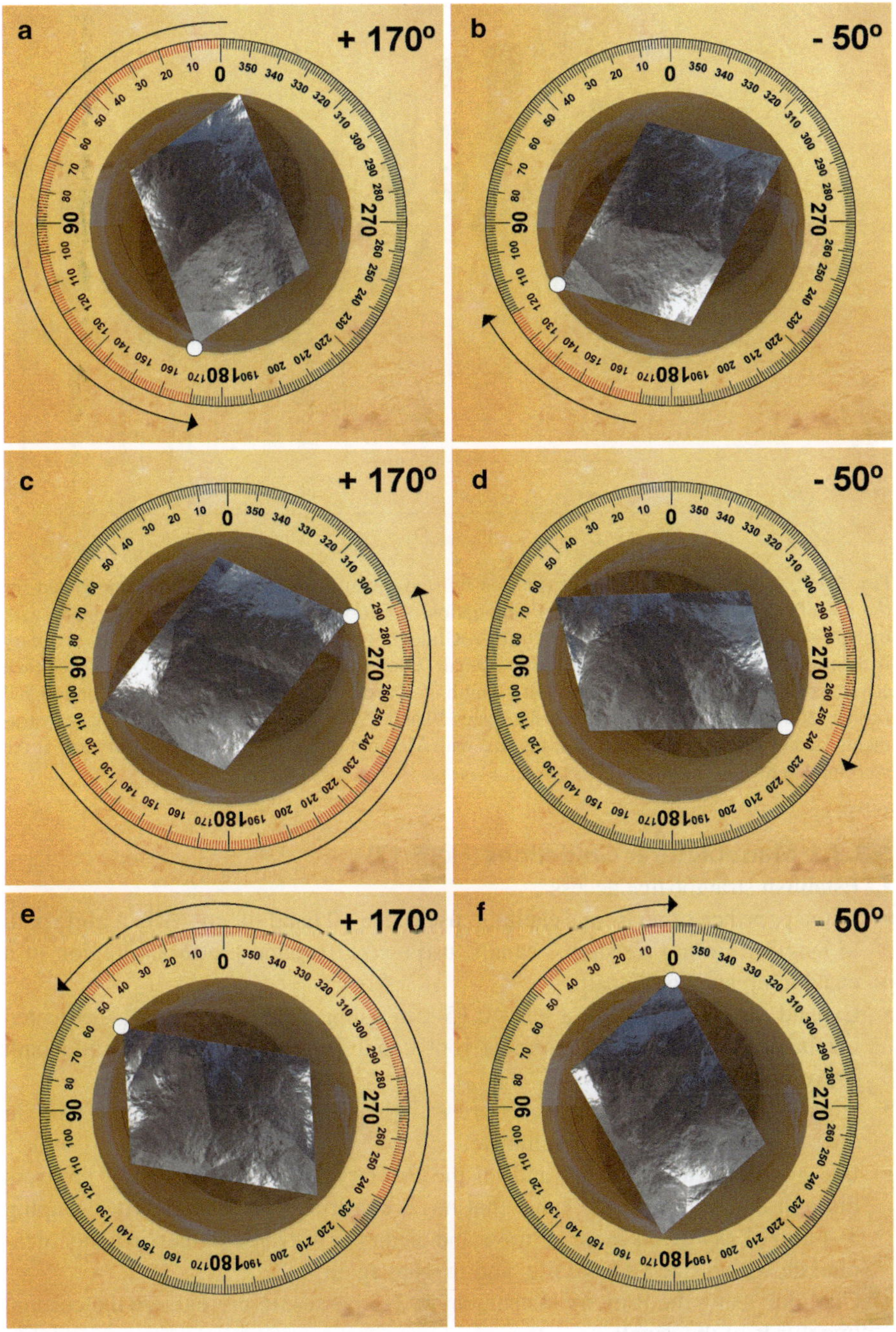

Fig. 5.16 Illustrative images demonstrating the complete 360° rotational effect of the reciprocating movement with a WaveOne Gold instrument adapted to a dedicated electric motor set at WAVEONE ALL motion, after (**a, c, e**) three cycles of 170° counterclockwise cut-off for the dentin followed by (**b, d, f**) a clockwise 50° movement

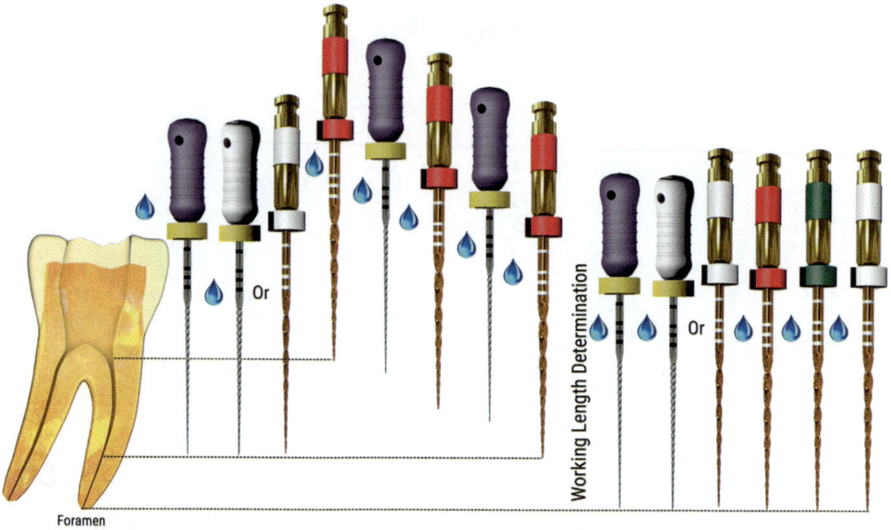

Fig. 5.17 Schematic illustration of the step-by-step manufacturer guidelines recommended for the use of the Wave-One Gold. Initial negotiation of two-third of the canal shall be made with manual K-file sizes 10 and 15 and a rotating ProGlider or Path NiTi instrument. Wave-One Primary is then used to explore the two-third of the canal, followed by a size 10 manual K-file after each advancement of 3–4 mm. At the two-third length, proceed with working length determination and further scouting and glide path with K-files sizes 10 and 15, ProGlider or Path Finder rotary instruments, and WaveOne Primary; Then, finalize with Medium or Large WaveOne instruments at the working length

5.3.3.1 Manufacturer Guidelines (Fig. 5.17)

- Establish straight-line access;
- In the presence of a viscous chelator, use a size 10 hand file to verify a glide path to length. In more restrictive canals, use a size 10 hand file in any region of a canal to create a glide path;
- Expand the glide path to at least 0.15 mm using either a manual or dedicated mechanical file, such as Pathfiles root canal or ProGlider rotary glide path instruments;
- Always initiate the shaping procedure with the Primary instrument (25/07 red) in the presence of sodium hypochlorite;
- Use gentle inward pressure and let the Primary instrument passively progress through any region of the canal that has a confirmed glide path. After shaping 3–4 mm of any given canal, remove and clean the instrument, then irrigate, recapitulate with a size 10 hand file, and irrigate again;
- Continue using the Primary instrument in 2–3 passes, to pre-enlarge the coronal two thirds of the canal;

- Use a brushing motion on the outstroke to eliminate coronal interferences or to enhance shaping results in canals that exhibit irregular cross-sections;
- In more restrictive canals, use a size 10 hand file in the presence of a viscous chelator to negotiate to the terminus of the canal. Gently work with the instrument until it is completely loose at length;
- Establish working length, confirm patency, and verify the glide path;
- Expand this glide path to at least 0.15 mm using a manual or mechanical glide path file;
- Use the Primary WaveOne Gold instrument to the full working length in one or more passes. Upon reaching length, remove the instrument to avoid over-enlargement of the foramen. Inspect the flutes next to the tip. If they are loaded with dentin chips, then shaping is complete. If the Primary instrument is loose at length with no dentin chips in the flutes, continue the shaping procedure with the Medium (35/06 green) and/or Large (45/05 white) instruments until flutes are loaded.
- If the PRIMARY file doesn't progress, then use the SMALL file (020/07 yellow) in one or more passes to working length and then re-attempt the PRIMARY file to working length;
- When the shaping is completed, proceed with 3-D disinfection protocols.

5.3.4 Race Evo R-Motion

R-Motion instruments are manufactured using a thermally treated NiTi alloy that exhibits greater flexibility and high resistance to cyclic fatigue. R-Motion presents a rounded triangular cross-section with sharp cutting edges and a thinner core with a new optimized tip (Table 5.1). According to the manufacturer, the exclusive R-Motion design and thinner core size significantly reduce the stress on dentin during root canal treatment by reducing the screwing effect, allowing better control of its progression into the root canal. The R-Motion system is composed of five instruments: R-Motion Glide (tip 15 and 0.03 taper), R-Motion 25 (tip 25 and 0.06 taper), R-Motion 30 (tip 30 and 0.04 taper), R-Motion 40 (tip 40 and 0.04 taper) and R-Motion 50 (tip 50 and 0.04 taper) (Fig. 5.18). According to the manufacturer, R-Motion instruments were designed to be used with standard asymmetric reciprocating modes in existing motors available on the market.

5.3.4.1 Manufacturer Guidelines (Fig. 5.19)

- Create straight-line access;
- Use an ISO 10 hand file to explore the canal;
- Determine the working length;
- Use the R-Motion Glider instrument applying gentle strokes of 2–3 mm to establish a glide path until the working length is reached. After three strokes, remove and clean the instrument, then irrigate; recapitulate with an ISO 10 hand file;

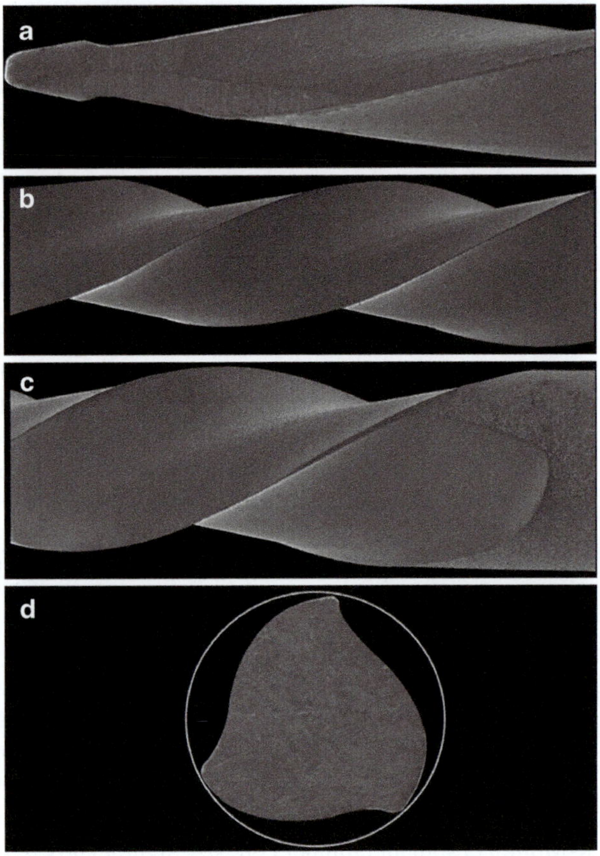

Fig. 5.18 Scanning electron microscopic images of the R-Motion instrument design showing its (**a**) conic truncated tip with transition curve, (**b**) the helical shaft, (**c**) the intermediary region, and (**d**) its rounded triangular symmetrical cross-section

- Select the R-Motion single-file shaping instrument which is best suited to the anatomy of the canal being treated. In most cases, and depending on your approach to apical preparation, the R-Motion 25 or 30 will be appropriate. If the radiographs do not allow you to clearly identify the anatomy of the canal, it can be gauged using hand files;
- Start the shaping procedure applying your usual irrigation/disinfection protocol;
- Use gentle strokes of 2–3 mm applying very light apical pressure to allow the R-Motion single-file shaping instrument to progress passively along the canal. After three strokes, remove and clean the instrument, then irrigate and recapitulate with an ISO size 10 hand file;
- Repeat the previous step until the R-Motion instrument reaches the working length. If necessary, a brushing motion may be applied to remove coronal interferences and/or ensure uniform shaping of irregular canals. Once the working length has been reached, remove the instrument to prevent over- enlargement of the foramen.

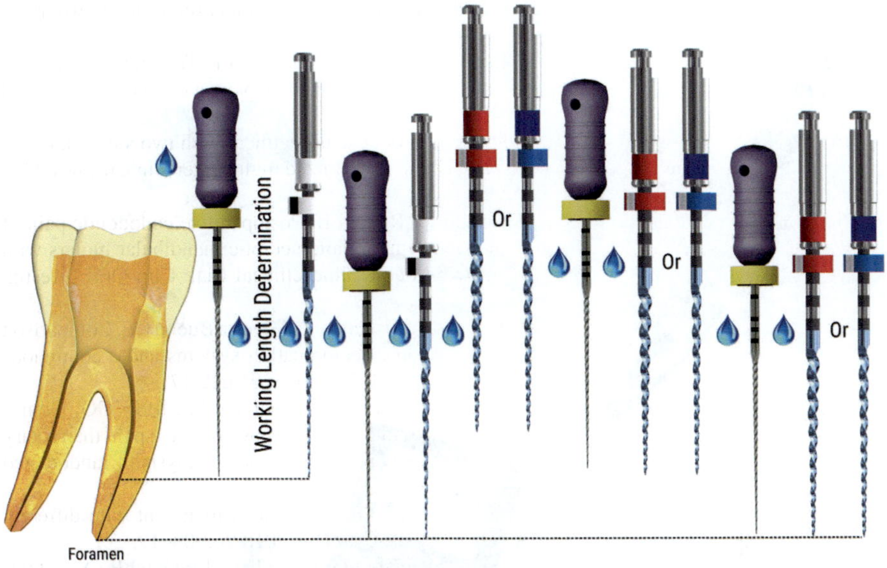

Fig. 5.19 Schematic illustration of the step-by-step manufacturer guidelines recommended for the use of the R-Motion reciprocating instrument. A size 10 K-file is used to explore the canal and determine the working length. Then, the R-Motion Glider initiate the glide path. A size 10 K-file must be used to recapitulate after every 3–4 mm of advancement until reaching the working length. Finally, R-Motion 25 or 30 is progressively used up to the working length, always recapitulating with a size 10 K-file

5.4 Reciprocating Motors

5.4.1 Dedicated Electronic Motors

There are several commercially available dedicated motors to perform the reciprocating movement that can be classified into three types:

- **Closed motors**: Devices that only execute previously recorded reciprocating movements and do not allow update or modification of their kinematics. Examples: X-Smart Plus (Dentsply Maillefer), TriAuto ZX2 (J Morita) and the Elements Motor (SybronEndo) (Fig. 5.20).
- **Closed motors, subject to update**: Devices that perform only recorded reciprocating movements registered in their libraries but, through an update, can be upgraded to new kinematics. Examples: VDW Silver (VDW), VDW Gold (VDW), VDW.CONNECT Drive (VDW), and X-Smart IQ (Dentsply) (Fig. 5.21). VDW and Dentsply motors offer a reciprocating movement in which the cutting is in a counterclockwise direction, completing a total rotation after three consecutive cycles. For this reason, the reciprocating movement is exclusive to endodontic instruments machined to cut in a counterclockwise direction, avoiding

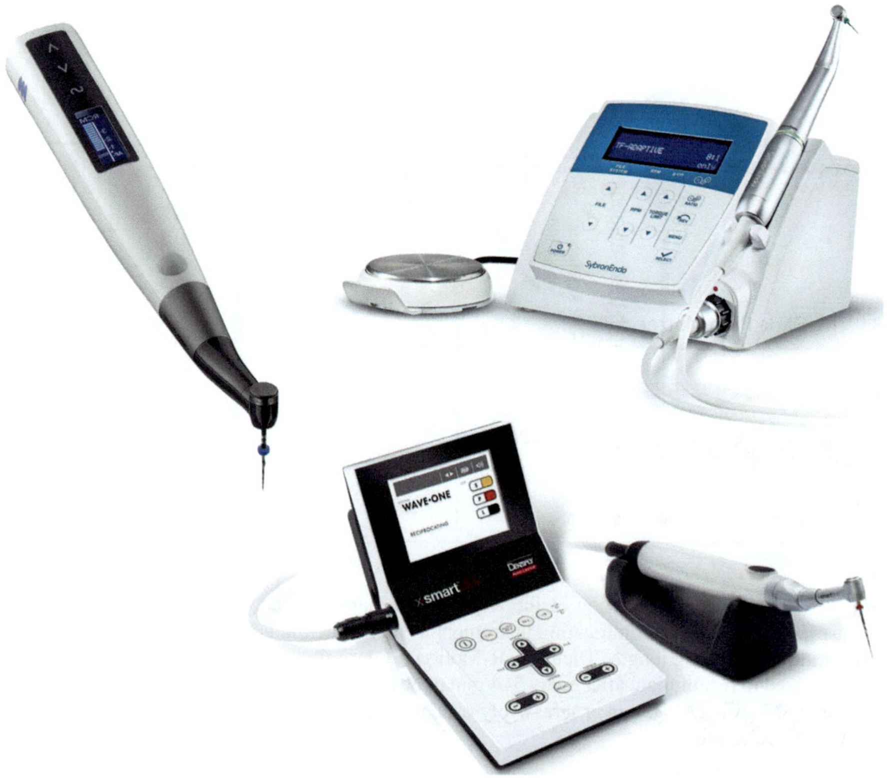

Fig. 5.20 X-Smart Plus (Dentsply Maillefer, Switzerland), TriAuto ZX2 (J Morita, Japan) and the Elements Motor (SybronEndo, USA) are examples of closed motors. These devices execute previously recorded reciprocating movements and do not allow update or modification of the instruments' kinematics

thus the use of instruments designed for continuous rotation in clockwise direction.

- **Open motors**: Devices that can be partially or totally programmed by the operator. The motor can be controlled to operate in different movements by setting clockwise and counterclockwise angles, torque and speed. Historically, it is worth to quote that the first open motors available on the market were the ATR motors (ATR, Italy), which demanded a time-consuming and complex set-up configuration to operate rotary NiTi instruments under reciprocating movement (Fig. 5.6). Examples of wireless open motors are C-Smart-Mini AP (Coxo), Endo Radar (Woodpecker), E-connect S (Eighteeth) and AI Motor (Woodpecker) (Fig. 5.22), while I-Endo Dual (Acteon) and Endo Pilot (Komet Dental) are wired open motors (Fig. 5.23). These open motors allow the use of continuous rotary instruments in reciprocating movement on a clockwise cutting angle. Nowadays, the advantages of reciprocating movement over continuous rotation are largely recognized, and open motors

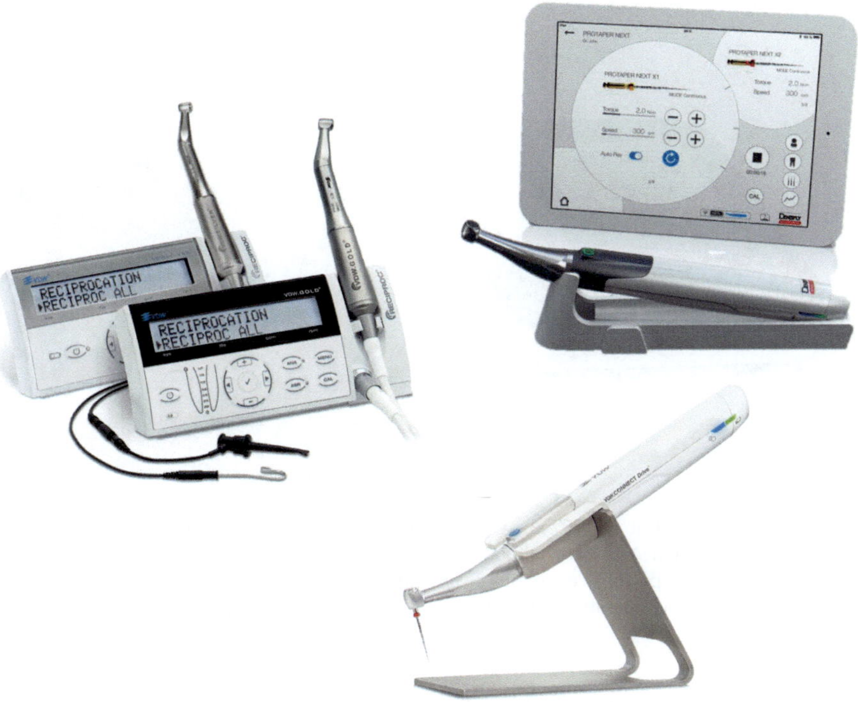

Fig. 5.21 VDW Silver, VDW Gold, VDW.CONNECT Drive (VDW, Germany) and X-Smart IQ (Dentsply Maillefer, Switzerland) are examples of closed motors, subject to update. These devices perform only recorded reciprocating movements registered in their libraries; however, their software can be updated with new kinematics

are no more than a clear indication of the ever-increasing popularity of reciprocating movement, since they allow for any instrument to be used under reciprocating kinematics.

5.4.2 Air-Driven Contra-Angle

To date, only the VDW Direct (VDW) fits within this category. It consists of a reducing contra-angle coupled with a low pneumatic or electric motor to make the reciprocating movement only with specific parameters of the Reciproc system. In other words, the manufacturer claims that this air-driven contra-angle is able to reciprocate 150° CCW and 30° CW. It is just a contra-angle, so it cannot be adjusted or updated to accommodate other systems (Fig. 5.24). The direct contra-angle makes it easier to switch to reciprocating movement since there is no need to acquire a specific reciprocating motor. Silva et al. [18] tested this device and demonstrated that instruments driven by direct contra-angle show a longer cyclic fatigue life than instruments driven by an electric torque-controlled motor, thus ensuring its safety.

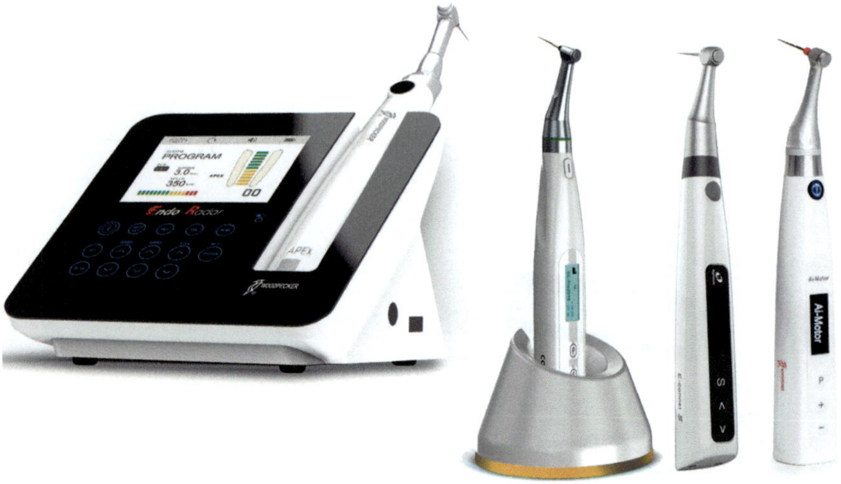

Fig. 5.22 C-Smart-Mini AP (Coxo, China), Endo Radar (Woodpecker, China), E-connect S (Eighteeth, China) and AI Motor (Woodpecker, China) are examples of wireless open motors. These devices can be partially or totally programmed, and the operator can control the motor to operate in different movements, setting clockwise and counterclockwise angles, torque and speed

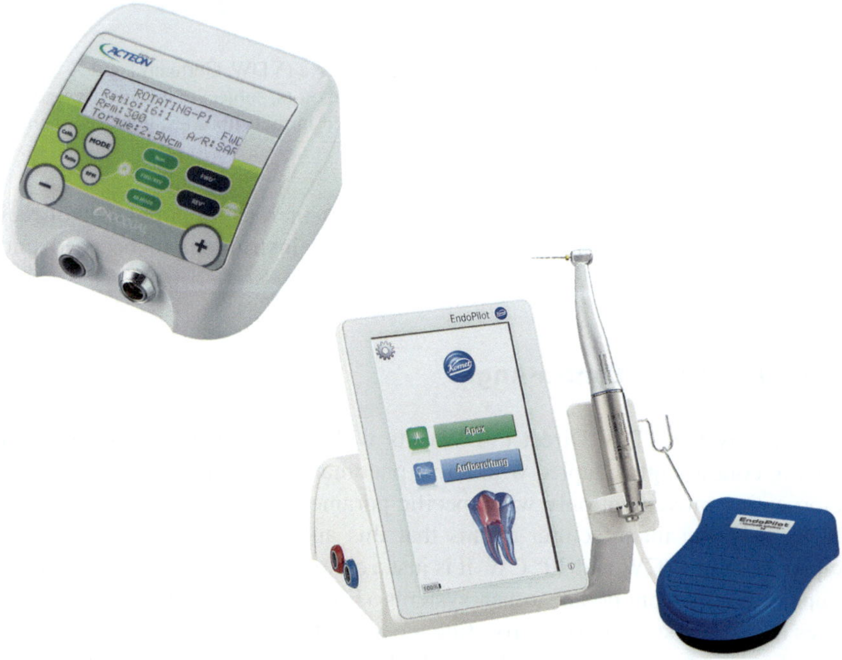

Fig. 5.23 I-Endo Dual (Acteon, France) and Endo Pilot (Komet Dental, Germany) are examples of wired open motors. These devices can be partially or totally programmed, and the operator can control the motor to operate in different movements, setting clockwise and counterclockwise angles, torque and speed

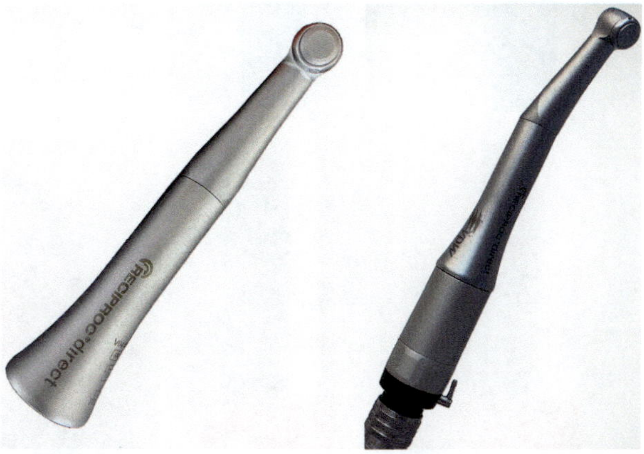

Fig. 5.24 Reciproc Direct air-driven contra-angle (VDW, Germany). This contra-angle is able to reciprocate 150° counterclockwise and 30° clockwise, such as the RECIPROC ALL motion set in the electric motor, at specific setting for Reciproc instruments

5.5 The R25: A Multitasking Single-File Instrument

5.5.1 Is Reciproc a Single-Use Instrument?

The number of times instruments can be used still remain as a highly controversial topic. The Reciproc instrument is commercially advertised as a single-file technique, which means that according to the manufacturer, the instruments must be discarded after each appointment, a recommendation confirmed by Kim et al. [19].

A root canal mechanically prepared with a single reciprocating instrument has a final shape that traditionally could only be obtained by a full sequence of rotary instrumentation, which means three or more instruments. Thus, logical reasoning dictates that an instrument able to shape the entire root canal alone is subjected to a high load of mechanical stress. On the contrary, conventional rotary multi-file systems involve more technical steps to provide a slower and more gradual mechanical canal enlargement and, therefore, the stress load is naturally distributed along the instruments' sequence. Based on this rationale, manufacturers suggest that reciprocating instruments are single-use. In fact, Reciproc is designed to be "forced single-use" instruments since a heat-sensitive plastic ring that surrounds the instrument shaft swells due to the sterilization process. As a consequence of the bigger size of the ring after sterilization, the instrument cannot be reinserted into the contra-angle (Fig. 5.25).

The practical advantage of the single-use approach is to improve the day-to-day workflow and provide a perception of safety by patients since only one packed-sterilized instrument is used per treatment. Yet the core argument in favor of single use is that the performance of the instrument would be critically compromised by reusing it. Besides, one can argue that there is no guarantee that the reciprocating motion programmed in the motor for a single use is able to keep the instrument action within its elastic range. Actually, it is reasonable to think that the interplay between the accumulated mechanical stress concentrated in a single and large reciprocating instrument and the effect of heating and cooling cycles during sterilization on the mechanical properties and resistance of endodontic instruments favor the single-use approach. However, none of these aspects are supported by current literature.

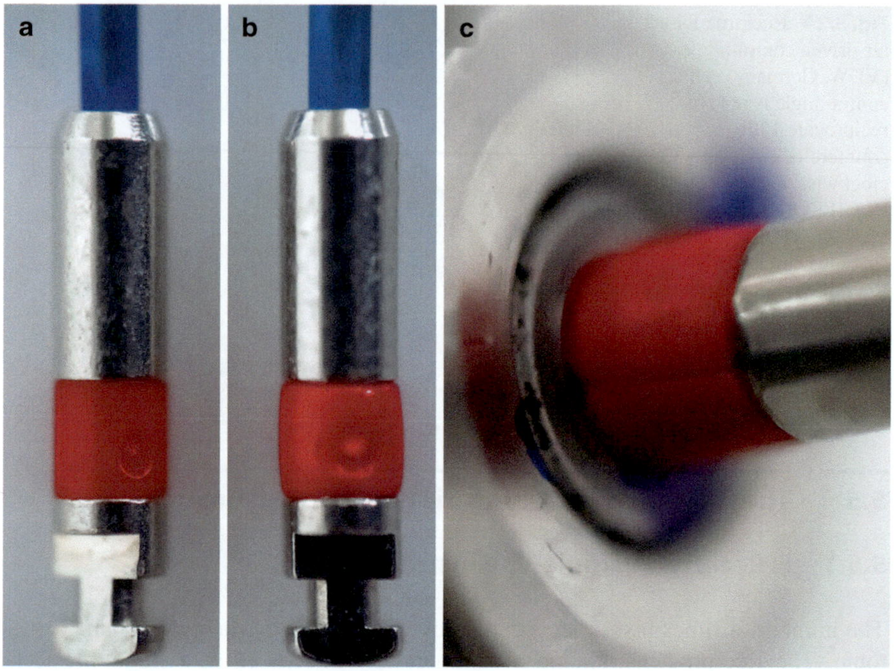

Fig. 5.25 Reciproc is designed to be a “forced single-use” instrument since a (**a**) heat-sensitive plastic ring that surrounds the instrument shaft (**b**) swells due to the sterilization process. As a consequence of the bigger size of the ring, (**c**) the instrument cannot be reinserted into the contra-angle

It was reported that changes in the mechanical properties of NiTi endodontic instruments after five cycles of commonly used sterilization procedures were insignificant [20]. In accordance, Silvaggio and Hicks [21] demonstrated that the sterilization process does not influence the resistance of NiTi rotary instruments. The impact of the cumulative effect of multiple uses of reciprocating instruments in clinics was investigated by Caballero-Flores et al. [22]. They prepared up to nine root canals using a single-file reciprocating system and reported no failure. As a matter of fact, the reuse of reciprocating instruments is a common practice adopted in several countries around the world for economic reasons [23]. Moreover, Bueno et al. [23] well described one interesting rationale on that topic: “... *it seems reasonable to assume that the wear suffered by an instrument when used in a tooth with only 1 canal is less than that observed when it is used in a tooth with 3 canals. Based on this reasoning, one could admit the possibility of using the same reciprocating instrument in more than 1 case, particularly in environments in which the high cost of instruments can hinder or preclude treatment altogether.*” Although the multiple use of reciprocating instruments has been related to a low fracture rate, a comparative analysis of two studies from the same research group clearly shows that single-use issue can provide lower fracture rates. The fracture rate was 0.84% considering the total number of teeth when reciprocating instruments were used to prepare up to three posterior teeth [23]. However, when reciprocating instruments were used once, no fractures were observed after root canal treatment of 750 maxillary and mandibular molars [24].

For the authors of this textbook, the single-use approach still seems to be advantageous over multiple use, not only for improvement in the operative workflow but mostly because the better scientific evidence and clinical performance of reciprocating instruments over the last decade were massively based on the single-use approach. Moreover, consistent concerns in the literature [25, 26] regarding the quality of cleanness and sterilization of used instruments drive some developed countries to request the adoption of a single disposable use requirement for any endodontic instrument (Fig. 5.26). However, it is totally understandable if clinicians embrace the multi-use approach for economic reasons.

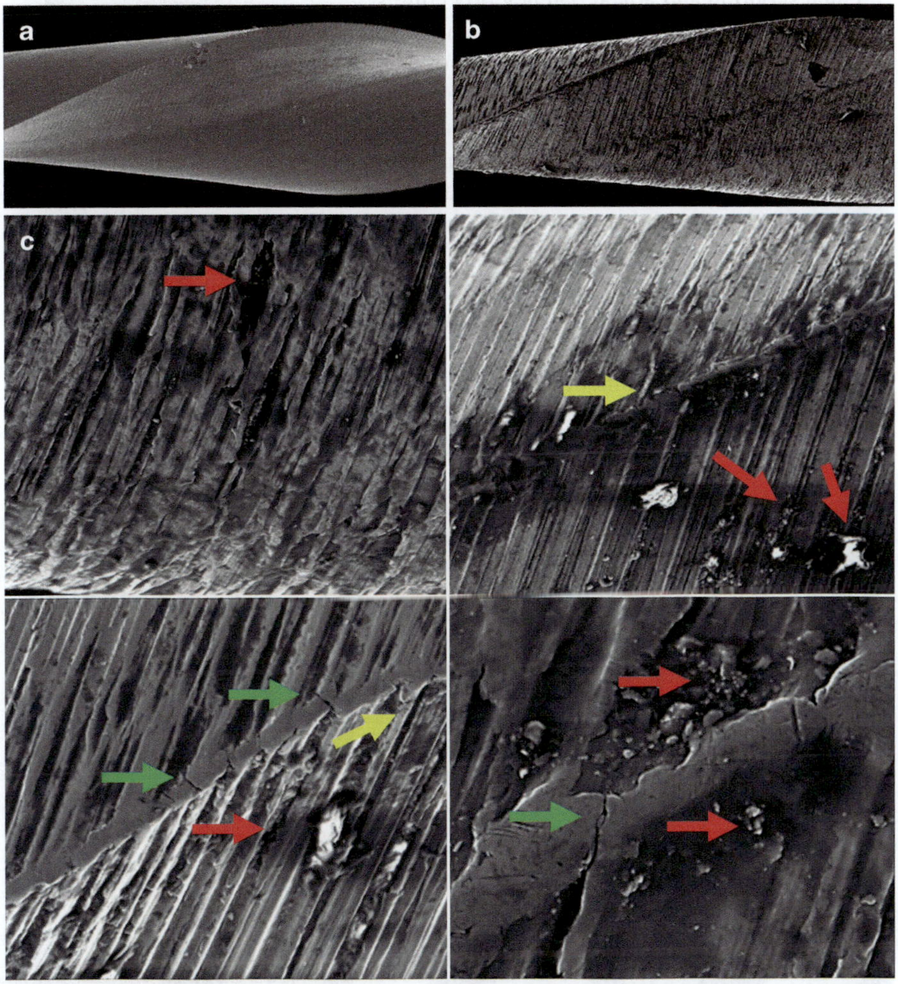

Fig. 5.26 Scanning electron microscopy of (**a**) an unused M-Wire Reciproc R25 instrument and (**b**) another Reciproc R25 instrument after use. (**c**) At high magnification, it is possible to observe the presence of debris (red arrows) on the surface of the instrument in (**b**) even after cleaning and sterilization procedures, the presence of several cracks on the instrument surface (green arrows), as well as, deformation at the lateral cutting edge (yellow arrows)

5.5.2 Reciprocation and the Coronal Preflaring Procedure

Coronal preflaring, canal scouting and glide path are early steps of the mechanical canal preparation. Coronal preflaring can be defined as an extension of the access cavity into the most coronal aspect of the canal space (Fig. 5.27). Flaring the coronal portion of a narrow, calcified, or difficult-to-access root canal affords several benefits by relocating the canal pathway, such as:

- Improving tactile sensation and control by removing calcifications and dentin overhangs, which allows further unimpeded access to the apical third to facilitate canal scouting and apical patency procedures;
- Facilitating larger instruments to reach the apical critical zone more loosely;
- Reducing procedural errors such as loss of working length and canal transportation;
- Optimizing infection control, considering that bacterial load is greater at the coronal and middle thirds of the canal. Thus, coronal preflaring allows the removal of most bacteria present in the canal space and deeper insertion of the irrigation needle in the earlier stages of Shaping for Cleaning procedures, optimizing irrigation and, consequently, improving infection control. The enlarged area created by coronal preflaring acts as an escape route for the irrigating solution, enabling better flow and reflux of the irrigating solution;
- Better control of postoperative pain due to less bacterial extrusion through the apical foramen;
- Better control of instrument fracture. According to Ehrhardt et al. [27], the use of an Mtwo system (VDW, Germany) after coronal preflaring results in a low fracture rate, even when reusing the instrument five times;

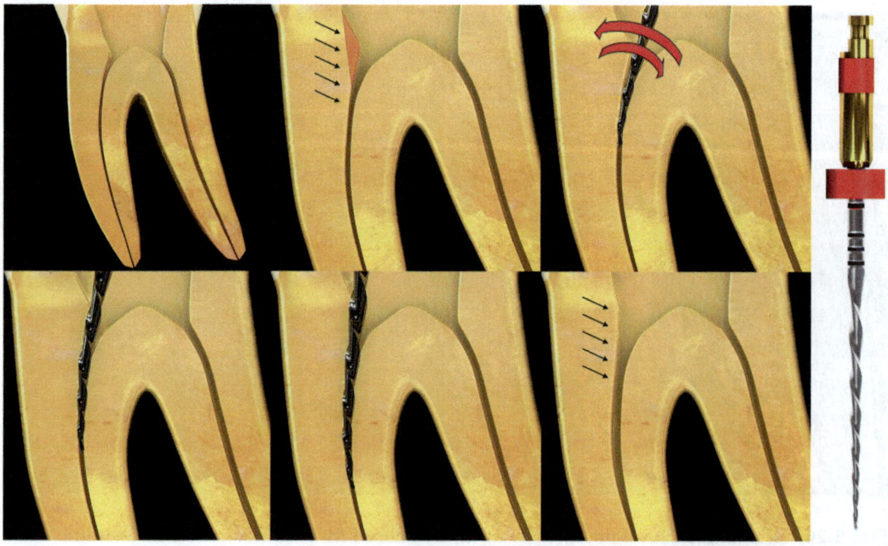

Fig. 5.27 Illustration of the coronal preflaring performed by the R25 instrument in a mesial canal of a maxillary molar demonstrating its ability to remove calcifications and dentin overhangs and allow further unimpeded access to the apical third, facilitating canal scouting and apical patency procedures

- Coronal preflaring leads to more accurate apical sizing [28, 29], and this information can be useful to define an appropriate final diameter for apical shaping.

Independently of all the aforesaid advantages of the preflaring procedure, overpreparation of canals by unbalanced enlargement of the coronal region through the use of large-tapered instruments can weaken the root [30, 31]. Ultimately, it can compromise the outcome of the root canal treatment due to the amount of dentinal tissue removed in this key and strategic structural region, the so-called pericervical dentin (PCD). The preservation of this region can be even more important to maintain the strength of endodontically treated teeth than a significant occlusal/cuspal reduction [32]. Overall, logical reasoning claims that the reduction of PCD implies in the weakening of the root structure and decreased resistance to vertical root fracture. Actually, the more tapered and flared is the root canal at the coronal region, the weaker the root resistance tends to be. PCD was defined by Clark and Khademi in their opinionated theoretical paper [33] as "*... the dentin near the alveolar crest. This critical zone, roughly 4 mm coronal to the crestal bone and extending 4 mm apical to it, is crucial to transferring load from the occlusal table to the root, and much of the PCD is irreplaceable.*" The authors moved ahead saying that no man-made material can compensate for the loss of tooth structure at the PCD area.

With the popularization of NiTi rotary instruments and the mentioned reasons, it is easy to understand the rapid influx of new instruments specifically designed to perform a better-balanced coronal preflaring procedure. The introduction of superelastic alloys associated with variable taper instruments (not following the ISO system) opened the way to new technical possibilities for coronal preflaring. Although several rotary NiTi instruments were specially designed to this task, such as Orifice Shapers from the ProFile system (Dentsply Tulsa Dental, USA) or Vortex orifice openers (Dentsply Tulsa Dental, USA), they have never really become popular, and none of them has become the archetypal instrument for the coronal preflaring procedure. On the other hand, variable regressive-taper reciprocating NiTi instruments are able to perform coronal preflaring and enlargement of the main root canal space in a significantly more conservative approach using the very same single instrument used for final shape. In fact, coronal preflaring with a single reciprocating instrument is done simultaneously with the canal scouting and presents at least four advantages:

- More conservative coronal preparation due to the regressive taper of the reciprocating instrument;
- Better technical workflow as a function of fewer transoperative stages and shortage of instruments used;
- Shorter learning curve;
- Improved safety by using reciprocating movement per se.

Thus, it is not erroneous to consider coronal preflaring performed with a single regressive-taper reciprocating instrument as an efficient technical approach, aligning the most up-to-date concepts of mechanical shaping and also emphasizing the preservation of irreplaceable dental tissues (Figs. 5.28 and 5.29).

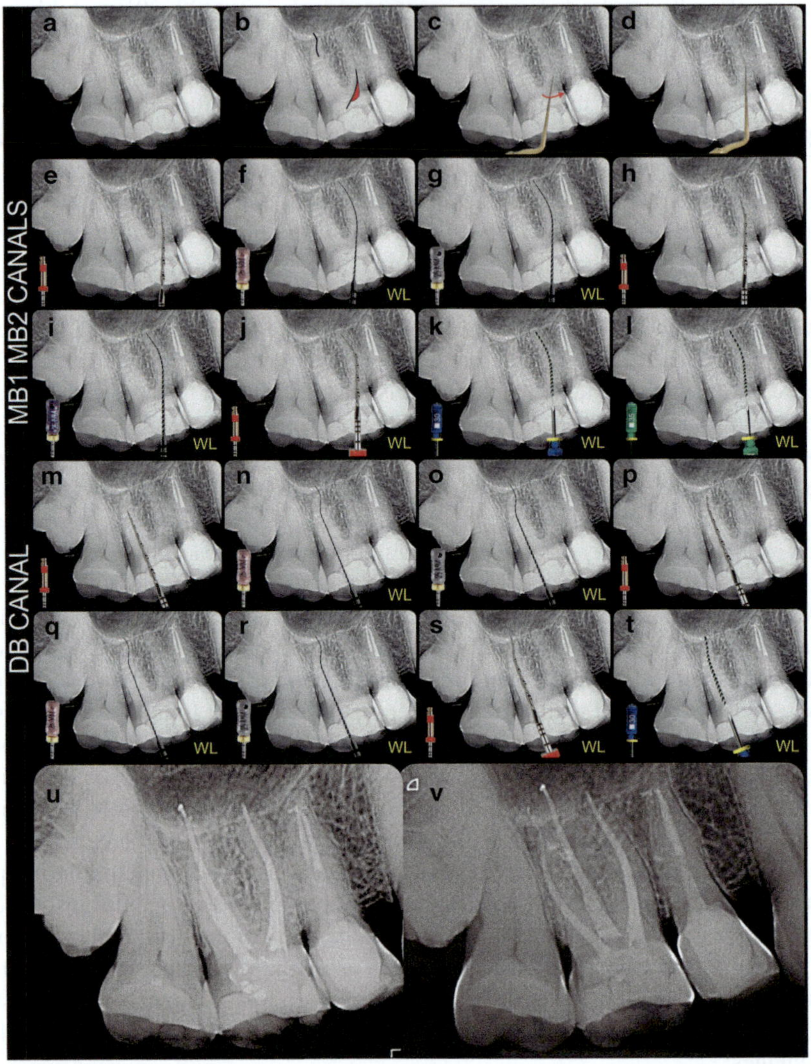

Fig. 5.28 Maxillary first right molar referred for endodontic treatment. (**a**) Preoperative radiograph showing narrow canals. (**b**) Observe the interference at the canal orifice of the mesial root (in red) and a double curvature at the apical portion of the DB canal. (**c, d**) Removal of the dentin at the orifice of the mesial canals with an ultrasonic tip. (**e**) Root canal preflaring with Reciproc R25 instrument up to the coronal portion of the mesial canals. (**f**) Scouting of the mesial canals with a size 06 K-file. (**g**) Working length determination with a size 10 K-file. (**h**) Enlargement of the mesial canals up to the middle third with Reciproc R25 instrument. (**i**) Glide path with a size 10 K-file. (**j**) Reciproc R25 up to the working length. (**k, l**) Apical enlargement with hand files sizes 30 and 35. (**m**) Preparation of the DB canal with Reciproc R25 up to the curvature. (**n, o**) Scouting of the canal up to working length with hand files sizes 06 and 08. (**p**) Reciproc R25 enlarged the first canal curvature, but did not advance beyond this point. (**q, r**) Glide path was performed with K-files sizes 06 and 08. (**s**) Reciproc R25 enlarging the DB canal up to the working length. (**t**) Final enlargement of the DB canal with a size 30 hand file. (**u, v**) Postoperative radiographs in different angulations

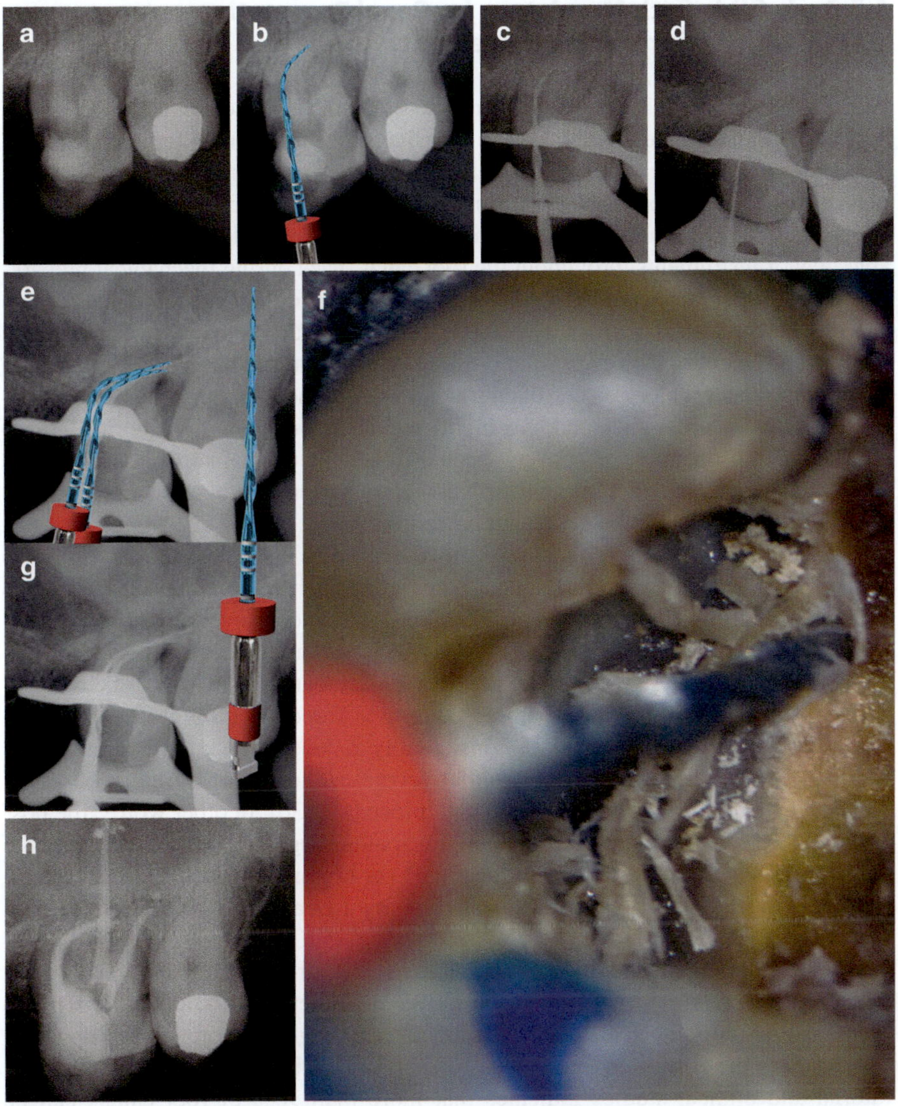

Fig. 5.29 (**a**) Asymptomatic maxillary second molar with narrow and curved mesial canals. (**b**) Preflaring procedure with the R25 instrument up to the middle third of the mesial canals. (**c, d**) After coronal flaring, canal scouting, apical patency and glide path procedures up to super loose K-file size 10. (**e–g**) Mechanical preparation of mesial canals with the Reciproc R25 instrument to the working length. (**h**) Immediate postoperative radiograph

5.5.3 Is Glide Path Mandatory for Canal Preparation with Reciprocating Movement?

As described in Chap. 3, glide path is commonly defined as a series of clinical procedural steps to pre-shape the canal space from its orifice to the main foramen [34, 35]. This procedure is done with either small SS hand files or a combination of small SS files and one small, tapered NiTi instrument. The objective of creating a glide path is to ensure that there is a free pathway with a minimal size to allow a safe and predictable flow of instruments throughout the root canal space during mechanical preparation [34, 35]. In other words, the glide path is a transoperative procedure that renders root canal shaping safer to rotary NiTi systems by reducing the risk of instrument binding and fracture. However, an interesting paradoxical situation is created as long as one important problem is controlled (fracture rate of the rotary instrument), another one emerges since the glide path is a highly technically demanding, laborious, time-consuming transoperative maneuver, which is frequently the main operative challenge of the treatment. Thus, the safe use of NiTi rotary systems embraces a considerable learning curve related to the glide path procedure.

The introduction of reciprocating movement with NiTi instruments in 2008 raised new perspectives on mechanical preparation of the root canal, and nowadays there is a well-built knowledge base showing its benefits over rotary movement [9–12, 14]. Yet, one peculiar point deserves special attention because it stands for its unique ability: to safely prepare the majority of root canals using only one reciprocating instrument without glide path. According to Yared [14], this ability is appealing because the learning curve is considerably reduced by simplification of the technique, while it reduces the potential for procedural errors usually observed when using hand files during the glide path procedure [36]. In other words, the possibility to explore the root canal without glide path in regular cases may become the mainspring feature to promote an educational paradigm shift related to canal shaping, as it drastically differs from the rotary's mainstream, in which the glide path maneuver is mandatory.

The best example is the first generation of the Reciproc instrument, the so-called classic Reciproc or the M-Wire Reciproc R25 instrument which, as function of the reciprocating motion per se, tends to follow the existing natural canal path up to the apex without the glide path for most cases [37]. Currently, evidence from both laboratorial and clinical studies indicates that more than 90% of root canals can be safely prepared with the M-Wire Reciproc R25 instrument without glide path [37–39], as a result of the interplay of three main factors: the reciprocation kinematics, the instrument's cross-section, and the heat-treated superelastic M-Wire alloy. Thus, the reciprocating movement prevents instrument fracture even without glide path as a consequence of the cyclical reversal of rotation, which drastically reduces the torsional stress on the instrument. Gathered with the reduced S-shaped cross-sectional metal mass that provides Reciproc with an enhanced cutting ability, the safety and efficiency of the R25 instrument without glide path can be easily explained.

However, it is important to understand that when the Reciproc system was launched in the late 2010s, there was no evidence to support its use without glide path for the majority of cases, but only and uniquely the manufacturer's claim. A radiography-based decision-making algorithm was developed by the manufacturer to guide clinicians in deciding whether it would be necessary to create a glide path prior the use of the Reciproc instrument. This decision-making algorithm was based on the initial X-ray as the starting point and encloses a clear orientation: if the canal is 100% visible on the initial X-ray and also if it is straight or shows moderate curvature, a priori, glide path is not required.

As time went by, extensive clinical and scientific knowledge was created about not only the Reciproc instrument but also the reciprocating movement, and experienced clinicians realized that the R25 is able to scout and shape much more challenging root canals than those described by the manufacturer's algorithm. It explains why the manufacturer's current usage recommendation no longer mentions the decision-making algorithm (https://www.vdw-dental.com/en/products/detail/reciproc/). The ongoing recommendation specifies the following: (1) after preparation of 2/3 of the working length with the R25, if an ISO 10 hand file goes straight to the length without being pre-curved, no glide path is needed and (2) whenever the R25 instrument presents some difficulty in advancing toward the apex, a glide path up to ISO 15 should be produced (Fig. 5.30). Overall, the current orientation has become

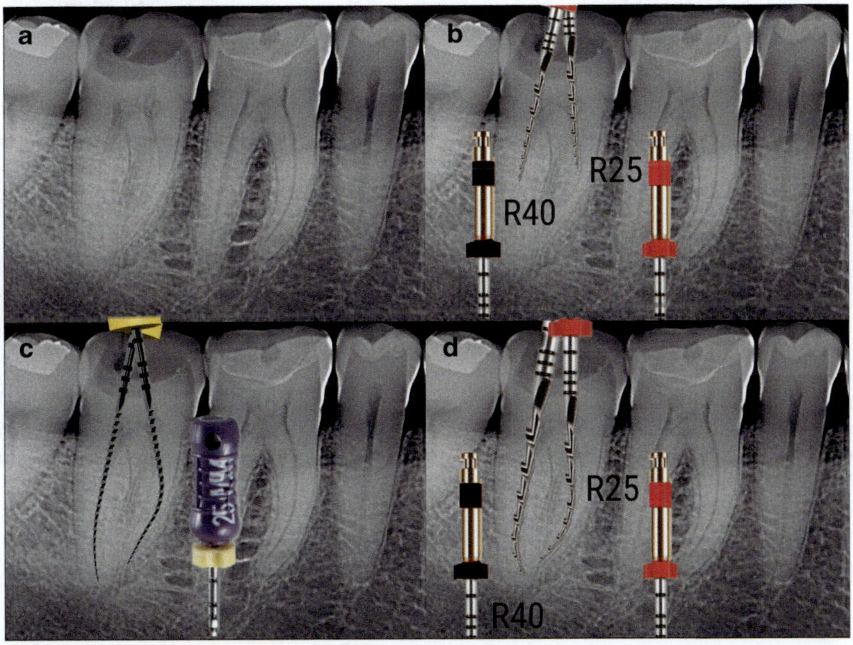

5.30 (**a**) Preoperative periapical radiograph of a mandibular right second molar referred for root canal treatment due to an irreversible pulpitis showing visible canals and moderate curvature of the mesial root. (**b**) Coronal enlargement was initially performed using Reciproc R40 in the distal canal and R25 in the mesial canals. (**c**) Then, working length was established with ISO size 10 K-files. (**d**) Final canal shaping was done with Reciproc R40 and R25 up to the working length in the distal and mesial canals, respectively. (**e**) Postoperative radiograph after root canal filling using the single cone technique

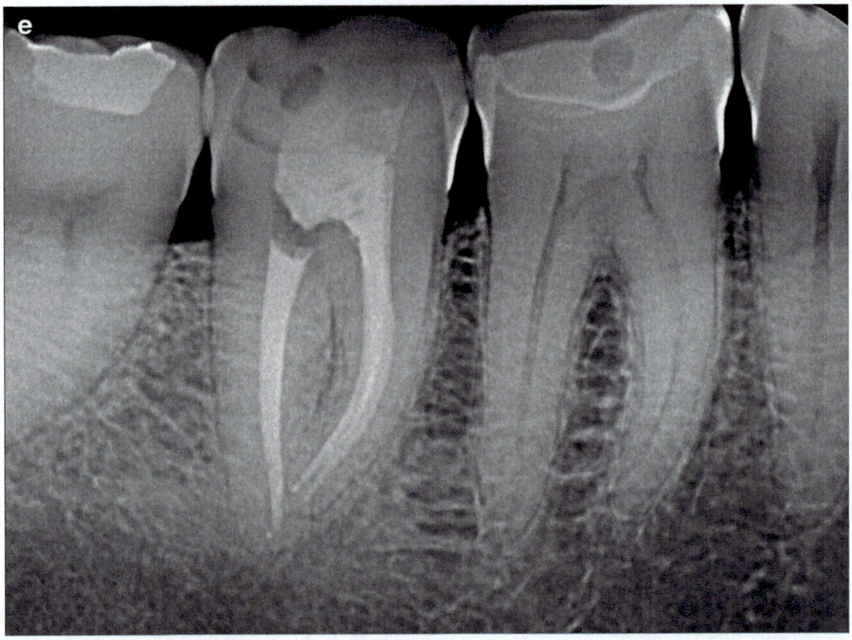

Fig. 5.30 (continued)

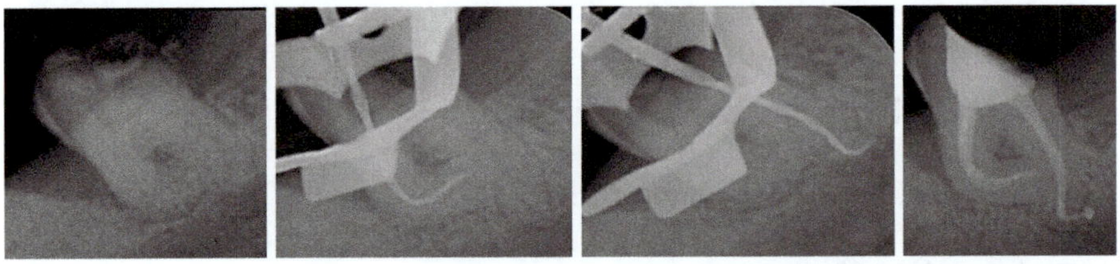

Fig. 5.31 Mandibular left second molar referred for root canal treatment due to an irreversible pulpitis showing no visible canals and severe curvature in the mesial and distal roots in the preoperative radiography. The Reciproc R25 instrument was used to shape the mesial and distal canals without glide path. Postoperative radiograph shows root canal filling using single cone technique. (Courtesy of Dr. Thodoris Mandas, Greece)

more inclusive inasmuch as the R25 instrument has been shown to scout and negotiate more challenging canals, such as curved root canals (Figs. 5.31, 5.32, and 5.33) and the MB2 canal of maxillary molars, in a high number of cases without glide path (Figs. 5.34 and 5.35). Once the canal orifice of the MB2 is located, another challenge faced by clinicians is to scout and negotiate this typically narrow, curved

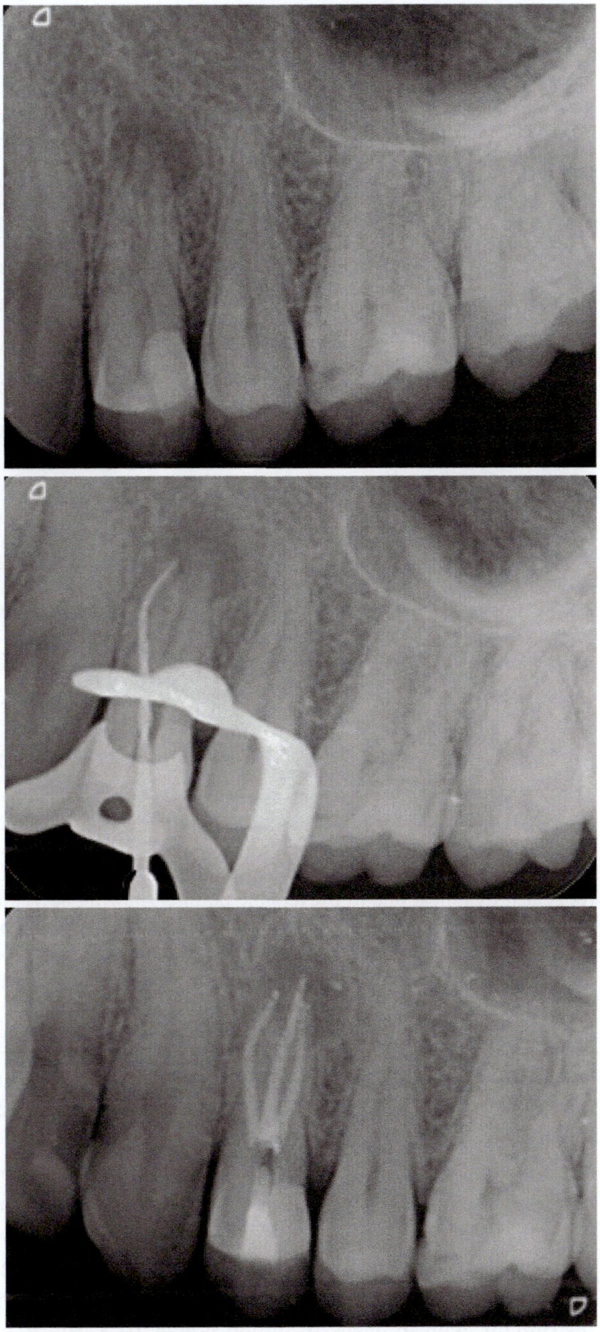

Fig. 5.32 Three-rooted maxillary left first premolar referred for root canal treatment due to pulp necrosis and apical periodontitis. The Reciproc R25 instrument was used to shape the canals without glide path. Root canals were filled with the single cone technique. (Courtesy of Dr. Thodoris Mandas, Greece)

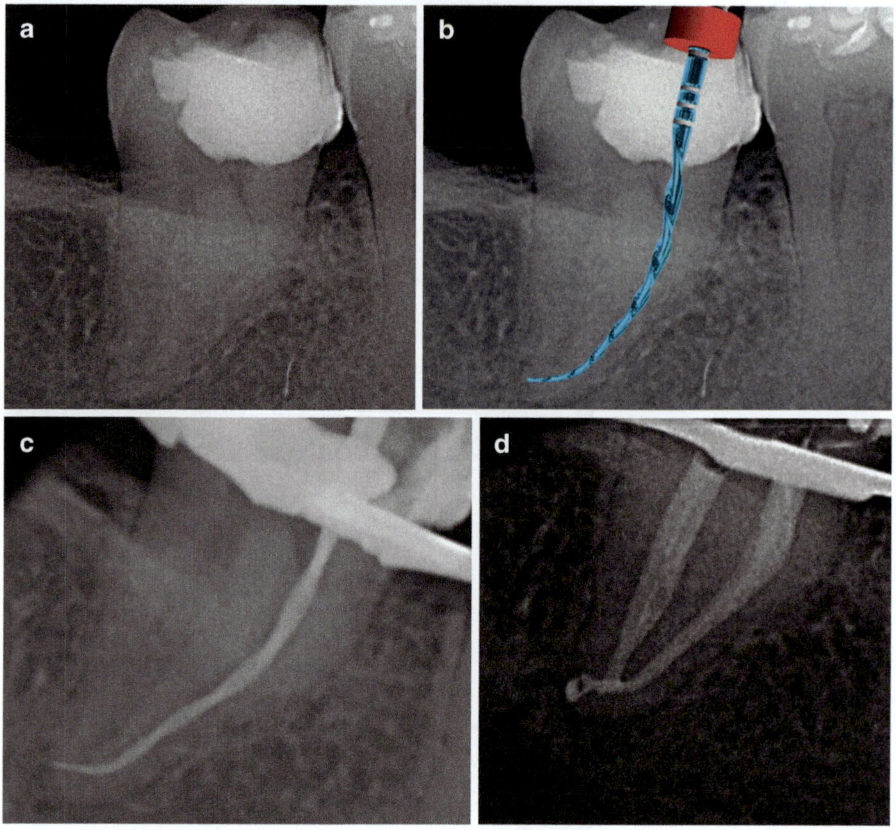

Fig. 5.33 (**a**) Preoperative periapical radiograph of a mandibular right third molar referred for root canal treatment due to irreversible pulpitis showing no visible canals and a long and curved mesial root. (**b**) Preoperative planning of mesial canal shaping procedure. (**c**) The Reciproc R25 was used to shape the canals without glide path. (**d**) Postoperative radiograph after root canal filling using the single cone technique. (Courtesy of Dr. Thodoris Mandas, Greece)

and intricate root canal. Zuolo et al. [39] conducted a prospective clinical study to verify the scouting ability of the Reciproc R25 instrument in 341 MB2 canals of maxillary molars. The authors showed that M-Wire R25 instruments were able to reach the working length in 85.63% of cases compared to 57.48% of cases using a conventional hand file, demonstrating the improved scouting efficiency of the R25. De-Deus et al. [40] also studied the scouting performance of the Reciproc Blue instrument in 250 root canals of extracted molars. In 50 canals in which a size 10 K-file was unable to reach the working length, the R25 Blue instrument succeeded in 47 of them. This result highlights the great scouting ability of the R25 instrument even in cases in which a size 10 K-file is unable to reach the working length. In summary, it may be said that canal enlargement using R25 instruments is a less sensitive procedure when compared with the technically demanding glide path procedure with hand or rotary instruments, rendering a more predictable

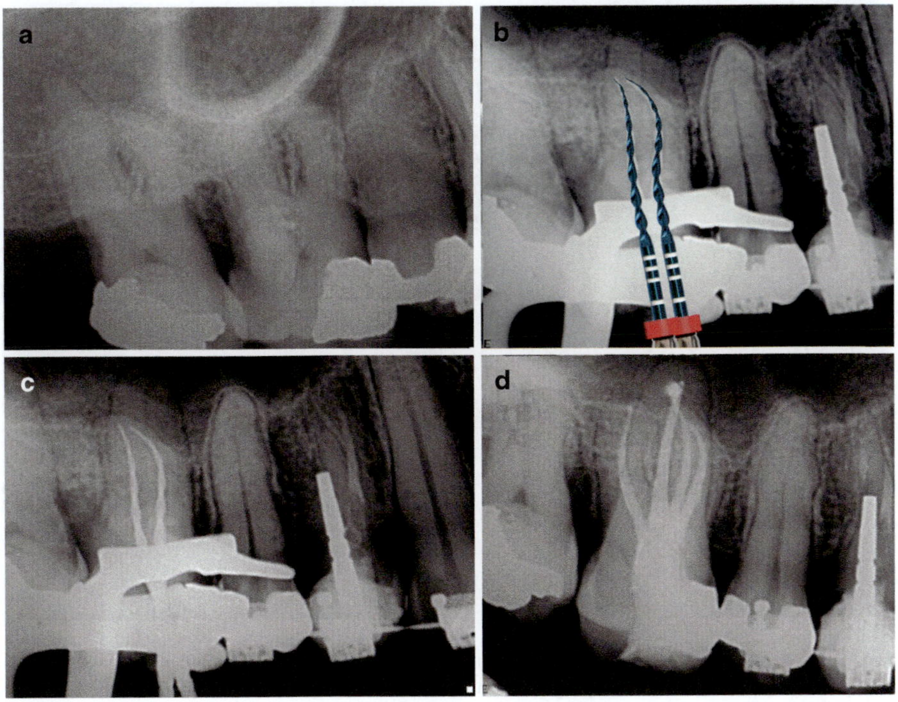

Fig. 5.34 (**a**) Symptomatic maxillary right first molar referred for root canal treatment. (**b**) Preoperative planning of the shaping procedure of the mesiobuccal canals (MB1 and MB2). (**c**) After scouting, MB1 and MB2 canals were enlarged with R25 instruments without glide path up to the WL. (**d**) Immediate postoperative radiograph

transoperative step and one less prone to error, even when performed by undergraduate students, which means that operator experience may not influence the incidence of fracture of reciprocating instruments [41].

5.5.4 Feedback of the R25 Instrument

In the long run, clinicians experienced with the Reciproc instrument naturally replaced the radiographic-based decision-making algorithm with the so-called "feedback of the R25 instrument." Feedback is a word that means the response to a particular request, process, activity or event and, in this particular case, can be used to refer to the specific ability of the R25 instrument to "respond" to the operator, giving a real time information about what is happening within the limits of its action in the root canal space. The R25 instrument is normally able to progressively advance toward the apex in a smooth and continuous way until reaching the main foramen. However, the inability of the R25 to continue advance at a certain level of the canal constitutes an important feedback that must be identified by the operator as a token signal of alert (Fig. 5.36). This intracanal obstacle indicates to the

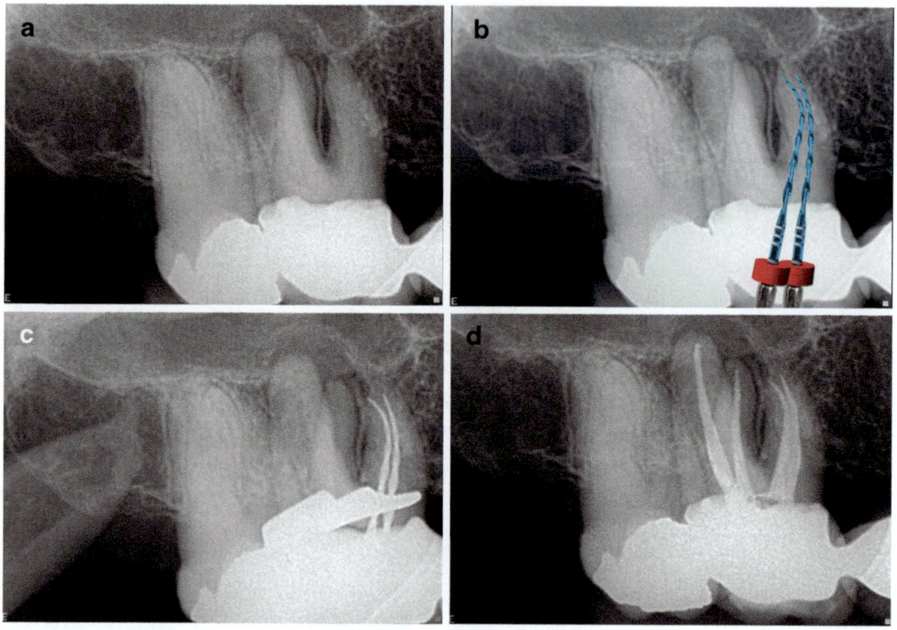

Fig. 5.35 (**a**) Asymptomatic maxillary right first molar referred for root canal treatment. (**b**) Preoperative planning of the shaping procedure of the mesiobuccal canals (MB1 and MB2). (**c**) Scouting and shaping procedures of the MB1 and MB2 with Reciproc R25 instruments without glide path up to the WL. (**d**) Immediate postoperative radiograph. (Courtesy of Dr. Evaldo Rodrigues, Brasil)

operator (feedback) a technical difficulty that may increase the risk of ledging or instrument separation. In other words, the R25 instrument is "saying" to the dentist that it needs help to finish the shaping procedure by creating a glide path. This unique feature of the R25 instrument to provide feedback to the operator in particular challenging situations is welcome as NiTi rotary instruments brought a critical loss of tactile sensitivity compared to manual instruments. When a rotary instrument confronts a difficulty in the apical advancement, its high rotational speed usually does not allow the operator to have tactile perception in time to avoid fracture of the instrument. The R25 instrument is the only motor-driven instrument able to provide accurate tactile feedback to the operator, thus facilitating the resolution of the case by another operative action route.

5.6 Finally, Low Risk of Fracture!

Instrument separation during shaping procedures with rotary NiTi systems is an undesired event that afflicts any clinician, even though previous studies have clearly demonstrated that the fracture of an instrument per se does not significantly alter the treatment prognosis [42–44]. Historically, to overcome this risk, a series of

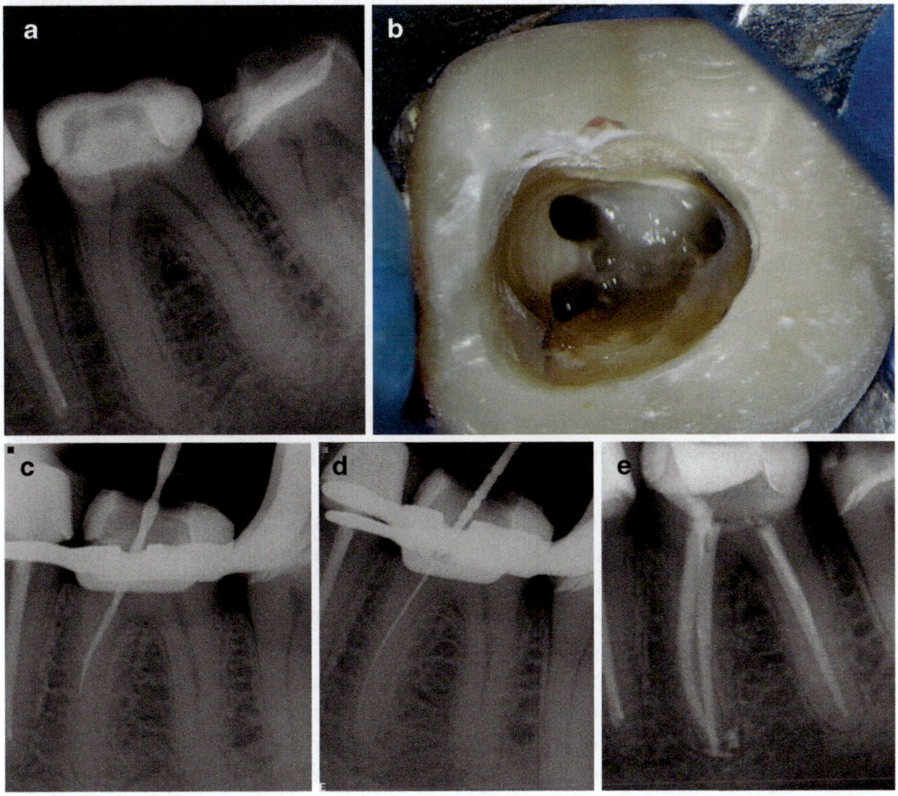

Fig. 5.36 (**a**) Symptomatic mandibular left first molar with narrow and long mesial canals referred for root canal treatment. (**b**) Occlusal view of the pulp chamber showing the root canal orifices after initial shaping procedures with the Reciproc R25 instrument. (**c**) The R25 instrument was able to progressively advance until the middle third when it suddenly stopped. The inability of this specific instrument to move forward to the apical direction is a kind of a feedback that must be identified by the operator as a token signal of alert as the instrument needs help to reach the apex. In other words, the R25 instrument is "saying" to the dentist that it needs help to finish the shaping procedure by creating a glide path. (**d**) Manual glide path to reach a super loose size 10 K-file up to the working length. (**e**) Immediate postoperative radiograph

modifications to the instruments have been suggested, including new NiTi alloys and variations in the design. However, despite such innovations, clinical studies still report a wide variation in the fracture rate. This means that it is not possible to predict the fracture of instruments driven in continuous rotation movement. To understand this statement, it is important to review some data widely explored in Chap. 4 of this textbook. Sattapan et al. [45] evaluated the type and frequency of defects after routine clinical use of NiTi Quantec Series 2000 instruments. Approximately 50% of them had visible defects, including fracture (21%) or defects without fracture (28%). Another clinical study demonstrated that during shaping procedures of 419 mandibular and maxillary molars using the ProFile system, 21 (5%) of the tested instruments fractured [46]. Patiño et al. [47] found a fracture rate of 26% when rotary NiTi instruments were used without a previous glide path as opposed to 12% when a glide path was performed. Wolcott et al. [48] evaluated the separation incidence of the ProTaper Universal rotary system in 4,652 root canals and observed an overall fracture rate of 2.4% with no significant difference over the first four uses. Inan and Gonulol [49] evaluated 593 Mtwo rotary instruments after clinical use and demonstrated that 25.8% of them showed some type of defect, with a fracture rate of 16.02%. In addition, Wu et al. [50] demonstrated an overall instrument separation incidence of 2.6%. Similar results were observed by Ehrhardt and colleagues [27] who reported a fracture rate of 1.98% when using Mtwo instruments for root canal preparation of mandibular and maxillary molars and premolars with previous coronal preflaring. These authors also observed a high deformation rate in instruments sizes 10/0.04 and 15/0.05.

The wide range of fracture rates reported in the literature (from 1.98% to 26%) highlights the unpredictability of this phenomenon in clinical practice and could certainly be related to multiple factors such as instrument design, number of uses, root canal anatomy, and operator experience. Nevertheless, among all of these studies, two common points may account for the fracture rate unpredictability: (1) the use of instruments in continuous rotation movement and (2) a variable number of reuses. Against this mainstream arises one of the most advantageous aspects of reciprocating movement: the improved security-efficiency binomial based on well-built scientific and clinical evidence. The first clinical study that evaluated the separation incidence of a reciprocating instrument (WaveOne) was performed over an 18-month period in which four experienced and calibrated endodontists performed endodontic treatment on posterior teeth. A total of 2,215 canals (711 teeth) were treated and only three instruments fractured (0.42% of cases) [51]. One may argue that these results are directly related to the experience of the clinicians; however, another clinical study assessed the fracture incidence of reciprocating systems when used by students in an endodontic undergraduate program and also showed low fracture rates [22]. In this study, 2,056 root canals from 826 teeth were included and the fracture rate was 0.84% and 0.93% for WaveOne and Reciproc systems, respectively. Shen et al. [52] also showed similar low fracture rates when single-use instruments were employed by endodontists and resident students. Out of 438 WaveOne instruments collected (from 438 cases), there were only two fractures (0.5%). As comparison between endodontists and students was performed, the authors concluded that fracture of these instruments was not influenced by operator experience—a unique feature of reciprocating movement. These results are in line with the study of Rodrigues et al. [38] that showed only three cases (0.44%) of fracture after canal preparation of 673 teeth with Reciproc instruments by four specialists in endodontics.

Even when instruments are reused, the safety of reciprocating movement is sustained. Bueno et al. [23] evaluated the fracture resistance of the Reciproc R25 and WaveOne Primary instruments according to the number of uses during the root canal preparation of posterior teeth. In this clinical study, three experienced specialists treated 358 posterior teeth (1,130 root canals) using 60 R25 instruments and 60 WaveOne Primary instruments. Each instrument was used in up to three teeth. After

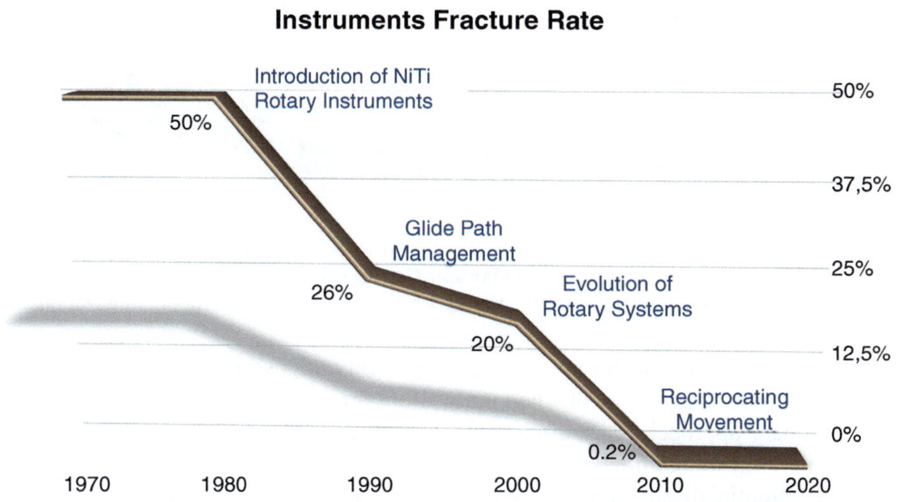

Fig. 5.37 Timeline illustration of the impact of technical advancements over the fracture rate of NiTi instruments along the recent history of root canal instrumentation technology. Observe that the glide path management and some specific advancements in the technology of rotary NiTi instruments, although have helped to control the fracture rate, the ultimate revolution in instrument separation control was given by the reciprocating movement

the first use, the instruments had their ABS O-ring removed and were sterilized in an autoclave between each use. In case of fracture or deformation during preparation, the instrument was discarded. The results of this study showed a low fracture rate of 0.84% (2 R25 and 1 WaveOne Primary instruments), all of them in mandibular molars.

More recently, Bueno et al. [24] in a prospective clinical study evaluated the incidence of fracture observed after root canal treatment of 750 maxillary or mandibular molars using WaveOne Gold instruments. Intracanal procedures were performed according to the manufacturer's recommendations, and each instrument was used in a single case. No instrument fracture was observed. Based on the aforementioned laboratorial and clinical studies, reciprocating movement can be considered safe if instruments are discarded after each appointment. Within these results, it seems fair and timely to say, FINALLY, LOW RISK OF FRACTURE! (Fig. 5.37).

5.7 Rational Approach for Reciprocating Preparation of Root Canals: A Clinical Perspective

Hans-Willi Herrmann

Almost three decades after the initial market launch there is no doubt that engine-driven rotary NiTi instruments not only have found their place in endodontics, but also led to a paradigm shift replacing more than 100-year prevailing standard of root canal preparation with hand files. The withdrawal of the hand instrumentation as the

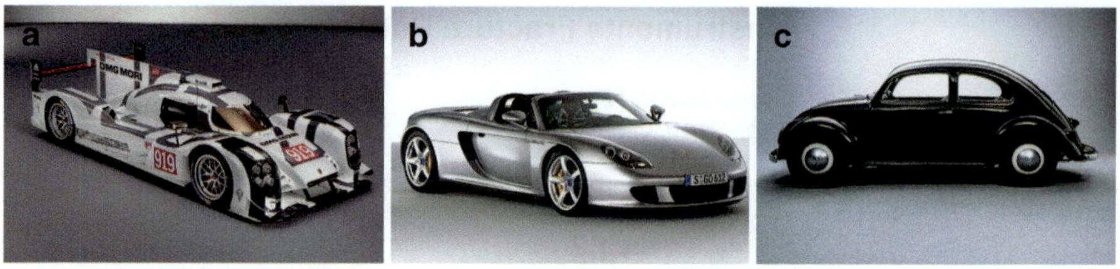

Fig. 5.38 Three types of cars designed by Ferdinand Porsche. (**a**) The Le Mans Porsche 919 Hybrid, a long-distance racing car. (**b**) The Porsche Carrera GT, a street-legal open sports convertible; and (**c**) a Volkswagen Beetle, an all-time automobile classic from the era of mobilization

gold standard, however, did not succeed overnight and a significant resistance had to be overcome. This is typical when innovations are created. At the beginning, most revolutionary approaches are often critically considered, taking an unsatisfactorily long time until things finally change. Given the existing practice-relevant difficulties and potential disadvantages of hand instrumentation, one would think that practitioners should be grateful for innovative new concepts. The opposite was the case. The strong criticism expressed firstly against the rotary and later, with similar vehemence, against the reciprocating instruments, seems to be conclusive and far exaggerated as expressed at the time of their respective commercialization.

So, how could this cognitive dissonance phenomenon be explained?

To answer this question, a real-life comparison used many times by this author in lectures and seminars is helpful and amazingly led to the same result. In this query, participants have to identify common features between the three main root canal preparation techniques (hand, rotary, and reciprocating) and three types of cars, all designed by Ferdinand Porsche: The Le Mans Porsche 919 Hybrid, a long-distance racing car (Fig. 5.38a), the Porsche Carrera GT, a street-legal open sports convertible (Fig. 5.38b), and a Volkswagen Beetle, an all-time automobile classic from the era of mobilization (Fig. 5.38c). As a result of this query, dentists in the audience unanimously decide for the VW Beetle as representing hand instrumentation. According to their opinion, this car was a worldwide standard in the past, but it is now obsolete, an outdated icon of automobile history, as poorly efficient and antiquated type of mobility that was discarded by technological progress. As far as the other two techniques are concerned, the respondents subsequently find it difficult to make a clear judgment. The assignment is individually different and non-uniform, a clear vote for one or the other technique does not want to appear.

Concerning the car selection, it seems that decision-making based on a rather emotional approach led to a fundamental misjudging. The way out of the aforementioned insoluble dilemma can be found if one is willing to allow a different way of looking at things, to replace the intuitively made emotions-based categorization with a rational examination, and to regard the Porsche long-distance sports car as a symbol of manual instrumentation. The Porsche 919 is a highly sophisticated machine that can only be driven efficiently and safely by a handful of specialists worldwide, who are able to push the car to its limit at maximum speed around a racetrack for the duration of the race at their physical and mental peak. Anyone who, nevertheless, tried it as a nonprofessional would probably fail catastrophically.

Apart from that, non-existing driving comfort, an extremely high noise level and exorbitant fuel consumption as well as a lack of road registration prohibit everyday use. So, the parallel to hand instrumentation is quite obvious. Only a very few dentists worldwide are able to carry out root canal preparation in complex situations using solely hand files, in a way that it does not only entirely matches the anatomical conditions, but also enables the root canals to be filled using warm gutta-percha techniques. The bottom line for hand preparation is that it is technique-sensitive, inefficient and therefore time-consuming, resulting in a fine line between success and failure.

The Porsche Carrera GT stands as a symbol for the continuous rotary preparation and thus represents the various facets of a technique simple at a first glance, but in reality, not free of problems. The Carrera GT appears as a modern, contemporary sports convertible with an impressive exterior design language, advertising as a car that can be handled by any driver with appropriate skills, since it is allowed to be moved in everyday traffic. However, we are dealing here with another pure-bred sports car. An automobile wolf in sheepskin. Similar to the Porsche 919, a detailed engagement with the topic and driving seminars given by racing specialists are mandatory to handle the car, comparable to hands-on courses for learning how to work with rotary instruments. After overcoming these obstacles, the driver is able to drive the car in regular traffic under normal conditions, i.e., clean, dry, straight road, adequate speed and acceleration. It changes, however, if extreme situations emerge abruptly, such as in the presence of fog, rain, bendy, and slippery road, combined with high speed. Then, unexpected situations, which are usually manageable for experienced drivers, can go beyond limits, leading from small accidents up to the total loss of the car and lives of the occupants. Again, the analogy to root canal preparation with rotary NiTi instruments is evident: after acquiring basic knowledge, better and faster results can be achieved with rotary techniques in simple situations (straight or slightly curved root canals, and uncomplicated canal anatomies), compared to hand instrumentation. Unforeseen difficulties, however, can either be mastered successfully, depending on the clinician's skills, or fatally lead to problems such as instrument fracture or ledge formation which, in worst cases, may end with tooth loss. In view of the previously described problems, many practitioners return to hand preparation, despite all the associated difficulties, or avoid switching to rotary techniques.

5.7.1 Main Reasons for Using Reciprocating Instruments

In the shadow of the sports cars, the VW Beetle is barely noticed. It has neither the nimbus nor the attractive looks of the prestigious Porsches. Nevertheless, the Beetle is one of the most successful cars ever produced and responsible for the global automobile mass mobilization after World War II. Its simple but reliable technology associated with its high suitability for everyday use led the Beetle to the most distant corners of the earth. Moreover, the small number of required switches makes it easier to get started than most other cars and, probably, every reader of this Chapter would be able to drive it safely in a road traffic after short training. So, what do make the reciprocating instruments the proverbial "VW Beetle" of engine-driven canal preparation? With these instruments it is possible to prepare the root canals more easily, quickly and safely than any rotary systems. This equally applies to the beginner as well as to the advanced user or even to the specialist. In fact, through their specific rotary movement the reciprocating systems eliminate the major disadvantages of continuously rotating instruments as they allow to successfully negotiate and prepare root canals with a small number of instruments or, in many cases, with a single instrument, reducing the risk of fracture to a minimum. But there is another important aspect to consider: instruments activated in reciprocating motion tend to find their own way apically through the root canal, preventing the instrument to work on the same level and not creating ledges. However, overpreparation may occur if the progression of the instrument does not stop as soon as the working length is reached. In some cases, depending on the anatomy of the root canal and the design, rotary instruments may unexpectedly be dragged into the canal, resulting in a significant change in length. On the other hand, the reciprocating movement, with its intentional "cut and relief" action, reduces the speed of apical advancement and standardizes it to a defined level. Sudden abrupt "screw-in" effect is an extremely rare incident.

5.7.2 A Simple and Easy to Learn Workflow

Root canal preparation with reciprocating instruments offers a number of advantages over the conventional rotary techniques for either beginner or skilled clinicians. This includes a faster, but nevertheless safe and simple structured, less stressful workflow using a minimum of instruments. For this reason, reciprocating instrumentation has been used as a standard preparation procedure in the authors practice limited to endodontics since 2006. They have completely replaced rotary systems over the years. Hand files are still used for scouting and to negotiate root canals, but are no longer required for canal preparation. By adopting this approach, it is possible to prepare a root canal with a single instrument size 25/0.08 like Reciproc R25, Reciproc Blue R25 (VDW, Germany) or WaveOne Gold PRIMARY (Dentsply, Switzerland) up to the working length.

In the workflow used by the author (Fig. 5.39), after initial scouting with an ISO size 10 hand file, a Reciproc R25 instrument is taken to approximately 3/4 of the estimated length of the root canal. In the next step, a small hand file is taken to working length, confirmed with an electronic apex locator. As an alternative to initial hand preparation, small reciprocating instruments like R-Pilot (VDW, Germany) or WaveOne Gold Glider (Dentsply, Switzerland) can be used in an engine-driven workflow to determine the working length. As it is possible to stop and restart the reciprocating motion any time without risk of torsional fracture, split second activation of the foot pedal or finger switch allows a very precise approach to the reference point within a fraction of a millimeter, a kind of precision that cannot be achieved with rotary instruments. In the next step, R25 instrument is then taken to the working length. If needed, based on apical gauging, increased apical preparation can be carried out with larger reciprocating instruments. To evaluate the possibility of such an approach, the "70-20-10" rule can be applied (Fig. 5.40). Based on this

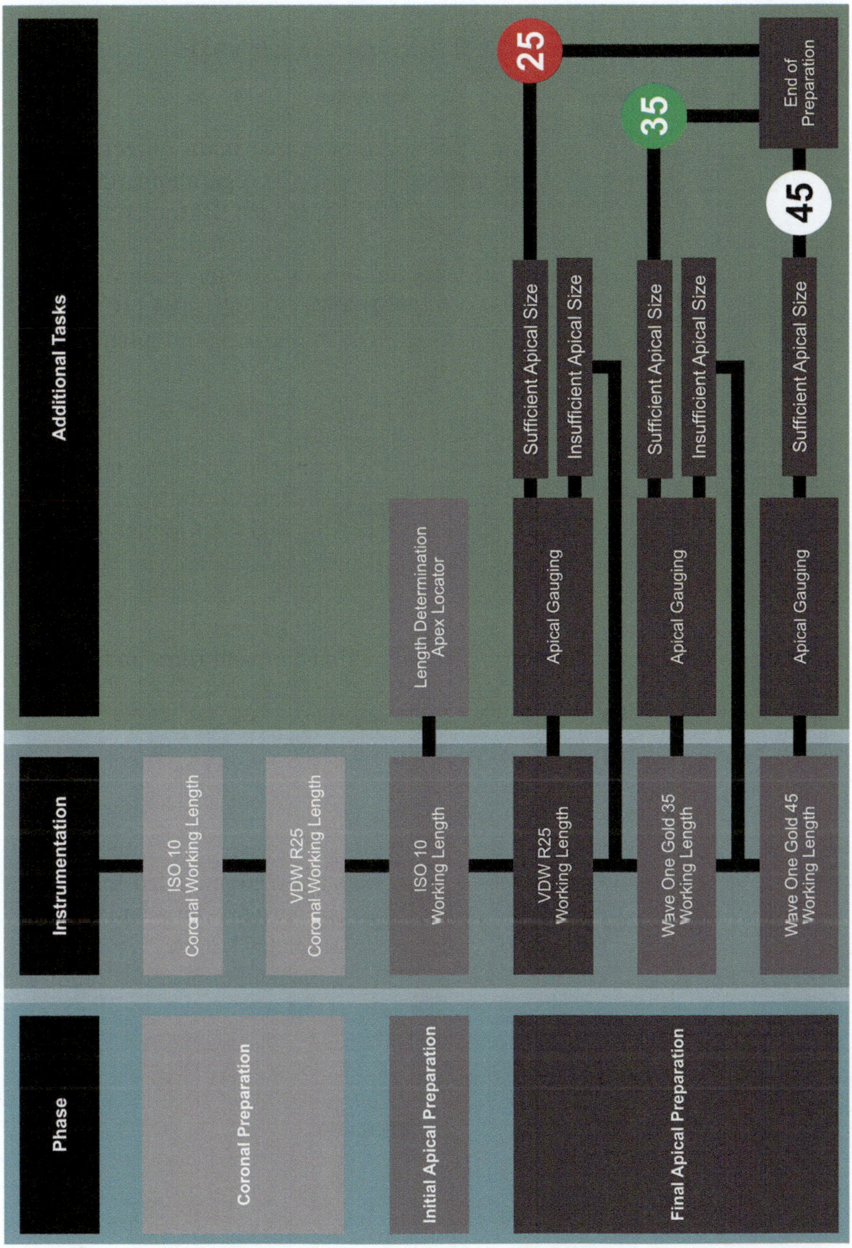

Fig. 5.39 Workflow for root canal preparation of simple cases using reciprocating instruments

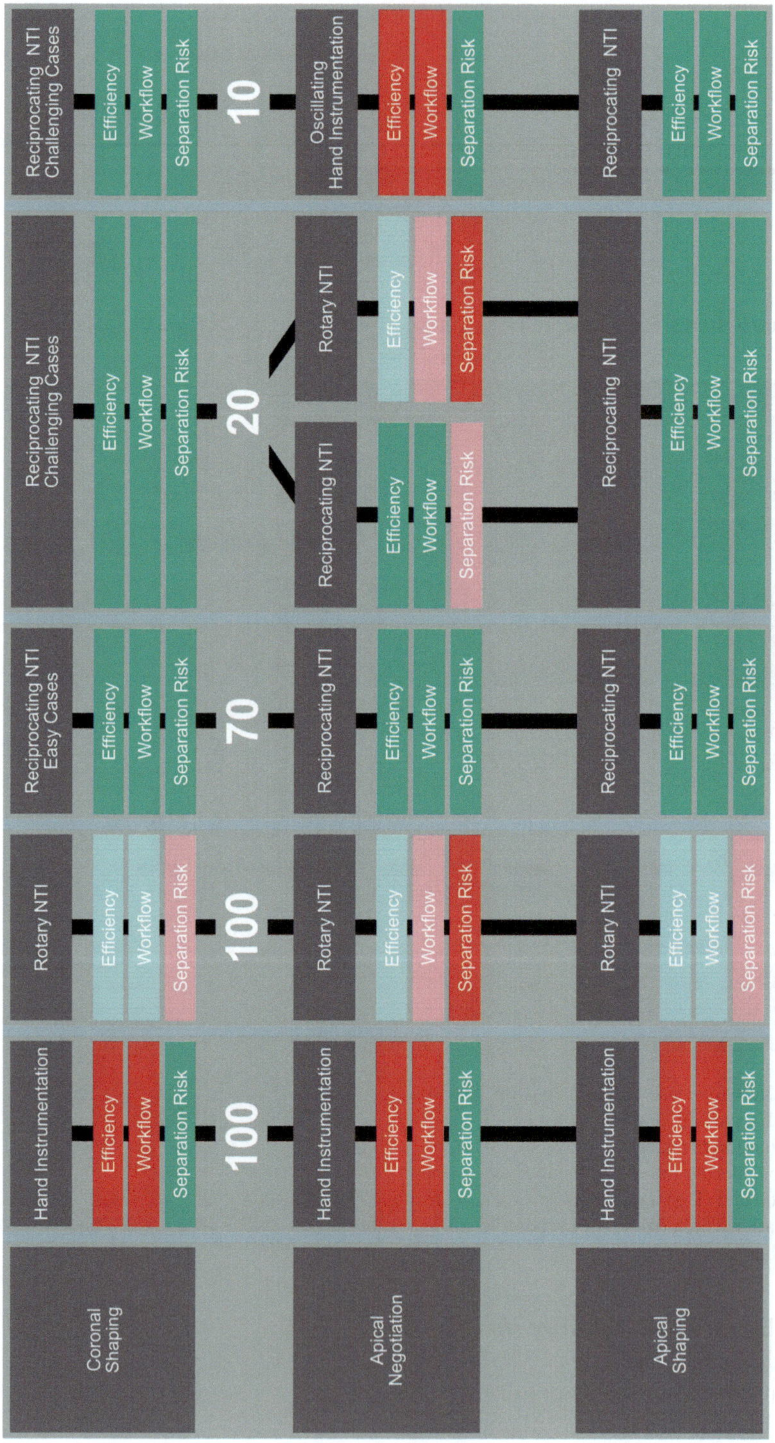

Fig. 5.40 Workflow to apply the "70-20-10" rule for root canal preparation

rule, it may be said that it is possible to prepare 70% of root canals with a single instrument to working length in such a fast and simple manner (Fig. 5.41). In 20% of the cases, this same approach is achievable, but requires significantly more time because of the necessary recapitulations. So, the experienced practitioner prefers a hybrid approach (Fig. 5.42) using smaller rotary or reciprocating instruments for the initial apical enlargement (Fig. 5.43) In the other 10% of the cases (for beginners), or 3–5% for experienced clinicians, it is not possible to carry out the treatment up to the working length with reciprocating or rotary instruments. In this situation, a time-consuming and technique-sensitive use of small hand files or engine-driven rotary instruments in an oscillating handpiece (TriAuto ZX2, J Morita, Japan) is unavoidable (Fig. 5.44). However, even in such challenging situations, the use of reciprocating instruments is advantageous. As the reciprocating instrument stops further penetration, as soon as it reaches an obstacle, it gives valuable feedback, indicating a difficult anatomical situation, an information that a rotary instrument does not deliver but has the potential risks of ledging or instrument fracture.

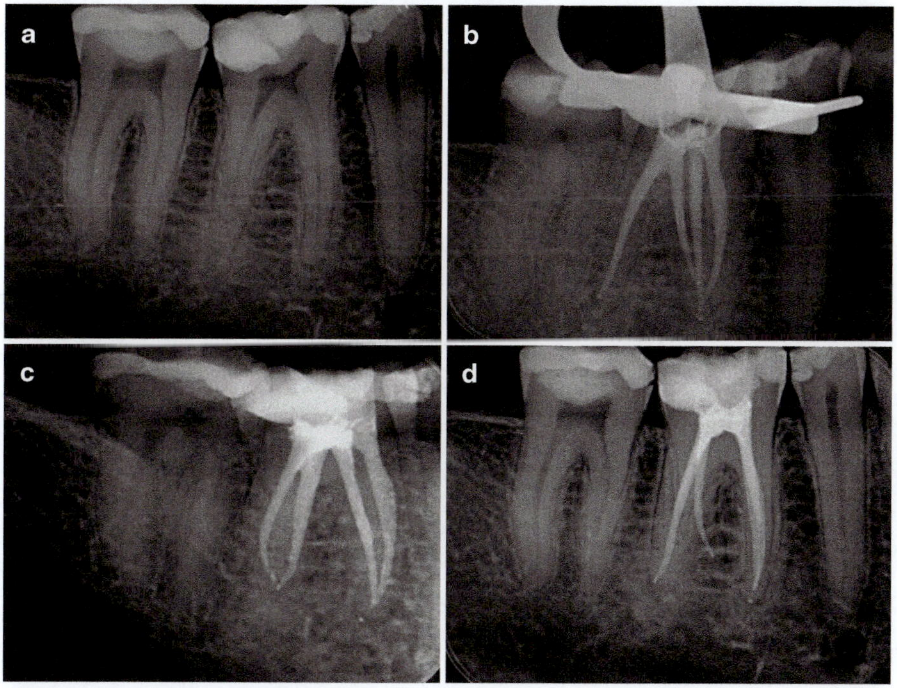

Fig. 5.41 (**a**) Symptomatic mandibular first right molar with radix entomolaris. A workflow for simple clinical situations as described in Fig. 5.40 was used. (**b, c**) Distal angled and mesial angled radiographs for backfill control. (**d**) Postoperative periapical radiograph showing root canals prepared with the Reciproc R25 and WaveOne Gold Medium instruments up to an apical size of 0.35 mm

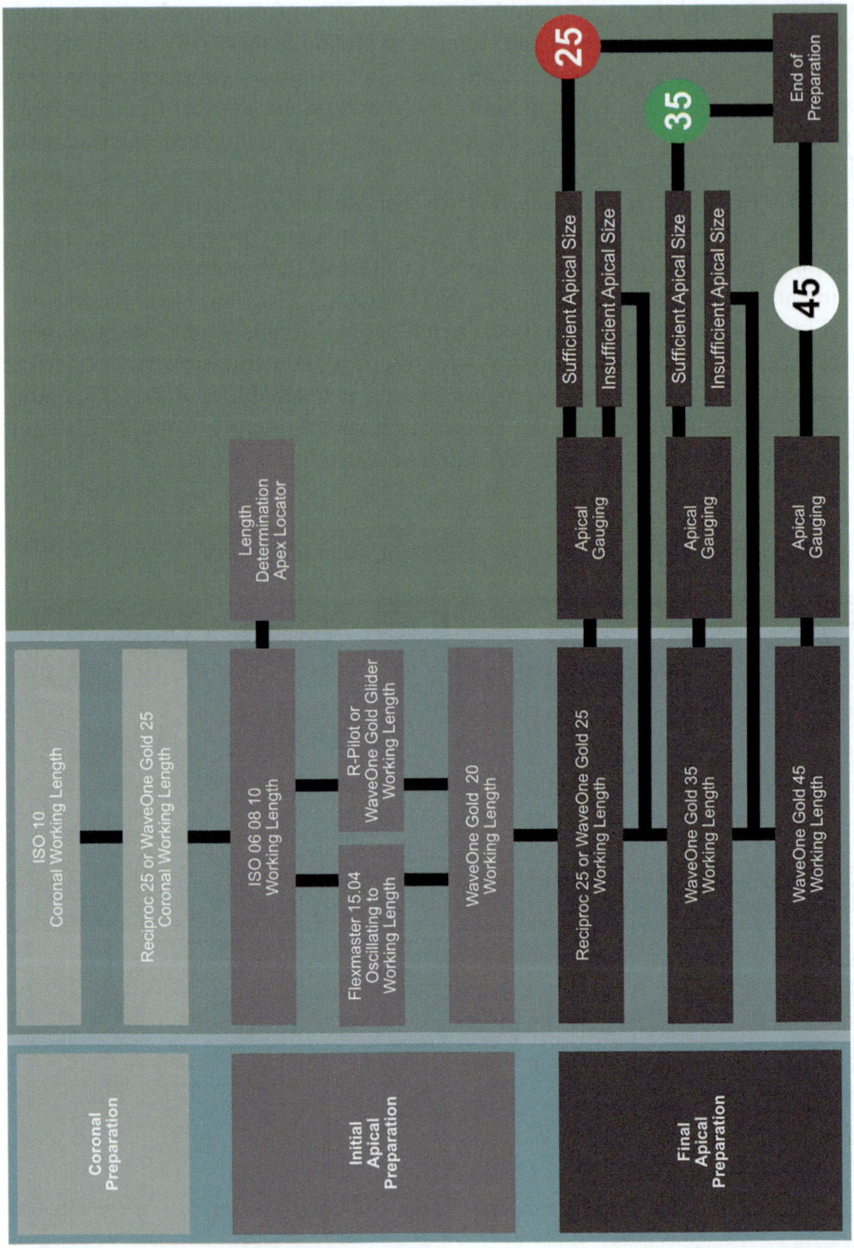

Fig. 5.42 Workflow for root canal preparation of complex cases (hybrid approach) using reciprocating instruments

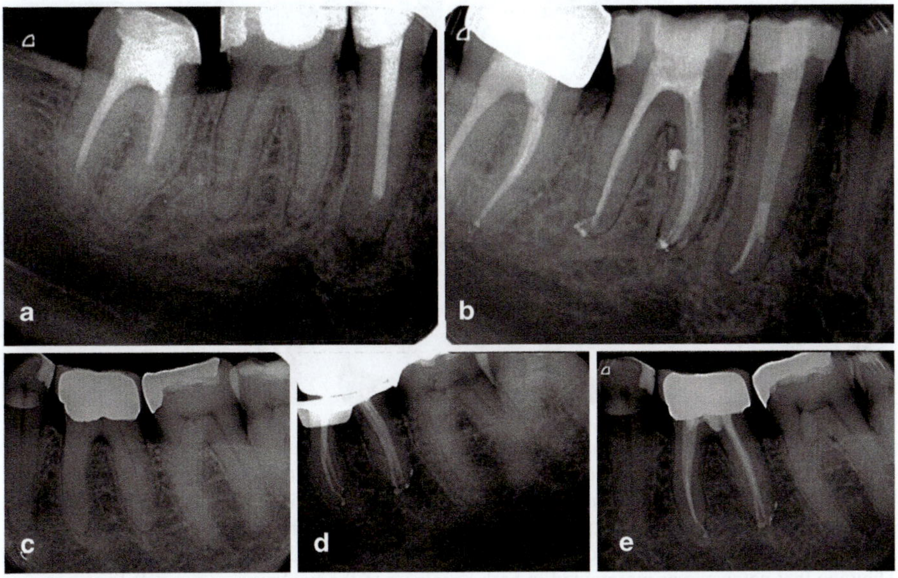

Fig. 5.43 (**a**) Mandibular right second premolar with insufficient root canal filling and asymptomatic apical periodontitis, mandibular right first molar with a deep restoration near to the pulp cavity and second molar with insufficient root canal filling. All teeth react normally on percussion. (**b**) Five months after retreatment of teeth 45 and 47, tooth 46 started to react clinically, so root canal treatment was also carried out. Postoperative radiograph shows the first molar prepared in a workflow as described in Fig. 5.40 with Reciproc R25 and WaveOne Gold Medium instruments up to 0.35 mm apically. Several lateral canals and isthmuses were filled using a warm vertical compaction technique. Second premolar already shows complete apical healing. The ledge in its apical third was bypassed with a prebent WaveOne Gold Small instrument, that was introduced manually and, after finding the original canal, was clipped into the handpiece for engine-driven glide path creation down to the working length. A fiber reinforced post was inserted after root canal filling. (**c**) Symptomatic mandibular left first molar with narrow and coronally obliterated root canals after initial treatment of the referring dentist who couldn't find the canal orifices. (**d**) Distal angled radiograph for backfill control shows apical preparation in mesial and distal canals up to sizes 0.35 mm and 0.45 mm, respectively. (**e**) Postoperative periapical radiograph shows the mandibular first molar prepared in a workflow used in challenging anatomies as described in Fig. 5.43. After coronal enlargement with the Reciproc R25 instrument, in the mesial canals the R-Pilot and WaveOne Gold Small instruments had to be used to reach the working length after initial hand instrumentation up to a ISO size 10 K-File. Final preparation was done with Reciproc R25 and WaveOne Gold Medium instruments. In the distal canals, the Reciproc R25 as well as the WaveOne Gold Medium and Large instruments were taken to the working length

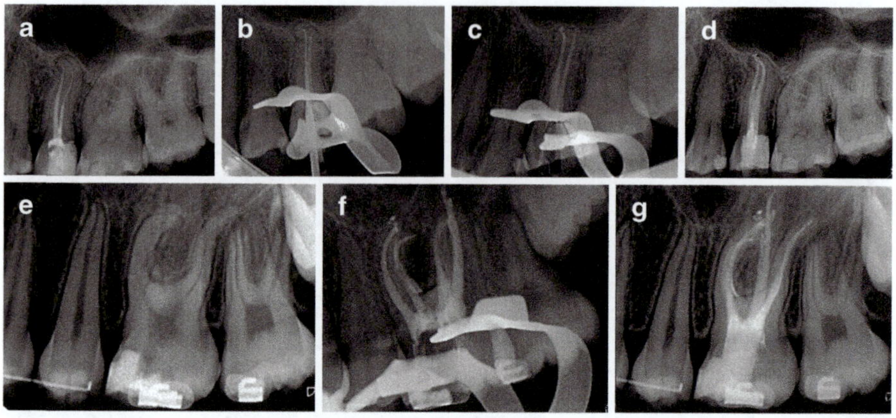

Fig. 5.44 (**a**) A symptomatic maxillary second left premolar with extremely narrow canals and separated instrument was referred for retreatment. (**b**) In the palatal canal, the R-Pilot instrument was taken to the working length, then detached from the handpiece with a gutta-percha master cone in the buccal canal for working length radiograph. The fragment was removed with the FragRemover device (FragRemover GbR, Germany). (**c**) Immediate postoperative radiograph showing that patency was maintained in both canals up to the final preparation. (**d**) Postoperative radiograph shows the root canals prepared apically up to 0.35 mm. (**e**) Symptomatic maxillary first left molar showing perforation of the pulp chamber floor referred for root canal treatment. The tooth has long and severely curved roots, complex anatomy with already strongly calcified canals. Long-time management with at least 20 hand instruments from sizes 06 to 10 in a crown-down/step-down combination of techniques were needed for initial negotiation. (**f**) Distal angled radiograph for backfill control shows multiple lateral canals and isthmuses filled. (**g**) Postoperative radiograph. The workflow described in Fig. 5.43 was used for apical preparation up to 0.35 mm in the buccal roots and 0.45 mm in the palatal root

5.8 Concluding Remarks: Reasons Why Reciprocation Is Not "More of the Same"

In the last decades, the endodontic field was drastically marked by two events: (1) a massive increase in the number of rotary systems ("more of the same" phenomenon) and (2) the emergence of asymmetric reciprocating systems. There are a series of consistent reasons that separate the reciprocating movement away from the "more of the same" phenomenon, such as:

- Very low fracture rate.
- Superb shaping ability.
- No glide path needed for the majority of cases.
- Simplified management of narrow/calcified canals.
- No need for a specific instrument for preflaring.
- Extreme efficiency for retreatment.
- Short learning curve.

Besides the number of advantages over the conventional rotary techniques for both beginner and advanced clinicians, there is a huge body of clinical experience and scientific evidence accumulated. Nowadays, a simple digital search in the PubMed database using the word Reciproc displays almost 1000 papers since 2010, meaning that Reciproc is the most studied instrument ever in the history of endodontics. Such a background frame settles reciprocating movement as the biggest development over the past 10 years in endodontics, moving far away from the "more of the same" phenomenon, which is the mainstream of rotary systems.

References

1. Hülsmann M, Peters OA, Dummer PMH. Mechanical preparation of root canals: shaping goals, techniques and means. Endod Topics. 2005;10:30–76.
2. Frank AL. An evaluation of the Giromatic endodontic handpiece. Oral Surg Oral Med Oral Pathol. 1967;24:419–21.
3. Schäfer E, Tepel J, Hoppe W. Properties of endodontic hand instruments used in rotary motion. Part 2. Instrumentation of curved canals. J Endod. 1995;21:493–7.
4. Gambarini G, Piasecki L, Miccoli G, Gaimari G, Di Giorgio R, Di Nardo D, et al. Classification and cyclic fatigue evaluation of new kinematics for endodontic instruments. Aust Endod J. 2019;45:154–62.
5. Lausten LL, Luebke NH, Brantley WA. Bending and metallurgical properties of rotary endodontic instruments. IV. Gates Glidden and Peeso drills. J Endod. 1993;19:440–7.
6. Luebke NH, Brantley WA. Physical dimensions and torsional properties of rotary endodontic instruments. 1. Gates Glidden drills. J Endod. 1990;16:438–41.
7. Klayman SM, Brilliant JD. A comparison of the efficacy of serial preparation versus Giromatic preparation. J Endod. 1975;1:334–7.
8. Molven O. A comparison of the dentin-removing ability of five root canal instruments. Scand J Dent Res. 1970;78:500–11.
9. Schulz-Bongert U, Weine FS, Schulz-Bongert J. Preparation of curved canals using a combined hand-filing, ultrasonic technique. Compend Contin Educ Dent. 1995;16:270, 2, 4 passim; quiz 86.
10. Weine FS, Kelly RF, Bray KE. Effect of preparation with endodontic handpieces on original canal shape. J Endod. 1976;2:298–303.
11. Weine FS, Kelly RF, Lio PJ. The effect of preparation procedures on original canal shape and on apical foramen shape. J Endod. 1975;1:255–62.
12. Roane JB, Sabala CL, Duncanson MG Jr. The "balanced force" concept for instrumentation of curved canals. J Endod. 1985;11:203–11.
13. Thompson NM. Development of a novel canal preparation technique using the torsional fatigue profile of the ProTaper(TM) F2 rotary instrument [Thesis (M Sc)]. Toronto: University of Toronto; 2006.
14. Yared G. Canal preparation using only one Ni-Ti rotary instrument: preliminary observations. Int Endod J. 2008;41:339–44.
15. Pereira ES, Gomes RO, Leroy AM, Singh R, Peters OA, Bahia MG, et al. Mechanical behavior of M-Wire and conventional NiTi wire used to manufacture rotary endodontic instruments. Dent Mater. 2013;29:e318–24.
16. De-Deus G, Silva EJ, Vieira VT, Belladonna FG, Elias CN, Plotino G, et al. Blue thermomechanical treatment optimizes fatigue resistance and flexibility of the Reciproc files. J Endod. 2017;43:462–6.

17. Silva EJNL, Hecksher F, Antunes HDS, De-Deus G, Elias CN, Vieira VTL. Torsional fatigue resistance of blue-treated reciprocating instruments. J Endod. 2018;44:1038–41.
18. Silva E, Vieira VTL, Gabina TTG, Antunes HDS, Lopes HP, De-Deus G. The impact of using a pneumatic contra-angle device on the lifespan of M-Wire- and Blue-treated instruments. Clin Oral Investig. 2019;23:617–21.
19. Kim JW, Ha JH, Cheung GS, Versluis A, Kwak SW, Kim HC. Safety of the factory preset rotation angle of reciprocating instruments. J Endod. 2014;40:1671–5.
20. Viana AC, Gonzalez BM, Buono VT, Bahia MG. Influence of sterilization on mechanical properties and fatigue resistance of nickel-titanium rotary endodontic instruments. Int Endod J. 2006;39:709–15.
21. Silvaggio J, Hicks ML. Effect of heat sterilization on the torsional properties of rotary nickel-titanium endodontic files. J Endod. 1997;23:731–4.
22. Caballero-Flores H, Nabeshima CK, Binotto E, Machado MEL. Fracture incidence of instruments from a single-file reciprocating system by students in an endodontic graduate programme: a cross-sectional retrospective study. Int Endod J. 2019;52:13–8.
23. Bueno CSP, Oliveira DP, Pelegrine RA, Fontana CE, Rocha DGP, Bueno C. Fracture incidence of WaveOne and Reciproc files during root canal preparation of up to 3 posterior teeth: a prospective clinical study. J Endod. 2017;43:705–8.
24. Bueno CSP, Oliveira DP, Pelegrine RA, Fontana CE, Rocha DGP, Gutmann JL, et al. Fracture incidence of WaveOne Gold files: a prospective clinical study. Int Endod J. 2020;53:1192–8.
25. Alapati SB, Brantley WA, Svec TA, Powers JM, Mitchell JC. Scanning electron microscope observations of new and used nickel-titanium rotary files. J Endod. 2003;29:667–9.
26. Sonntag D, Peters O. Effect of prion decontamination protocols on nickel-titanium rotary surfaces. J Endod. 2007;33:442–6.
27. Ehrhardt IC, Zuolo ML, Cunha RS, De Martin AS, Kherlakian D, Carvalho MC, et al. Assessment of the separation incidence of mtwo files used with preflaring: prospective clinical study. J Endod. 2012;38:1078–81.
28. Schmitz Mda S, Santos R, Capelli A, Jacobovitz M, Spanó JC, Pécora JD. Influence of cervical preflaring on determination of apical file size in mandibular molars: SEM analysis. Braz Dent J. 2008;19:245–51.
29. Vanni JR, Santos R, Limongi O, Guerisoli DM, Capelli A, Pecora JD. Influence of cervical preflaring on determination of apical file size in maxillary molars: SEM analysis. Braz Dent J. 2005;16:181–6.
30. Isom TL, Marshall JG, Baumgartner JC. Evaluation of root thickness in curved canals after flaring. J Endod. 1995;21:368–71.
31. Kessler JR, Peters DD, Lorton L. Comparison of the relative risk of molar root perforations using various endodontic instrumentation techniques. J Endod. 1983;9:439–47.
32. Reeh ES, Messer HH, Douglas WH. Reduction in tooth stiffness as a result of endodontic and restorative procedures. J Endod. 1989;15:512–6.
33. Clark D, Khademi J. Modern molar endodontic access and directed dentin conservation. Dent Clin N Am. 2010;54:249–73.
34. Plotino G, Nagendrababu V, Bukiet F, Grande NM, Veettil SK, De-Deus G, et al. Influence of negotiation, glide path, and preflaring procedures on root canal shaping-terminology, basic concepts, and a systematic review. J Endod. 2020;46:707–29.
35. West J. Endodontic update 2006. J Esthet Restor Dent. 2006;18:280–300.
36. Pasqualini D, Bianchi CC, Paolino DS, Mancini L, Cemenasco A, Cantatore G, et al. Computed micro-tomographic evaluation of glide path with nickel-titanium rotary PathFile in maxillary first molars curved canals. J Endod. 2012;38:389–93.
37. De-Deus G, Arruda TE, Souza EM, Neves A, Magalhaes K, Thuanne E, et al. The ability of the Reciproc R25 instrument to reach the full root canal working length without a glide path. Int Endod J. 2013;46:993–8.
38. Rodrigues E, De-Deus G, Souza E, Silva EJ. Safe mechanical preparation with reciprocation movement without glide path creation: result from a pool of 673 root canals. Braz Dent J. 2016;27:22–7.

39. Zuolo ML, Carvalho MC, De-Deus G. Negotiability of second mesiobuccal canals in maxillary molars using a reciprocating system. J Endod. 2015;41:1913–7.
40. De-Deus G, Cardoso ML, Belladonna FG, Cavalcante DM, Simoes-Carvalho M, Souza EM, et al. Performance of Reciproc blue R25 instruments in shaping the canal space without glide path. J Endod. 2019;45:194–8.
41. Muñoz E, Forner L, Llena C. Influence of operator's experience on root canal shaping ability with a rotary nickel-titanium single-file reciprocating motion system. J Endod. 2014;40:547–50.
42. McGuigan MB, Louca C, Duncan HF. The impact of fractured endodontic instruments on treatment outcome. Br Dent J. 2013;214:285–9.
43. McGuigan MB, Louca C, Duncan HF. Clinical decision-making after endodontic instrument fracture. Br Dent J. 2013;214:395–400.
44. Ungerechts C, Bårdsen A, Fristad I. Instrument fracture in root canals—where, why, when and what? A study from a student clinic. Int Endod J. 2014;47:183–90.
45. Sattapan B, Nervo GJ, Palamara JE, Messer HH. Defects in rotary nickel-titanium files after clinical use. J Endod. 2000;26:161–5.
46. Al-Fouzan KS. Incidence of rotary ProFile instrument fracture and the potential for bypassing in vivo. Int Endod J. 2003;36:864–7.
47. Patiño PV, Biedma BM, Liebana CR, Cantatore G, Bahillo JG. The influence of a manual glide path on the separation rate of NiTi rotary instruments. J Endod. 2005;31:114–6.
48. Wolcott S, Wolcott J, Ishley D, Kennedy W, Johnson S, Minnich S, et al. Separation incidence of protaper rotary instruments: a large cohort clinical evaluation. J Endod. 2006;32:1139–41.
49. Inan U, Gonulol N. Deformation and fracture of Mtwo rotary nickel-titanium instruments after clinical use. J Endod. 2009;35:1396–9.
50. Wu J, Lei G, Yan M, Yu Y, Yu J, Zhang G. Instrument separation analysis of multi-used ProTaper Universal rotary system during root canal therapy. J Endod. 2011;37:758–63.
51. Cunha RS, Junaid A, Ensinas P, Nudera W, Bueno CE. Assessment of the separation incidence of reciprocating WaveOne files: a prospective clinical study. J Endod. 2014;40:922–4.
52. Shen Y, Coil JM, Mo AJ, Wang Z, Hieawy A, Yang Y, et al. WaveOne rotary instruments after clinical use. J Endod. 2016;42:186–9.

6 Scientific and Educational Aspects of Reciprocating Movement

Erick Souza, Emmanuel J. N. L. Silva, Gustavo De Deus, Marco A. Versiani, and Mario Zuolo

6.1 Introduction

The broad support of the literature on the efficiency and safety of reciprocating movement and its wide acceptance has stimulated the commercial emergence of new systems from different manufacturers. The objectives of this chapter are to provide an overview of the literature regarding the advantages and disadvantages of reciprocating motion compared to continuous rotation, and to discuss the educational aspects related to this topic.

6.2 Scientific Aspects of Reciprocating Movement

6.2.1 Cyclic Fatigue Resistance

Reciprocating movement was developed to reduce the incidence of instrument breakage. Because instruments in reciprocating movement travel a shorter circumferential distance than a rotary instrument during cutting action, they are subjected

E. Souza (✉)
Federal University of Maranhão, São Luis, Brazil
e-mail: erickmsouza@uol.com.br

E. J. N. L. Silva
Fluminense Federal University, Grande Rio University, Rio de Janeiro State University, Niterói, Brazil

G. De Deus
Fluminense Federal University, Niterói, Brazil

M. A. Versiani
Dental Specialty Center, Brazilian Military Police, Minas Gerais, Brazil

M. Zuolo
Dental School of APCD – FAOA, São Paulo, Brazil

G. De Deus et al. (eds.), *Shaping for Cleaning the Root Canals*,
https://doi.org/10.1007/978-3-030-84617-6_6

to lower stress values [1]. Consequently, a greater resistance to fatigue is expected when instruments are used in reciprocating movement as opposed to continuous rotation (Fig. 6.1). The first study published on this topic [2] pointed out the role of reciprocating movement in the prevention of instrument separation, as an extended cyclic fatigue life of the F2 ProTaper instrument was observed when reciprocating. These results were later confirmed by a plethora of studies [3–7], supporting that the reciprocating movement per se extends the resistance to cyclic fatigue of all tested instruments (Figs. 6.2 and 6.3).

Altering the amplitude of reciprocation also has a significant influence on the cyclic fatigue life of NiTi instruments. For example, by changing a 90° CW and

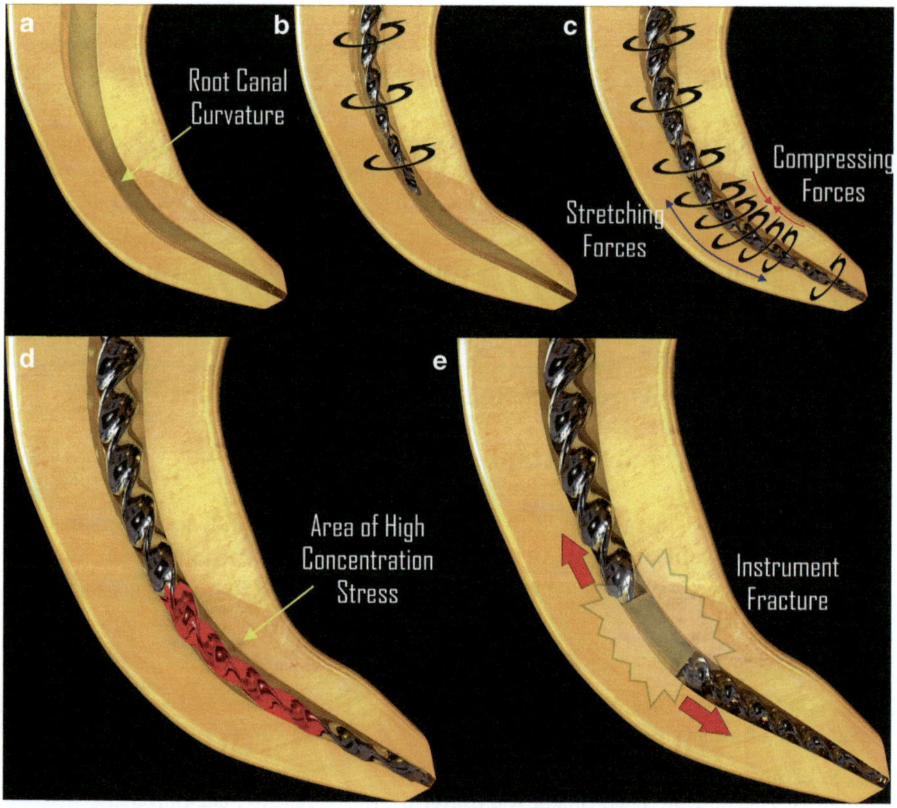

Fig. 6.1 Schematic representation of rotary NiTi instrument fracture by cyclic fatigue during clinical use. (**a**, **b**) A rotary NiTi instrument is activated in continuous rotation at a constant speed and torque value in a curved root canal. (**c**, **d**) When the instrument reaches the curvature, one half of its shaft on the outside of the curve is submitted to a tension force, whereas the other half (inside the curve) to compression (red area). (**e**) This repeated tension–compression cycles developed at the point of maximum flexure increase the cyclic fatigue of the instrument, generating microcracks on its surface, which spread until a catastrophic failure occurs and the instrument breaks as a consequence of metal fatigue

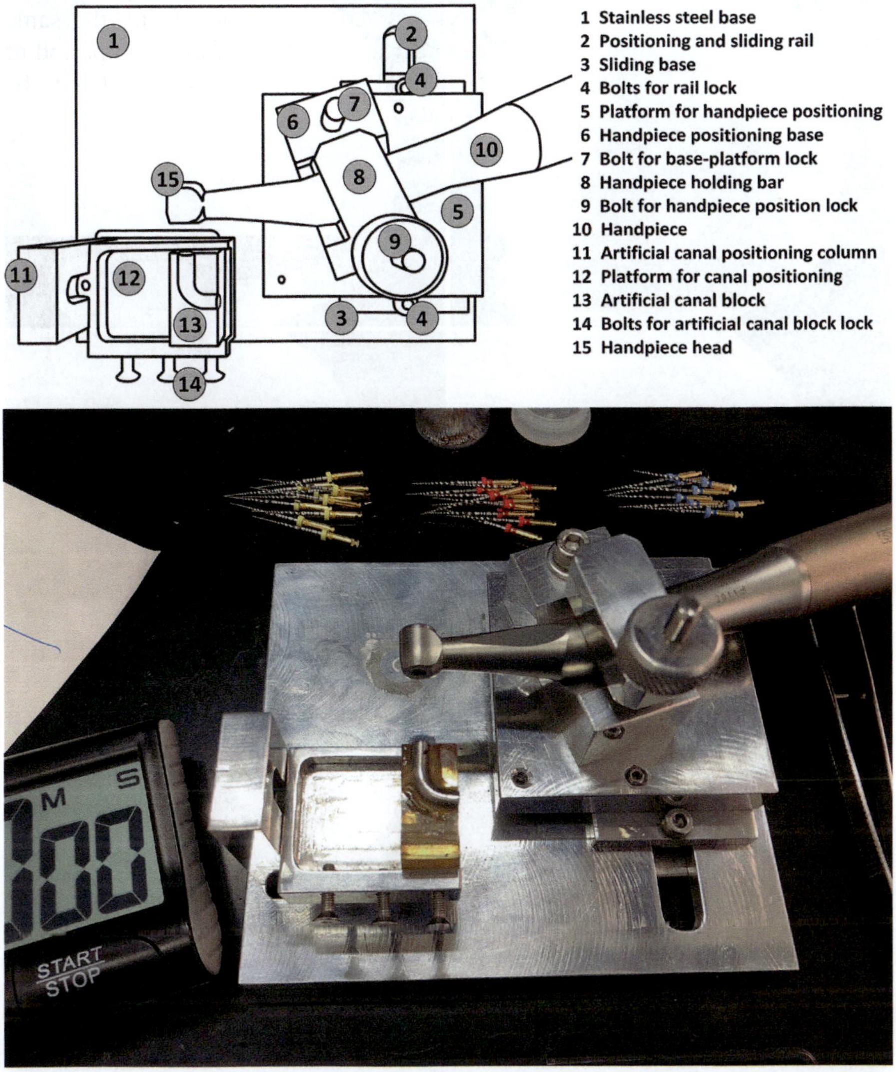

Fig. 6.2 A custom-made device to perform the cyclic fatigue resistance test. This device allows a reproducible assessment of an instrument rotating loose inside an artificial curved canal until fracture occurs. The block containing the artificial canal is connected to a main frame to which a mobile support for the handpiece is also connected, aiming to allow precise and reproducible placement of the instruments to the same depth inside the artificial canal

30° CCW rotation angles (angle of progression for each reciprocation cycle = 60°) to a 120° CW and 30° CCW (angle of progression for each reciprocation cycle = 90°), the resistance to cyclic fatigue is reduced [8]. Fatigue life also decreases when increasing reciprocating amplitude in symmetric stationary reciprocation, i.e., using the same clockwise and counterclockwise angles (symmetric

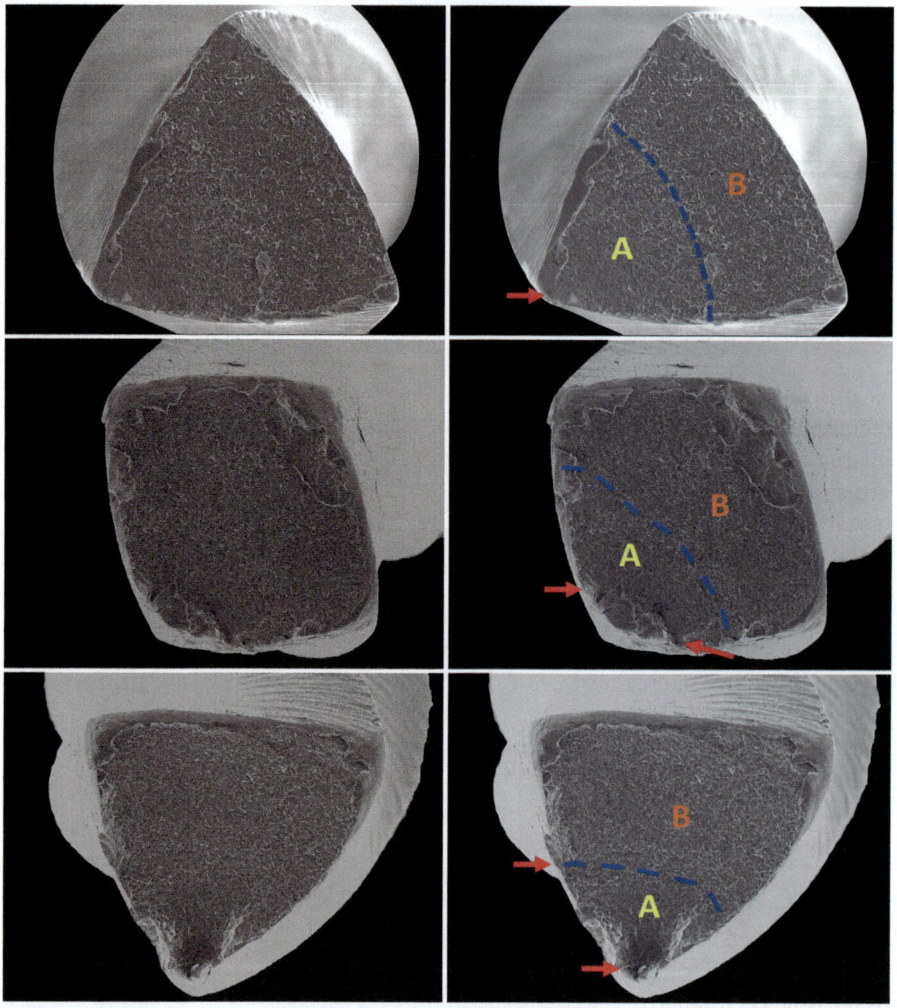

Fig. 6.3 Representative scanning electron microscopy images of fractured surfaces of NiTi instruments after cyclic fatigue resistance test (×250 original magnification). The cross-sectional images revealed typical morphological features of the ductile nature of the ultimate catastrophic failure in which are depicted the crack initiation area(s) (red arrows), (**A**) the fatigue propagation area, and (**B**) the fast fracture zone with numerous dimples

motion) [9]. Furthermore, asymmetric reciprocating movement yields a longer fatigue life compared to symmetric stationary reciprocating motion [9]. In symmetric progressive reciprocating movement, the most critically strained locations move forward to new locations during the periodic angular increment instead of remaining stationary. This effectively distributes fatigue damage to different points on the circumference of the instrument, reducing the detrimental effect of localized damage.

6.2.2 Torsional Resistance

The most used methodology to evaluate the torsional resistance of endodontic instruments is based on ISO Specification 3630-1 [10] (Fig. 6.4). It basically consists of clamping the instrument at its tip maintaining rotation of instrument's shank in clockwise direction until the fracture occurs. The torque load and the angular rotation at the moment of fracture are obtained and data can be compared among tested instruments (Figs. 6.5 and 6.6). Therefore, the ISO methodology allows the evaluation of characteristics related to the instrument's metallurgy and design, but is not suitable to compare different kinematics.

As previously described in Chap. 5, the rationale of reciprocating movement is based on a series of experiments to estimate the maximum rotational angle before the development of plastic deformation. Working in a counterclockwise or clockwise angulation below the elastic limit of the instrument dramatically reduces the possibility of instrument fracture by torsional forces. This is the basis of the reciprocating movement and the explanation for the reduced fracture rates observed in these instruments.

6.2.3 Cutting Efficiency

The ability of an instrument to efficiently remove dentin depends on a complex interrelationship of different aspects related to its design including the number and depth of flutes, cross-sectional area and format, helical and rake angle, configuration of the tip, metallurgical properties, and surface treatment (Fig. 6.7). At a first

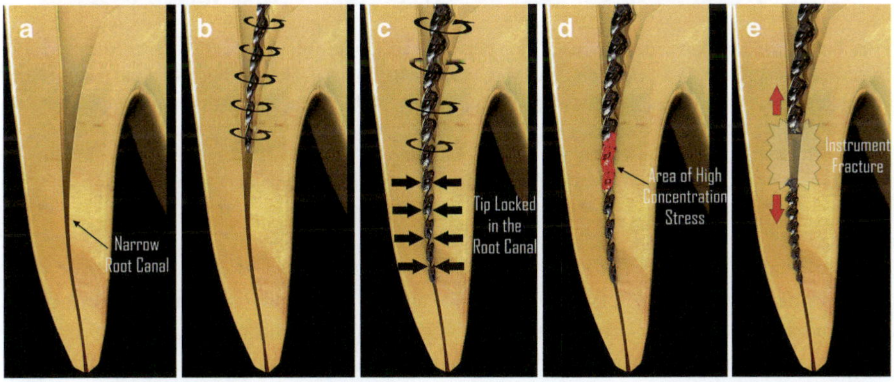

Fig. 6.4 Schematic representation of a NiTi instrument fracture by torsional fatigue during clinical use. (**a, b**) A rotary NiTi instrument is activated in continuous rotation at a constant speed and torque value in a narrow canal. (**c, d**) When the instrument reaches the narrowest part of the canal, its tip (or another part of the instrument) is locked while the shank continues the movement. (**e**) When the elastic limit of the metal is exceeded by the torque exerted by the handpiece (red area), fracture of the tip becomes inevitable

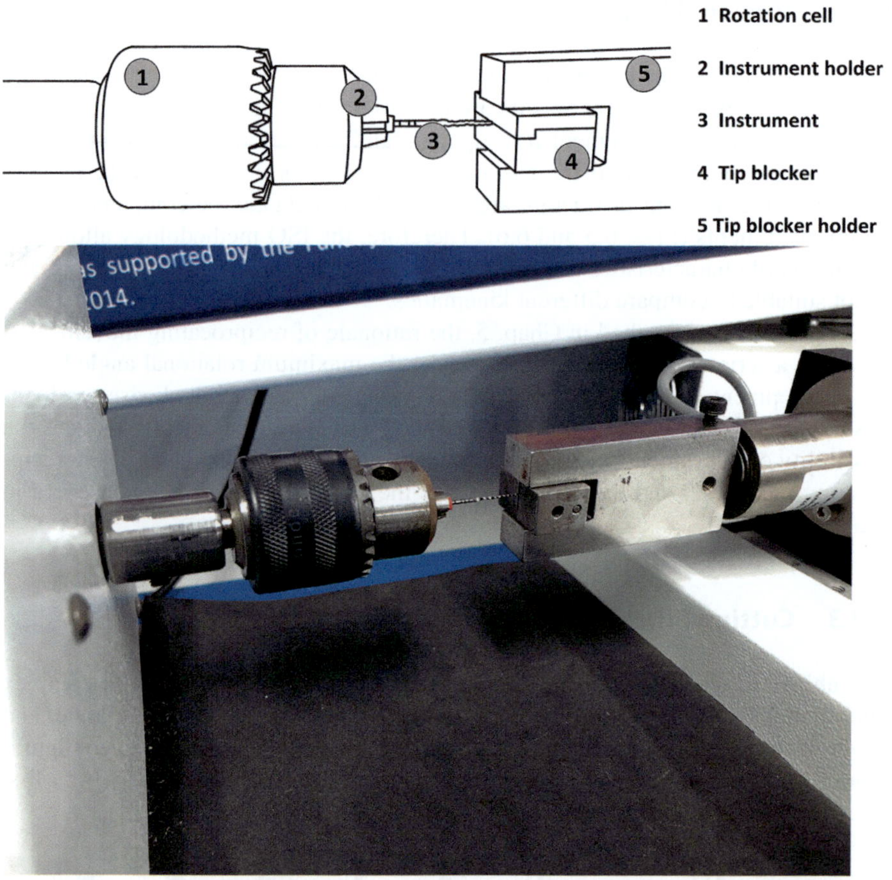

Fig. 6.5 Custom-made device used to perform torsional resistance test according to the Specification ISO 3630-1 [10]. In this device, each instrument is clamped in its apical 3 mm using a chuck connected to a torque-sensing load cell. The shaft of the instrument is fastened into an opposing chuck able to be rotated with a geared motor. Instruments are rotated either clockwise or counterclockwise on a constant pace (two rotations per minute) until rupture. The maximum torque (in N.cm) and angle of rotation (°) prior to fracture are determined with this test

glance, it seems logical to believe that alternating angles, such as in reciprocating movement, might negatively influence the cutting efficiency of an instrument when compared to continuous rotation. However, when the same instrument is used in continuous rotary or reciprocating movement, no differences in cutting efficiency has been observed [11, 12] (Fig. 6.8). Moreover, when the cutting ability of glide path instruments was compared, reciprocating instruments (R-Pilot and WaveOne Gold Glider) showed better results than those in continuous rotation (HyFlex EDM Glidepath File and One G) [13]. Therefore, it might be concluded that instruments under reciprocating movement have a better or at least similar cutting efficiency than when rotating (Fig. 6.9).

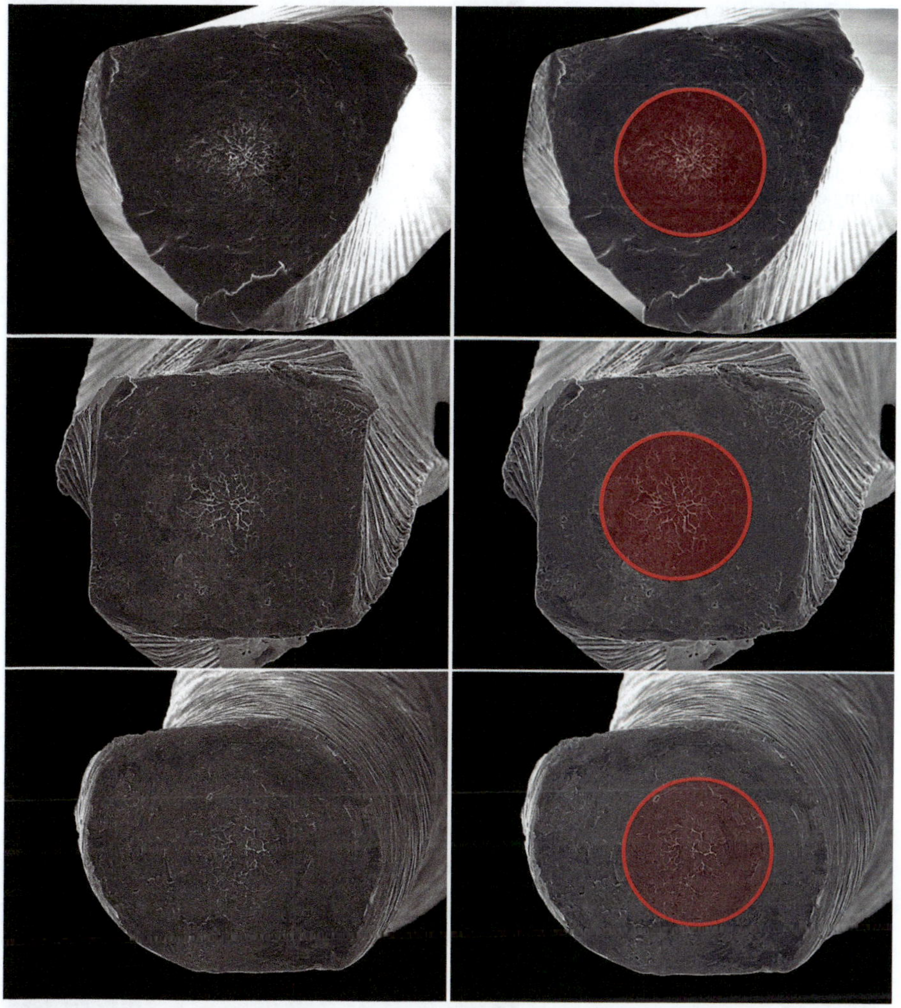

Fig. 6.6 Representative scanning electron microscopy images of the fractured surfaces of NiTi instruments after torsional resistance test (×250 original magnification). The cross-sectional images revealed typical features of the torsional fracture, with concentric abrasion marks and fibrous dimples from the torsional center (red areas)

6.2.4 Shaping Ability

Adequate preparation, preserving the original canal shape, can be obtained with contemporary NiTi instruments activated under reciprocating movement as the result of an interplay of different factors: the reciprocation kinematics, the instrument's cross-section, and the heat-treated alloy. In fact, several studies have demonstrated excellent shaping and centering ability outcomes of reciprocating instruments [14–17].

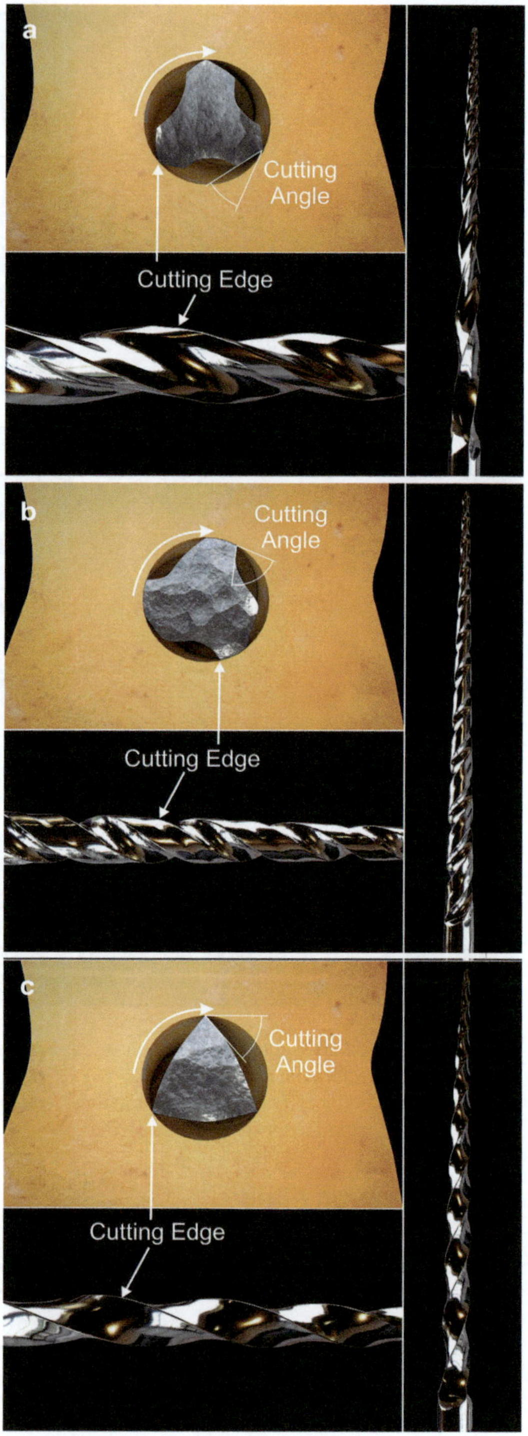

Fig. 6.7 Schematic representation of the cutting angle and cutting edge of (**a**) ProTaper F3, (**b**) K3 Endo, and (**c**) ProTaper Universal NiTi instruments. During root canal preparation, the cutting angle is the angle formed by the cutting edge of the instrument and the surface to be cut (dentin)

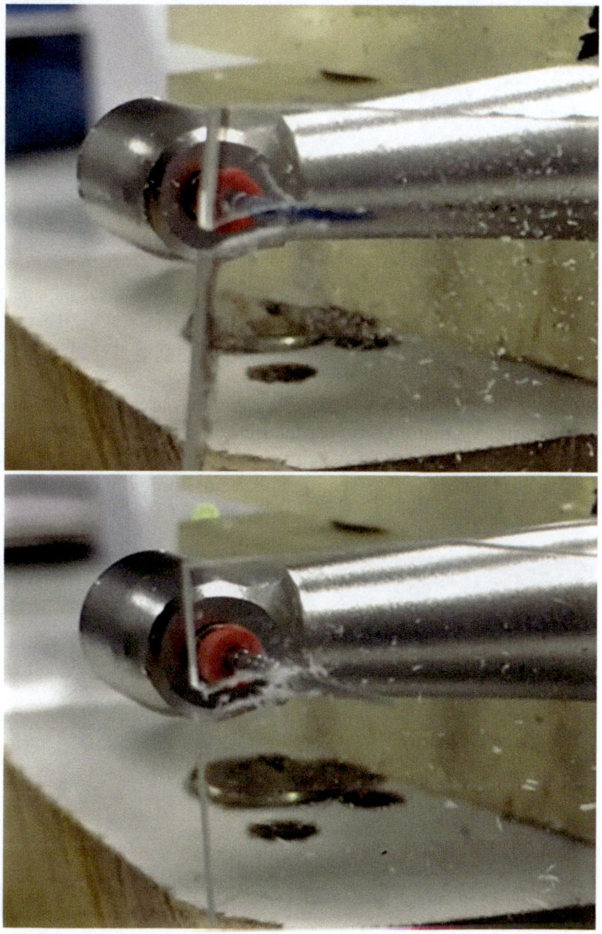

Fig. 6.8 Reciproc Blue (above) and M-Wire (below) Reciproc instruments during progressive cutting of a Plexiglas block illustrating the testing device to assess the cutting ability

The shaping ability of some rotary instruments, such as FlexMaster, ProTaper, Mtwo, ProFile, and RaCe used in continuous rotation, is also well documented with favorable results. Recent studies showed that the use of these instruments in reciprocation resulted in centering and shaping abilities similar to continuous rotation [18–20].

After the introduction of NiTi instruments specifically designed to operate under reciprocating movement, numerous studies have compared those systems with different types of NiTi instruments used in continuous rotation. In general, reciprocating systems have similar shaping ability and can preserve the original anatomy compared not only to those activated in continuous rotation [15, 17, 21], but also with the SAF system operated with an up/down vibration [22, 23].

A few studies confirmed that the use of a small-sized K-file followed by a more flexible and less tapered NiTi rotary instrument for glide path ensures a better respect to the original canal anatomy, minimizing procedural errors and

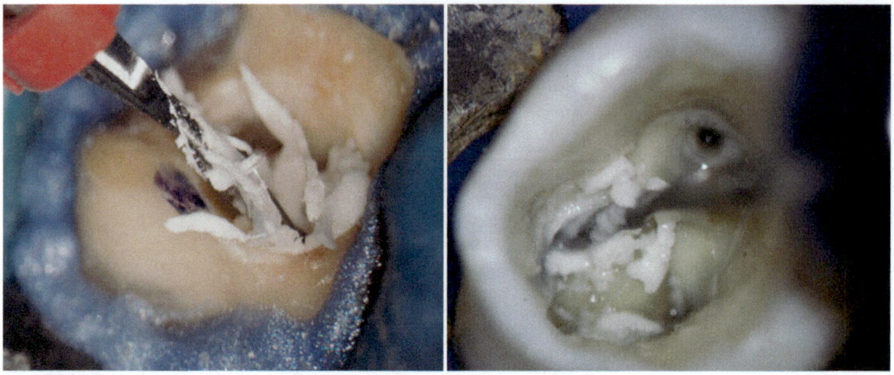

Fig. 6.9 Clinical images of the root canal preparation of a mandibular molar using Reciproc R25 instrument. A great amount of dentinal chips (pieces of dentin) are coming out from the canal space as a consequence of the cutting ability of this instrument, which is a result of the interplay between its S-shape cross-section and the reciprocating motion

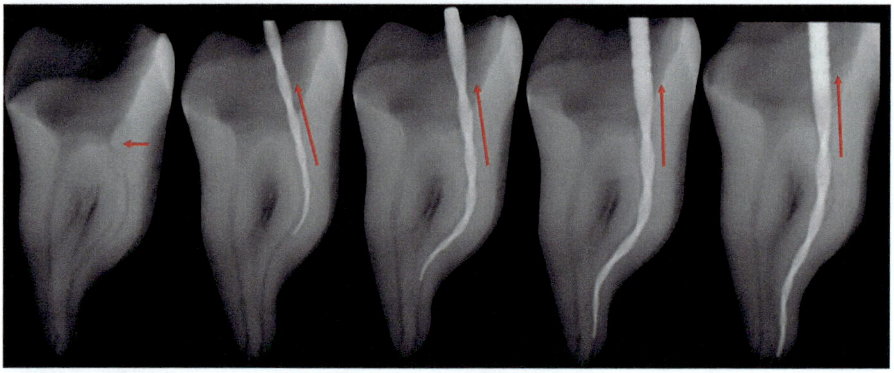

Fig. 6.10 Sequence of radiographic images showing the ability of the Reciproc instrument to advance toward the apex in a mesial root canal of a mandibular molar with double curvature. Red arrows indicate the changes in insertion angle of the instrument: as deeper the instrument goes, as straighter the insertion angle becomes

requiring fewer pecking motions to reach the working length [24–26]. While WaveOne instruments require a glide path prior to their use, as recommended by the manufacturer, and can reach the working length with fewer pecking motions after this preliminary enlargement [24–26], the Reciproc instruments, on the contrary, do not require glide path. These instruments are able to reach the working length in a high frequency in straight and curved canals, without a glide path as demonstrated by *in vitro* [27] (Fig. 6.10) and *in vivo* [28] (Fig. 6.11) studies. In addition, Reciproc instruments are more efficient in reaching the working length in the MB2 canal without any prior instrumentation compared to an initial scouting with small stainless-steel files [29].

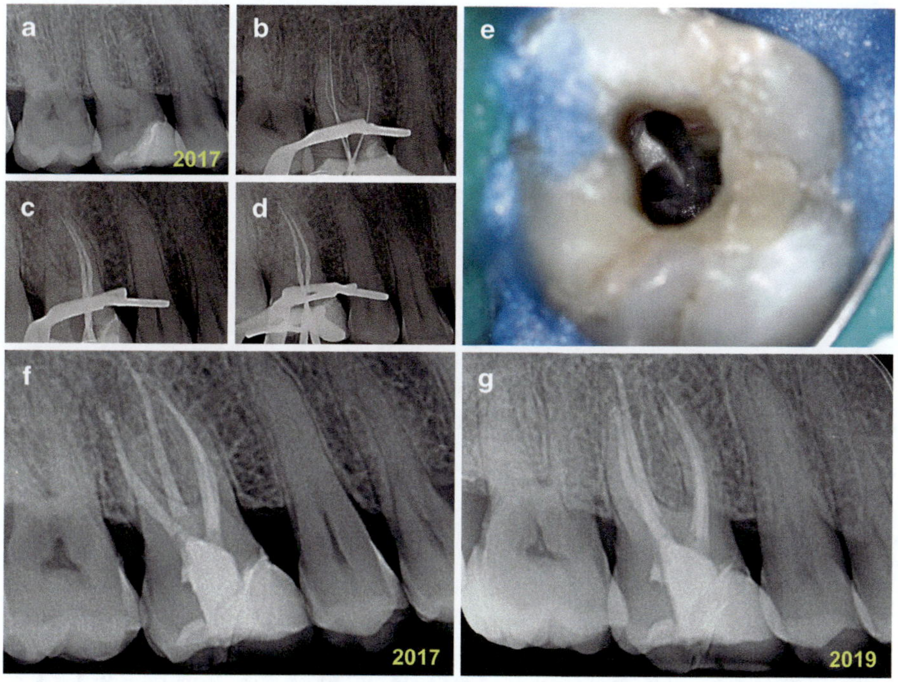

Fig. 6.11 (**a**) Preoperative radiograph of a maxillary right first molar referred for root canal treatment due to irreversible pulpitis. (**b**) Working length determination with hand files. (**c**, **d**) Angled radiographic views showing Reciproc R25 instruments at the working length of the mesiobuccal canals. (**e**) Pulp chamber floor observed under microscope showing the mesiobuccal canals orifices after preparation with Reciproc R25 instruments. (**f**) Immediate postoperative radiograph. (**g**) Two-year follow-up radiograph

The research on the shaping ability associated with reciprocation is exhaustive. In summary, the kinematics does not appear to affect the quality of root canal preparation (Fig. 6.12) since a sound research methodology is followed. For example, the tested instruments should be similar in size and dimensions, and the experimental groups should be paired according to the canal configuration, length, volume, geometry, surface area, and curvature. In this way, kinematics seem to have a neglectable influence on shaping ability (Fig. 6.12).

6.2.5 Microcrack Formation

The idea that preparation using reciprocating motion induces dentinal defects is based on the rationale that using only a single, large-tapered instrument to prepare uninstrumented root canals without any prior enlargement (glide path) would cause high amounts of stress on tooth structure leading to microcrack formation and propagation. However, this argument was established by studies

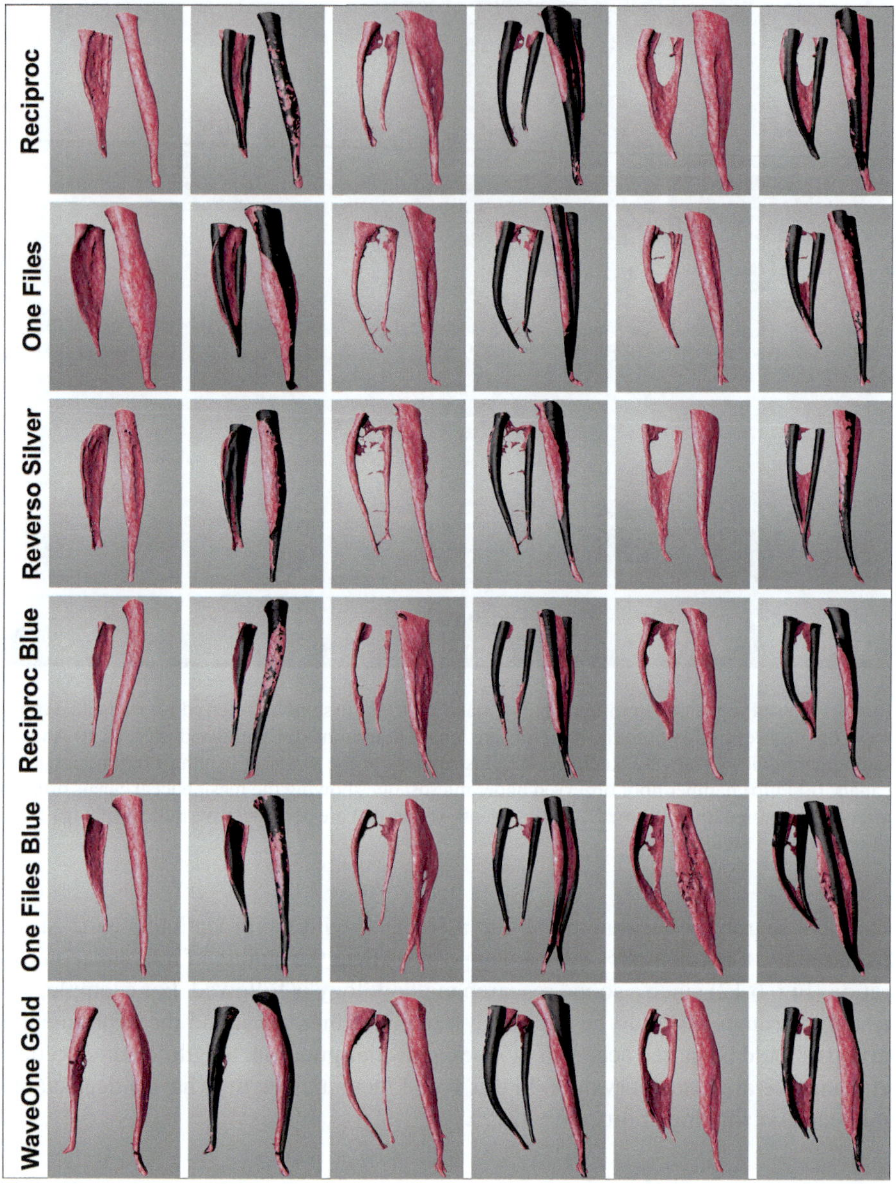

Fig. 6.12 Micro-CT models of 18 anatomically matched canals of mandibular molars prepared with six different reciprocating systems depicting their root canal systems before (surface textured to simulate pulp tissue) and after (in black) preparation. It is possible to observe, by the remaining untouched canal areas (in pink) after preparation, that none of the shaping protocols were able to prepare the entire surface area of the root canal

based on root sectioning methods and direct observation under optical microscopy [30–33] (Figs. 6.13 and 6.14). These methods undoubtedly have a major drawback related to the destructive nature of the experiment. The control groups, which used unprepared teeth, seemed to validate these results because no dentinal defects could be detected; however, they do not take into account the potential damage produced by the interplay among three sources of stresses on the root dentin [34]:

1. The mechanical preparation.
2. The chemical attack with sodium hypochlorite-based irrigation.
3. The sectioning procedure per se.

As time went by, it was demonstrated that the adequate methodology to study microcracks is the nondestructive micro-CT technology. By using this method, De-Deus et al. [34] found a clear lack of causal relationship between the development of dentinal microcracks and canal preparation with either rotary or

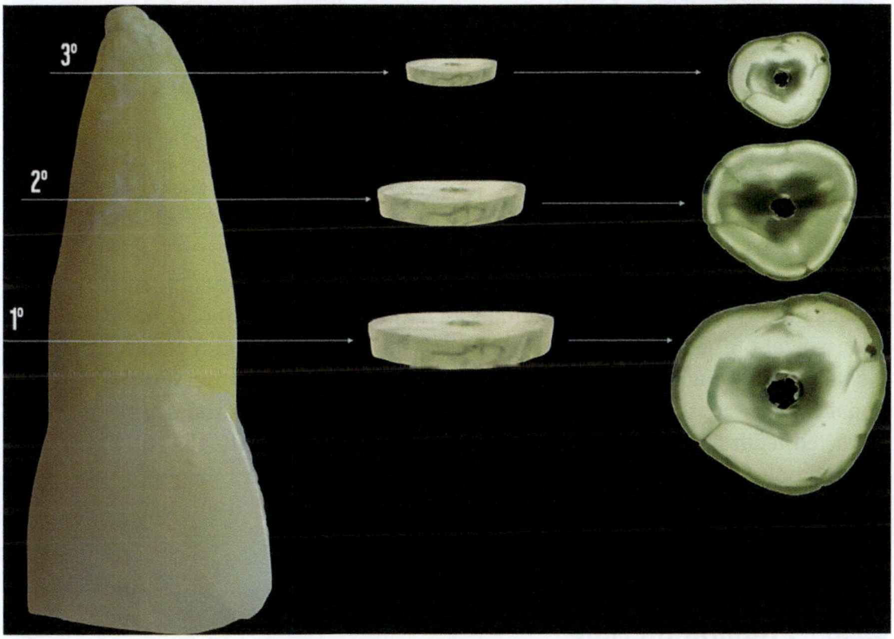

Fig. 6.13 Cross-sectioning method for the study of dentinal cracks in a maxillary incisor. This method comprises the use of a thin diamond blade to progressively saw the tooth under low speed and profuse water irrigation to minimize heating and further damages to the dental structure. An important limitation of the conventional sectioning technique is not only the evaluation of a few slices per tooth, with the real possibility of missing several previous defects along the root, but also the impossibility to assess microcracks and craze lines on the longitudinal axis of the root, as the vertical extension of such defects would provide better knowledge of the connection between the size of the dentinal defect and its potential to develop into a vertical root fracture

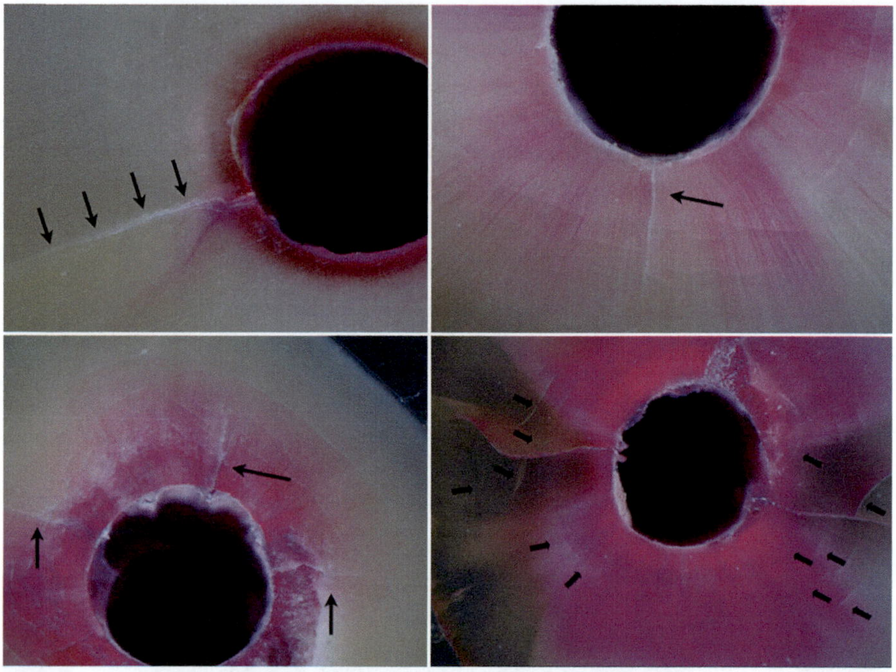

Fig. 6.14 Representative optical microscopy cross-section images showing the presence of dentinal microcracks (black arrows) after canal preparation. These are the type of images that give rise to the concern that dentinal defects may be caused by endodontic procedures such as root canal preparation and obturation

reciprocating systems (Fig. 6.15). This conclusion was later confirmed by other studies [35–39] using the same method. In addition, it was further demonstrated, by the association between the micro-CT analytical platform and a cadaveric experimental model, that the so-called root dentinal microcracks observed in cross-sectional images are indeed a phenomenon that belongs to the framework of stored/extracted teeth mostly caused by dehydration [35, 37, 38, 40] (Fig. 6.16). In other words, root dentinal microcracks are not a true clinical phenomenon, and as such, all of the concerns regarding a possible relationship between mechanical preparation and the development of root defects can be dismissed.

6.2.6 Preparation Time

Several studies have reported that the use of reciprocating instruments reduces the overall shaping time compared with rotary systems [15, 41–43]. In fact, this reduction in preparation time is most likely related to the reduced number of instruments associated with the reciprocating technique (as recommended by manufacturers),

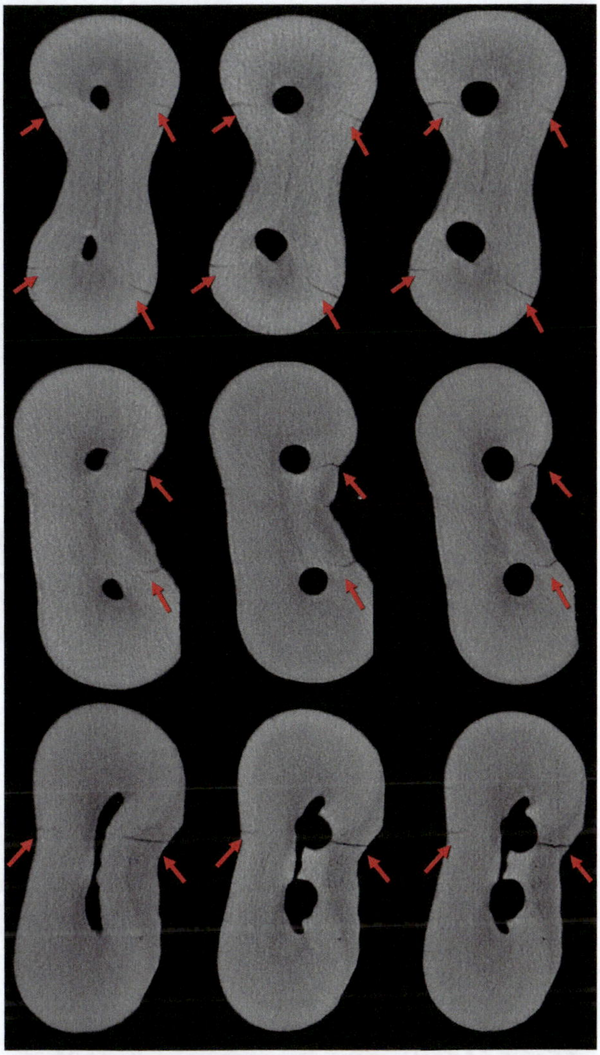

Fig. 6.15 Representative micro-CT cross-section images of mesial roots of mandibular molars showing the presence of dentinal microcracks (red arrows) before and after canal preparation with BioRace (above), WaveOne (middle), and Reciproc (below) systems. It is possible to observe that all microcracks were already present in the sound canals before preparation, which means that the mechanical shaping per se did not cause the dentinal defects

than the kinematics per se. When comparing different systems, several studies concluded that the shaping time with Reciproc was significantly shorter than with WaveOne [15, 42, 44]. Moreover, one study reported that there was a linear inverse relationship between decreasing the reciprocating range (angle of progression) of WaveOne instruments and the time needed to reach the working length [45]. The shorter preparation time related to reciprocating systems is in line with the general idea of this textbook: an adequate and refined cleaning process is necessary after the fast-pace root canal shaping (Fig. 6.17).

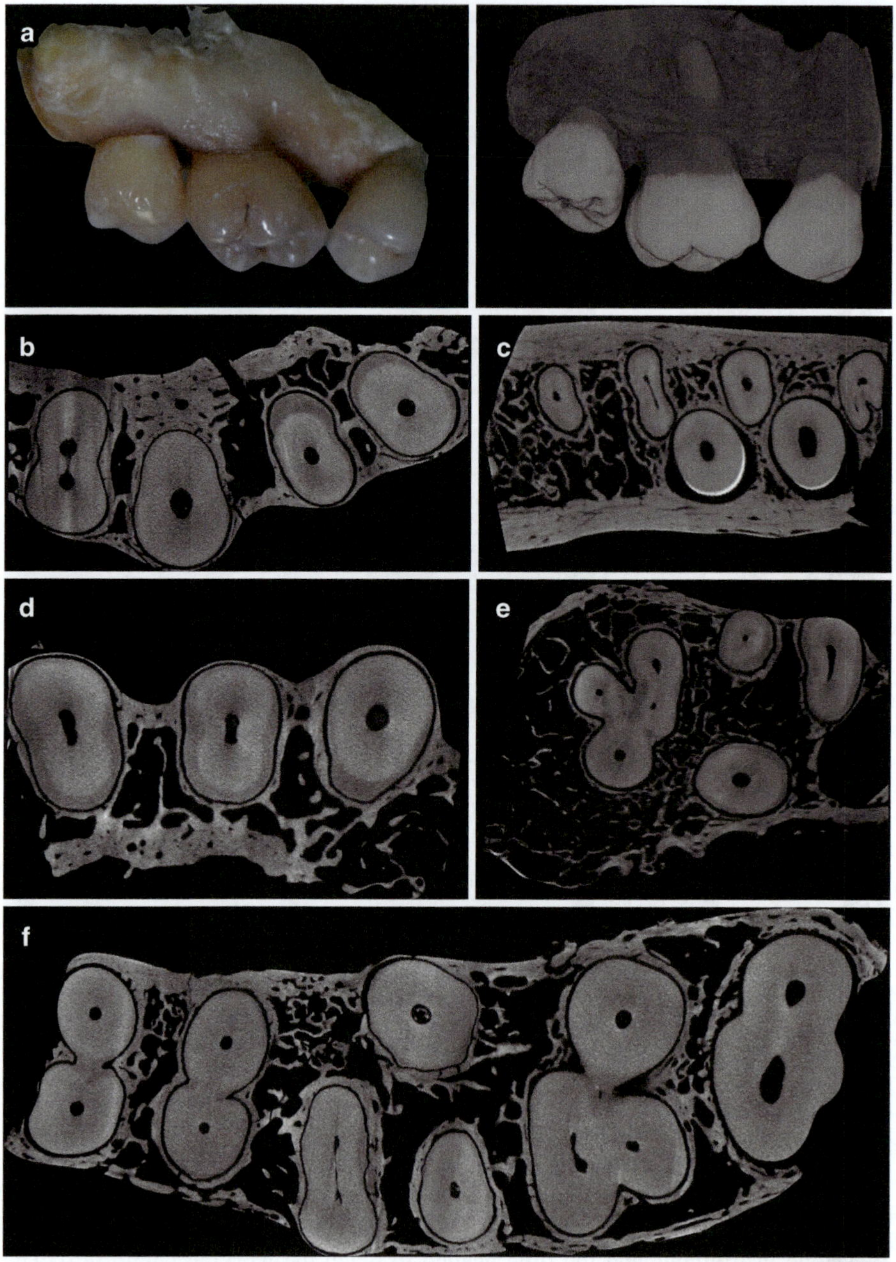

Fig. 6.16 (**a**) Real image and micro-CT 3D model of a maxillary bone-block of a fresh cadaver. (**b–f**) Typical cross-sectional micro-CT images of maxillary bone-blocks containing premolar and molar teeth in which is possible to observe the dentinal tissue without defects

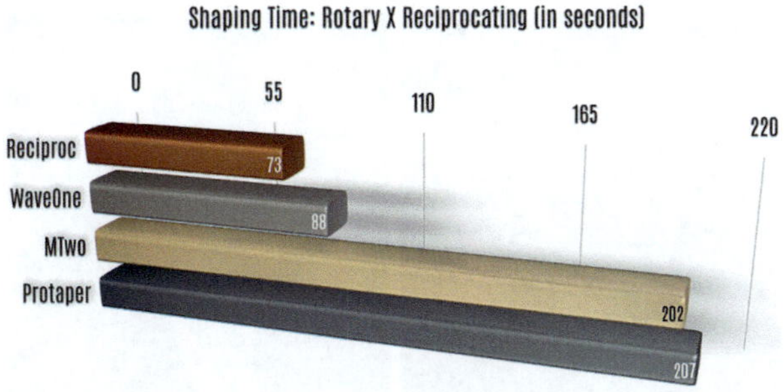

Fig. 6.17 Preparation time with different instruments activated in rotary or reciprocating motion in maxillary incisors. (Adapted from Bürklein and Schäfer [42])

6.2.7 Accumulated Hard Tissue Debris and Debris Extrusion

Accumulation of debris in the lateral extensions of root canals and apically extruded debris have been extensively studied topics. It has been speculated that reciprocating movement and the single-file technique may facilitate the occurrence of these events. Despite a micro-CT study reported that WaveOne led to more debris accumulation than ProTaper, especially in the isthmuses and fins of mandibular molar canals [46], several other studies could not determine differences when reciprocating or rotary instruments were compared [47–49]. Taken together, these results suggest that the instrument design, irrigation protocols, and operator are more decisive for the accumulation of hard tissue debris than the number of instruments used or their kinematics (Fig. 6.18).

The worldwide rise of reciprocating systems also led to another potential drawback: single-file mechanical preparation cutting significant amounts of dentin in short periods of time would be more prone to force debris, dentin chips, irrigants, remaining pulp tissue, bacteria, and their by-products through the apex. The basis for this assumption is the clinical impression that reciprocation is an overall forceful movement, which may act as a mechanical piston, pumping debris and irrigants through the apex. However, at least to some measure, this assumption may not have a well-built background, since reciprocation tries to mimic a balanced force kinematics technique, which is well known as being a pressureless movement pushing less material into the periapical tissues [50, 51] (Fig. 6.19).

Extrusion of debris may happen because the flutes of reciprocating instruments are designed to remove them only in a single direction. In the framework of rotary motion, the forward movement continually removes dentinal debris to the coronal direction. This means that, theoretically, kinematics would play a role in packing debris into the irregular areas of the root canal space and/or pushing them beyond the apex as a consequence of the backward movement (relief angle). The counterargument claims that multi-file rotary systems are prone to extrude more debris and irrigants as a function of more technical steps (insertions and withdrawals of the instruments) necessary to shape the canal.

Several studies have tried to shed some light on this topic [41, 42, 47–49, 52, 53], but the existing research results remain inconclusive. Despite some studies reported

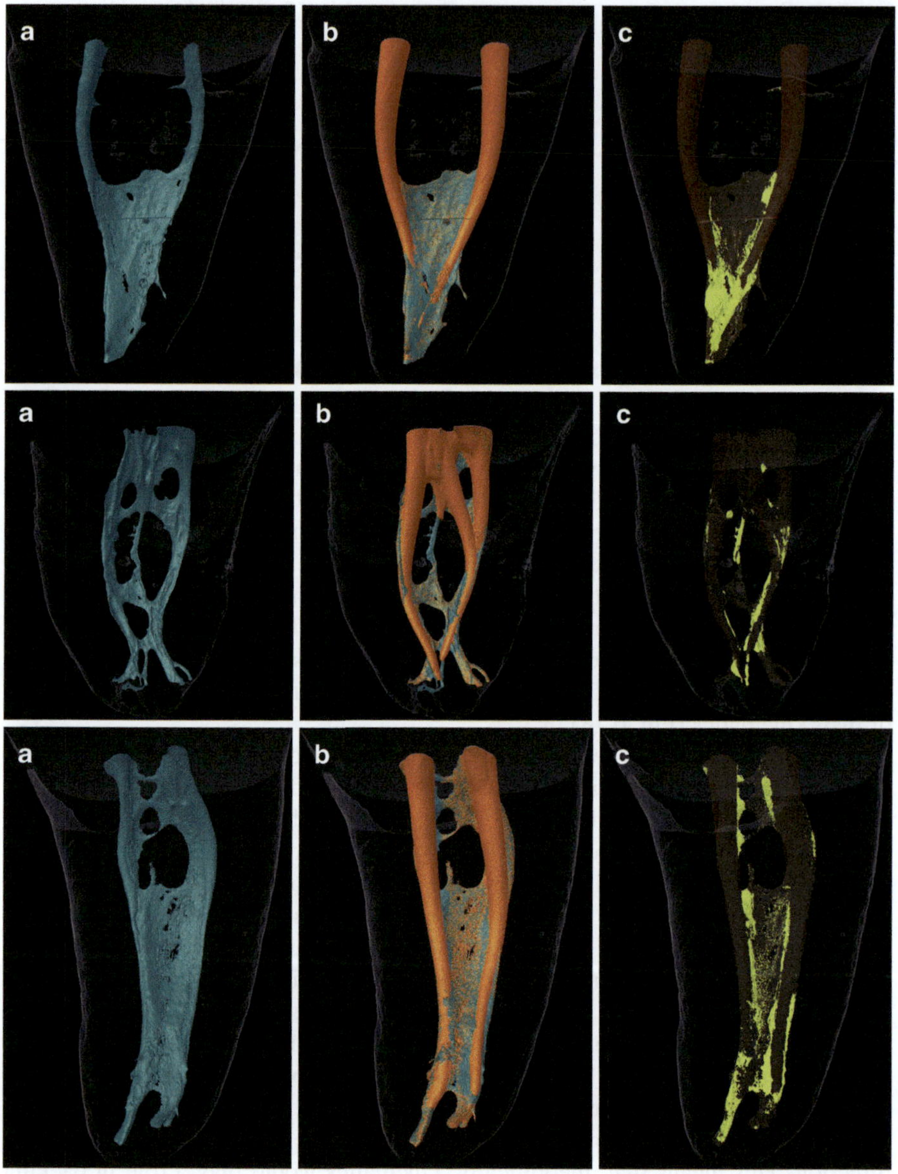

Fig. 6.18 Three-dimensional micro-CT models depicting the internal anatomy of three mesial roots of mandibular molars (**a**) before (in green) and (**b**) after (in orange) chemomechanical preparation of root canals with ProTaper Next rotary instruments. Canals were irrigated with 1 mL of 2.5% sodium hypochlorite after each instrument using a 27-G needle adapted to a 3-mL syringe. (**c**) The presence of accumulated hard-tissue debris in irregularities of the canal anatomy created by the mechanical preparation can be seen in yellow

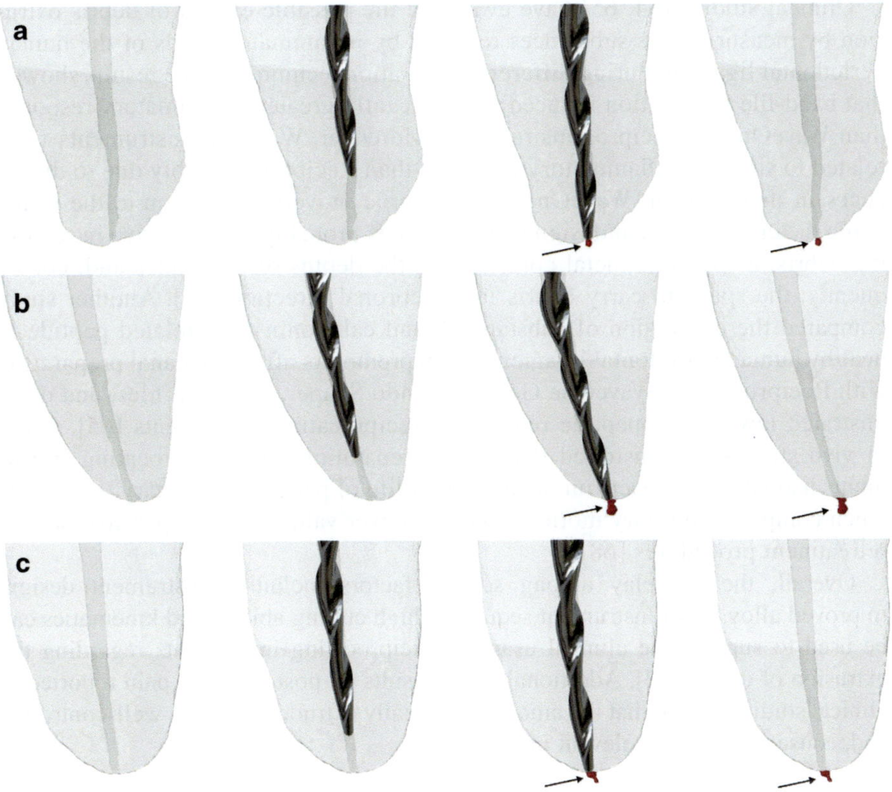

Fig. 6.19 Micro-CT models of (**a–c**) three mandibular canines demonstrating the apical extrusion of debris (in red) caused by the preparation of the root canals with NiTi instruments

more debris extrusion associated with reciprocating (Reciproc and WaveOne) rather than rotary instruments (ProTaper and Mtwo) [41, 42, 53], other studies showed no difference [47–49, 52] or observed less debris extrusion using reciprocating motion [50, 51, 54]. A favorable input in terms of debris extrusion was reported for the F2 ProTaper used in reciprocating motion [55] and for the WaveOne which were significantly better than the ProTaper Universal [56]. Other authors found that the use of both WaveOne and Reciproc systems minimized the extrusion of bacteria [57] and reduced the extrusion of debris [50, 51, 54] compared to multi-file rotary systems regardless of the irrigation protocol or the size of apical preparation [58]. Some results showed that reciprocating instruments were associated with less debris extrusion even during retreatment procedures in comparison to continuous rotary multi-file systems [59–61], while another study reported that the Reciproc system extruded significantly more debris than rotary retreatment NiTi instruments [62]. A comprehensive review of the literature [63] concluded that kinematics have no influence on the accumulation and extrusion of dentinal debris. Therefore, there is no robust evidence that instruments working in reciprocating motion extrude more debris than in continuous rotation.

Clinical studies [64, 65] have evaluated the possible effects of debris extrusion by measuring the substances released by inflammatory cells of the human periodontal ligament during different preparation techniques. The results showed that hand-file preparation induced a significantly greater inflammatory response than WaveOne or Reciproc instruments. Moreover, WaveOne instruments were related to stronger inflammatory reactions than Reciproc, possibly due to differences in their design. WaveOne and Reciproc movements are quite the same, while the cross-sectional design of WaveOne is probably less effective in removing debris, as its large metal core reduces the depths of the blades and, consequently, the space to carry debris in the coronal direction [66]. Another study compared the expression of substance P and calcitonin gene-related peptide in healthy human periodontal ligaments from premolars after root canal preparation with Reciproc Blue, WaveOne Gold, XP-endo Shaper, and hand files, and demonstrated lower neuropeptide release for reciprocating instruments [65]. Other in vivo studies demonstrated that canal preparation with reciprocating instruments had similar impacts on the quality of life of patients in primary treatments when compared to rotary motion [67], and lower values of postoperative pain in retreatment procedures [68].

Overall, the interplay among several factors including instrument design, improved alloy, short instrument sequence, high cutting ability, and kinematics can be used to support the clinical usage of reciprocating instruments regarding the extrusion of debris [63]. Additionally, the results on postoperative pain reported in clinical studies restate that the amount of apically extruded debris is well-controlled and, consequently, not relevant in practice.

6.2.8 Disinfection Ability: Reduction of Bacterial Load and Toxins

Chemomechanical preparation has an important role in reducing bacteria from the root canal system. However, even after preparation, the anatomical complexities of the root canals can accumulate remnants of pulp tissue, necrotic debris, and bacterial biofilm which may result in persistent infection and treatment failure [69]. The effectiveness of cleaning root canals using reciprocating instruments was investigated in terms of removal of endotoxins and cultivable bacteria to promote disinfection [70–73]. The results confirmed the ability of different instruments to promote significant bacterial and endotoxin reduction, but none of them were able to completely disinfect the root canal system [70, 73, 74], once no bacteria-free root canals were observed in either primary treatment or retreatment.

One concern about the use of single-file reciprocating systems is the reduced overall preparation time that could compromise the process of root canal cleaning and disinfection. However, the mechanical action of endodontic instruments on dentin, together with copious irrigation, is more critical for bacterial and endotoxin removal than the number of instruments used in a sequence. Although some reports demonstrated better reduction of bacterial load associated with rotary instruments [75–77], most of the studies showed that the single-file reciprocating technique

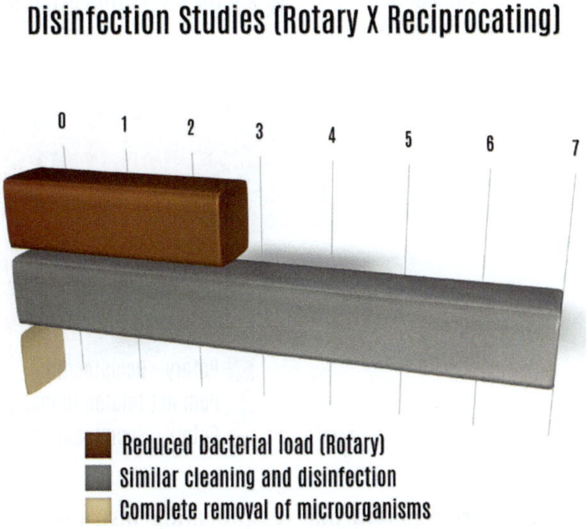

Fig. 6.20 Number of studies comparing reciprocating and rotary motions according to disinfection markers. Rotary was superior to reciprocation in three studies regarding reduction of bacterial load, while reciprocating was similar to rotary in seven studies on cleaning and disinfection. No study demonstrated a complete removal of bacteria from root canals associated with any given instrumentation technique

achieved similar cleaning [15, 52] and disinfection efficacy [70–72, 78, 79] than those of rotary multi-instrument systems. The differences among these studies seem to be related to the irrigation protocol (volume of irrigant and intracanal contact time) than with the mechanical preparation itself.

The most evaluated reciprocating instruments, WaveOne and Reciproc, have been found to be effective in the eradication of *Enterococcus faecalis* from root canals [78, 80]. In general, when comparing the antibacterial efficacy of WaveOne and/or Reciproc instruments with different rotary systems (BioRace [73], Mtwo [70–72], ProTaper [71, 72, 79], RaCe [71]), it was shown that all systems are highly effective in reducing the total bacterial counts [70–73, 79] and endotoxin levels [70–72, 79] (Fig. 6.20).

Taken together, these results emphasize the idea highlighted in this textbook that shaping procedures should always be followed by an adequate cleaning and disinfection protocol, as none of the systems available for either continuous rotation or reciprocating movement can completely remove microorganisms from the root canal. Therefore, the importance of optimal chemical disinfection is re-emphasized.

6.2.9 Clinical Performance: Postoperative Pain

Mild postoperative pain often occurs following endodontic treatment, regardless of the instrumentation technique adopted, and generally does not require any additional treatment [81]. Postoperative pain has been associated with insufficient canal debridement, hyperocclusion, the presence of apical periodontitis, and the extrusion of infected debris to the periapical tissues [82]. Comparisons of postoperative pain between rotary and reciprocating systems have shown conflicting findings. Some studies associate reciprocating instruments with worse postoperative pain [83–85],

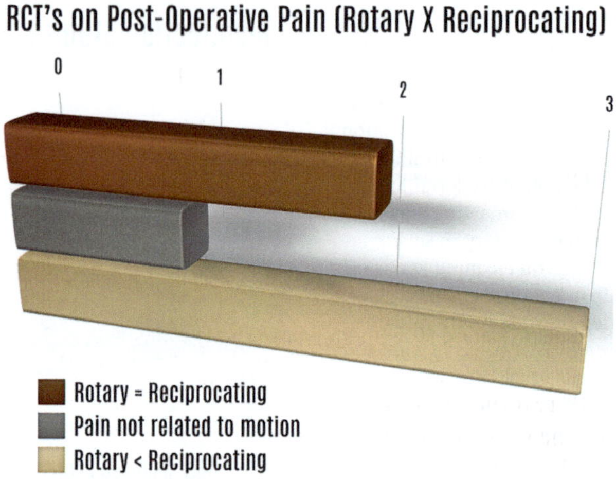

Fig. 6.21 Number of randomized clinical trials (RCT's) comparing reciprocating to rotary motion regarding postoperative pain

while others reported that reciprocating instruments caused less pain than rotary [86, 87]. In addition, one study demonstrated a total lack of effect stemming from kinematics (single-file reciprocating or single-file rotary) on postoperative pain [88] (Fig. 6.21).

A systematic review and meta-analysis indicated that rotary motion has a negative impact on postoperative pain after endodontic treatment and revealed that a larger number of patients complained of severe pain 48 h after treatment under rotary motion compared to reciprocating [89]. In another review reported the use of rotary instruments was related to a lower incidence of postoperative pain in comparison to reciprocating systems [90]. Other systematic review reported conflicting results between engine-driven instruments with different kinematics, given the low quality of evidence and contrasting findings. Among those studies, several types of instruments were tested and the difference in the results might be due to other methodological reasons rather than the motion itself [91]. The heterogeneity in the findings of these studies indicates that there is no definitive answer associating the high incidence and intensity of postoperative pain with instrument kinematics (Fig. 6.22).

6.3 Educational Aspects of Reciprocating Movement

The inception of reciprocating movement has brought new perspectives to endodontic education. Essentially, the possibility of using a single instrument to achieve the final shape of the root canal without the need of a previous glide path [27, 28] and under a neglectable risk of fracture [1, 6, 27, 28] has filled a gap which has long existed in the educational process of root canal preparation: the steep learning curve to safely and predictably enlarge the canal space using stainless-steel instruments. It is acknowledged that students face difficulties while attempting to learn how to

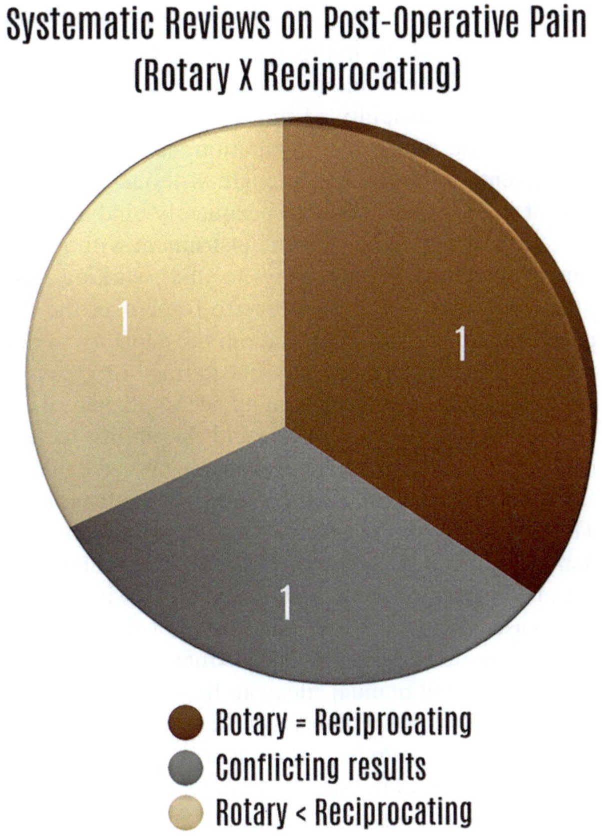

Fig. 6.22 Number of systematic reviews comparing reciprocating to rotary motion regarding postoperative pain

prepare the root canal. The request to fully understand how an endodontic manual file safely operates inside the root canal turns out to be the greatest educational challenge since it embraces the need to develop very specific tactile perceptions that can only be achieved after a long-term practice driven by a great dose of self-didactics. As wisely observed by John West [92]: "*when treating endodontic patients, you know what you want: confidence, consistency and control, but you should not disregard what you need: skills, skills and skills.*" No other step of root canal therapy requires more development of very specific and highly sensitive skills than root canal preparation.

The process of learning any technique is recognized to be meticulous and requires prudence along the step-by-step development of very specific technical abilities usually aligned with a long and tough educational curve, a lot of attention, and intense dedication of the apprentice [93]. Learning root canal preparation is even more complex since, for the first time in the learning progression of a dental student, the manual maneuver made with an instrument cannot be directly visualized, meaning that the only practical information and feedback to the student come from an indirect tactile sense given by the instrument itself [94], which takes time to learn and understand its significance. As examples, we can point out the difficulty of any endodontic apprentice in mastering the various phases of the root canal preparation, such as scouting with small stainless-steel instruments up to a desired length without instrument distortion; the determination of the first instrument to adequately bind at the working length to start shaping; the ability to withdraw the instrument without its complete removal from the canal, returning it precisely to the working length while avoiding over-instrumentation; the use of precise force over the instruments to obtain the best performance without deformation; the capacity to determine when an instrument is seriously deformed and/or prone to fracture; the recognition of the moment when the instrumentation is adequately accomplished; the identification that the apical enlargement size is sufficient; and the ability to learn how to pre-curve instruments, how to operate bent files inside curved canals, recognizing when specially sized files are required for scouting difficult narrow and/or curved canals [94]. This is just a short summary of the situations in which self-tactile sense is demanded from the student. These abilities cannot be actually grasped in theory, but only experienced by practice, being also influenced by the specific anatomy of each case, the quality and conditions of the instruments, and the student's own level of manual skills. This means that the learning process of endodontic instrumentation using manual files can be very frustrating, resulting in an experience that is usually filled with accidents and technical intercurrences faced by many (or a non-negligible number of) students.

Overall, most of the specific abilities required for manual instrumentation are not prerequisites when learning canal preparation with reciprocating instruments, since they have the unique ability to advance safely toward the working length, which makes it easier to be learned even by beginners [95]. Among the reciprocating systems, the ability of the Reciproc instrument to inflex the learning curve of root canal preparation deserves to be highlighted as it combines (1) an optimal cutting efficiency that allows a unique advancement of the instrument inside the root canal [27, 28], (2) a negligible fracture rate, which is well documented in the literature [1, 6, 27, 28], and (3) the possibility of using a pneumatic dedicated contra-angle to operate the instrument (Fig. 6.23), reducing the need to purchase expensive motors to apply the technique. Moreover, its technical simplicity can be assured even in root canals of moderately complexity, using an algorithm that includes the scouting of the canal with a size 10 hand file as a token of strong confidence to enlarge the canal with the Reciproc R25 instrument (size 25, taper 0.08v), without glide path in the majority of the cases [27, 28]. The ability of this instrument turns out to be the decisive educational breakthrough that allows the use of mechanically driven NiTi instruments by undergraduated students, ultimately adding safety, confidence, and optimal technical results to an expedited learning curve for root canal preparation, an experience that could not be entirely applied to rotary movement due to its

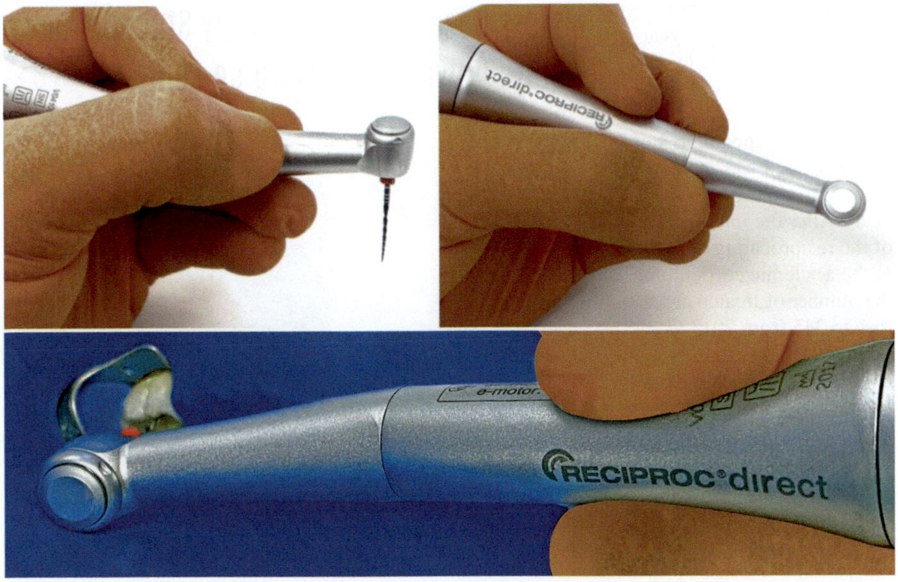

Fig. 6.23 Reciproc R25 instrument adapted to the VDW Reciproc Direct pneumatic contra-angle coupled to a low-speed handpiece during root canal preparation of a mandibular molar

hard-to-accomplish glide path procedure required for all cases, and the high incidence of instrument fracture [24, 26, 28], especially among apprentices.

Educational experiences with reciprocating movement with undergraduate students have already successfully passed the test of time. In the last decade, some dental schools in Brazil documented a significant rise in the number of molar cases done by students (Figs. 6.24 and 6.25), with a negligible fracture rate (Fig. 6.26) and a clear increase in the technical quality of root canal preparation (Figs. 6.27, 6.28, 6.29, and 6.30). Considering that the technical quality of root canal preparation is of concern, the introduction of reciprocating movement into the curriculum of undergraduates has helped to reduce the overall feeling of failure that commonly stirs a large number of students. The increase in self-confidence is important in a technically demanding specialty such as endodontics. It helps to reduce significantly the first phase of the learning curve as proposed by Strauss and Sayles [96], that is, the frustrating step which, when teaching the traditional stainless steel-based education, takes almost the entire period of learning. In this sense, reciprocating movement provides the necessary reduction in technical sensitivity to rapidly overcome the first frustrating phase by progressively increasing the technical quality until the student reaches the so-called false platform (Fig. 6.31a–c) in which the professor's role is to progressively increase the complexity of cases so that the apprentice can reach the apex of knowledge (Fig. 6.31d), where they can be considered adequately qualified for seeing patients after graduation. When stainless-steel-based instrumentation dominates undergraduate education, many students are unable to even reach the

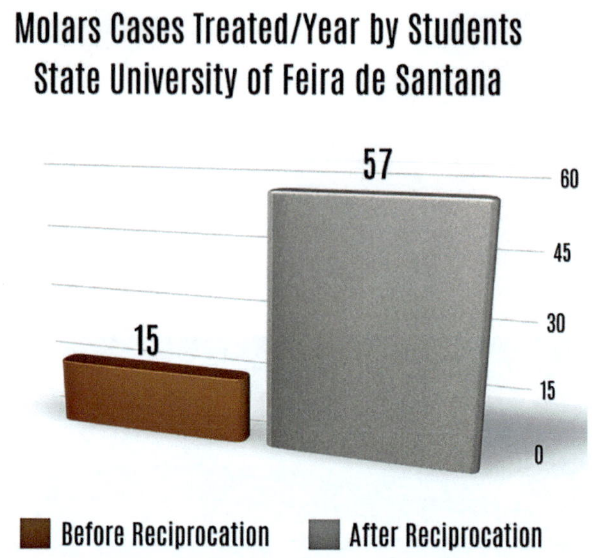

Fig. 6.24 Percentage of molar teeth treated per year on the undergraduate level at the State University of Feira de Santana, Brazil. From 2010 to 2012, the number of molars treated was lower than 45 cases (or almost 15 per year). After the introduction of the reciprocating technique in the academic curriculum, the number of treated cases rose to 345 from 2013 to 2019, which means approximately 57 cases per year. (Data courtesy of Dr. Evaldo Rodrigues, Brazil)

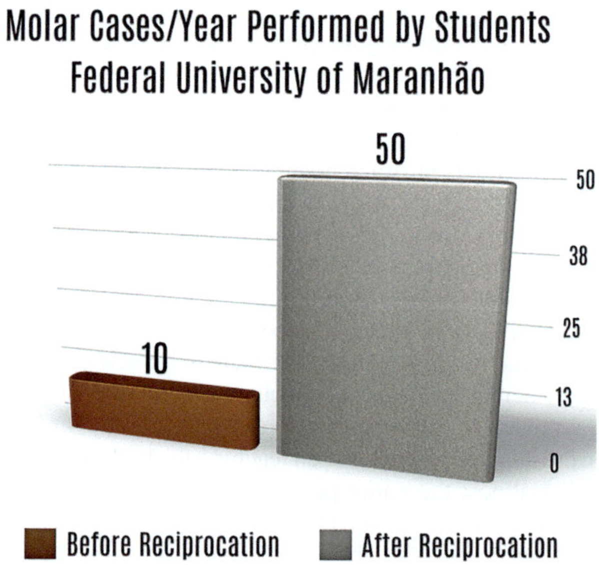

Fig. 6.25 Similar profile of Fig. 6.24 recorded in a discipline dedicated only to root canal treatment of molar teeth performed by undergraduate students at the Federal University of Maranhão, Brazil, in which the reciprocating protocol was introduced in 2013. The mean number increased from 10 cases per year to 50 endodontic treatments of molars per year, a raise of about 500%

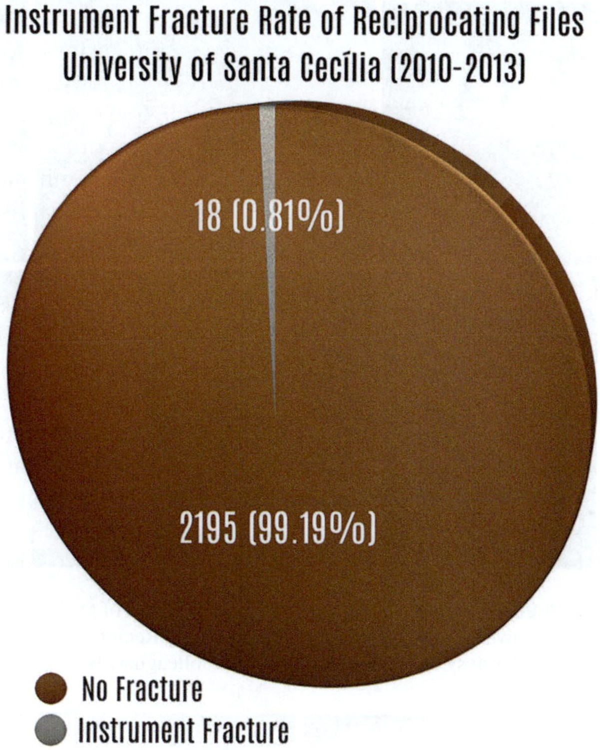

Fig. 6.26 Number of root canals treated by undergraduate students at the University of Santa Cecília (Brazil), from February 2013 to December 2015, in which reciprocating protocol was also introduced in clinical practice. From a total of 2,213 root canals (1,102 teeth), only 18 (0.81%) had instrument fracture. In just two cases, fracture occurred during the first use of the instrument. (Unpublished data. Courtesy of Dr. Giulio Gavini and colleagues, Brazil)

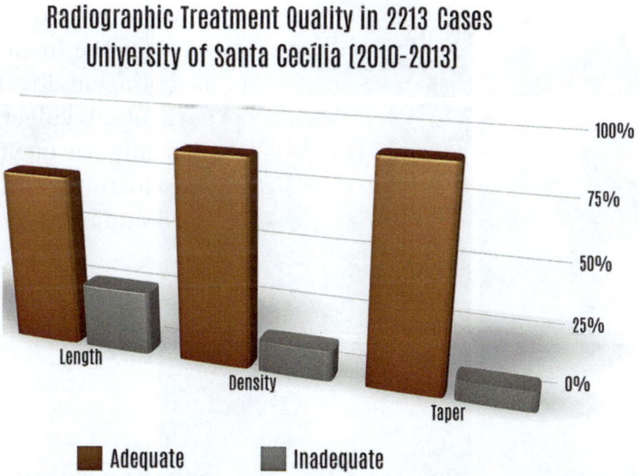

Fig. 6.27 Percentage adequacy to radiographic quality after canal preparation with reciprocating instruments and final obturation with single cone technique performed by undergraduate students of the University of Santa Cecília (Brazil). The frequency of root canals categorized as adequate regarding preparation length, canal taper, and obturation density is highly significantly. (Unpublished data. Courtesy of Dr. Giulio Gavini and colleagues, Brazil)

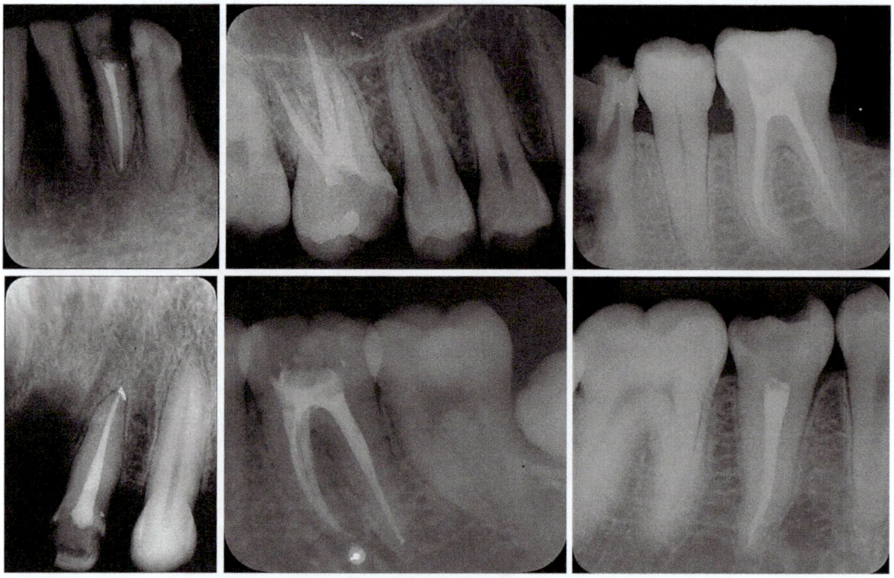

Fig. 6.28 Root canal treatments in different groups of teeth performed by undergraduate students of the University of Santa Cecília (Brazil) using Reciproc System and single cone obturation technique. (Courtesy of Dr. Giulio Gavini and colleagues, Brazil)

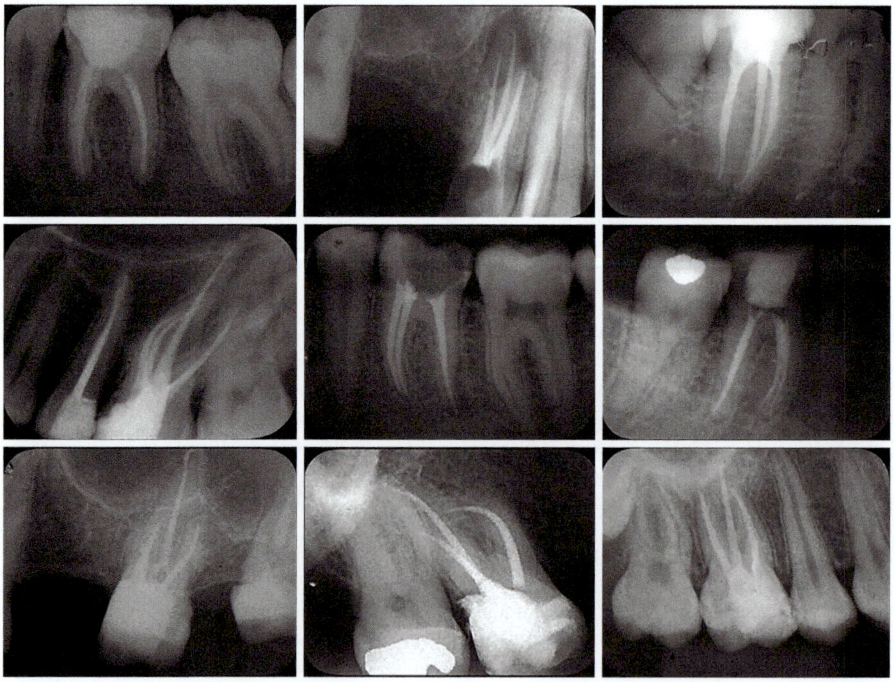

Fig. 6.29 Root canal treatments in different groups of teeth performed by undergraduate students of the State University of Feira de Santana (Brazil) using Reciproc System and single cone obturation technique. (Courtesy of Dr. Evaldo Rodrigues)

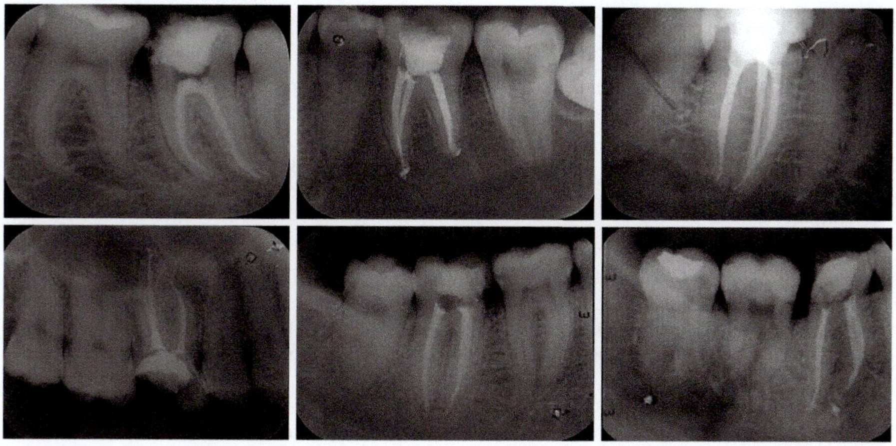

Fig. 6.30 Root canal treatments in different groups of teeth performed by undergraduate students of the Federal University of Maranhão (Brazil) using Reciproc System and single cone obturation technique

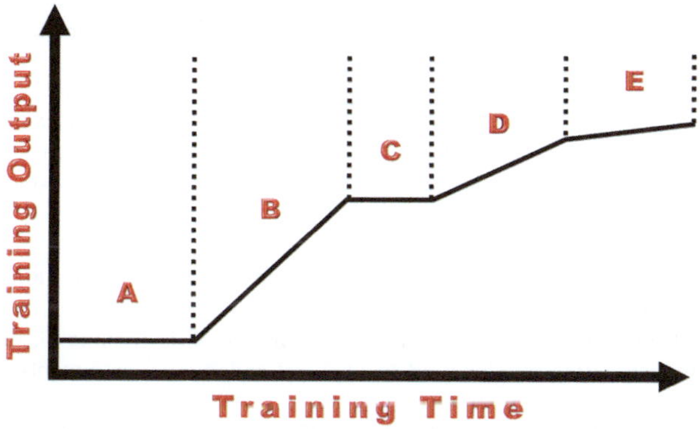

Fig. 6.31 Learning curve. (Adapted from Strauss and Sayles [96]). (**A**) Frustrating phase—it is the most difficult phase in which several errors are prone to happen. (**B**) Progressive results—it starts when the student gets a progressive understanding on how the technique works. As a rule of thumb, the more complex the technique, the longer will be the frustrating phase and progressive phases. (**C**) False platform—it represents the moment when the student gets a false perception of acquaintance. At this phase, the job of the instructor is to keep on increasing the complexity of the cases. (**D**) Apex of knowledge—that is when the acquaintance is reached. In less complex techniques, this level can be reached faster. (**E**) Retraining period—a necessary lifetime dedication to maintain the acquired acquaintanceship

false platform phase, as simple cases take most of the timeframe dedicated to endodontic practice. In this sense, the inception of reciprocating movement in the undergraduate curriculum ultimately has a relevant social impact by releasing onto the market more qualified and trained professionals able to solve cases of moderate complexity using an intuitive, easy to learn, and implement technique that allows optimal results even in the hands of newly graduated nonspecialist dentists.

References

1. Plotino G, Ahmed HM, Grande NM, Cohen S, Bukiet F. Current assessment of reciprocation in endodontic preparation: a comprehensive review—part II: properties and effectiveness. J Endod. 2015;41:1939–50.
2. De-Deus G, Moreira EJ, Lopes HP, Elias CN. Extended cyclic fatigue life of F2 ProTaper instruments used in reciprocating movement. Int Endod J. 2010;43:1063–8.
3. Gavini G, Caldeira CL, Akisue E, Candeiro GT, Kawakami DA. Resistance to flexural fatigue of Reciproc R25 files under continuous rotation and reciprocating movement. J Endod. 2012;38:684–7.
4. Kiefner P, Ban M, De-Deus G. Is the reciprocating movement per se able to improve the cyclic fatigue resistance of instruments? Int Endod J. 2014;47:430–6.
5. Lee W, Hwang YJ, You SY, Kim HC. Effect of reciprocation usage of nickel-titanium rotary files on the cyclic fatigue resistance. Aust Endod J. 2013;39:146–50.
6. Pedulla E, Grande NM, Plotino G, Gambarini G, Rapisarda E. Influence of continuous or reciprocating motion on cyclic fatigue resistance of 4 different nickel-titanium rotary instruments. J Endod. 2013;39:258–61.
7. Vadhana S, SaravanaKarthikeyan B, Nandini S, Velmurugan N. Cyclic fatigue resistance of RaCe and Mtwo rotary files in continuous rotation and reciprocating motion. J Endod. 2014;40:995–9.
8. Gambarini G, Rubini AG, Al Sudani D, Gergi R, Culla A, De Angelis F, et al. Influence of different angles of reciprocation on the cyclic fatigue of nickel-titanium endodontic instruments. J Endod. 2012;38:1408–11.
9. Shin CS, Huang YH, Chi CW, Lin CP. Fatigue life enhancement of NiTi rotary endodontic instruments by progressive reciprocating operation. Int Endod J. 2014;47:882–8.
10. ISO. International Organization for Standardization ISO 3630-1. Dental root canal instruments: part 1-files, reamers, barbed broaches, rasps, paste carriers, explorers and cotton broaches. Geneva: International Organization for Standardization; 1992.
11. Gambarini G, Giansiracusa Rubini A, Sannino G, Di Giorgio G, Piasecki L, Al-Sudani D, et al. Cutting efficiency of nickel-titanium rotary and reciprocating instruments after prolonged use. Odontology. 2016;104:77–81.
12. Giansiracusa Rubini A, Plotino G, Al-Sudani D, Grande NM, Sonnino G, Putorti E, et al. A new device to test cutting efficiency of mechanical endodontic instruments. Med Sci Monit. 2014;20:374–8.
13. Pedulla E, Leanza G, La Rosa GRM, Gueli AM, Pasquale S, Plotino G, et al. Cutting efficiency of conventional and heat-treated nickel-titanium rotary or reciprocating glide path instruments. Int Endod J. 2020;53:376–84.
14. Abu Haimed AS, Abuhaimed TS, Dummer PE, Bryant ST. The root canal shaping ability of WaveOne and Reciproc versus ProTaper Universal and Mtwo rotary NiTi systems. Saudi Endod J. 2017;7:8–15.
15. Bürklein S, Hinschitza K, Dammaschke T, Schäfer E. Shaping ability and cleaning effectiveness of two single-file systems in severely curved root canals of extracted teeth: Reciproc and WaveOne versus Mtwo and ProTaper. Int Endod J. 2012;45:449–61.
16. Franco V, Fabiani C, Taschieri S, Malentacca A, Bortolin M, Del Fabbro M. Investigation on the shaping ability of nickel-titanium files when used with a reciprocating motion. J Endod. 2011;37:1398–401.
17. Navos BV, Hoppe CB, Mestieri LB, Bottcher DE, So MV, Grecca FS. Centering and transportation: in vitro evaluation of continuous and reciprocating systems in curved root canals. J Conserv Dent. 2016;19:478–81.
18. Giuliani V, Di Nasso L, Pace R, Pagavino G. Shaping ability of waveone primary reciprocating files and ProTaper system used in continuous and reciprocating motion. J Endod. 2014;40:1468–71.

19. Hwang YH, Bae KS, Baek SH, Kum KY, Lee W, Shon WJ, et al. Shaping ability of the conventional nickel-titanium and reciprocating nickel-titanium file systems: a comparative study using micro-computed tomography. J Endod. 2014;40:1186–9.
20. Jin SY, Lee W, Kang MK, Hur B, Kim HC. Single file reciprocating technique using conventional nickel-titanium rotary endodontic files. Scanning. 2013;35:349–54.
21. Berutti E, Chiandussi G, Paolino DS, Scotti N, Cantatore G, Castellucci A, et al. Canal shaping with WaveOne Primary reciprocating files and ProTaper system: a comparative study. J Endod. 2012;38:505–9.
22. Versiani MA, Leoni GB, Steier L, De-Deus G, Tassani S, Pecora JD, et al. Micro-computed tomography study of oval-shaped canals prepared with the Self-adjusting File, Reciproc, WaveOne, and ProTaper universal systems. J Endod. 2013;39:1060–6.
23. Zuolo ML, Zaia AA, Belladonna FG, Silva E, Souza EM, Versiani MA, et al. Micro-CT assessment of the shaping ability of four root canal instrumentation systems in oval-shaped canals. Int Endod J. 2018;51:564–71.
24. Berutti E, Paolino DS, Chiandussi G, Alovisi M, Cantatore G, Castellucci A, et al. Root canal anatomy preservation of WaveOne reciprocating files with or without glide path. J Endod. 2012;38:101–4.
25. Dhingra A, Nagar N, Sapra V. Influence of the glide path on various parameters of root canal prepared with WaveOne reciprocating file using cone beam computed tomography. Dent Res J (Isfahan). 2015;12:534–40.
26. Zheng L, Ji X, Li C, Zuo L, Wei X. Comparison of glide paths created with K-files, PathFiles, and the ProGlider file, and their effects on subsequent WaveOne preparation in curved canals. BMC Oral Health. 2018;18:152.
27. De-Deus G, Arruda TE, Souza EM, Neves A, Magalhaes K, Thuanne E, et al. The ability of the Reciproc R25 instrument to reach the full root canal working length without a glide path. Int Endod J. 2013;46:993–8.
28. Rodrigues E, De-Deus G, Souza E, Silva EJ. Safe mechanical preparation with reciprocation movement without glide path creation: result from a pool of 673 root canals. Braz Dent J. 2016;27:22–7.
29. Zuolo ML, Carvalho MC, De-Deus G. Negotiability of second mesiobuccal canals in maxillary molars using a reciprocating system. J Endod. 2015;41:1913–7.
30. Bürklein S, Tsotsis P, Schäfer E. Incidence of dentinal defects after root canal preparation: reciprocating versus rotary instrumentation. J Endod. 2013;39:501–4.
31. Kosti E, Zinelis S, Lambrianidis T, Margelos J. A comparative study of crack development in stainless-steel hedstrom files used with step-back or crown-down techniques. J Endod. 2004;30:38–41.
32. Liu R, Hou BX, Wesselink PR, Wu MK, Shemesh H. The incidence of root microcracks caused by 3 different single-file systems versus the ProTaper system. J Endod. 2013;39:1054–6.
33. Shemesh H, Bier CA, Wu MK, Tanomaru-Filho M, Wesselink PR. The effects of canal preparation and filling on the incidence of dentinal defects. Int Endod J. 2009;42:208–13.
34. De-Deus G, Silva EJ, Marins J, Souza E, Neves Ade A, Goncalves Belladonna F, et al. Lack of causal relationship between dentinal microcracks and root canal preparation with reciprocation systems. J Endod. 2014;40:1447–50.
35. Cavalcante DM, De-Deus G, Belladonna FG, Simoes-Carvalho M, Carvalhal JCA, Souza EM, et al. Do pre-existing microcracks play a role in the fracture resistance of roots in a laboratory setting? Int Endod J. 2020;53(11):1506–15.
36. De-Deus G, Belladonna FG, Souza EM, Silva EJ, Neves Ade A, Alves H, et al. Micro-computed tomographic assessment on the effect of Protaper Next and Twisted File Adaptive systems on dentinal cracks. J Endod. 2015;41:1116–9.
37. De-Deus G, Cavalcante DM, Belladonna FG, Carvalhal J, Souza EM, Lopes RT, et al. Root dentinal microcracks: a post-extraction experimental phenomenon? Int Endod J. 2020;53:137–42.
38. De-Deus G, Cesar de Azevedo Carvalhal J, Belladonna FG, Silva E, Lopes RT, Moreira Filho RE, et al. Dentinal microcrack development after canal preparation: a longitudinal in situ micro-computed tomography study using a cadaver model. J Endod. 2017;43:1553–8.

39. Bayram HM, Bayram E, Ocak M, Uygun AD, Celik HH. Effect of ProTaper Gold, Self-Adjusting File, and XP-endo Shaper instruments on dentinal microcrack formation: a micro-computed tomographic study. J Endod. 2017;43:1166–9.
40. Arashiro FN, De-Deus G, Belladonna FG, Cavalcante DM, Coelho MS, Silva E, et al. Dentinal microcracks on freshly extracted teeth: the impact of the extraction technique. Int Endod J. 2020;53:440–6.
41. Burklein S, Benten S, Schafer E. Quantitative evaluation of apically extruded debris with different single-file systems: Reciproc, F360 and OneShape versus Mtwo. Int Endod J. 2014;47:405–9.
42. Bürklein S, Schäfer E. Apically extruded debris with reciprocating single-file and full-sequence rotary instrumentation systems. J Endod. 2012;38:850–2.
43. You SY, Bae KS, Baek SH, Kum KY, Shon WJ, Lee W. Lifespan of one nickel-titanium rotary file with reciprocating motion in curved root canals. J Endod. 2010;36:1991–4.
44. Saber Sel D. Abu El Sadat SM. Effect of altering the reciprocation range on the fatigue life and the shaping ability of WaveOne nickel-titanium instruments. J Endod. 2013;39:685–8.
45. Saber SE, Nagy MM, Schäfer E. Comparative evaluation of the shaping ability of ProTaper Next, iRaCe and Hyflex CM rotary NiTi files in severely curved root canals. Int Endod J. 2015;48:131–6.
46. Robinson JP, Lumley PJ, Cooper PR, Grover LM, Walmsley AD. Reciprocating root canal technique induces greater debris accumulation than a continuous rotary technique as assessed by 3-dimensional micro-computed tomography. J Endod. 2013;39:1067–70.
47. Kirchhoff AL, Fariniuk LF, Mello I. Apical extrusion of debris in flat-oval root canals after using different instrumentation systems. J Endod. 2015;41:237–41.
48. Kocak S, Kocak MM, Saglam BC, Turker SA, Sagsen B, Er O. Apical extrusion of debris using self-adjusting file, reciprocating single-file, and 2 rotary instrumentation systems. J Endod. 2013;39:1278–80.
49. Kucukyilmaz E, Savas S, Saygili G, Uysal B. Assessment of apically extruded debris and irrigant produced by different nickel-titanium instrument systems. Braz Oral Res. 2015;29:1–6.
50. De-Deus G, Neves A, Silva EJ, Mendonca TA, Lourenco C, Calixto C, et al. Apically extruded dentin debris by reciprocating single-file and multi-file rotary system. Clin Oral Investig. 2015;19:357–61.
51. Lu Y, Chen M, Qiao F, Wu L. Comparison of apical and coronal extrusions using reciprocating and rotary instrumentation systems. BMC Oral Health. 2015;15:92.
52. De-Deus G, Marins J, Silva EJ, Souza E, Belladonna FG, Reis C, et al. Accumulated hard tissue debris produced during reciprocating and rotary nickel-titanium canal preparation. J Endod. 2015;41:676–81.
53. Surakanti JR, Venkata RC, Vemisetty HK, Dandolu RK, Jaya NK, Thota S. Comparative evaluation of apically extruded debris during root canal preparation using ProTaper, Hyflex and Waveone rotary systems. J Conserv Dent. 2014;17:129–32.
54. Arslan H, Doganay E, Alsancak M, Capar ID, Karatas E, Gunduz HA. Comparison of apically extruded debris after root canal instrumentation using Reciproc((R)) instruments with various kinematics. Int Endod J. 2016;49:307–10.
55. De-Deus G, Brandao MC, Barino B, Di Giorgi K, Fidel RA, Luna AS. Assessment of apically extruded debris produced by the single-file ProTaper F2 technique under reciprocating movement. Oral Surg Oral Med Oral Pathol Oral Radiol Endod. 2010;110:390–4.
56. Karatas E, Ersoy I, Gunduz HA, Uygun AD, Kol E, Cakici F. Influence of instruments used in root canal preparation on amount of apically extruded debris. Artif Organs. 2016;40:774–7.
57. Tinoco JM, De-Deus G, Tinoco EM, Saavedra F, Fidel RA, Sassone LM. Apical extrusion of bacteria when using reciprocating single-file and rotary multifile instrumentation systems. Int Endod J. 2014;47:560–6.
58. Silva EJ, Teixeira JM, Kudsi N, Sassone LM, Krebs RL, Coutinho-Filho TS. Influence of apical preparation size and working length on debris extrusion. Braz Dent J. 2016;27:28–31.
59. Dincer AN, Er O, Canakci BC. Evaluation of apically extruded debris during root canal retreatment with several NiTi systems. Int Endod J. 2015;48:1194–8.

60. Silva EJ, Sa L, Belladonna FG, Neves AA, Accorsi-Mendonca T, Vieira VT, et al. Reciprocating versus rotary systems for root filling removal: assessment of the apically extruded material. J Endod. 2014;40:2077–80.
61. Uzunoglu E, Turker SA. Impact of different file systems on the amount of apically extruded debris during endodontic retreatment. Eur J Dent. 2016;10:210–4.
62. Canakci BC, Ustun Y, Er O, Genc Sen O. Evaluation of apically extruded debris from curved root canal filling removal using 5 nickel-titanium systems. J Endod. 2016;42:1101–4.
63. Pedrinha VF, Brandao J, Pessoa OF, Rodrigues PA. Influence of file motion on shaping, apical debris extrusion and dentinal defects: a critical review. Open Dent J. 2018;12:189–201.
64. Caviedes-Bucheli J, Moreno JO, Carreno CP, Delgado R, Garcia DJ, Solano J, et al. The effect of single-file reciprocating systems on substance P and calcitonin gene-related peptide expression in human periodontal ligament. Int Endod J. 2013;46:419–26.
65. Caviedes-Bucheli J, Rios-Osorio N, Rey-Rojas M, Laguna-Rivero F, Azuero-Holguin MM, Diaz LE, et al. Substance P and calcitonin gene-related peptide expression in human periodontal ligament after root canal preparation with Reciproc Blue, WaveOne Gold, XP EndoShaper and hand files. Int Endod J. 2018;51:1358–66.
66. Webber J, Machtou P, Pertot WJ, Kuttler S, Ruddle CJ, West J. The WaveOne single-file reciprocating system. Roots. 2011;7:28–33.
67. Oliveira PS, da Costa KNB, Carvalho CN, Ferreira MC. Impact of root canal preparation performed by ProTaper Next or Reciproc on the quality of life of patients: a randomized clinical trial. Int Endod J. 2019;52:139–48.
68. Garcia-Font M, Duran-Sindreu F, Morello S, Irazusta S, Abella F, Roig M, et al. Postoperative pain after removal of gutta-percha from root canals in endodontic retreatment using rotary or reciprocating instruments: a prospective clinical study. Clin Oral Investig. 2018;22:2623–31.
69. Ricucci D, Siqueira JF Jr, Bate AL, Pitt Ford TR. Histologic investigation of root canal-treated teeth with apical periodontitis: a retrospective study from twenty-four patients. J Endod. 2009;35:493–502.
70. Cavalli D, Toia CC, Flores Orozco EI, Khoury RD, Cardoso F, Alves MC, et al. Effectiveness in the removal of endotoxins and microbiological profile in primary endodontic infections using 3 different instrumentation systems: a randomized clinical study. J Endod. 2017;43:1237–45.
71. Marinho AC, Martinho FC, Goncalves LM, Rabang HR, Gomes BP. Does the Reciproc file remove root canal bacteria and endotoxins as effectively as multifile rotary systems? Int Endod J. 2015;48:542–8.
72. Martinho FC, Gomes AP, Fernandes AM, Ferreira NS, Endo MS, Freitas LF, et al. Clinical comparison of the effectiveness of single-file reciprocating systems and rotary systems for removal of endotoxins and cultivable bacteria from primarily infected root canals. J Endod. 2014;40:625–9.
73. Neves MA, Provenzano JC, Rôças IN, Siqueira JF Jr. Clinical antibacterial effectiveness of root canal preparation with reciprocating single-instrument or continuously rotating multi-instrument systems. J Endod. 2016;42:25–9.
74. Siddique R, Nivedhitha MS. Effectiveness of rotary and reciprocating systems on microbial reduction: a systematic review. J Conserv Dent. 2019;22:114–22.
75. Gazzaneo I, Vieira GCS, Perez AR, Alves FRF, Goncalves LS, Mdala I, et al. Root canal disinfection by single- and multiple-instrument systems: effects of sodium hypochlorite volume, concentration, and retention time. J Endod. 2019;45:736–41.
76. Krokidis A, Bonfanti C, Cerutti AC, Barabanti N, Panopoulos P. Rotary versus reciprocating shaping files in bacterial elimination from long oval canals. Aust Endod J. 2018;44:240–4.
77. Vasconcelos L, Midena RZ, Minotti PG, Pereira TC, Duarte MAH, Andrade FB. Effect of ultrasound streaming on the disinfection of flattened root canals prepared by rotary and reciprocating systems. J Appl Oral Sci. 2017;25:477–82.
78. Machado ME, Nabeshima CK, Leonardo MF, Reis FA, Britto ML, Cai S. Influence of reciprocating single-file and rotary instrumentation on bacterial reduction on infected root canals. Int Endod J. 2013;46:1083–7.

79. Martinho FC, Freitas LF, Nascimento GG, Fernandes AM, Leite FR, Gomes AP, et al. Endodontic retreatment: clinical comparison of reciprocating systems versus rotary system in disinfecting root canals. Clin Oral Investig. 2015;19:1411–7.
80. Nabeshima CK, Caballero-Flores H, Cai S, Aranguren J, Borges Britto ML, Machado ME. Bacterial removal promoted by 2 single-file systems: Wave One and One Shape. J Endod. 2014;40:1995–8.
81. Cicek E, Kocak MM, Kocak S, Saglam BC, Turker SA. Postoperative pain intensity after using different instrumentation techniques: a randomized clinical study. J Appl Oral Sci. 2017;25:20–6.
82. Seltzer S, Naidorf IJ. Flare-ups in endodontics: I. Etiological factors. J Endod. 1985;11:472–8.
83. Krithikadatta J, Sekar V, Sudharsan P, Velumurugan N. Influence of three Ni-Ti cleaning and shaping files on postinstrumentation endodontic pain: a triple-blinded, randomized, controlled trial. J Conserv Dent. 2016;19:311–6.
84. Nekoofar MH, Sheykhrezae MS, Meraji N, Jamee A, Shirvani A, Jamee J, et al. Comparison of the effect of root canal preparation by using WaveOne and ProTaper on postoperative pain: a randomized clinical trial. J Endod. 2015;41:575–8.
85. Zand V, Milani AS, Hassani Dehkharghani A, Rahbar M, Tehranchi P. Treatment of necrotic teeth using two engine-driven systems and patient's postoperative pain: a double-blind clinical trial. Iran Endod J. 2016;11:267–72.
86. Neelakantan P, Sharma S. Pain after single-visit root canal treatment with two single-file systems based on different kinematics—a prospective randomized multicenter clinical study. Clin Oral Investig. 2015;19:2211–7.
87. Shokraneh A, Ajami M, Farhadi N, Hosseini M, Rohani B. Postoperative endodontic pain of three different instrumentation techniques in asymptomatic necrotic mandibular molars with periapical lesion: a prospective, randomized, double-blind clinical trial. Clin Oral Investig. 2017;21:413–8.
88. Kherlakian D, Cunha RS, Ehrhardt IC, Zuolo ML, Kishen A, da Silveira Bueno CE. Comparison of the incidence of postoperative pain after using 2 reciprocating systems and a continuous rotary system: a prospective randomized clinical trial. J Endod. 2016;42:171–6.
89. Martins CM, De Souza Batista VE, Andolfatto Souza AC, Andrada AC, Mori GG, Gomes Filho JE. Reciprocating kinematics leads to lower incidences of postoperative pain than rotary kinematics after endodontic treatment: a systematic review and meta-analysis of randomized controlled trial. J Conserv Dent. 2019;22:320–31.
90. Sun C, Sun J, Tan M, Hu B, Gao X, Song J. Pain after root canal treatment with different instruments: a systematic review and meta-analysis. Oral Dis. 2018;24:908–19.
91. Spohr AR, Sarkis-Onofre R, Pereira-Cenci T, Pappen FG, Dornelles Morgental R. A systematic review: effect of hand, rotary and reciprocating instrumentation on endodontic postoperative pain. G Ital Endod. 2019;33:24–34.
92. West J. Endodontic predictability: "are you making the right decisions"? Dent Today. 2010;29:90, 2–5.
93. Kahneman D. Thinking, fast and slow. 1st pbk. ed. New York: Farrar, Straus and Giroux; 2013.
94. Souza E, Rodrigues E, De-Deus G, Zuolo ML, Silva EJNL, Versiani MA. Movimento reciprocante e a curva de aprendizado do preparo mecânico. In: De-Deus G, EJNL S, Souza E, Versiani MA, Zuolo ML, editors. O movimento reciprocante na endodontia. São Paulo: Quintessence Publishing; 2017. p. 213–32.
95. Silva E, Belladonna FG, Carapia MF, Muniz BL, Rocha MS, Moreira EJL. Micro-computed tomographic evaluation of canal retreatments performed by undergraduate students using different techniques. Restor Dent Endod. 2018;43:e5.
96. Strauss G, Sayles L. Los problemas humanos de la dirección. Manual do treinamento na empresa moderna. São Paulo: Atlas; 1971.

Shaping for Cleaning in Retreatment Cases

7

Mario Zuolo, Emmanuel J. N. L. Silva, Erick Souza, Gustavo De Deus, and Marco A. Versiani

7.1 Introduction

Endodontic treatment is an effective method for maintaining natural teeth in the oral cavity and, from the patient's perspective, endodontic care could be considered as an improvement in their life quality [1]. However, as it may happen with other dental procedures, root canal treatment can also fail. Endodontic failures are usually managed by two approaches: (a) retreatment, a nonsurgical procedure carried out by removing filling materials from the root canal, followed by cleaning, shaping, and a new filling procedure; or (b) surgery, carried out by the surgical exposure of the apical portion of the tooth through an osteotomy, surgical removal of the lesion, and commonly, removal of the root end, retrograde preparation, disinfection, and filling of the apical portion of the root canal [2].

M. Zuolo (✉)
Dental School of APCD – FAOA, São Paulo, Brazil
e-mail: mlzuolo@uol.com.br

E. J. N. L. Silva
Fluminense Federal University, Grande Rio University, Rio de Janeiro State University, Niterói, Brazil

E. Souza
Federal University of Maranhão, São Luis, Brazil

G. De Deus
Fluminense Federal University, Niterói, Brazil

M. A. Versiani
Dental Specialty Center, Brazilian Military Police, Minas Gerais, Brazil

G. De Deus et al. (eds.), *Shaping for Cleaning the Root Canals*,
https://doi.org/10.1007/978-3-030-84617-6_7

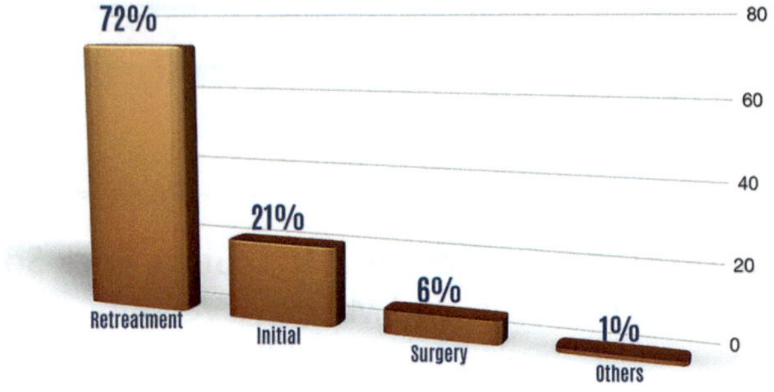

Fig. 7.1 Percentage of endodontic treatments performed in 5,346 teeth at a private practice in São Paulo, Brazil, from 2005 to 2015

In recent years, there has been an increased interest in endodontic retreatment observed by an overload of related literature with more than 480 papers published in the last 10 years (PubMed search on March 15, 2020). There is also a perceived concern of patients looking to keep their natural teeth, as observed in many dental practices around the world. As an example, in a private clinical practice in São Paulo, Brazil, with three chairs dedicated exclusively to endodontics, a total of 5,346 teeth were treated from 2005 to 2015. Retreatment cases represented 72% of the cases (Fig. 7.1). These findings point out that a specialist in endodontics should be prepared for a high prevalence of retreatment cases in daily practice.

The purpose of this chapter is to discuss retreatment of conventional cases filled with gutta-percha and sealer, excluding the management of procedural errors, using selected scientific evidences and our clinical expertise coupled with up-to-date technology. The most relevant clinical and scientific aspects of this topic are highlighted, and clinical protocols for retreatment, using the Shaping for Cleaning concept, are also proposed.

7.1.1 Predictability of the Initial Endodontic Treatment

Outcome in endodontics remains a controversial point of discussion in the literature. Several clinical trials and systematic literature reviews have been published in the last years aiming to establish a success rate or predictability of primary endodontic treatment [3–10]. A systematic review conducted by Ng et al. [9] investigated the probability of success after initial endodontic treatment and demonstrated success rates ranging from 31 to 100%. Such discrepancies were related to differences in the variables evaluated in each study: criteria for success/failure, follow-up period, clinical technique, geographical location, operator skills, among others. Preoperative absence of periapical radiolucency, root filling with no voids, root filling extending 2 mm short of the radiographic apex, and satisfactory coronal restoration were found to significantly improve the outcome of primary root canal treatment [11]. This review also emphasized that, although the influence of preoperative pulp and periapical status of the teeth on treatment outcome is usually well explored in most of studies, important issues such as the influence of treatment techniques have been poorly investigated.

7.1.2 Success and Clinical Practice

Dentists traditionally rely on a combination of clinical evaluation and periapical radiographs as reference standards to evaluate the presence or absence of endodontic disease [12]. From a clinical point of view, the use of two-dimensional periapical radiographs has been the standard method to detect the presence or confirm the absence or regression of apical lesions. This imaging exam associated with clinical examinations to seek for clinical signs and symptoms of infection/inflammation is widely used. Follow-up clinical studies have shown that root canal treatment applying these criteria and modern principles of practice can yield favorable outcomes with healing rates above 90% [10].

However, Patel et al. [12], in an interesting editorial published in the *International Endodontic Journal*, called our attention to what they named as "*The elephant in the room*." This concept means that with the advent of high-resolution 3D imaging systems, such as small field of view (FOV) cone-beam computed tomography (CBCT), periapical radiolucencies can be detected more frequently than with the conventional two-dimensional periapical radiographic method. This perception is reinforced by several other studies with a systematic review of endodontic outcome studies revealing that CBCT imaging has twice the odds of detecting a periapical lesion than traditional periapical radiograph [13]. A study by Al-Nuaimi et al. [14], for instance, evaluating treatment outcome of 354 teeth, identified a great discrepancy in the detection of pretreatment (baseline) radiolucencies between periapical radiographs and CBCT (188 vs. 264, respectively).

Taken together, these findings led us to an important reflection: The need for endodontic retreatment will certainly be increased in the near future with the use of new 3D imaging technologies for diagnostic purposes. Thus, more than ever, clinicians should be well acquainted with the best concepts and techniques for performing this procedure as a result of an inevitable increase in the demand for endodontic retreatment.

7.1.3 Purpose of Retreatment

The aim of a new intervention in the root canal is to render the endodontically treated tooth functional and asymptomatic, by achieving the complete repair of the supporting tissues [2]. The main objective in retreatment cases is the removal of the etiologic agent responsible for the failure of the endodontic treatment—in most cases of microbiologic nature, arising from an intra-canal infection—and preserving the maximum of the healthy dental structure as possible, so a final restoration can be properly done. Therefore, the success of endodontic retreatment will depend on proper disinfection and reduction of bacterial load which is not simple considering the higher technical and demanding challenges compared to the primary treatment.

7.1.4 The Filling Materials

Gutta-percha remains the most commonly used filling material and is widely accepted in endodontic practice. Because gutta-percha does not combine physically or chemically with dentin, generally this material is used together with an endodontic sealer. The most common groups of sealers include: zinc oxide-eugenol-based sealers, resin-based sealers, silicone-based sealer, calcium hydroxide-based sealers and, more recently, calcium-silicate-based sealers, usually referred to as bioceramics. Gutta-percha cones come in variable shapes and tapers and are employed using cold techniques such as lateral condensation or plasticized by heated condensers and/or thermo-compactors [2]. Thus, in most of retreatment cases, the dentist must be prepared to remove a mass of filling material composed of gutta-percha and sealer introduced into canals by a variety of different techniques. The proper removal of the gutta-percha and sealer is paramount to achieve dentinal walls free of debris, allowing the instruments and irrigants to reach areas that are possibly infected and thus permitting the healing process to initiate.

7.2 When Is Retreatment Possible?

After a proper diagnosis of a failed initial case, there are some questions that should be answered before making the decision about retreating an endodontically treated tooth:

(a) *How many times has the tooth undergone endodontic procedures? Or, can I improve the previous treatment?*

There is an important difference when dealing with retreatment cases where the initial treatment was poor and did not meet the acceptable technical standards resulting in lack of intra-radicular infection control [15]. Teeth with inadequate canal preparation, incorrect working length, unprepared canals, and/or inadequate filling, with only one previous intervention, are the most suitable cases for retreatment (Fig. 7.2). On the other hand, if a tooth was treated more than once, or has a radiographic or CBCT image of well-prepared and filled canals, the retreatment should be evaluated with caution. Despite the most common cause of failure is related to intracanal infection, there are other reasons such as extra-radicular infection represented by the presence of biofilms outside the canal. Nevertheless, there are also some reports suggesting that nonmicrobial factors, such as true cysts, cholesterol crystals, and other extrinsic causes like materials that may be inadvertently extruded apically and cause a foreign body reaction, might be related to endodontic failure, perpetuating periradicular lesions [15]. However, Siqueira et al. [16] previously stated that "in most of these cases it is very difficult to rule out the concomitant presence of infection as the cause of disease." In other words, today it remains difficult to confirm that technical mishaps were exclusively the cause of a treatment failure. Well-treated cases with apical lesions could be also related to complex anatomies, cracked

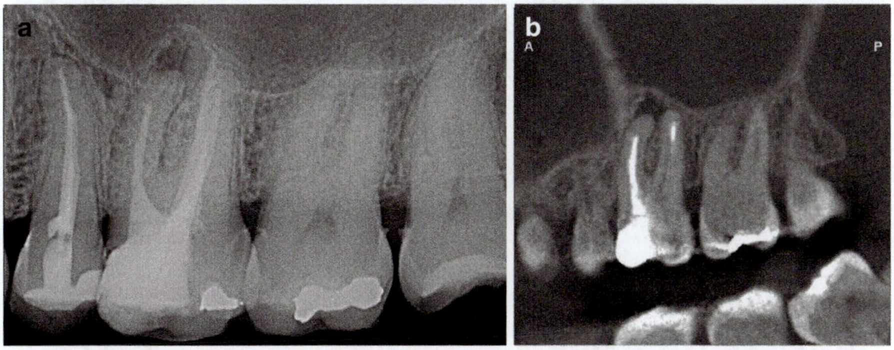

Fig. 7.2 (**a**) Radiographic and (**b**) tomographic images of a maxillary left first molar in which the root canal treatment does not meet acceptable standards, with an incomplete preparation of the mesiobuccal canals and chronic apical periodontitis

roots or extraradicular biofilms, and orthograde retreatment may not be the ideal therapeutic option (Fig. 7.3).

(b) *When was the last endodontic intervention performed on the tooth?*

Treatments completed less than 1 year previously may provide poor clinical evidence for assessing outcome, except in cases associated with pain or any other clinical sign or symptom of inflammation or infection. Molven et al. [17] clearly demonstrated the potential of late changes in the periapical status after a long follow-up. The authors also emphasized that late periapical changes are usually associated with more successes than failures. Thus, in cases of short follow-ups with no clinical signs or symptoms, it is recommended to continuous monitoring the patient, rather than carry out a prompty retreatment.

(c) *Is the tooth restorable?*

The contemporary literature clearly establishes that the success of endodontic treatment is related to bacterial control and the presence of adequate restoration [18–23]. Aquilino and Caplan [18] evaluated 400 teeth 2 years after the endodontic treatment and observed that, when clinical parameters such as tooth group and caries were controlled, the non-crowned teeth had a failure rate six times higher than teeth crowned just after the endodontic intervention. Lazarski et al. [21] used the database from the University of Washington to study the outcome of root canal treatment and observed that the group of teeth with the highest rate of extraction after endodontic treatment was the one without adequate restoration (11.2%) when compared to those adequately restored (2.5%).

Clinical parameters, such as cusp protection for posterior teeth, adequate proximal contacts, remaining dental structure (especially in marginal ridge regions), the use of an intra-radicular post for prosthetic crown retention only in cases of extensive dental tissue loss, cementation of prosthetic pieces onto remaining sound dental tissue using the ferrule concept, and correct occlusal balance to prevent functional overload, should be observed for all cases considered for retreatment [18–23].

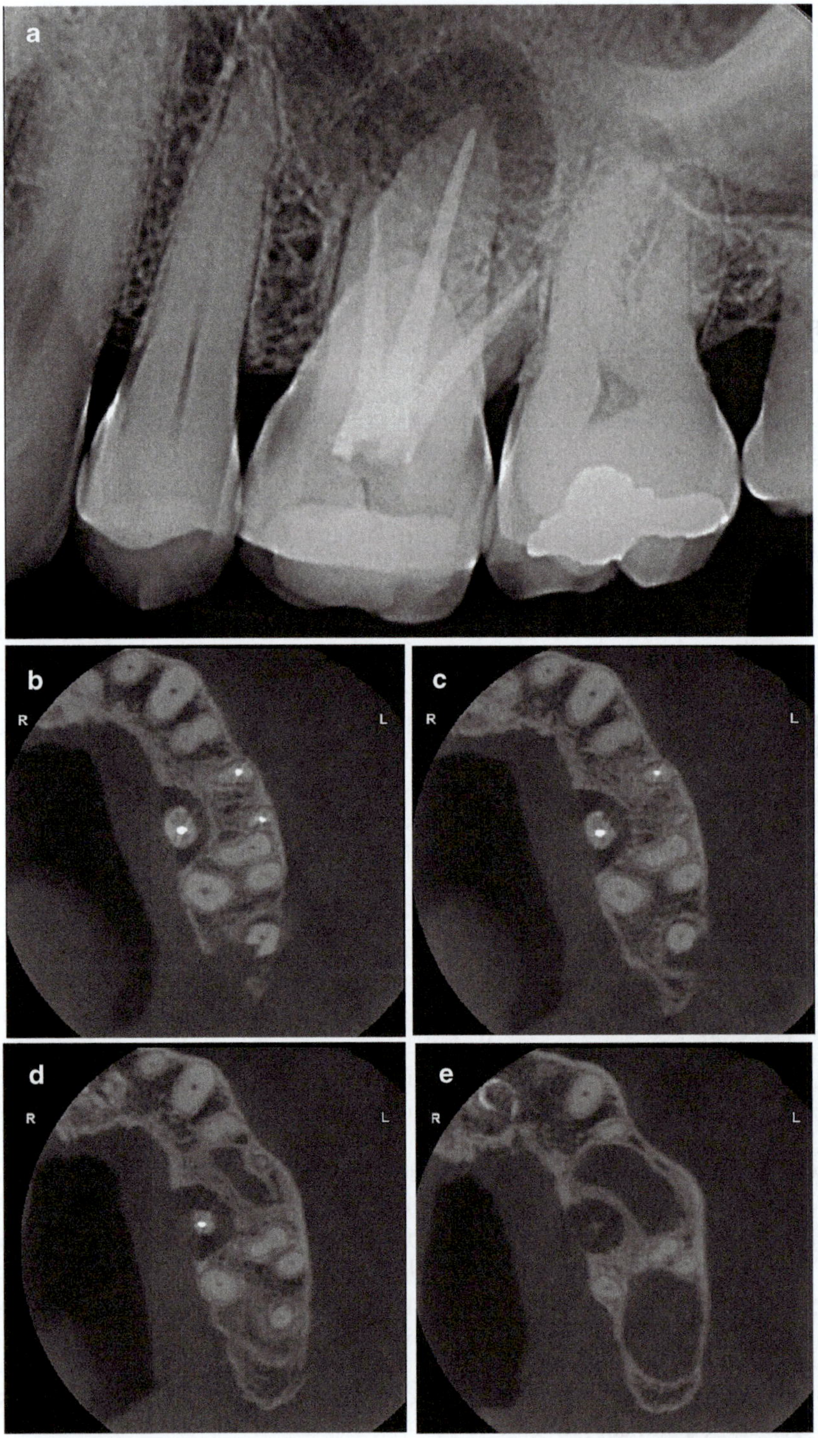

Fig. 7.3 (**a**) Radiograph of a maxillary left first molar showing a failed root canal treatment that could be acceptable from a technical perspective. (**b–e**) Four axial tomographic images of the apical third of the palatal root showing an extensive bone loss

The literature clearly points to the fact that teeth with exiguous remaining dental structure preventing adequate restorations should not be considered as candidates for endodontic retreatment, especially when they serve as abutment for fixed or removable dentures (Fig. 7.4). Finally, clinicians often postpone the final restoration to await the resolution of an apical lesion: this approach should be considered part of the past of endodontics. Acknowledging the importance of an adequate final restoration after completion of endodontic retreatment should thus be stressed, and patients warned about its relevance for prognosis [2].

(d) *What is the periodontal condition of the tooth?*

Signs of periodontal disease represented by marginal bone loss in the alveolar ridge may be a negative predictive factor for endodontically treated teeth [24, 25]. Periodontal disease is not a contraindication to retreatment, but when coupled with other negative predictors, it may restrict the indication for retreatment. So, teeth with doubtful periodontal prognosis should be evaluated with extreme caution before endodontic retreatment (Fig. 7.5).

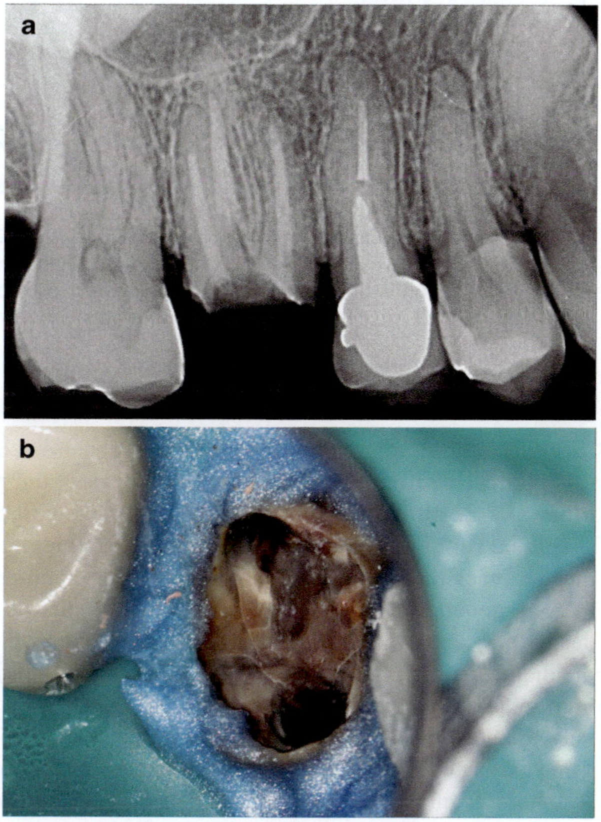

Fig. 7.4 (**a**) Preoperative radiograph of a maxillary right first molar referred for retreatment showing incomplete canal treatment and apical lesion. (**b**) After decay removal, inspection of the pulp chamber floor with magnification and adequate illumination showed several fracture lines. The tooth was referred for extraction since no sound dentin was available for proper prosthetic rehabilitation

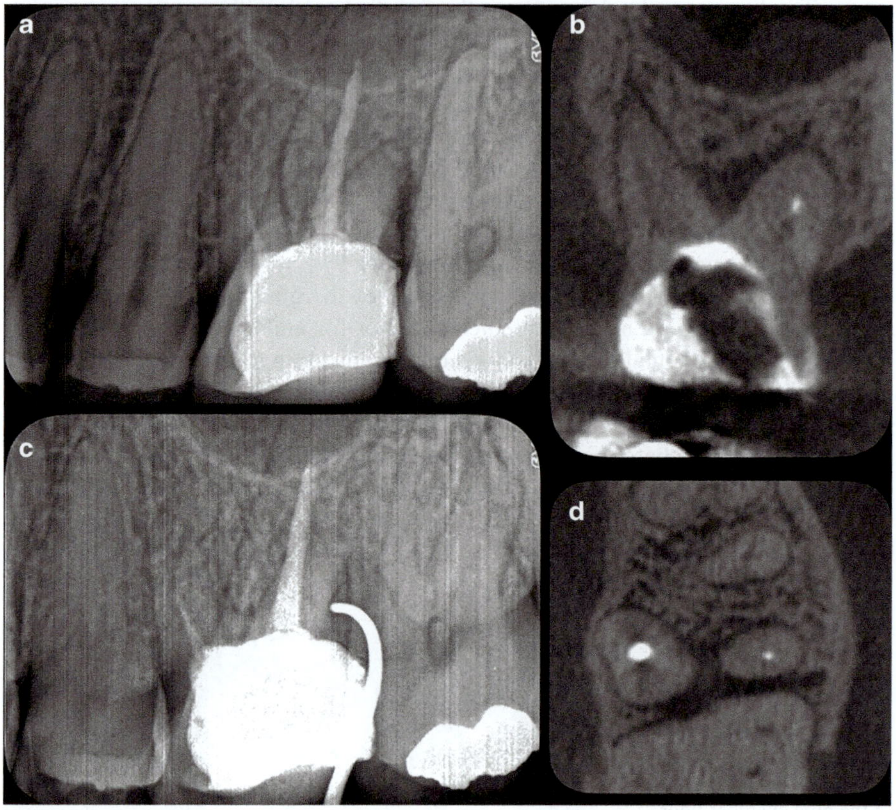

Fig. 7.5 Maxillary left first molar in which retreatment was not indicated because of periodontal reasons. (**a**) Preoperative radiograph. (**b**) Coronal tomographic image depicting great bone loss at the furcation area. (**c**) Radiograph indicating a furcation defect degree 2 at the distal aspect of the distobuccal root. (**d**) Axial tomographic image showing bone loss at the distal aspect of the tooth

7.2.1 Access Preparation and Retreatment

It is not within the scope of this chapter to discuss access cavity preparation, but it is interesting to note that in retreatment cases, the procedure is generally performed on teeth with extensive restorations or with a full crown in position. It should be kept in mind that the access in retreatment cases must be made without interferences that could jeopardize the proper canal reshaping and disinfection.

As a general rule we should consider removing all previous restorations and decay before starting retreatment procedures. Inspection with magnification for the diagnosis of fracture lines in the enamel and dentin is mandatory. There is a high incidence of these fractures in the crown, and their position and extension may dictate not only the kind of adequate restoration after retreatment, but in some cases could be also a contraindication for the procedure [26–28] (Fig. 7.6). Another advantage of a proper access cavity is the inspection of the pulp chamber floor aiming to locate a missed or extra canal, another very frequent finding in retreatment cases, as well as, the location of narrow and calcified canals (Fig. 7.7). Knowledge of the internal and external anatomies will guide the location of all canals present in a dental element and, coupled with the CBCT exam, will assist the clinician in the diagnosis and localization of these canals in selected cases (Fig. 7.8).

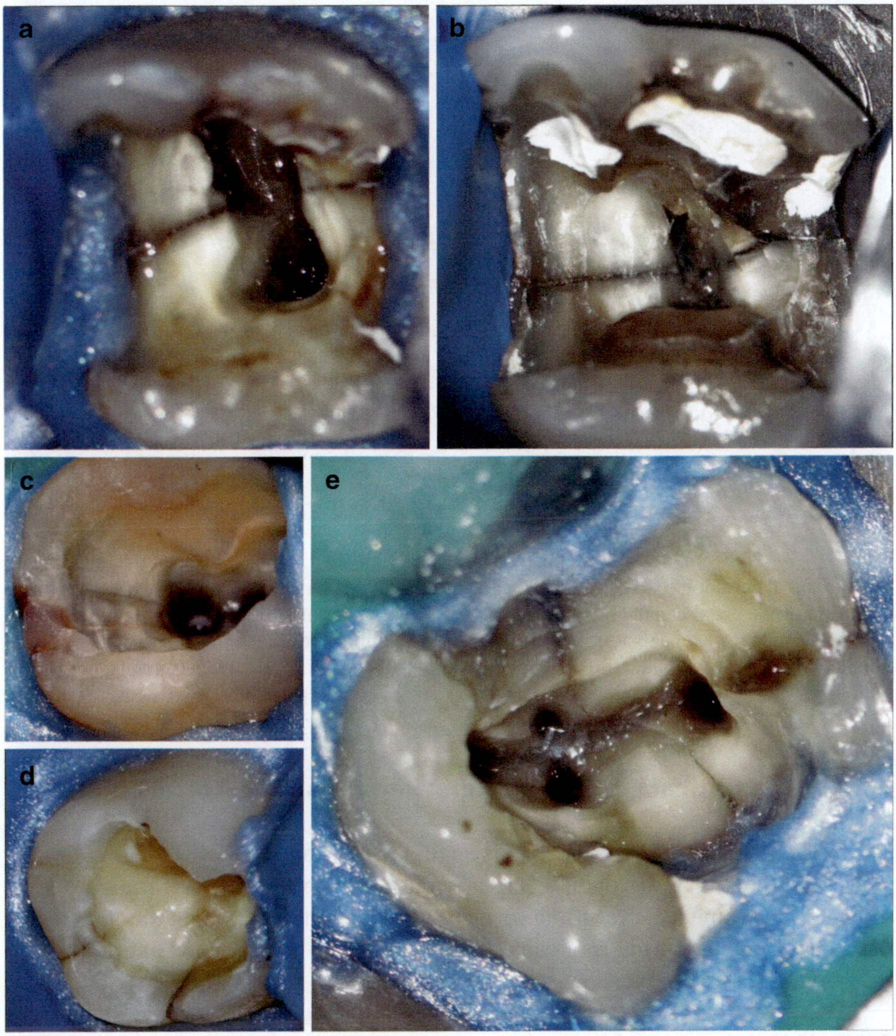

Fig. 7.6 Dentinal cracks with distinct locations and extensions observed under microscope after the removal of restorations of (**a**) a maxillary right first molar, (**b**) a maxillary right second molar, (**c**) a mandibular right first molar, (**d**) a mandibular right first molar, and a (**e**) maxillary left second molar

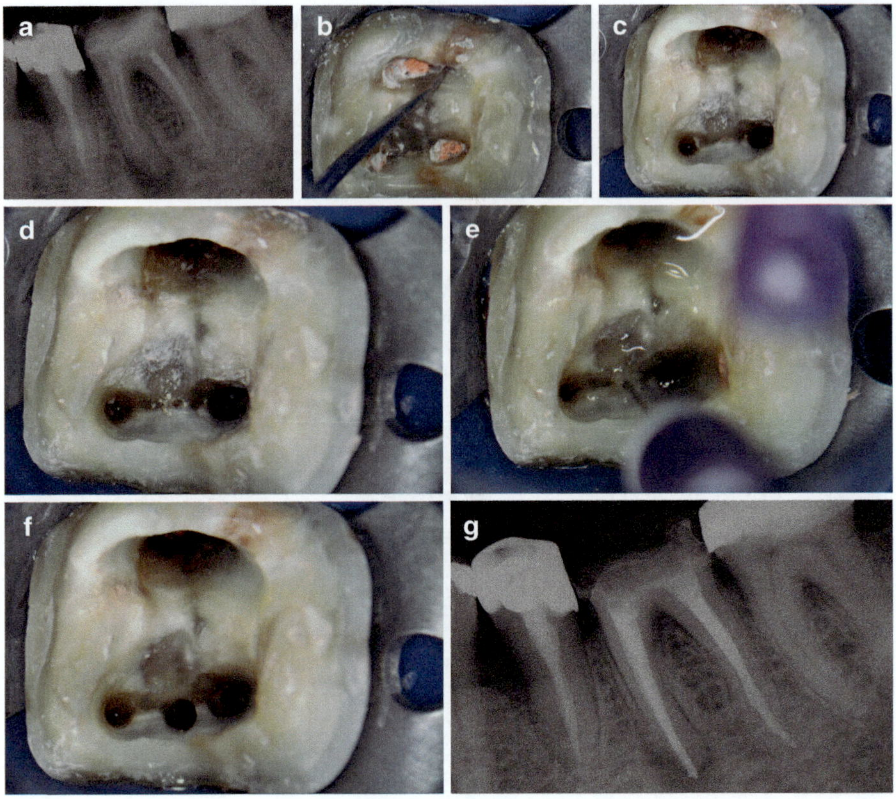

Fig. 7.7 (**a**) Preoperative radiograph of a previously treated mandibular left first molar with chronic apical periodontitis. (**b**) Access opening and canal orifice location. Observe the unprepared extension of the distal canal. (**c**) After removal of filling material, a small amount of gutta-percha in between the mesial canals was observed. (**d–f**) After removal of the remnants of gutta-percha, a middle mesial canal was identified, scouted with a size 10 K-file, and shaped. (**g**) Postoperative radiograph after filling the entire canal system. (Courtesy Dr. Leandro Pereira, Brazil)

7.2.2 The Critical Last Millimeters: Regaining the Apical Patency

The success of the retreatment depends on finding the natural path of root canals usually compromised by iatrogenic causes such as transportation, perforation, ledge, separated instruments, overfilling, or any other event that prevents the location of the apical foramen during root canal reshaping. These mishaps prevent proper disinfection of the whole canal system [2].

As there is a positive correlation between intracanal infection and endodontic failure [29], it is reasonable to affirm that cleaning the root canals in their whole extension is crucial to improve the prognosis. This was demonstrated in a prospective clinical trial assessing the success rate of 452 teeth submitted to endodontic retreatment. In this study, Gorni and Gagliani [30] concluded that, after a 2-year

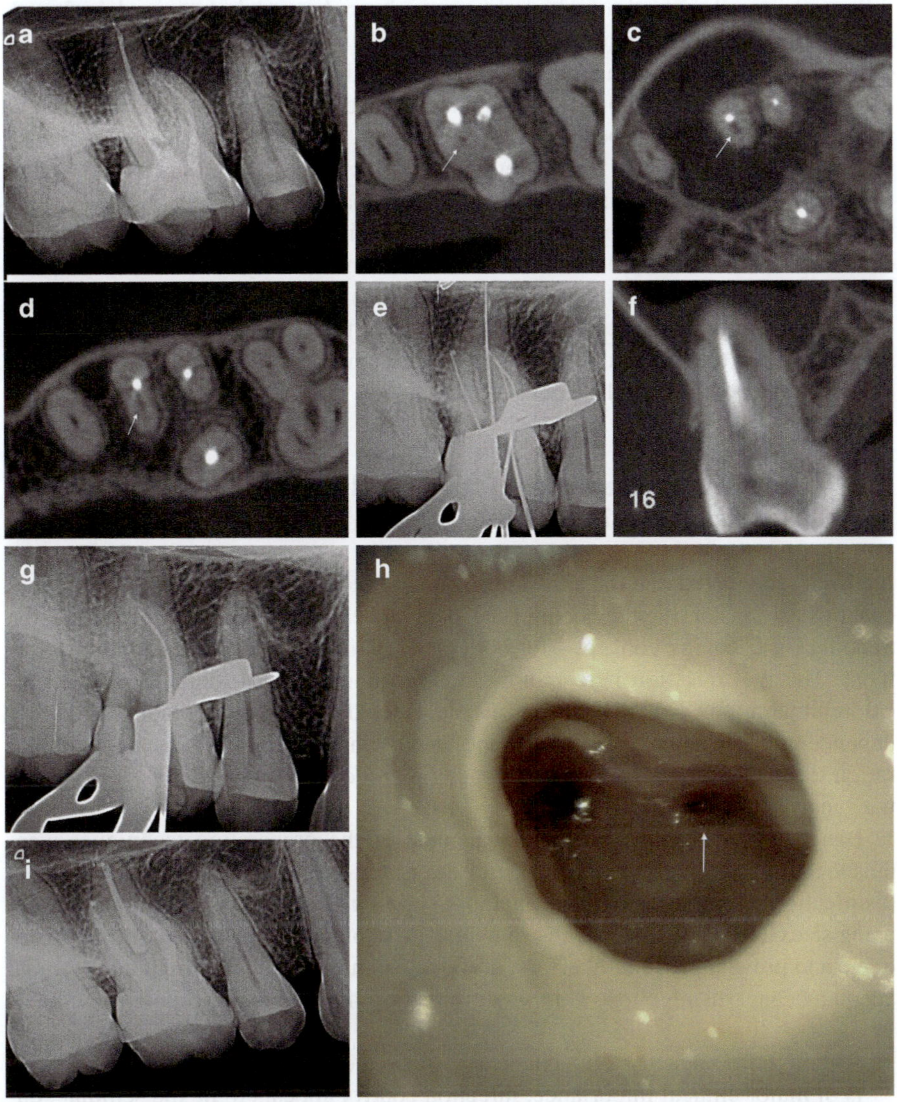

Fig. 7.8 (**a**) Maxillary right first molar referred for retreatment due to signs and symptoms of inflammation. (**b–d**) Axial tomographic images of the coronal, middle, and apical thirds, respectively, depicting the presence of a missed canal in the mesiobuccal root. (**e**) Measurement of canal lengths using size 10 K-files in each one of the four root canals. (**f**) Parasagittal tomographic image showing the missed mesiobuccal canal. (**g**) Radiograph showing the location of the missed canal. (**h**) Clinical view of the pulp chamber after preparation of both mesiobuccal canals. The white arrow indicates the orifice of the missed canal. (**i**) Postoperative radiograph

follow-up period, in teeth in which the original canal anatomy remained unaltered, and patency regained, success rate reached 87%. In contrast, the success rate in cases in which the foramen could not be located—those with altered anatomy—was around 47%, clearly demonstrating the importance of controlling intracanal infection during endodontic procedures.

Then, the best scenario for the retreatment procedure is when the final 3–4 mm of the canal is accessible and can be properly prepared, while the worst scenario is when a blockage prevents achieving patency. In clinical practice, these two parameters should be carefully evaluated before intervention in order to detect the presence of mishaps and deviations of the original canal path (Fig. 7.9). But sometimes, only an accurated clinical exploration can depict the case and determine the next steps regarding the choice of endodontic retreatment, apical surgery, or extraction of the involved tooth (Fig. 7.10).

7.2.3 Anatomical Diameter of the Apical Foramen: To Enlarge or Not to Enlarge?

It is well recognized that the apical third is one of the most relevant area of the root canal when considering the need for mechanical debridement and disinfection—the Shaping for Cleaning concept—for both primary treatment and endodontic retreatment. The real question here is how to determine the final diameter of the apical repreparation. The master apical file elected for instrumentation is highly dependent on the apical topology (shape) and diameter of the root canal, the preparation technique and the presence of bacteria and/or biofilm at the last 3–4 mm of the canals [2].

Baugh and Wallace [31] stated that most of the preparation techniques were developed based on concerns related to the filling stage rather than the root canal disinfection. According to these authors, minimal apical preparation, generally using sizes 25/0.02 or 30/0.02 instruments, are enough to perform the filling procedures and prevent procedural errors; however, such enlargement might not promote adequate canal disinfection. This way of thinking has two major problems:

1. Although the capacity to mechanically shape the apical portion of the root canal is of major clinical importance, infection control appears to be the seminal condition to trigger the healing process and determine the treatment outcome.
2. The anatomical diameter of original foramen is larger than dentists can determine clinically, and literature reports diameters varying from 0.20 to 0.70 mm, depending on the group of teeth.

For these reasons, there is a strong consensus in the endodontic literature that larger apical preparations translate into greater elimination of bacteria and debris compared to more conservative apical enlargement, especially in retreatment cases. In the presence of apical periodontitis, in which it is likely the existance of bacteria at the apical portion of the canals, the need to perform larger apical preparations, as

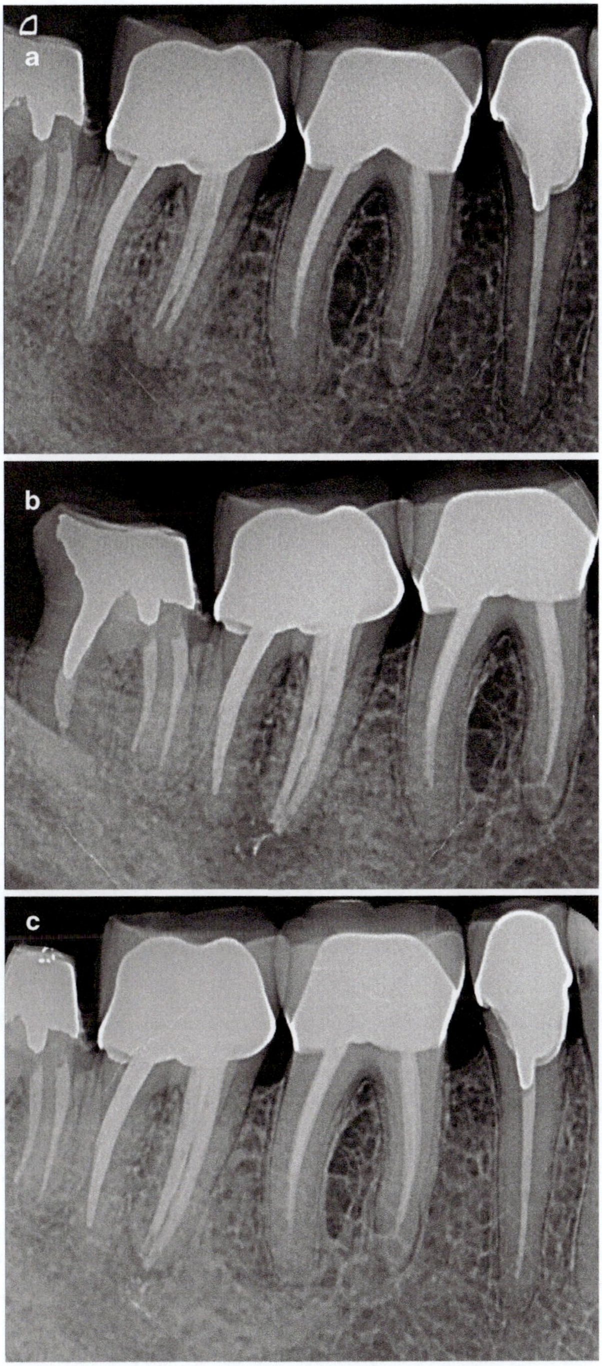

Fig. 7.9 (**a**) Radiograph showing a mandibular right second molar with chronic apical periodontitis, canal deviation, and incorrect vertical extention of the filling procedure. (**b**) Immediate postoperative radiograph after re-shaping and re-filling. (**c**) A 14-month follow-up period depicting the apical healing

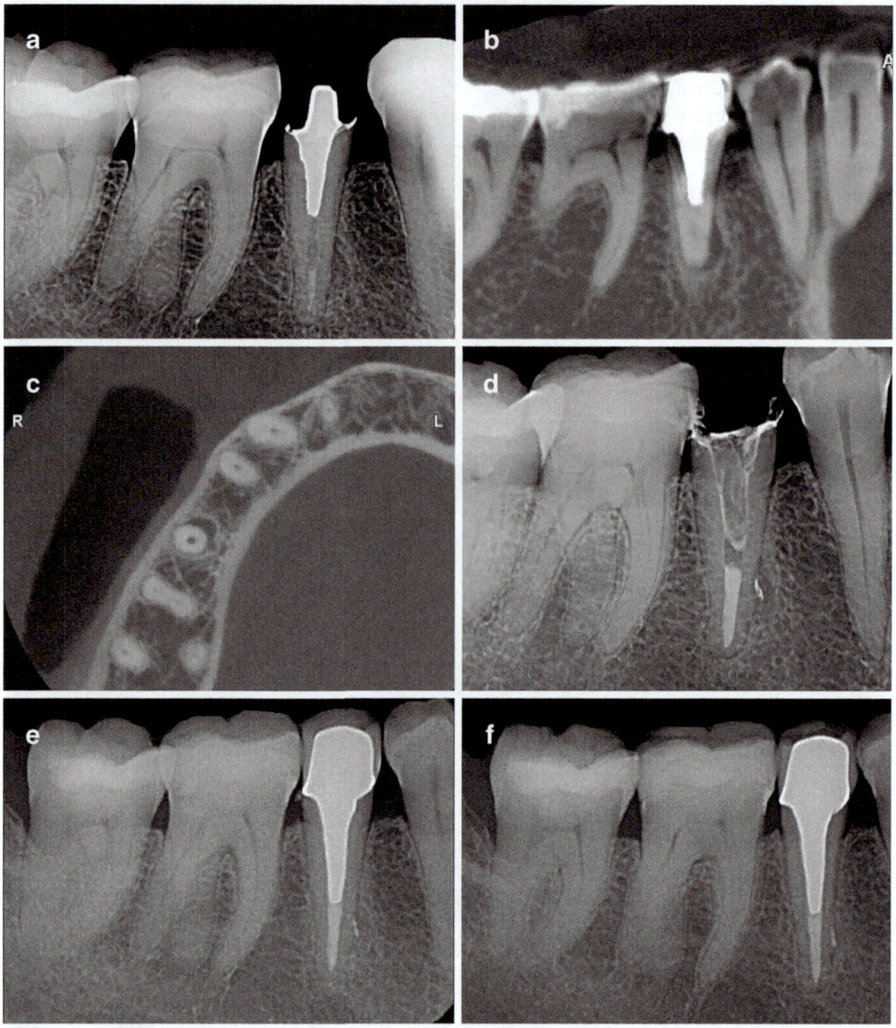

Fig. 7.10 (**a**) Radiographic image of a mandibular right second premolar showing a lateral root lesion. Main patient's complaint was discomfort on biting and the possible etiological causes were a vertical root fracture or a lateral canal. (**b**) Parasagittal tomographic image showed a lateral lesion with apical extension. (**c**) Axial tomographic image at the center of the lesion in which no fracture or lateral canal could be observed. Treatment plan was to remove the post and, if no fracture was observed, perform the retreatment. (**d**) Immediate postoperative radiograph of the tooth with a provisional restoration in which is possible to observe a lateral canal filled with sealer. (**e, f**) One- and two-years follow-up of the tooth with final restoration in position and bone formation

well as, the enlargement of the apical foramen seem obvious. These approaches allow to improve disinfection, cleansing, and also increase the flux of irrigants in this region [32–38]. Fornari et al. [37] used mesiobuccal curved root canals of maxillary molars prepared with rotary instruments to assess the influence of the preparation size on the cleansing of the apical third and concluded that the apical enlargement with files sizes 40/0.02 and 45/0.02 promoted a substantial reduction in the residual debris compared to small enlargements (30/0.02 and 35/0.02). In a clinical trial involving 40 patients, Card et al. [35] concluded that increasing the apical canal to a size 60 for molars and size 80 for premolars yields bacteria-free canals even in the presence of apical periodontitis. Alves et al. [33] in a clinical trial comparing single- and multiple-instrument systems concluded that, despite the system, large apical preparations ranging from 40/0.04,0.06 and 50/0.04,0.05 promoted levels of disinfection above 95%. Aminoshariae and Kulild [34] performed a systematic review of healing outcomes in endodontics and concluded that the best available clinical evidence suggested that, for patients with teeth with necrotic pulp and periapical lesions, large apical preparations would result in an increased healing outcome in terms of clinical and radiographic evaluations.

Based on this body of evidence, it is reasonable to conclude that, in retreatment cases with periapical lesion, a master apical file with sizes between 35/0.04 and 80/0.02 should be used, respecting the anatomy of each group of teeth to promote adequate cleansing and disinfection of the apical portion of the canal. Clinically, we can consider as a rule that the final instrument should be 3–4 times greater than the initial file [39, 40]. As an initial file, we should consider the file that binds at the working length and carries dentin in the final 3–4 mm of the instrument, as demonstrated in Fig. 7.11.

Finally, it is important to point out that foraminal enlargement and maintenance of apical patency does not increase the degree of postoperative pain, as shown in many studies [41–43].

7.3 Effects of Gutta-Percha Removal in the Canal Walls

The effects of retreatment protocols in the canal walls can be analyzed from two perspectives: (1) the effect of the chemical substances in the molecular structure of the dentin; and (2) the mechanical defects created during the removal of gutta-percha from the canals.

A great number of chemical solutions have been recommended to be used for canal retreatment. During retreatment procedures, for example, radicular and coronal dentin are exposed to gutta-percha solvents. The use of solvents such as chloroform, eucalyptol, orange oil, halothane, and others is still very popular. Such solvents may alter the chemical composition and microhardness of the dentinal surface and affect its interaction with materials used for coronal restoration [44–47]. For this reason, it might be speculated that the use of solvents negatively affect the dentinal structure, as well as, the final restoration of the tooth, and their use should be limited to the minimum possible amount for the removal of gutta-percha.

From the mechanical point of view, root canal deviations caused by attempting to remove the filling materials from the canal walls should be avoided during retreatment. This topic will be discussed later in this chapter. However, another mechanical problem that should be considered in retreatment is the potential

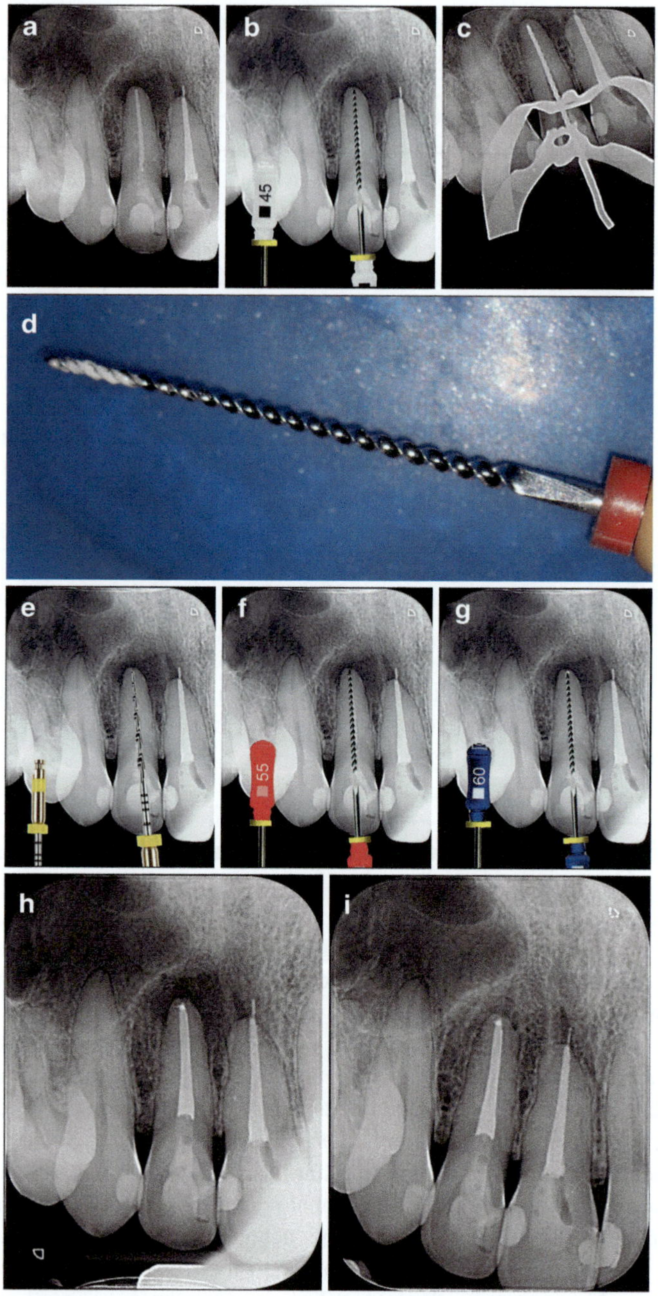

Fig. 7.11 Apical enlargement procedure. (**a**) Preoperative radiograph of a maxillary right lateral incisor with apical periodontitis. (**b, c**) The first instrument that cut the dentin at the working length was a size 45 K-file. (**d**) View of the instrument with the aid of a microscope allowed to observe 4 mm of its tip covered with dentinal debris. (**e**) Apical preparation was initially performed with a Reciproc R50 instrument followed by (**f**) a size 55 manual K-file. (**g**) Final apical enlargement was done with a size 60 manual K-file. (**h**) Postoperative radiograph and (**i**) 20-month follow-up showing the apical healing and a normal periodontal ligament space

development of defects such as microcracks and dentin fractures. Shemesh et al. [48], using extracted teeth, compared the effect of a rotary instrument (ProTaper Retreatment), Gates–Glidden burs, and Hedströem files on canal walls and concluded that all of them could significantly damage the root by creating cracks and fractures. These defects were also reported by other authors when evaluating the root canal preparation with different instruments [49, 50]. However, we need to interpret these results with skepticism since dentinal microcracks were analyzed based on root-sectioning methods and direct observation with a stereomicroscope. De-Deus and colleagues [51, 52] reported no causal relationship between canal preparation with rotary/reciprocating systems and microcrack formation using a noninvasive micro-CT model in which the specimens were evaluated at the same position before and after canal preparation, without sectioning the root. In another study, a lack of causal relationship was also observed between mechanical preparation and formation of microcracks during endodontic retreatment using the noninvasive micro-CT model [53]. Although these findings suggest that it is unlikely that retreatment procedures can cause the development of dentinal microcracks, future studies using nondestructive analytical tools in a fresh-cadaver model should attempt to shed more light on this topic.

7.3.1 Getting Rid of the Bulk-Filling Material: Solvent, Burs, and Files

Many techniques for removing root canal fillings have been proposed in the literature. Taken together, there is a consensus that it is impossible to remove completely all the remnants of gutta-percha and sealers from the root canals, especially those attached to root canal walls. The main objective during retreatment is to get rid of the maximum amount of the initial filling material, allowing instruments and irrigants to reach untouched areas of the canal, including isthmuses and irregularities in order to significantly reduce the intracanal infection [2].

Solvents are the most widely employed technique for removing gutta-percha and sealer from root canals. The softened gutta-percha can be penetrated by instruments and burs and then be removed with the aid of larger instruments. All proposed techniques for gutta-percha removal include the use of some kind of solvent, and several studies evaluated their cytotoxicity and their effects on the gutta-percha dissolution [54–56]. In the last years, micro-CT technology has been also used to evaluate filling material remnants after different retreatment protocols [57–59]. Despite the use of solvents is a very popular method for retreatment, its use deserves some reflections as the softened filling material can be constantly forced against irregularities of the root canal walls, especially into isthmus areas and the oval portions of narrowed canals (Fig. 7.12). Rossi-Fedele and Ahmed [59], in a systematic review, discussed the effectiveness of different instrumentation procedures in removing root canal filling materials assessed by micro-CT and concluded that solvents enhanced the penetration of files, but hindered the root canal cleaning.

With the current technology and knowledge, the use of solvents cannot improve filling material removal from canals and isthmuses. In fact, the use of solvents might

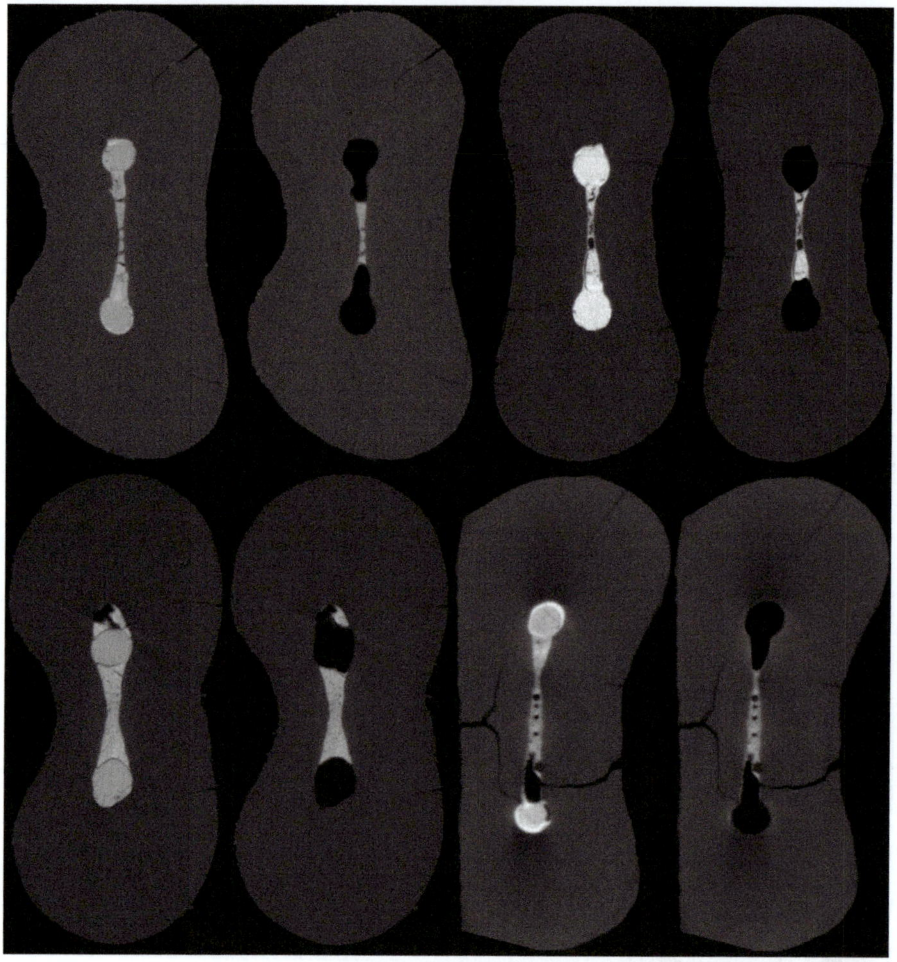

Fig. 7.12 Micro-CT cross-sections of four mesial roots of mandibular molars after root canal filling and after retreatment procedure demonstrating the presence of remnants of filling material in the isthmus areas

corroborate negatively in adequate cleaning procedures during root canal retreatment. For this reason, our advice is to start retreatment without solvents and, when necessary, confine their use to small amounts and only at the apical portion of the canal. Chloroform and orange oil are the most used and recommended solvents to be used in clinical practice.

At the coronal canal third, Gates-Glidden or Peeso drills are common instruments used to initiate the removal of filling materials. These low-speed drills allow effective gutta-percha removal due to their unique design, mechanical action, and heat generation [2]. On the other hand, the large diameter of these burs, ranging from 0.70 to 1.50 mm, can promote unnecessary removal of intra-radicular dentin, especially in the medial-distal aspect of flattened canals. Therefore, their use should be limited to large canals, and efforts should be made to only touch the filling materials, and not the dentinal walls.

A great variety of endodontic instruments, made with different alloys and design used manually or driven by electric motors with different kinematics have been proposed to increase the effectiveness of gutta-percha removal during retreatment. Again, it is important to emphasize that the literature points out that none of them are completely effective in removing all filling materials [54]. Therefore, it can be stated that the method of gutta-percha removal is a matter of personal preference. The effects of diverse instruments and systems for gutta-percha removal and for canal reshaping procedures will be further discussed in this chapter.

Along with these instruments, ultrasonic inserts or tips can be used as a non-rotary method for removing filling materials using piezoelectric oscillations [60]. The use of these kinds of inserts, associated with magnification and illumination, allows a more controlled removal of the dental structure, increasing the prepared surface areas especially in oval-shaped canals [61]. A wide variety of smooth and diamond tips with different sizes and length, straight or angulated inserts, are available on the market and can be used for all steps of root canal treatment and retreatment (Fig. 7.13). A combination of ultrasonic inserts, reciprocating instruments, and hand files will be discussed at the end of this chapter as a proposed clinical protocol for retreatment.

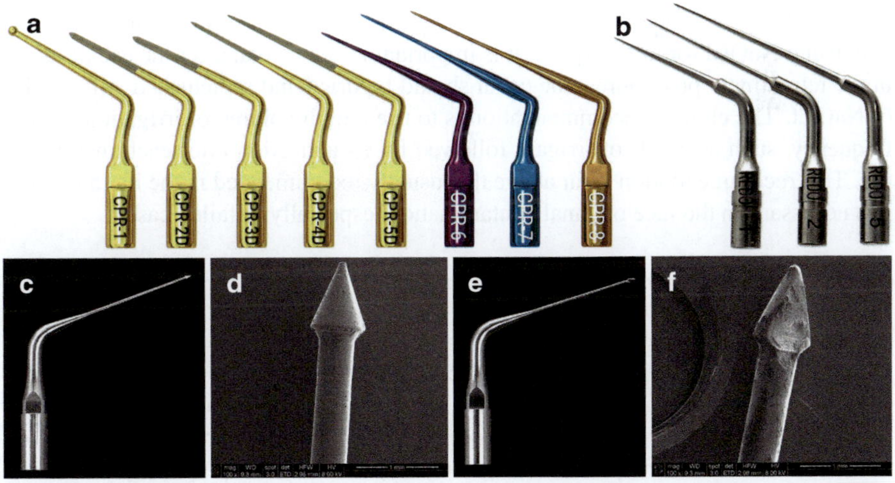

Fig. 7.13 Ultrasonic tips. (**a**) CPR (Obtura Spartan, USA) numbers 2–5 (diamond-coated surface) and 6–8 (titanium alloy). (**b**) Smooth inserts with different diameters and lengths (VDW, Germany). (**c**) Flatsonic insert (Helse, Brazil). (**d**) Scanning electron microscopy from the tip of the Flatsonic instrument showing its conic form. (**e**) Clearsonic insert (Helse, Brazil). (**f**) Scanning electron microscopy from Clearsonic tip depicting its arrow-shape

7.3.2 Challenges: Oval Canals, Irregularities, and Isthmuses

One of the major challenges is how to clean adequately the untouched canal walls, especially in the presence of gutta-percha remnants and sealer that can preclude access to infected areas at the canal walls. As discussed in Chap. 2, the activation of irrigant solutions seems to be an alternative to fullfil this purpose [62, 63]. This is also true for retreatment procedures.

In fact, the interchange irrigation using EDTA and NaOCl is a good alternative for retreatment, and the irrigant of choice to initiate the procedure is 17% EDTA aqueous solution, for two reasons:

1. Chelating solutions have a slight dissolving effect on most sealers.
2. Chelating solutions dissolve the inorganic components from the root canal walls facilitating the mechanical removal of filling materials.

Besides, chelating solutions can help disinfection since they can interfere with biofilm cohesion. A 10% citric acid solution has similar properties to 17% EDTA and can be an option for irrigation when associated with NaOCl [63]. Once the bulk of gutta-percha is removed, the canals need to be disinfected and the use of sodium hypochlorite (NaOCl) in high concentrations (2.5–5.25%) is the first choice because of its broad antimicrobial spectrum and outstanding effect on biofilm, as well as, its capacity to dissolve necrotic tissue remnants [62]. The use of sonic and ultrasonic activation of the irrigant has gained popularity among specialists and has been proven to enhance disinfection and debris removal. As a final irrigation, in order to flush the debris out of the canal, when irrigation with high pressure is needed to remove debris from the canal walls, saline solution can be used. High pressure with saline solution is safer than using NaOCl for this purpose. It is important to notice that after the use of saline in the retreatment procedures, the canal should be dried and replenished with EDTA or NaOCl. The clinical recommendation is to use a high volume of irrigation in high frequency, such as 5 mL of irrigant followed by its activation after each instrument use. This recommendation is far above that usually recommended in the literature, but it is necessary in the face of canal contamination, especially in failed cases.

7.4 Root Canal Reshaping

During retreatment, it is impossible to separate the removal of gutta-percha phase from the reshaping canal step since both are carried out simultaneously. An extensive body of literature shows the impossibility of completely removing all filling material remnants from previous treatment even after reshaping [59]. So, when evaluating the effects of canal reshaping, it is important to consider the following:

- Reshaped canals are generally widened in the same direction of the initial preparation when the same instrumentation technique is used. The clinical significance of this finding is that, ideally, reshaping should be conducted with a

distinct technique [64, 65]. From a practical point of view, this is possible only when the same professional retreats his/her own cases.
- Patency and apical enlargement are positively correlated with periapical healing [8].
- The maintenance of as much of the original morphology of root canals as possible during retreatment, avoiding procedural errors such as canal deviations, ledges, perforations, and broken instruments, is positively associated with clinical success [30].
- Excessive dentin removal should be prevented to avoid weakening of the root and increase the risk of vertical root fracture [66].
- Some manufacturers developed rotary instrumentation systems specifically designed for endodontic filling removal, but they do not have good performance compared with conventional instruments [59].
- The use of the crown-down preparation concept, which starts the removal of filling materials, by widening the coronal and middle thirds before preparing the apical third, is the most suitable approach for attaining the objectives of root canal reshaping in retreatment cases [2].

7.4.1 Vertical Extent of Instrumentation

The vertical extent of instrumentation and filling in primary endodontic treatment is a controversial topic, resulting in endless discussions between academicians and clinicians. In cases of apical periodontitis, in which bacteria and biofilm are spread throughout the root canal system, including the apical portion [29], it seems logical that the vertical extent of the preparation should be set the nearest as possible to the apical foramen [2, 67].

Today, there is no doubt about the superiority of electronic apex locators in determining the working length over the traditional radiographic method. Apex locators that work by impedance difference allow the precise location of the apical foramen, enabling the practitioner to respect the anatomical and morphological limits of the canal, providing greater predictability to the endodontic treatment [68].

7.4.2 Which Is the Best File for Retreatment?

As discussed before, the complete removal of the filling material from the canal space, regardless of the instrument or technique, is not possible. Manual, rotary, or reciprocating instruments can be used for this purpose, basically with the same results. Therefore, the technique used for endodontic retreatment can be considered a personal preference.

The development of the asymmetric reciprocating movement allowed an effective approach for the removal of root filling materials and represents our preferred technique for retreatment because of its simplicity, efficacy, and low incidence of procedural errors. The use of a reciprocating instrument for retreatment was first described by Zuolo et al. [69]. The authors compared the percentage of filling material found on the canal walls after performing different retreatment techniques. The use of a reciprocating instrument resulted in an overall gutta-percha removal of 95%. A great number of authors also support that the reciprocating movement is safe and effective for this purpose [2, 31, 70–84]. The reciprocating movement is also faster than manual or rotary instruments for gutta-percha removal [69, 82, 84]. Silva et al. [83] demonstrated that the reciprocating technique performed by undergraduate students was the most effective and less time-consuming in the removal of gutta-percha than rotary or manual techniques. Together, these results emphasize the efficacy and simplicity of this technique for endodontic retreatment. Clinically, we have seen that the use of Reciproc instruments usually remove gutta-percha in large fragments, especially at the coronal and middle portions of the canal, and is associated with less time required to take out the bulk of filling materials (Fig. 7.14).

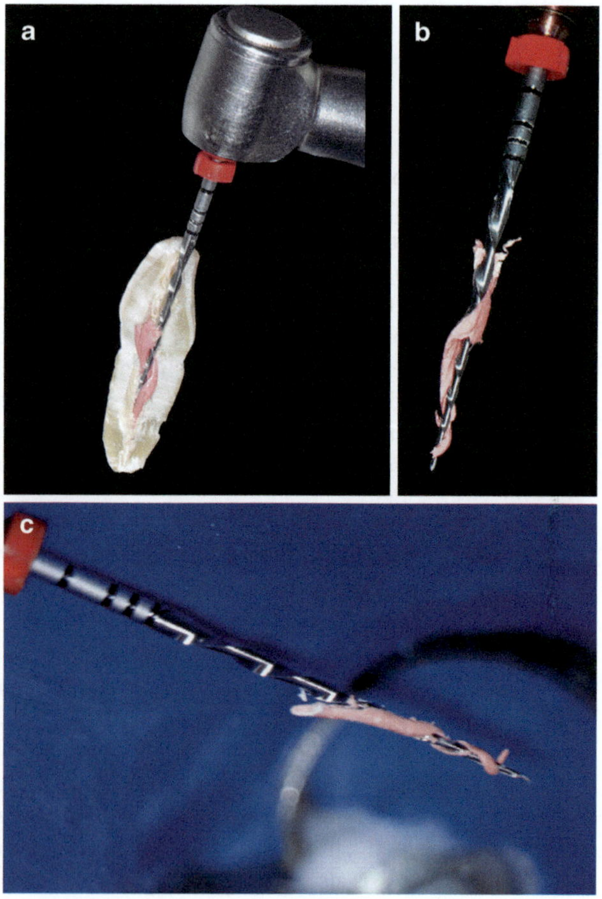

Fig. 7.14 (**a**) Reciproc R25 M-wire instrument removing filling material from the root canal of an extracted endodontically-treated tooth. The tooth was split in halves to facilitate visualization of the efficiency of the R25 instrument to imbricate into the filling material. (**b**) The filling material in (**a**) was almost entirely removed from the root canal by the R25 instrument. (**c**) Clinical image showing the removal of filling material with the R25 M-wire instrument

The safety of the reciprocating movement has also been tested to evaluate transportation in curved canals. Rödig et al. [82] showed no procedural errors such as canal blockage, ledge, or perforation in the preparation of 60 curved canals with Reciproc instruments. Nevares et al. [79] compared Reciproc and ProTaper Next for reshaping mesial root canals of molar with severe curvature and reported no significant difference between the two systems regarding the remaining of filling materials, volume of dentin removed, or apical transportation. Bago et al. [70] tested four retreatment NiTi systems and showed that Reciproc M-Wire and ReciprocBlue instruments were effective in removing filling materials from curved canals of extracted teeth compared to WaveOne Gold and ProTaper retreatment systems.

Extrusion of debris should be avoided during the removal of filling material as it has been associated to some retreatment techniques or instruments. Silva et al. [85] compared the rotary and reciprocating techniques regarding the extrusion of debris and observed that Reciproc and WaveOne systems resulted in less extrusion of debris than the ProTaper retreatment system. Other authors confirmed these results [86, 87]. In addition, Comparin et al. [88] found that reciprocating and continuous rotary systems were equivalent regarding the incidence, intensity, and duration of postoperative pain after endodontic retreatment.

7.4.3 Interappointment Medication: Actual Scientific Status

The use of a chemical solution as an inter-appointment dressing with the main objective to control intracanal infection and prevent postoperative pain is widely employed in endodontics. Calcium hydroxide stands out as being the most common medication used with this objective [2]. However, a great number of authors, based on the results of randomized clinical trials using human teeth and systematic literature reviews, have stated that, at least for primary endodontic infections, no scientific evidence supports the use of a two-visit approach to enhance outcome or to prevent postoperative pain [89–95].

Zehnder and Paqué [63] emphasized that in retreatment cases the removal of all filling materials from the canals and the reshaping step can be time-consuming in such a way that it may be advisable to postpone the filling procedure to a second visit. But there is no evidence to suggest that retreatment of simple cases could or should not be performed in one visit [96]. On the other hand, some authors prefer to routinely use a second visit for retreatment cases [97–99].

In the case of two or more appointments, calcium hydroxide should be the first choice as intracanal medication because of its antimicrobial effect and tissue-dissolving capacity [100, 101]. Furthermore, calcium hydroxide should be used because of its good compatibility with sodium hypochlorite. Indeed, calcium hydroxide powder can even be mixed with the NaOCl irrigant used beforehand to obtain an intervisit dressing with combined short- and long-term antimicrobial power. Mixing pure calcium hydroxide powder with sodium hypochlorite solution used for irrigation will save chair time because the sodium hypochlorite contained in the aqueous phase will continue to act on the canal microbiota, at least for some time [63]. Nowadays, various brands have pre-manipulated calcium hydroxide pastes with easy-to-handle devices that facilitate the material insertion and clinical use.

Finally, we should point out that the removal of calcium hydroxide in the beginning of the second visit is not easy and the use of chelating agents and agitation of the solution should be employed, but the complete removal of the calcium hydroxide paste from the canals and irregularities is also unlikely to occur [102, 103].

7.5 Suggested Clinical Protocol

7.5.1 Case Planning: Anatomical Knowledge with 3D Visualization of the Canals

Our proposed retreatment protocol is focused on three main objectives: (1) removal of the bulk-filling material from the canal; (2) regain apical patency; and (3) canal reshaping at the established working length. Before starting the clinical procedures, the dentist should determine a treatment plan based on the familiarity with the external and internal anatomies of each group of teeth. Radiographic images and, when possible and properly indicated [104], high-resolution CBCT images should be used. The treatment plan should also include:

- Recognition of the inclination of the tooth in the jaw.
- Recognition of particular anatomic details of each root, i.e., the number of canals, the shape of the roots, the cross-sectional shape of the canals at each third, the presence of curvatures, the apical ending, and the foramen position.
- Type of filling material and its relation with the anatomy and its adaptation degree to the canal walls.
- Presence of mishaps and deviations in the original canal anatomy.
- Presence and position of the lesion and its relationship with roots and adjacent dental structures.
- Presence of root resorptions.

7.5.2 Instruments and Materials

The use of the following materials and instruments are recommended for retreatment procedures: K-type hand files, a reciprocating system, ultrasonic inserts, magnification and illumination of the operative field, NaOCl 2.5%, 17% aqueous EDTA, saline solution, and an apparatus/system for the agitation/activation of the irrigants.

7.5.3 New Instruments and Approaches to Deal with the Remaining Gutta-Percha

As discussed, no instrument/technique can render canals 100% free of filling materials in retreatment cases. For this reason, new commercial products and instruments are continuously appearing on the market, some of them with scarce literature to support their use. Among them, we can highlight the following that can be useful for retreatment:

The XP-endo Finisher (FKG Dentaire, Switzerland) was recently introduced for use as a supplementary step to improve root canal cleaning. It consists of a size 25 tip and a nontapered rotary NiTi instrument made of a special alloy (MaxWire; Martensite Austenite Electropolish Flex, FKG Dentaire). The instrument changes its shape according to the temperature. At room temperature, in its martensitic phase (M-phase), it is straight. However, when submitted to body temperatures, it changes to the austenitic phase (A-phase) and assumes a spoon-like shape of 1.5 mm depth in the final 10 mm of its length. According to the manufacturer, when the instrument is placed inside the canal in rotation mode, the A-phase shape allows the instrument to access and clean areas that other instruments might not be able to reach, without damaging dentin or altering the original canal shape. The XP-endo Finisher R (FKG Dentaire) is a new variation of the XP-endo Finisher and was developed for retreatment. The instrument displays a larger core diameter (tip size 30) and variations in its tip, making it stiffer and therefore more aggressive. These changes aimed to increase its effectiveness in touching and displacing root-filling materials that remain after the use of conventional techniques [84]. The XP-endo Finisher family seems to perform very well as an adjunct tool to improve the removal of filling materials. Silva et al. [84] demonstrated that XP-Endo Finisher and XP-Endo Finisher R were equally effective in the additional removal of remaining filling material from straight oval-shaped root canals. Similar findings were observed by Aksel et al. [105] in the mesial root of mandibular first molars filled with bioceramic sealers and Alves et al. [106] in the removal of filling materials from curved canals.

Lasers have also been indicated for retreatment procedures and literature has evidence that Nd:YAG and Er:YAG lasers can be used to remove filling remnants. The application of lasers in retreatment procedures relies mainly on the thermal effect of irradiation [107–109]. An example is the photon-induced photoacoustic streaming (PIPS), a laser-activated irrigation system device that uses a very low-power source, at energy levels below those reported in the literature (20 mJ), to rapidly pulse laser light energy, which is absorbed by the molecules within the irrigant. This transfer of energy results in a series of rapid and powerful shock waves capable of forcefully propelling the irrigant throughout the root canal system with no thermal effects on the dentinal surface [110, 111].

Keleş et al. [112] used micro-CT imaging to investigate the use of Er:YAG laser-based photon-induced photoacoustic streaming (PIPS) in the endodontic retreatment by assessing its efficacy in removing filling remnants from oval-shaped canals after retreatment with rotary instruments. These authors concluded that, overall, filling residues were located mainly at the apical third and in canal irregularities after retreatment procedures. A comparison between the supplementary tested protocols showed that Er:YAG laser application resulted in a higher removal of filling remnants than PIPS. However, considering the 95% confidence interval of each group, the effect size of the difference of the percentage volume of the remaining filling materials after rotary preparation and laser application was small, suggesting that the improvement in the removal of filling materials by the laser may not be substantial in clinical terms. In a clinical setup, if not properly controlled, the interaction between the laser energy and the root canal walls can cause an increase in the temperature to the point that the tooth may be lost or have the surrounding soft tissues damaged.

The GentleWave System (Sonendo Inc., USA) is another device that was developed as an innovative way to clean and disinfect the root canal system after minimal mechanical shaping. According to the manufacter, before its use, patency must be obtained with sizes 10 and 15 K-files, and the apical preparation should only be enlarged up to a size 20. The so-called multisonic ultra-cleaning technology uses fluid dynamics, acoustic energy, and tissue dissolution chemistry to clean and disinfect the root canal system. A broad spectrum of acoustic energy is delivered to all anatomic features inside the canals. It is an innovative technology, and to date, there is a scarcity of data on its efficacy reported by independent and unbiased research groups. Despite the promising initial results related to tissue dissolution and treatment of primary infections [113–115], the impact of this technology in endodontic retreatment still do not look promising. Wright et al. [116] compared irrigation with the side-vented needle (positive pressure irrigation), EndoVac (negative pressure irrigation), and GentleWave (multisonic energy) for the removal of residual filling materials from the root canal system and observed no differences among groups. Therefore, it is yet to be confirmed whether the GentleWave system is able to disinfect and remove tissue debris in the presence of residual filling material during endodontic retreatment.

7.5.4 Main Clinical Protocol

The suggested clinical protocol is subjected to variations dictated by dental anatomy and uses the crown-down concept of canal preparations. Basically, it can be divided into three steps.

7.5.4.1 Removal of the Bulk Filling Material (Fig. 7.15)

After proper access and orifice canal location, the filling materials just below the canal entrance should be removed with an arrowhead ultrasonic tip (Clearsonic Tip; Helse Ultrasonic, USA) or another ultrasonic insert compatible with the anatomy of the canal. The aim of this procedure is to touch only the filling material; of course, this can be performed with other devices, such as small Gates-Glidden burs. At this stage, irrigation is performed with 17% EDTA solution delivered by a short 27-gauge needle, under high volume and pressure. Always activate the irrigant with sonic or ultrasonic tips to flush out the remnants of gutta-percha and sealer. Use

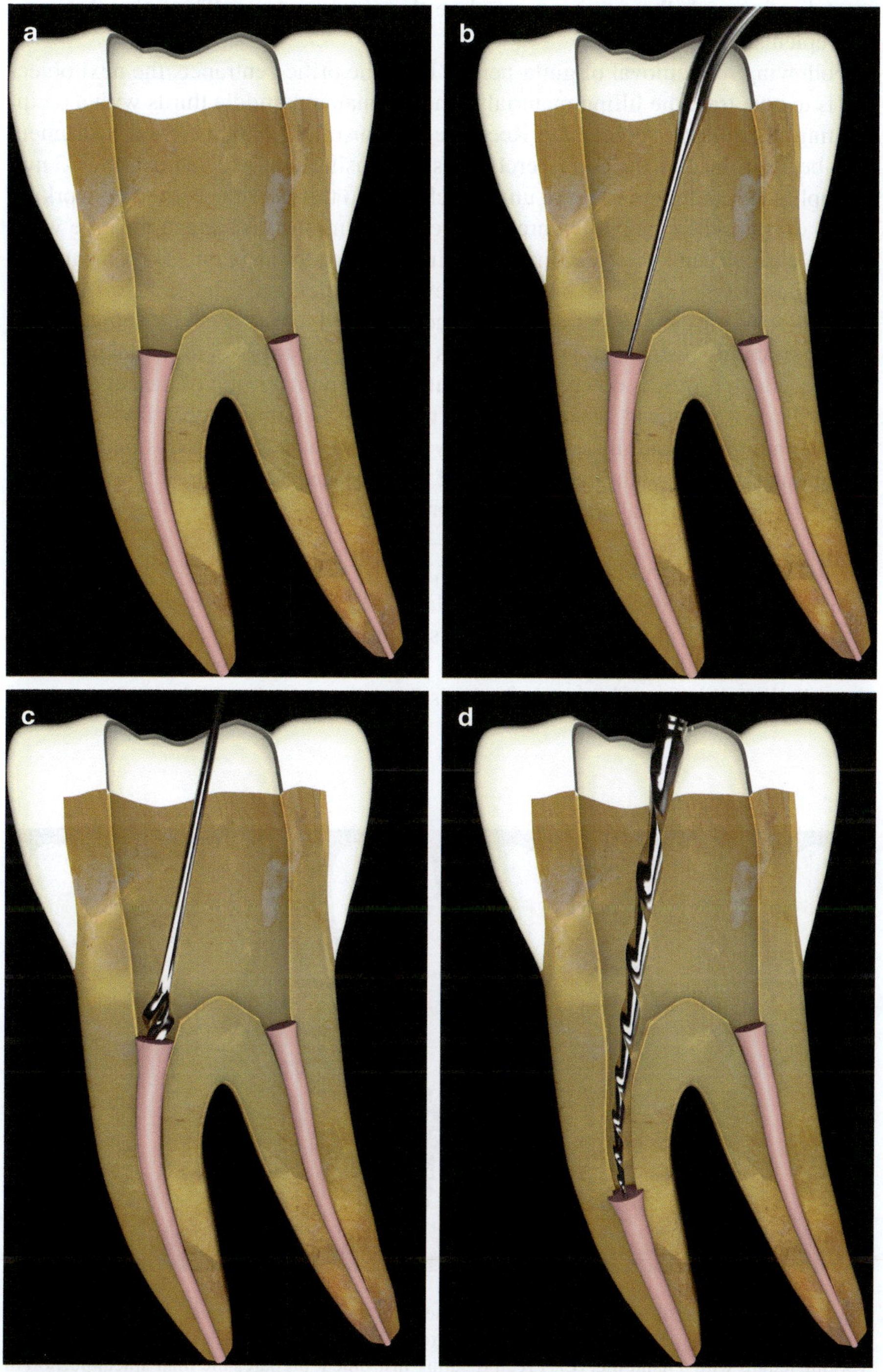

Fig. 7.15 Schematic illustration of the retreatment protocol in a mandibular molar (Part 1). (**a**) Access preparation. (**b**) Removal of the bulk filling material from the coronal thirds using an ultrasonic insert or (**c**) a GG bur (size 2). (**d**) Removal of the filling material from the middle third with a reciprocating instrument using a light apical pressure

magnification and illumination to explore the canal anatomy. Then, dry the canal and replenish it with EDTA.

Following the removal of gutta-percha from the orifice entrance, the next objective is to penetrate the filling material at the coronal and middle thirds with a reciprocating instrument, such as the Reciproc R25 or other. The preferred instrument must be positioned on the gutta-percha mass and, using small movements of 1–3 mm in amplitude, go down the canal until reaching two thirds of the estimated working length or up to the canal curvature. After each 3 mm, the instrument must be withdrawn, cleaned, and the canal irrigated. In addition, the irrigant solution must be also agitated with sonic or ultrasonic devices. Under magnification, inspect the cleanliness of the canal walls. It is also recommended to use brush movements with the reciprocating instrument to avoid areas with low intra-root dentin thickness. The main idea is to progress down the canal with the coronal portion of the canal free of debris. Do not go ahead if you see small remnants of gutta-percha. Try to remove them with an adequate ultrasonic tip. Dry the canal with suction tips and perform irrigation/activation with great volume of solution and be prepared to explore the final portion of the canal and establish working length.

7.5.4.2 Regain Apical Patency (Fig. 7.16a, b)

After drying the clean canal, start to use NaOCl 2.5% delivered by a 30-gauge side-vented needle. Do not use excessive pressure at this time. The apical third should be explored with K-type hand files sizes 10 or 15, initially without solvent. Use controlled clockwise and counterclockwise movements with the hand files toward

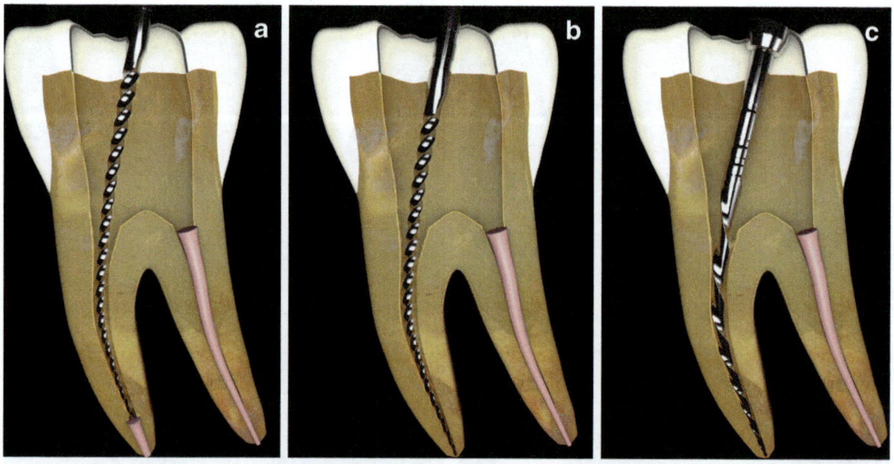

Fig. 7.16 Schematic illustration of the retreatment protocol in a mandibular molar (Part 2). (**a**) Removal of the filling remnants of the apical third with a hand instrument. (**b**) Determination of working length with a hand file. (**c**) A reciprocating instrument prepares the final apical portion of the canal to a size 25/0.06 or 0.08 taper

the apical portion and establish working length near the foramen with an apex locator reading at "0" or "0.5" mark. If resistance is present, a drop of solvent must be used to facilitate the exploration of the apical canal, preventing the risk of canal deviations. After using the solvent, irrigate and dry the canals to eliminate softened gutta-percha from the walls. Saline solution irrigation can be performed after the use of solvent for mechanical debris removal. The saline solution can also be delivered with a 30-gauge needle with pressure. If used, the saline solution should be removed with suction tips and the canal replenished again with sodium hypochlorite. There is no doubt that this stage is time-consuming, especially in canals in which the anterior filling is positioned close to the apical foramen. Canals with moderate or strong curvatures, roots with marked tapering, and thin apical areas with rounded canal cross-section are also a challenge. Take your time here. Discard deformed files and always use new ones. Stiff files like C Pilot (VDW, Germany) can be a great option to reach the foramen. Once working length is established, perform the glide path at least with a size 15 hand file and proceed to the enlargement of the apical portion.

7.5.4.3 Reshaping the Canals at the Established Working Length (Fig. 7.16c)

Bring the reciprocating instrument of choice back to the scenario again. The reciprocating instrument should be used at the working length with gentle apical movements of 1–2 mm of amplitude without forcing the instrument. In case of resistance, return to the glide path instrument or use another drop of solvent if necessary; however, always after the use of the solvent, irrigate the canal in order to prevent the slurry material precluding further cleaning. Dry the canal and irrigate again with NaOCl delivered with a 30-gauge needle with no pressure. Apical enlargement should be performed based on canal anatomy and in the first instrument that cuts dentin at the apical portion, generally the final 3–4 mm of the canal. Enlarge the canal with an ISO file at least three sizes larger than the initial instrument. After apical preparation, final irrigation should be performed, and the solution must be sonically or ultrasonically agitated for 1 min in each canal. A final flush with 5 mL of saline solution could be performed with the objective of washing out debris. Dry the canal and finish the case with proper filling or place an intracanal dressing of calcium hydroxide mixed with NaOCl or any other calcium hydroxide-based material.

7.6 Final Considerations

Retreatment procedures are generally not an easy task, demanding a well-trained operator working in a controlled environment with the aid of technology. While some cases may be easy to do, others present a real challenge for the dentist. If one considers cases with posts to be removed, ledges, apical deviations, broken files, and so on, sometimes it would be simply impossible to achieve the requirements of proper Shaping for Cleaning (Figs. 7.17, 7.18, and 7.19).

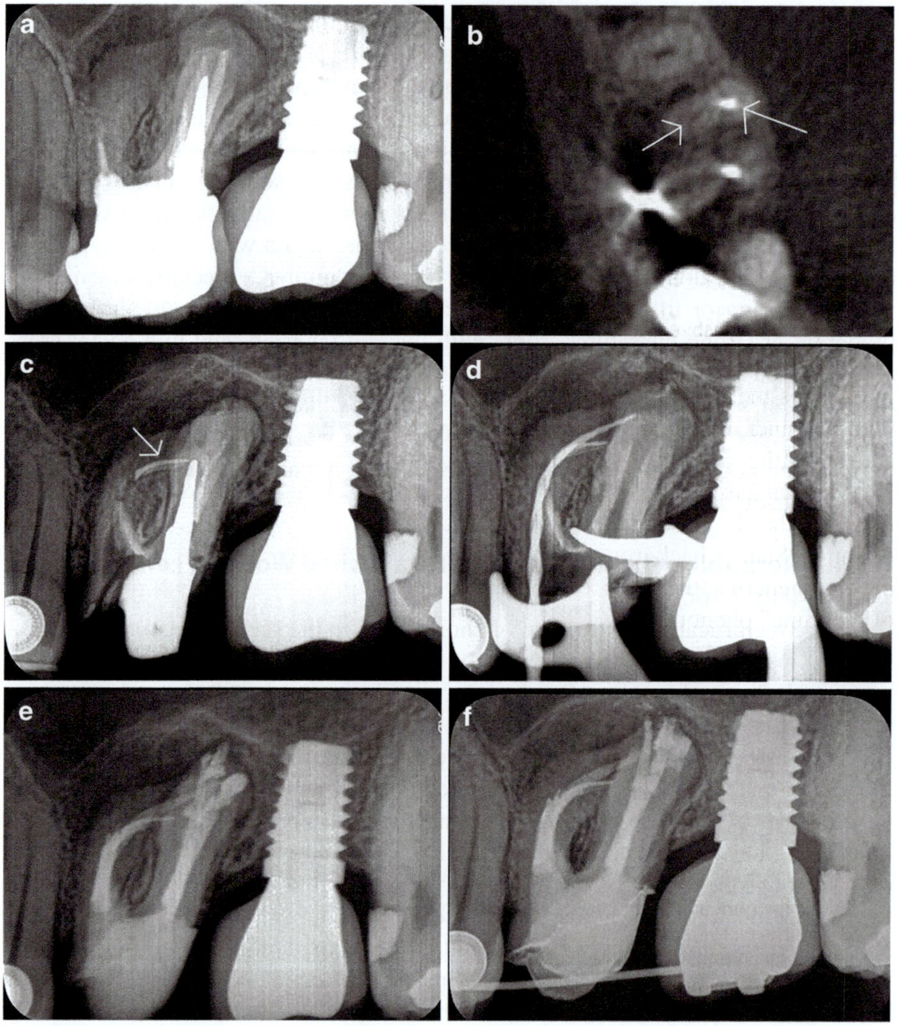

Fig. 7.17 Clinical case showing iatrogenic mishaps during the retreatment procedure in a maxillary first left molar. (**a**) Preoperative radiograph. (**b**) Axial tomographic image highlighting the presence of two canals in the mesiobuccal root (arrows). (**c**) A size 10 K-file was fractured after the curvature of the MB2 canal during scouting procedure. Another size 10 K-file was used to bypass and regain access. The canal was manually enlarged up to a size 20 K-file. Then, a Reciproc R25 instrument was used in an attempt to reach the working length, but it also fractured. (**d**) MB1 canal was prepared with Reciproc R25 and the fractured instruments were left in the MB2 canal. (**e**) Immediate postoperative radiograph of filling procedures. (**f**) Six-month follow-up showing the lack of bone healing

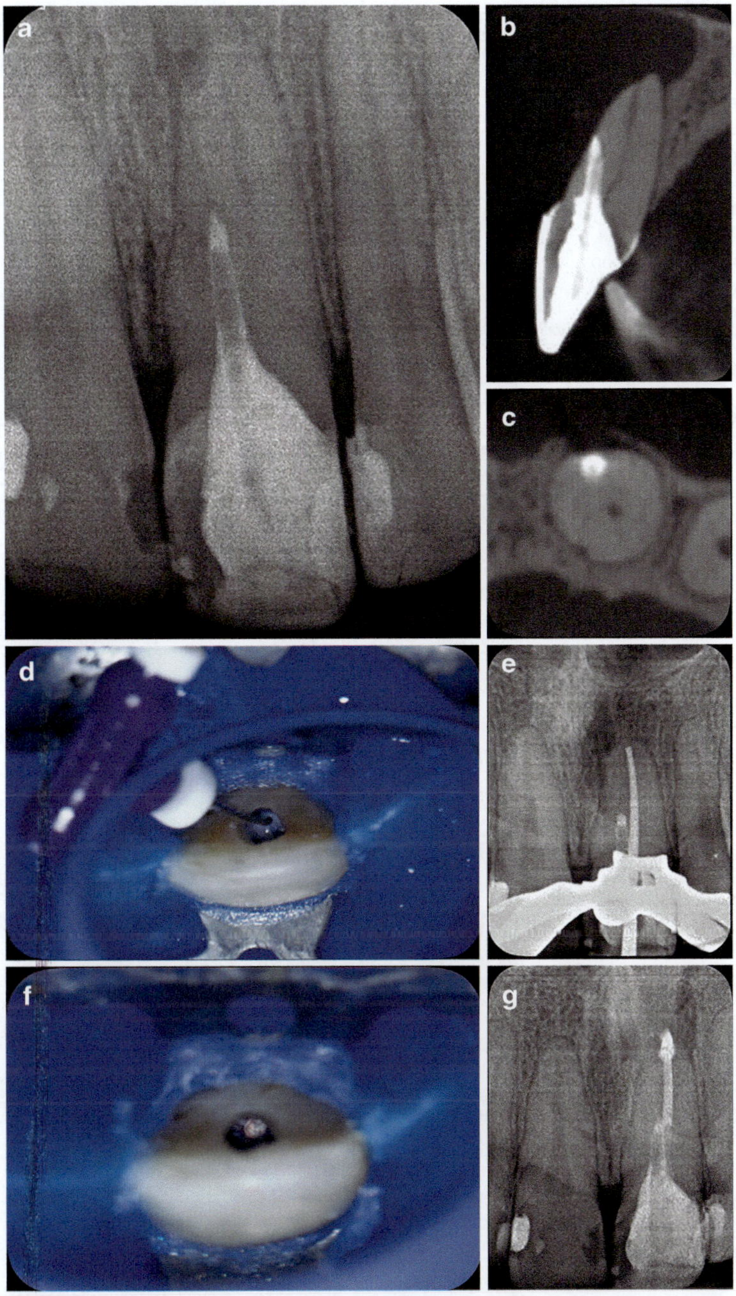

Fig. 7.18 Clinical case illustrating the importance of tomographic examination for diagnosis before retreatment procedure in a maxillary left central incisor. (**a**) Preoperative radiograph suggesting the presence of a post deviated to the mesial side of the root. (**b, c**) Sagittal and axial tomographic images demonstrating that the post was deviated towards the buccal aspect of the root. (**d**) Access preparation and location of the original root canal path without removing the post. (**e**) Trans-operative radiograph for cone fit. (**f, g**) Root canal was filled with gutta-percha and AH Plus sealer

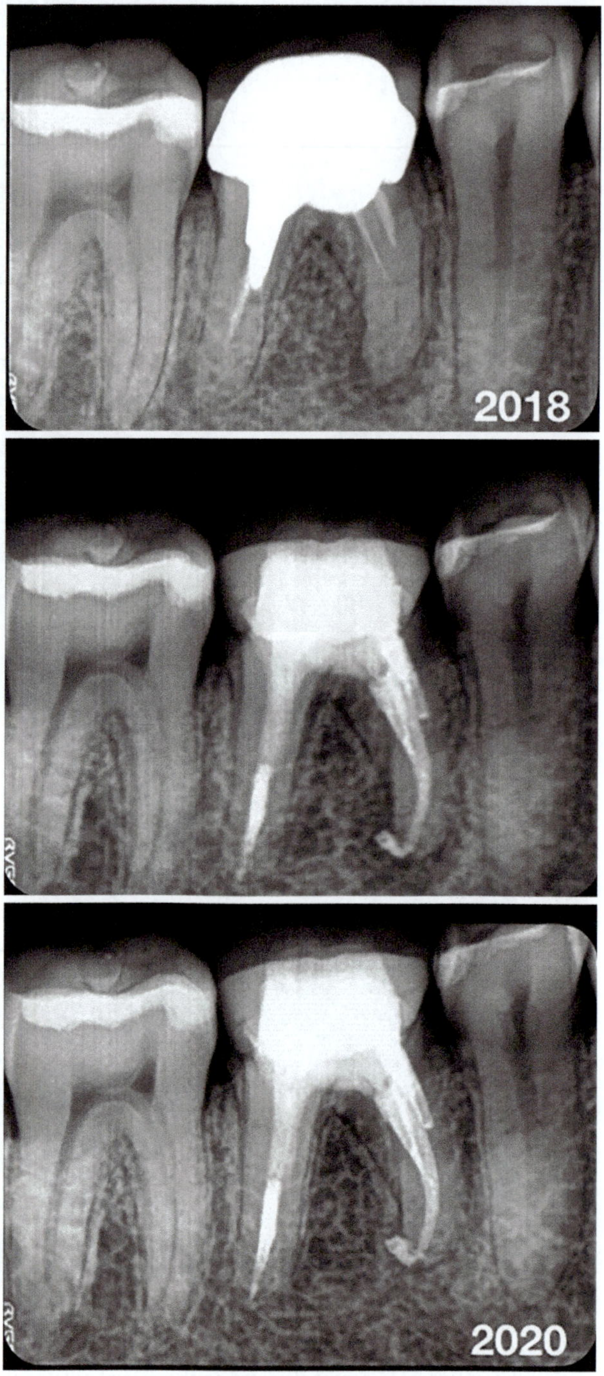

Fig. 7.19 Retreatment of a mandibular right first molar having an iatrogenic ledge at the mesial root. (Top) Preoperative radiograph suggesting the presence of ledge in the mesial canals. (Middle) Original canal path was located under microscopy, re-shaped with Reciproc R25 instrument and filled. (Bottom) Two-year follow-up radiograph showing the healing of the apical lesion

7.6.1 How to Determine the Outcome in Retreatment Cases

From all classifications of "success or failure"—and keeping in mind the previous comment on "the elephant in the room" [12]—we can evaluate the outcome of retreatment as proposed by Friedman and Mor [4], but modified by Zuolo et al. [2]:

7.6.1.1 Healing: Grouped into Two Types

- Complete: absence of clinical and radiographic signs of apical periodontitis. Periodontal ligament space should be visualized in the radiograph or in a CBCT scan, especially for molar teeth (Figs. 7.20 and 7.21).
- Incomplete: owing to the dynamic nature of the repair process, regression of radiolucent areas along with the absence of clinical signs of inflammation or infection can be interpreted as an ongoing healing response or progression (Figs. 7.22, 7.23, and 7.24).

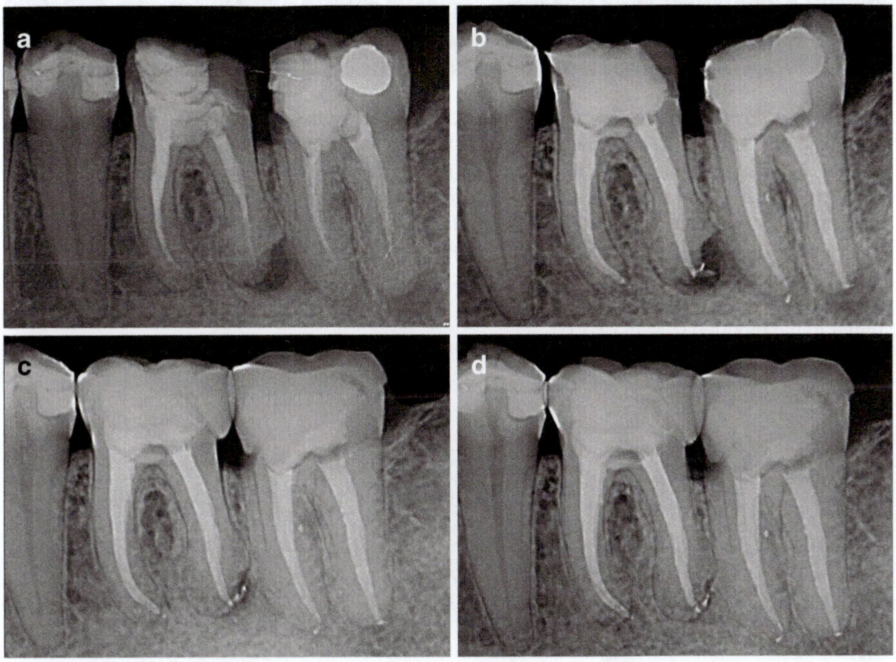

Fig. 7.20 (**a**) Preoperative radiograph showing the presence of apical periodontitis in previously treated mandibular first and second left molars. (**b**) Immediate postoperative radiography after retreatment of both teeth. (**c, d**) 1- and 4-year radiographic follow-up showing new bone formation at the periapical area and the integrity of the periodontal ligament space

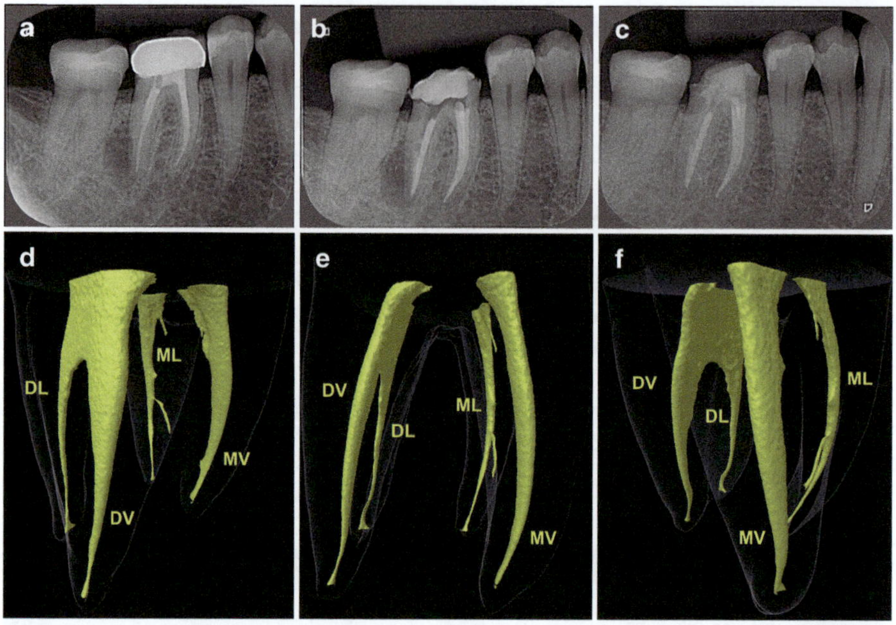

Fig. 7.21 (**a**) Preoperative radiograph of a mandibular first right molar with apparent well-treated canals showing a large lesion related to the distal root. (**b**) Immediate postoperative radiograph after retreatment procedure. Note that root canals were reshaped at the apical third after establishing a new working length. Besides, a missed canal was found at the distal root and properly prepared and filled. (**c**) At a 17-month follow-up, it was possible to observe the complete healing of the apical lesion, as well as, the normality of the periodontal ligament space. (Courtesy of Dr. Maria Cristina de Carvalho, Brazil) (**d–f**) Different views of a 3D model acquired by the micro-CT technology of a mandibular molar showing the presence of two independent canals in each root similar to the reported case in (**a–c**)

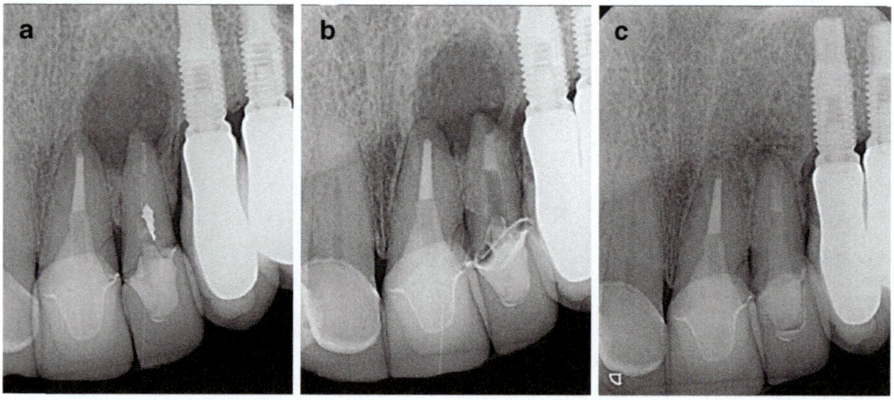

Fig. 7.22 Incomplete healing (scar tissue). (**a**) Preoperative radiograph of a maxillary left lateral incisor with a previously treated root canal in which it is possible to see a broken post and a large periapical lesion. (**b**) Immediate postoperative radiograph after using an apical MTA plug to seal the foramen, followed by post space preparation. (**c**) A 13-month follow-up showing the reduction in size of the apical lesion. (Courtesy of Dr. Maria Cristina de Carvalho, Brazil)

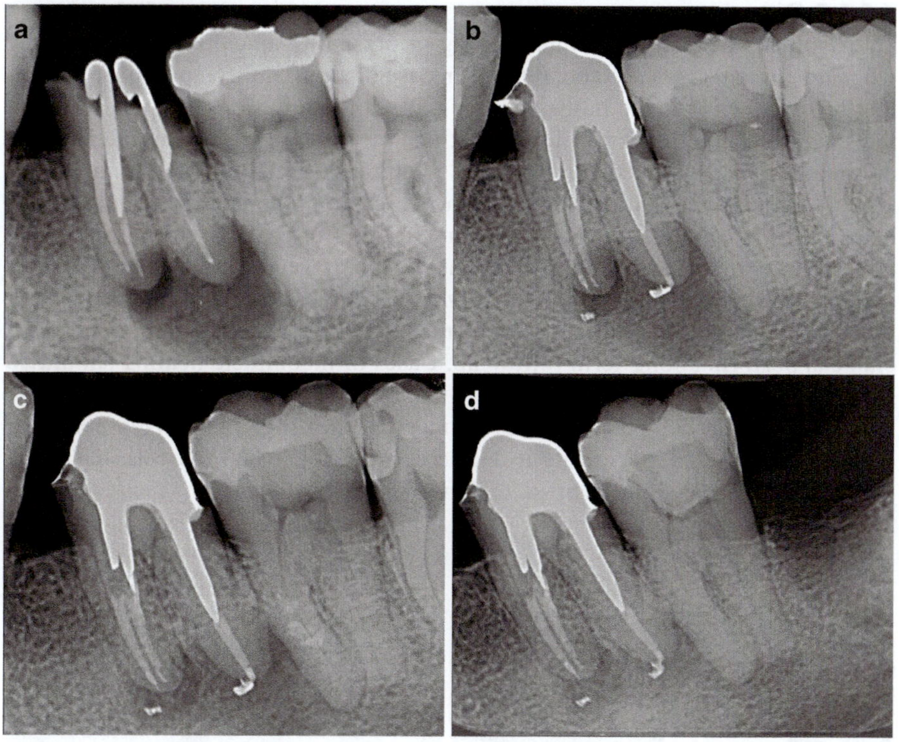

Fig. 7.23 Incomplete healing (scar tissue). (**a**) Preoperative radiograph of a mandibular first left molar with a large periapical lesion. (**b**) Radiographic examination after retreatment and post insertion. (**c**) 12-month and (**d**) 7-year follow-up show the reduction of the lesion, but without a complete healing

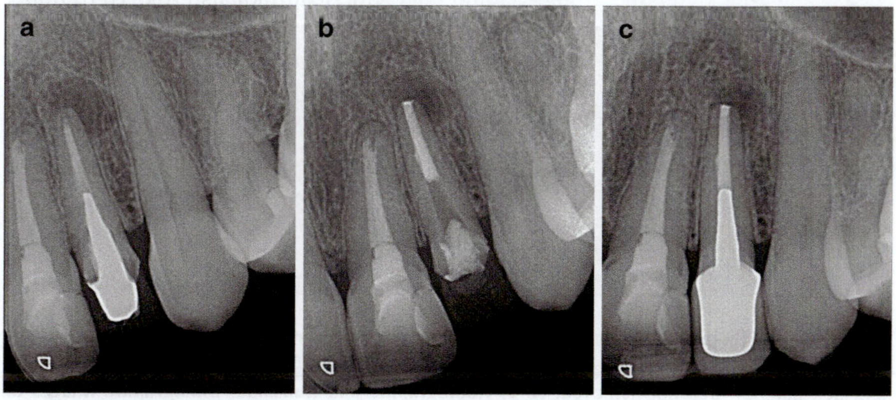

Fig. 7.24 Uncertain healing. (**a**) Preoperative radiograph of a maxillary left lateral incisor which had a post in a previously treated root canal. (**b**) Root canal retreatment was performed after post removal. (**c**) At the 13-month follow-up, it is possible to see a reduction in the bone lesion. Considering the patient was asymptomatic, another follow-up must be considered. (Courtesy of Dr. Maria Cristina de Carvalho, Brazil)

7.6.1.2 Disease

To establish whether there is developing or persisting apical bone lesion, even when no clinical signs are apparent; or in case of signs and symptoms of inflammation or infection, even in the absence of radiographic signs of apical disease, the suggested timeline for follow-up is: wait at least 12 months in the absence of clinical signs, even in the presence of symptoms of inflammation or infection. Patients should be comfortable, with no chief complaint. Cases classified as healed after 12 months with a correct restoration in position do not need any other follow-up. However, long-term outcomes are welcomed, although, generally, this is a patient decision. Clinically, it can be observed that it is very likely that the patient will be back for the treatment of another tooth and then the clinician can perform a long-term follow-up. Cases of incomplete healing should be followed for more than 12 months, when a new evaluation using the same parameter should be made. In cases of uncertain healing, a follow-up period of 4 years is advisable, according to Halse et al. [117], when the case has to be judged as healed or failure (Figs. 7.25 and 7.26).

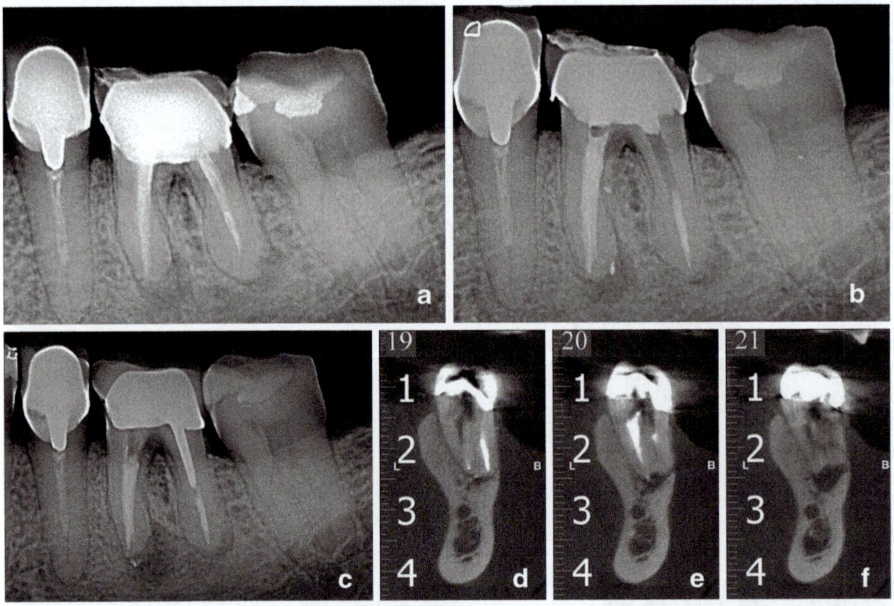

Fig. 7.25 (**a**) Preoperative radiograph showing the failure of a retreatment procedure in a mandibular first left molar. (**b**) Immediate postoperative radiograph after a new retreatment procedure in which patency was not achieved. (**c**–**f**) Radiographic and transaxial tomographic images at 9-month follow-up showing the enlargement of the periapical lesion. Clinically, the patient complained of pain to percussion

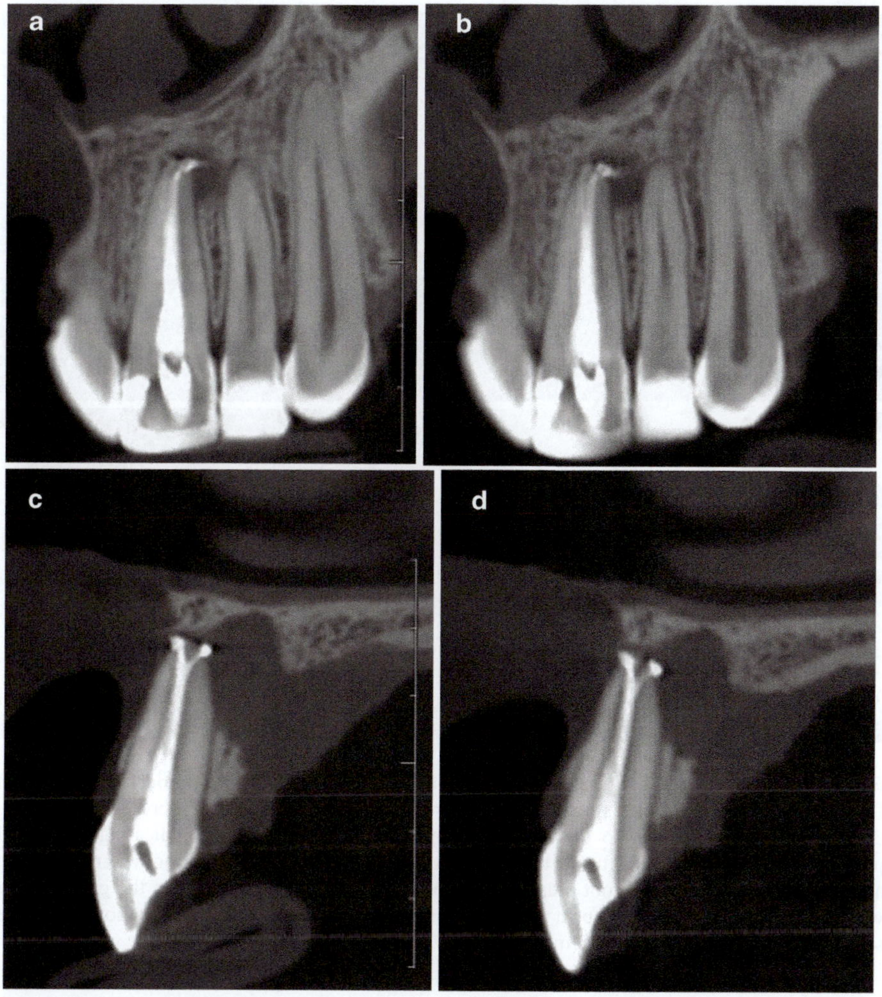

Fig. 7.26 Short-term unsatisfactory endodontic retreatment of a maxillary left central incisor. Transaxial (**a**, **b**) and parasagittal (**c**, **d**) tomographic images showing the presence of a large apical lesion just after the retreatment procedure (**a–c**) as well as at 5-month follow–up (**b–d**). After 5 months, the patient still complained of pain upon chewing, and there was the presence of a palatal edema. Tooth was referred for extraction. (Courtesy Dra. Priscila Fernandes, Brazil)

7.6.2 Selective Root Canal Retreatment

Recently, a new retreatment technique, referred to as "selective root retreatment" was presented as a "conservative" technique in which multirooted teeth have retreatment performed in only single root or roots that clearly show periapical pathosis, as demonstrated by CBCT, while leaving the other root(s) with no visible

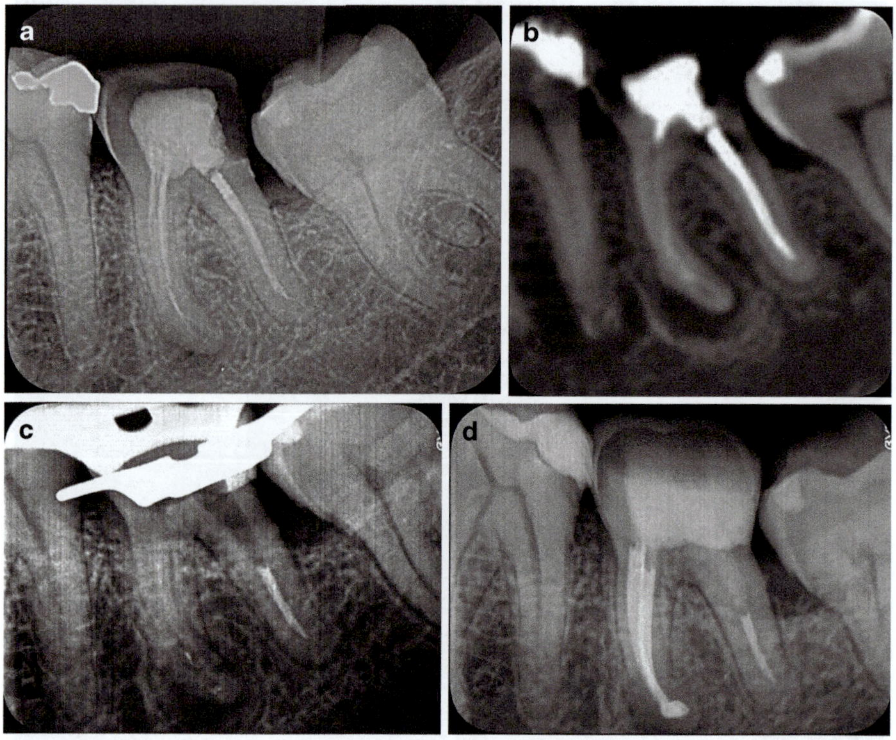

Fig. 7.27 Mandibular left second molar in which a selective retreatment approach was used. (**a**) Initial radiograph indicating a fractured instrument in the mesial canal and the presence of an apical radiolucency associated to this root. (**b**) Sagittal tomographic image indicating the apical pathology associated with the mesial root, and not to the distal. (**c**) The mesial root was re-accessed and re-shaped and the distal root prepared for post placement. The condition of the gutta-percha was verified while preparing for post to certify no sign of solubilization. (**d**) Final radiograph of the selective retreatment and post assembled

or perceived pathosis untouched [118]. Although it seems a promising proposal, it is based only on a few case reports and, in the light of current scientific evidence, it should not be a reasonable option of choice for endodontic retreatment. Further investigations and reports on long-term success rates using this conservative technique should be performed before indicating this modality as a treatment option (Figs. 7.27 and 7.28).

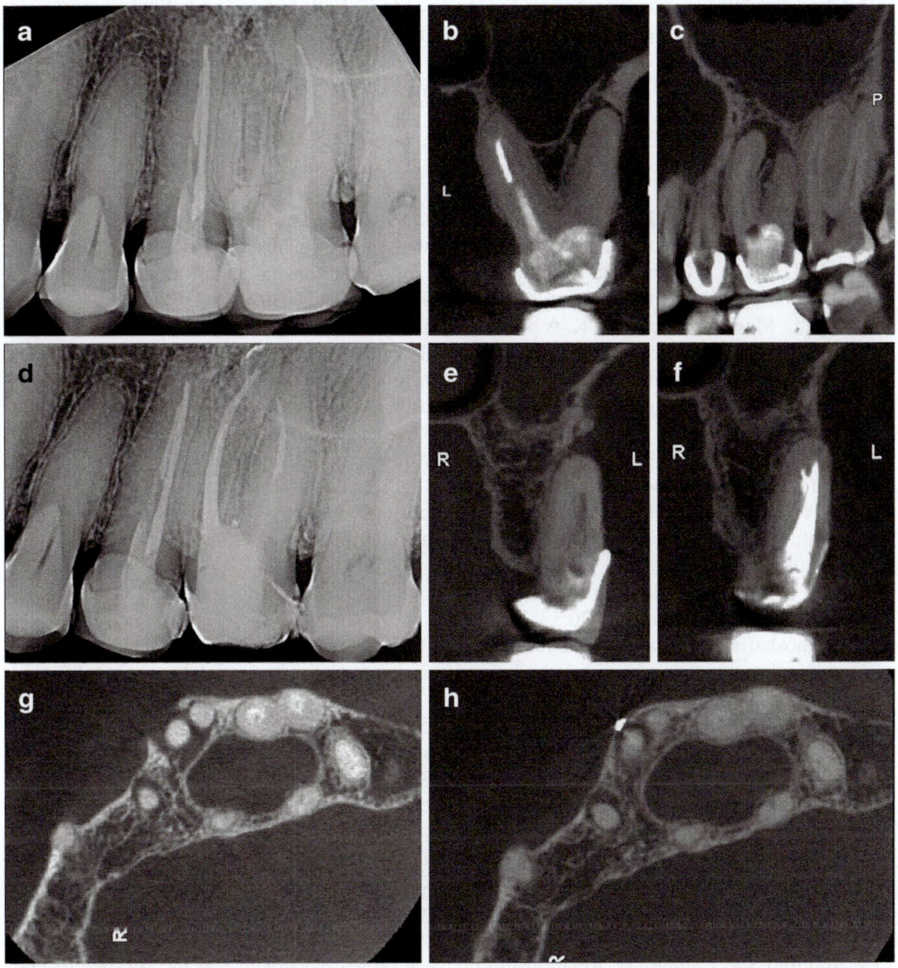

Fig. 7.28 Selective retreatment of a maxillary left first molar. Patient's chief complaint was pain to palpation at the mesiobuccal root region that also had a discreet edema; (**a**–**c**) Preoperative radiographic and tomographic images show that only the palatal canal was treated, and there was a lesion restricted to the periapical area of the mesiobuccal root, and a calcified distobuccal canal. (**d**) Immediate postoperative radiograph show the selective retreatment of the mesiobuccal canal only. (**e**–**h**) Axial and transaxial tomography images comparing the conditions of the periapical area of the mesiobuccal root (**e** and **g**) before and (**f** and **h**) after a 10-month follow up, with bone healing and cortical formation

References

1. Liu P, McGrath CBA, Cheung GSP. Improvement in oral health–related quality of life after endodontic treatment: a prospective longitudinal study. J Endod. 2014;40:805–10.
2. Zuolo ML, Kherlakian D, Mello JE Jr, Carvalho MC, Fagundes MI. Reintervention in endodontics. 1st ed. São Paulo: Quintessence; 2017.

3. Chércoles-Ruiz A, Sánchez-Torres A, Gay-Escoda C. Endodontics, endodontic retreatment, and apical surgery versus tooth extraction and implant placement: a systematic review. J Endod. 2017;43:679–86.
4. Friedman S, Mor C. The success therapy: healing and functionality. J Calif Dent J. 2004;32:493–503.
5. Imura N, Pinheiro ET, Gomes BPFA, Zaia AA, Ferraz CCR, Souza-Filho FJ. The outcome of endodontic treatment: a retrospective study of 200 cases performed by a specialist. J Endod. 2007;33:1278–82.
6. Jacob CB, Stover S, Eichmiller F, Bhagavatula P. Outcomes of primary endodontic therapy provided by endodontic specialists compared with other providers. J Endod. 2014;42:702–5.
7. Ng YL, Mann V, Gulabivala K. Tooth survival following non-surgical root canal treatment: a systematic review of the literature. Int Endod J. 2010;43:171–89.
8. Ng YL, Mann V, Gulabivala K. A prospective study of the factors affecting outcomes of non-surgical root canal treatment: part 1: periapical health. Int Endod J. 2011;44:583–609.
9. Ng YL, Mann V, Rahbaran S, Lewsey J, Gulabivala K. Outcome of primary root canal treatment: systematic review of the literature—part 1. Effects of study characteristics on probability of success. Int Endod J. 2007;40:921–39.
10. Rotstein I, Salehrabi R, Forrest JL. Endodontic treatment outcome: survey of oral health care professionals. J Endod. 2006;32:399–403.
11. Ng YL, Mann V, Rahbaran S, Lewsey J, Gulabivala K. Outcome of primary root canal treatment: systematic review of the literature—part 2. Influence of clinical factors. Int Endod J. 2008;41:6–31.
12. Patel S, Arias A, Whitworth J, Mannocci F. Outcome of endodontic treatment—the elephant in the room. Int Endod J. 2020;53:291–7.
13. Aminoshariae A, Kulild JC, Syed A. Cone-beam computed tomography compared with intraoral radiographic lesions in endodontic outcome studies: a systematic review. J Endod. 2018;44:1626–31.
14. Al-Nuaimi N, Patel S, Davies A, Bakhsh A, Foschi F, Mannocci F. Pooled analysis of 1-year recall data from three root canal treatment outcome studies undertaken using cone beam computed tomography. Int Endod J. 2018;51(Suppl 3):e216–e26.
15. Siqueira JF Jr. Aetiology of root canal treatment failure: why well-treated teeth can fail. Int Endod J. 2001;34:1–10.
16. Siqueira JF Jr, Rocas IN, Ricucci D, Hulsmann M. Causes and management of post-treatment apical periodontitis. Br Dent J. 2014;216:305–12.
17. Molven O, Halse A, Fristad I, MacDonald-Jankowski D. Periapical changes following root-canal treatment observed 20-27 years postoperatively. Int Endod J. 2002;35:784–90.
18. Aquilino SA, Caplan DJ. Relationship between crown placement and the survival of endodontically treated teeth. J Prosthet Dent. 2002;87:256–63.
19. Dammaschke T, Steven D, Kaup M, Ott KH. Long-term survival of root-canal-treated teeth: a retrospective study over 10 years. J Endod. 2003;29:638–43.
20. De Backer H, Van Maele G, Decock V, Van den Berghe L. Long-term survival of complete crowns, fixed dental prostheses, and cantilever fixed dental prostheses with posts and cores on root canal-treated teeth. Int J Prosthodont. 2007;20:229–34.
21. Lazarski MP, Walker WA 3rd, Flores CM, Schindler WG, Hargreaves KM. Epidemiological evaluation of the outcomes of nonsurgical root canal treatment in a large cohort of insured dental patients. J Endod. 2001;27:791–6.
22. Mindiola MJ, Mickel AK, Sami C, Jones JJ, Lalumandier JA, Nelson SS. Endodontic treatment in an American Indian population: a 10-year retrospective study. J Endod. 2006;32:828–32.
23. Schwartz RS, Robbins JW. Post placement and restoration of endodontically treated teeth: a literature review. J Endod. 2004;30:289–301.
24. Ørstavik D, Qvist V, Stoltze K. A multivariate analysis of the outcome of endodontic treatment. Eur J Oral Sci. 2004;112:224–30.

25. Stassen IG, Hommez GM, De Bruyn H, De Moor RJ. The relation between apical periodontitis and root-filled teeth in patients with periodontal treatment need. Int Endod J. 2006;39:299–308.
26. Clark DJ, Sheets CG, Paquette JM. Definitive diagnosis of early enamel and dentin cracks based on microscopic evaluation. J Esthet Restor Dent. 2003;15:391–401.
27. Kang SH, Kim BS, Kim Y. Cracked teeth: distribution, characteristics, and survival after root canal treatment. J Endod. 2016;42:557–62.
28. Tan L, Chen NN, Poon CY, Wong HB. Survival of root filled cracked teeth in a tertiary institution. Int Endod J. 2006;39:886–9.
29. Ricucci D, Siqueira JF Jr. Biofilms and apical periodontitis: study of prevalence and association with clinical and histopathologic findings. J Endod. 2010;36:1277–88.
30. Gorni FG, Gagliani MM. The outcome of endodontic retreatment: a 2-yr follow-up. J Endod. 2004;30:1–4.
31. Baugh D, Wallace J. The role of apical instrumentation in root canal treatment: a review of the literature. J Endod. 2005;31:333–40.
32. Albrecht LJ, Baumgartner JC, Marshall JG. Evaluation of apical debris removal using various sizes and tapers of ProFile GT files. J Endod. 2004;30:425–8.
33. Alves FR, Rocas IN, Almeida BM, Neves MA, Zoffoli J, Siqueira JF Jr. Quantitative molecular and culture analyses of bacterial elimination in oval-shaped root canals by a single-file instrumentation technique. Int Endod J. 2012;45:871–7.
34. Aminoshariae A, Kulild JC. Master apical file size—smaller or larger: a systematic review of healing outcomes. Int Endod J. 2015;48:639–47.
35. Card SJ, Sigurdsson A, Ørstavik D, Trope M. The effectiveness of increased apical enlargement in reducing intracanal bacteria. J Endod. 2002;28:779–83.
36. de Souza Filho FJ, Benatti O, de Almeida OP. Influence of the enlargement of the apical foramen in periapical repair of contaminated teeth of dog. Oral Surg Oral Med Oral Pathol. 1987;64:480–4.
37. Fornari VJ, Silva-Sousa YT, Vanni JR, Pécora JD, Versiani MA, Sousa-Neto MD. Histological evaluation of the effectiveness of increased apical enlargement for cleaning the apical third of curved canals. Int Endod J. 2010;43:988–94.
38. McGurkin-Smith R, Trope M, Caplan D, Sigurdsson A. Reduction of intracanal bacteria using GT rotary instrumentation, 5.25% NaOCl, EDTA, and $Ca(OH)_2$. J Endod. 2005;31:359–63.
39. Mickel AK, Chogle S, Liddle J, Jones JJ. The role of apical size determination and enlargement in the reduction of intracanal bacteria. J Endod. 2007;33:21–3.
40. Pérez AR, Alves FRF, Marceliano-Alves MF, Provenzano JC, Gonçalves LS, Neves AA, et al. Effects of increased apical enlargement on the amount of unprepared areas and coronal dentine removal: a micro-computed tomography study. Int Endod J. 2018;51:684–90.
41. Abdulrab S, Rodrigues JC, Al-Maweri SA, Halboub E, Alqutaibi AY, Alhadainy H. Effect of apical patency on postoperative pain: a meta-analysis. J Endod. 2018;44:1467–73.
42. Silva EJ, Menaged K, Ajuz N, Monteiro MR, Coutinho-Filho TS. Postoperative pain after foraminal enlargement in anterior teeth with necrosis and apical periodontitis: a prospective and randomized clinical trial. J Endod. 2013;39:173–6.
43. Yaylali IE, Demirci GK, Kurnaz S, Celik G, Kaya BU, Tunca YM. Does maintaining apical patency during instrumentation increase postoperative pain or flare-up rate after nonsurgical root canal treatment? A systematic review of randomized controlled trials. J Endod. 2018;44:1228–36.
44. Demirbuga S, Pala K, Topcuoglu HS, Cayabatmaz M, Topcuoglu G, Ucar EN. Effect of different gutta-percha solvents on the microtensile bond strength of various adhesive systems to pulp chamber dentin. Clin Oral Investig. 2017;21:627–33.
45. Erdemir A, Eldeniz AU, Belli S. Effect of gutta-percha solvents on mineral contents of human root dentin using ICP-AES technique. J Endod. 2004;30:54–6.
46. Erdemir A, Eldeniz AU, Belli S. Effect of the gutta-percha solvents on the microhardness and the roughness of human root dentine. J Oral Rehabil. 2004;31:1145–8.

47. Kaufman D, Mor C, Stabholz A, Rotstein I. Effect of gutta-percha solvents on calcium and phosphorus levels of cut human dentin. J Endod. 1997;23:614–5.
48. Shemesh H, Roeleveld AC, Wesselink PR, Wu MK. Damage to root dentin during retreatment procedures. J Endod. 2011;37:63–6.
49. Hin ES, Wu MK, Wesselink PR, Shemesh H. Effects of self-adjusting file, Mtwo, and ProTaper on the root canal wall. J Endod. 2013;39:262–4.
50. Liu R, Hou BX, Wesselink PR, Wu MK, Shemesh H. The incidence of root microcracks caused by 3 different single-file systems versus the ProTaper system. J Endod. 2013;39:1054–6.
51. De-Deus G, Belladonna FG, Souza EM, Silva EJ, Neves Ade A, Alves H, et al. Micro-computed tomographic assessment on the effect of Protaper Next and Twisted File Adaptive systems on dentinal cracks. J Endod. 2015;41:1116–9.
52. De-Deus G, Silva EJ, Marins J, Souza E, Neves Ade A, Goncalves Belladonna F, et al. Lack of causal relationship between dentinal microcracks and root canal preparation with reciprocation systems. J Endod. 2014;40:1447–50.
53. Yilmaz A, Helvacioglu-Yigit D, Gur C, Ersev H, Kiziltas Sendur G, Avcu E, et al. Evaluation of dentin defect formation during retreatment with hand and rotary instruments: a micro-CT study. Scanning. 2017;2017:4868603.
54. Chutich MJ, Kaminski EJ, Miller DA, Lautenschlager EP. Risk assessment of the toxicity of solvents of gutta-percha used in endodontic retreatment. J Endod. 1998;24:213–6.
55. Hunter KR, Doblecki W, Pelleu GB Jr. Halothane and eucalyptol as alternatives to chloroform for softening gutta-percha. J Endod. 1991;17:310–1.
56. Kaplowitz GJ. Evaluation of Gutta-percha solvents. J Endod. 1990;16:539–40.
57. Campello AF, Almeida BM, Franzoni MA, Alves FRF, Marceliano-Alves MF, Rocas IN, et al. Influence of solvent and a supplementary step with a finishing instrument on filling material removal from canals connected by an isthmus. Int Endod J. 2019;52:716–24.
58. de Siqueira ZA, Zuolo ML, da Silveira Bueno CE, Chu R, Cunha RS. Evaluation of the efficacy of TRUShape and Reciproc file systems in the removal of root filling material: an ex vivo micro-computed tomographic study. J Endod. 2016;42:315–9.
59. Rossi-Fedele G, Ahmed HM. Assessment of root canal filling removal effectiveness using micro-computed tomography: a systematic review. J Endod. 2017;43:520–6.
60. Iqbal MK. Nonsurgical ultrasonic endodontic instruments. Dent Clin N Am. 2004;48:19–34.
61. De-Deus G, Simoes-Carvalho M, Belladonna FG, Cavalcante DM, Portugal LS, Prado CG, et al. Arrowhead design ultrasonic tip as a supplementary tool for canal debridement. Int Endod J. 2020;53:410–20.
62. Zehnder M. Root canal irrigants. J Endod. 2006;32:389–98.
63. Zehnder M, Paqué F. Disinfection of the root canal system during root canal re-treatment. Endod Topics. 2011;19:58–73.
64. Wilcox LR, Swift ML. Endodontic retreatment in small and large curved canals. J Endod. 1991;17:313–5.
65. Wilcox LR, Van Surksum R. Endodontic retreatment in large and small straight canals. J Endod. 1991;17:119–21.
66. Ganesh A, Venkateshbabu N, John A, Deenadhayalan G, Kandaswamy D. A comparative assessment of fracture resistance of endodontically treated and re-treated teeth: an in vitro study. J Conserv Dent. 2014;17:61–4.
67. Wu MK, Wesselink PR, Walton RE. Apical terminus location of root canal treatment procedures. Oral Surg Oral Med Oral Pathol Oral Radiol Endod. 2000;89:99–103.
68. ElAyouti A, Dima E, Ohmer J, Sperl K, von Ohle C, Lost C. Consistency of apex locator function: a clinical study. J Endod. 2009;35:179–81.
69. Zuolo AS, Mello JE Jr, Cunha RS, Zuolo ML, Bueno CE. Efficacy of reciprocating and rotary techniques for removing filling material during root canal retreatment. Int Endod J. 2013;46:947–53.
70. Bago I, Suk M, Katic M, Gabric D, Anic I. Comparison of the effectiveness of various rotary and reciprocating systems with different surface treatments to remove gutta-percha and an epoxy resin-based sealer from straight root canals. Int Endod J. 2019;52:105–13.

71. Bernardes RA, Duarte MAH, Vivan RR, Alcalde MP, Vasconcelos BC, Bramante CM. Comparison of three retreatment techniques with ultrasonic activation in flattened canals using micro-computed tomography and scanning electron microscopy. Int Endod J. 2016;49:890–7.
72. Crozeta BM, Silva-Sousa YT, Leoni GB, Mazzi-Chaves JF, Fantinato T, Baratto-Filho F, et al. Micro-computed tomography study of filling material removal from oval-shaped canals by using rotary, reciprocating, and adaptive motion systems. J Endod. 2016;42:793–7.
73. De-Deus G, Belladonna FG, Zuolo AS, Cavalcante DM, Simoes Carvalho M, Marinho A, et al. 3-dimensional ability assessment in removing root filling material from pair-matched oval-shaped canals using thermal-treated instruments. J Endod. 2019;45:1135–41.
74. De-Deus G, Belladonna FG, Zuolo AS, Simoes-Carvalho M, Santos CB, Oliveira DS, et al. Effectiveness of Reciproc Blue in removing canal filling material and regaining apical patency. Int Endod J. 2019;52:250–7.
75. Fruchi Lde C, Ordinola-Zapata R, Cavenago BC, Hungaro Duarte MA, Bueno CE, De Martin AS. Efficacy of reciprocating instruments for removing filling material in curved canals obturated with a single-cone technique: a micro-computed tomographic analysis. J Endod. 2014;40:1000–4.
76. Kaloustian MK, Nehme W, El Hachem C, Zogheib C, Ghosn N, Mallet JP, et al. Evaluation of two shaping systems and two sonic irrigation devices in removing root canal filling material from distal roots of mandibular molars assessed by micro CT. Int Endod J. 2019;52:1635–44.
77. Marfisi K, Mercade M, Plotino G, Clavel T, Duran-Sindreu F, Roig M. Efficacy of Reciproc and Profile instruments in the removal of gutta-percha from straight and curved root canals ex vivo. J Oral Maxillofac Res. 2015;6:e1.
78. Martins MP, Duarte MA, Cavenago BC, Kato AS, da Silveira Bueno CE. Effectiveness of the ProTaper Next and Reciproc systems in removing root canal filling material with sonic or ultrasonic irrigation: a micro-computed tomographic study. J Endod. 2017;43:467–71.
79. Nevares G, de Albuquerque DS, Freire LG, Romeiro K, Fogel HM, Dos Santos M, et al. Efficacy of ProTaper NEXT compared with Reciproc in removing obturation material from severely curved root canals: a micro-computed tomography study. J Endod. 2016;42:803–8.
80. Özyürek T, Demiryürek EO. Efficacy of different nickel-titanium instruments in removing gutta-percha during root canal retreatment. J Endod. 2016;42:646–9.
81. Rios Mde A, Villela AM, Cunha RS, Velasco RC, De Martin AS, Kato AS, et al. Efficacy of 2 reciprocating systems compared with a rotary retreatment system for gutta-percha removal. J Endod. 2014;40:543–6.
82. Rödig T, Reicherts P, Konietschke F, Dullin C, Hahn W, Hülsmann M. Efficacy of reciprocating and rotary NiTi instruments for retreatment of curved root canals assessed by micro-CT. Int Endod J. 2014;47:942–8.
83. Silva E, Belladonna FG, Carapia MF, Muniz BL, Rocha MS, Moreira EJL. Micro-computed tomographic evaluation of canal retreatments performed by undergraduate students using different techniques. Restor Dent Endod. 2018;43:e5.
84. Silva E, Belladonna FG, Zuolo AS, Rodrigues E, Ehrhardt IC, Souza EM, et al. Effectiveness of XP-endo Finisher and XP-endo Finisher R in removing root filling remnants: a micro-CT study. Int Endod J. 2018;51:86–91.
85. Silva EJ, Sa L, Belladonna FG, Neves AA, Accorsi-Mendonca T, Vieira VT, et al. Reciprocating versus rotary systems for root filling removal: assessment of the apically extruded material. J Endod. 2014;40:2077–80.
86. Dincer AN, Er O, Canakci BC. Evaluation of apically extruded debris during root canal retreatment with several NiTi systems. Int Endod J. 2015;48:1194–8.
87. Lu Y, Wang R, Zhang L, Li HL, Zheng QH, Zhou XD, et al. Apically extruded debris and irrigant with two Ni-Ti systems and hand files when removing root fillings: a laboratory study. Int Endod J. 2013;46:1125–30.
88. Comparin D, Moreira EJL, Souza EM, De-Deus G, Arias A, Silva E. Postoperative pain after endodontic retreatment using rotary or reciprocating instruments: a randomized clinical trial. J Endod. 2017;43:1084–8.

89. Kvist T, Molander A, Dahlen G, Reit C. Microbiological evaluation of one- and two-visit endodontic treatment of teeth with apical periodontitis: a randomized, clinical trial. J Endod. 2004;30:572–6.
90. Manfredi M, Figini L, Gagliani M, Lodi G. Single versus multiple visits for endodontic treatment of permanent teeth. Cochrane Database Syst Rev. 2016;12:CD005296.
91. Molander A, Warfvinge J, Reit C, Kvist T. Clinical and radiographic evaluation of one- and two-visit endodontic treatment of asymptomatic necrotic teeth with apical periodontitis: a randomized clinical trial. J Endod. 2007;33:1145–8.
92. Penesis VA, Fitzgerald PI, Fayad MI, Wenckus CS, Begole EA, Johnson BR. Outcome of one-visit and two-visit endodontic treatment of necrotic teeth with apical periodontitis: a randomized controlled trial with one-year evaluation. J Endod. 2008;34:251–7.
93. Sathorn C, Parashos P, Messer H. Antibacterial efficacy of calcium hydroxide intracanal dressing: a systematic review and meta-analysis. Int Endod J. 2007;40:2–10.
94. Sathorn C, Parashos P, Messer H. The prevalence of postoperative pain and flare-up in single- and multiple-visit endodontic treatment: a systematic review. Int Endod J. 2008;41:91–9.
95. Weiger R, Rosendahl R, Lost C. Influence of calcium hydroxide intracanal dressings on the prognosis of teeth with endodontically induced periapical lesions. Int Endod J. 2000;33:219–26.
96. Ng YL, Mann V, Gulabivala K. Outcome of secondary root canal treatment: a systematic review of the literature. Int Endod J. 2008;41:1026–46.
97. Erdem Hepsenoglu Y, Eyuboglu TF, Ozcan M. Postoperative pain intensity after single-versus two-visit nonsurgical endodontic retreatment: a randomized clinical trial. J Endod. 2018;44:1339–46.
98. He J, White RK, White CA, Schweitzer JL, Woodmansey KF. Clinical and patient-centered outcomes of nonsurgical root canal retreatment in first molars using contemporary techniques. J Endod. 2017;43:231–7.
99. Riis A, Taschieri S, Del Fabbro M, Kvist T. Tooth survival after surgical or nonsurgical endodontic retreatment: long-term follow-up of a randomized clinical trial. J Endod. 2018;44:1480–6.
100. Hasselgren G, Olsson B, Cvek M. Effects of calcium hydroxide and sodium hypochlorite on the dissolution of necrotic porcine muscle tissue. J Endod. 1988;14:125–7.
101. Zehnder M, Grawehr M, Hasselgren G, Waltimo T. Tissue-dissolution capacity and dentin-disinfecting potential of calcium hydroxide mixed with irrigating solutions. Oral Surg Oral Med Oral Pathol Oral Radiol Endod. 2003;96:608–13.
102. Marques-da-Silva B, Alberton CS, Tomazinho FSF, Gabardo MCL, Duarte MAH, Vivan RR, et al. Effectiveness of five instruments when removing calcium hydroxide paste from simulated internal root resorption cavities in extracted maxillary central incisors. Int Endod J. 2020;53:366–75.
103. Wigler R, Dvir R, Weisman A, Matalon S, Kfir A. Efficacy of XP-endo finisher files in the removal of calcium hydroxide paste from artificial standardized grooves in the apical third of oval root canals. Int Endod J. 2017;50:700–5.
104. Patel S, Brown J, Semper M, Abella F, Mannocci F. European Society of Endodontology position statement: use of cone beam computed tomography in endodontics: European Society of Endodontology (ESE) developed by. Int Endod J. 2019;52:1675–8.
105. Aksel H, Kucukkaya Eren S, Askerbeyli Ors S, Serper A, Ocak M, Celik HH. Micro-CT evaluation of the removal of root fillings using the ProTaper Universal Retreatment system supplemented by the XP-Endo Finisher file. Int Endod J. 2019;52:1070–6.
106. Alves FR, Marceliano-Alves MF, Sousa JC, Silveira SB, Provenzano JC, Siqueira JF Jr. Removal of root canal fillings in curved canals using either reciprocating single- or rotary multi-instrument systems and a supplementary step with the XP-Endo Finisher. J Endod. 2016;42:1114–9.
107. Blum JY, Peli JF, Abadie MJ. Effects of the Nd:YAP laser on coronal restorative materials: implications for endodontic retreatment. J Endod. 2000;26:588–92.

108. Farge P, Nahas P, Bonin P. In vitro study of a Nd:YAP laser in endodontic retreatment. J Endod. 1998;24:359–63.
109. Viducic D, Jukic S, Karlovic Z, Bozic Z, Miletic I, Anic I. Removal of gutta-percha from root canals using an Nd:YAG laser. Int Endod J. 2003;36:670–3.
110. Lloyd A, Uhles JP, Clement DJ, Garcia-Godoy F. Elimination of intracanal tissue and debris through a novel laser-activated system assessed using high-resolution micro-computed tomography: a pilot study. J Endod. 2014;40:584–7.
111. Ordinola-Zapata R, Bramante CM, Aprecio RM, Handysides R, Jaramillo DE. Biofilm removal by 6% sodium hypochlorite activated by different irrigation techniques. Int Endod J. 2014;47:659–66.
112. Keleş A, Arslan H, Kamalak A, Akcay M, Sousa-Neto MD, Versiani MA. Removal of filling materials from oval-shaped canals using laser irradiation: a micro-computed tomographic study. J Endod. 2015;41:219–24.
113. Haapasalo M, Wang Z, Shen Y, Curtis A, Patel P, Khakpour M. Tissue dissolution by a novel multisonic ultracleaning system and sodium hypochlorite. J Endod. 2014;40:1178–81.
114. Molina B, Glickman G, Vandrangi P, Khakpour M. Evaluation of root canal debridement of human molars using the GentleWave system. J Endod. 2015;41:1701–5.
115. Sigurdsson A, Garland RW, Le KT, Rassoulian SA. Healing of periapical lesions after endodontic treatment with the GentleWave procedure: a prospective multicenter clinical study. J Endod. 2018;44:510–7.
116. Wright CR, Glickman GN, Jalali P, Umorin M. Effectiveness of gutta-percha/sealer removal during retreatment of extracted human molars using the GentleWave system. J Endod. 2019;45:808–12.
117. Halse A, Molven O, Fristad I. Diagnosing periapical lesions—disagreement and borderline cases. Int Endod J. 2002;35:703–9.
118. Nudera WJ. Selective root retreatment: a novel approach. J Endod. 2015;41:1382–8.

Managing Canal Anatomies in the Context of Shaping for Cleaning Proposal

8

Marco A. Versiani, Emmanuel J. N. L. Silva, Erick Souza, Gustavo De Deus, and Mario Zuolo

8.1 The Importance of Anatomical Knowledge of Root Canals in Clinical Practice

Root canal anatomy is the foundation of the art and science of endodontic therapy and subsequent posttreatment healing [1]. Thereby, a thorough knowledge of the most common morphological variations of all groups of teeth is a basic requirement to perform endodontic treatment. However, the ability to understand and to anticipate the internal anatomy of teeth prior to treatment is still a challenge for many clinicians who confront this issue every day as they peer into access openings and search for canal orifices. Indeed, human dentition presents a wide range of anatomical variations in each tooth type, which differ greatly among populations, within populations, and even in the same individual [2], making its overall knowledge sometimes complex. In the past, a lot of research work were done on this subject, and the findings have had a noteworthy influence on clinical practice and dental

M. A. Versiani (✉)
Dental Specialty Center, Brazilian Military Police, Minas Gerais, Brazil
e-mail: marcoversiani@yahoo.com

E. J. N. L. Silva
Fluminense Federal University, Grande Rio University, Rio de Janeiro State University, Niterói, Brazil

E. Souza
Federal University of Maranhão, São Luis, Brazil

G. De Deus
Fluminense Federal University, Niterói, Brazil

M. Zuolo
Dental School of APCD – FAOA, São Paulo, Brazil

G. De Deus et al. (eds.), *Shaping for Cleaning the Root Canals*,
https://doi.org/10.1007/978-3-030-84617-6_8

education. In fact, the history of endodontics as a dental specialty is relatively recent and was born from an improved understanding of the morphology and biology of teeth [3]. For instance, although anatomy is the oldest scientific discipline of medicine, with the first documented dissections on the human body carried out as early as the third century B.C. in Alexandria [4], the first printed image of the root canal was published almost 1900 years later, in one of the of seven books written by Andreas Vesalius (1514–1564) entitled *De Humani Corporis Fabrica* ("On the Fabric of the Human Body") [5]. In Chapter XI, there is a drawing of a sectioned two-rooted mandibular molar showing its internal anatomy: the pulp chamber and two root canals (Fig. 8.1a). Since then, and until the first half of the nineteenth century, only few authors have published new anatomical aspects of the internal anatomy of teeth [3], although the world has witnessed the rise of dentistry as a distinct profession, with its own practitioners, techniques, standards, and specific literature devoted to dental science. At the end of the nineteenth century, some researchers finally realized the need for in-depth research on tooth morphology, and some initial studies were performed to highlight the number and configuration of root canals by sectioning teeth in different directions [6–9]. But it was only at the early twentieth century that new three-dimensional methods were developed to evaluate the internal anatomy of teeth [10–13], enabling a profound and comprehensive understanding of the complexity of the root canal system (Fig. 8.1b–e) and its relation with the

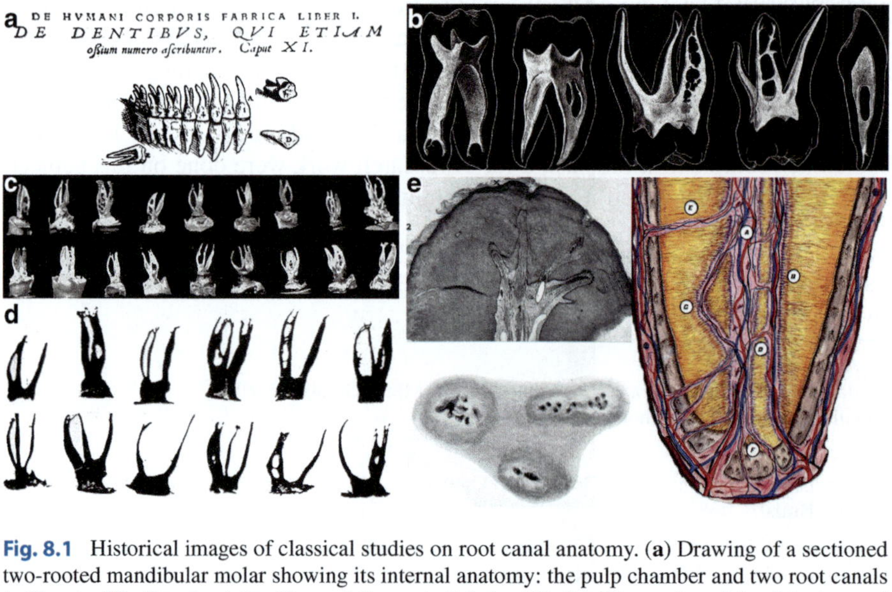

Fig. 8.1 Historical images of classical studies on root canal anatomy. (**a**) Drawing of a sectioned two-rooted mandibular molar showing its internal anatomy: the pulp chamber and two root canals in Chapter XI of the book *De Humani Corporis Fabrica [5]*. (**b**) 3D metal models of the internal anatomy of different teeth obtained by Preiswerk (1903) [13]. (**c**) 3D models of the internal anatomy of teeth obtained by Fisher using collodion solution (1907) [10]. (**d**) Canal shapes of mandibular molars obtained by injecting vulcanite into the canal systems by Hess (1925) [20]. (**e**) The complexity and unpredictability of the root canal morphology that led Guido Fischer (1877–1959) [10] to conceive the term root canal system. (Courtesy of Dr. Nicola Perrini, Italy [3]. Published with permission)

periapical tissues, forming the baseline for the biological basis of endodontic treatment. Actually, the conception of pulp and periodontal tissue as a continuum allowed the association between the endodontic disease and the periapical host immune response, as well as, the therapeutic significance of the apical terminus. Furthermore, leveraging on current knowledge, it is recognized that effective nonsurgical root canal treatment and endodontic surgery require a thorough knowledge of tooth morphology and canal anatomy [14]. In summary, a deep knowledge of root canal anatomy is essential for the clinician in order to explain the treatment plan to a patient, to properly examine radiological imaging of teeth and surrounding structures, to detect all canal orifices and to perform invasive procedures by avoiding iatrogenic injuries during pulp chamber access, canal instrumentation, or post-space preparation procedures. Unfortunately, these are only the preliminary steps because some of the therapeutic issues associated with complex canal morphologies still remain as challenges, as depicted in this chapter.

8.2 Applied Anatomy: What We Really Need to Know About Each Group of Teeth

At the end of the twentieth century, technological advancements enabled a considerable range of techniques that were successfully employed to visualize the anatomy of human teeth, including nondestructive three-dimensional tools such as conventional medical computed tomography, magnetic resonance microscopy, tuned-aperture computed tomography, optical coherence tomography, volumetric or cone beam-computed tomography (CBCT), and the high-resolution X-ray micro-computed tomography (micro-CT) [15]. Innovative image technologies such as CBCT and micro-CT allowed the study of the root canal system by reconstructing digital cross sections of the teeth into 3D volumes. These volumes can be used to generate computerized images that can be manipulated, sectioned, prepared, dissected, and measured to reveal both internal and external morphologies, without destroying the original specimens (Fig. 8.2a). Nowadays, CBCT and micro-CT have been considered the most important and accurate research tools for the study of root canal anatomy. While CBCT allows the possibility of performing in vivo studies using large populations with relatively low cost, addressing the influence of several variables such as ethnicity, aging, and gender on anatomical variations of different populations, micro-CT can be applied in the study of specific anatomical features, thereby permitting the accurate assessment of qualitative and quantitative morphological parameters such as volume, surface area, diameter, geometry, and cross-sectional appearance. Acquired data from hundreds or thousands of slices can be plotted on graphs using automatic computational tools, before or after any endodontic procedure (Fig. 8.2b) [16]. In the next sections, the results of anatomical studies using CBCT and micro-CT technologies will be described, as well as, the discussion on the influence of root canal complexities on shaping, cleaning, and filling procedures, providing a thorough in-depth background knowledge on this subject.

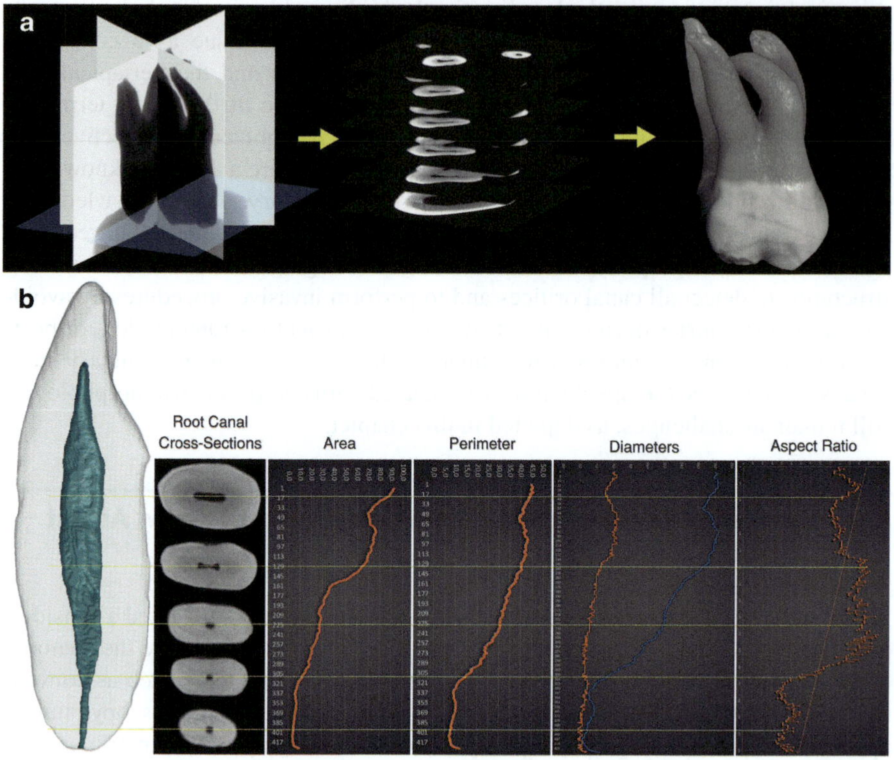

Fig. 8.2 Micro-CT acquisition and analysis of a maxillary molar tooth. (**a**) The projection data of a tooth is obtained from multiple directions and used as input for a reconstruction algorithm that computes a 3D image of its internal anatomy without destroying the original specimen. (**b**) 2D quantitative parameters (area, perimeter, diameters, and aspect ratio) of the root canal of a mandibular incisor acquired from 421 slices and plotted on graphs using an automatic computational tool

8.2.1 Root Canal Complexities: Rule or Exception?

The root canal is the portion of the pulp canal space within the root of the tooth limited by the pulp chamber and the foramen that usually follows the external outline of the root (Fig. 8.3a). It can be subdivided into the main canal, which is mostly cleaned by mechanical means, and lateral components such as isthmuses, fins, accessory canals (furcation, lateral, and secondary canals), and some recesses of flattened- and oval-shaped canals (Fig. 8.3b–e). In longitudinal section, canals are usually broader buccolingually than in the mesiodistal plane, but it may also show different shapes at different levels of the root. However, at the apical third, it is usually rounder or slightly oval in shape in comparison with the middle and coronal thirds. It is worth pointing out that some factors can modify the anatomy of the pulp chamber and root canals, such as aging, caries, peri-radicular pathologies, and occlusion [17]. In teeth with physiologic wear or other irritations, for example, the continuous dentin formation

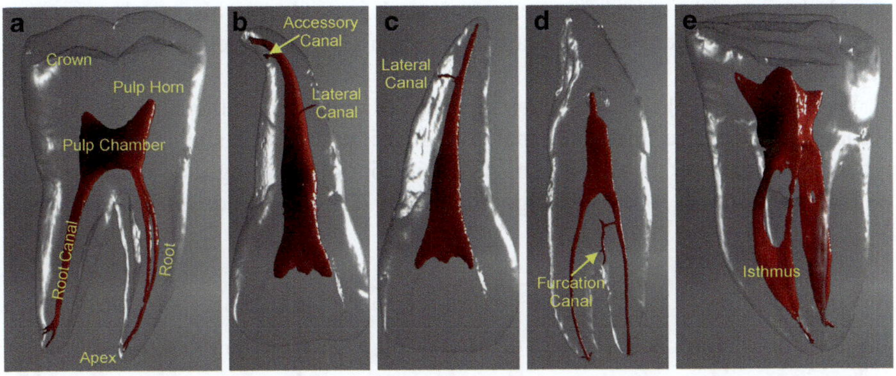

Fig. 8.3 Root canal components. (**a**) The root canal is the portion of the pulp canal space within the root of the tooth limited by the pulp chamber and the foramen that usually follows the external outline of the root. The root canal can be subdivided into the main canal(s) and (**b**–**e**) lateral components composed by isthmuses, fins, accessory canals (furcation, lateral, and secondary canals), and some recesses of flattened- and oval-shaped canals

(either physiologic or reactionary) by primary odontoblasts may result in a decrease of the pulpal space dimensions, which, in some cases, can compromise root canal treatment [18]. Taken together, these components create a complex environment in which bacteria originated from the oral cavity can invade, spread throughout, and hide from disinfection procedures. Thus, the answer to the question on the title of this subsection is that the complexities within the root canal system are more rule than exception, and these complexities may hinder residual bacteria and debris within isthmuses, lateral canals, apical ramifications, and recesses from oval/flattened canals, which ultimately can compromise the treatment outcome. By the way, the complexity and unpredictability of root canal morphology were the main reasons that led the German dentist Guido Fischer (1877–1959) to conceive the term *Kanalsystem* back in 1907 [10], which today is widely known as the "root canal system" (Fig. 8.1e).

8.2.2 One Root Means a Single Canal?

Since the first systematic studies on root canal anatomy performed by Hess and colleagues in the first half of the twentieth century [19–21] (Fig. 8.1d), it became clear that teeth have an intricate canal system rather than a simplified morphology. Sadly, this knowledge has been largely disregarded and dentists remain obsessed with the old concept of a root canal as a hollow tube that has to be cleaned and shaped, eventually appearing as pleasant white lines on postoperative radiographs. Besides, in endodontics, there still exists a misconception of thinking that "one root equals one canal," although this has been shattered by a number of classic papers that demonstrate the opposite. In fact, several studies classified and described the morphology of multiple canals in a broad-diameter root. This multiple-canal configuration may divide, combine, and separate as it forms in root closure toward the various morphologies of the apical foramen terminus. It is prudent to assume that any root that requires treatment may contain more than one canal per root, until proved otherwise.

Weine et al. [22], using sectioning and radiographic methods, were the first authors to categorize different canal configurations within a single root into four types, depending on the division of the main root canal along its course from the pulp chamber to the root apex (Fig. 8.4a). In 1972, Piñeda and Kuttler [23], based

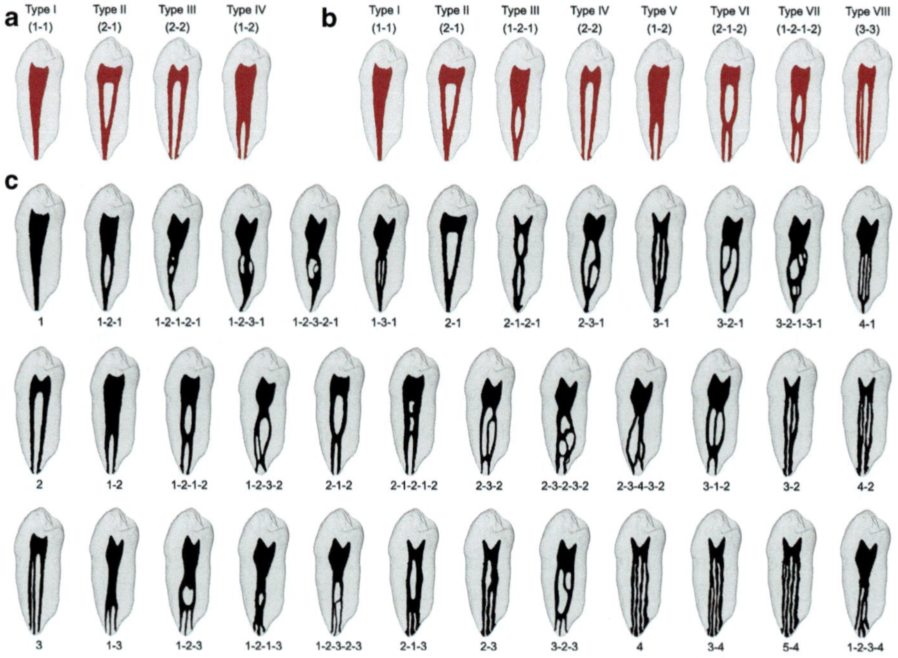

Fig. 8.4 Root canal configuration systems. (**a**) Diagrammatic representations of Weine's classification for root canal morphology. Type I: A single canal from pulp chamber to the apex (1-1 configuration); Type II: Two separate canals leaving the chamber but merging short of the apex to form a single canal (2-1 configuration); Type III: Two distinct canals from pulp chamber to the apex (2-2 configuration); Type IV: A single canal leaving the chamber and dividing into two separate canals at the apex (1-2 configuration). (**b**) Diagrammatic representations of Vertucci's classification for root canal morphology. Type I: A single canal from pulp chamber to the apex (1-1 configuration); Type II: Two separate canals leaving the chamber, but merging short of the apex to form a single canal (2-1 configuration); Type III: A single canal that divides into two and subsequently merges to exit as one (1-2-1 configuration); Type IV: Two distinct canals from pulp chamber to the apex (2-2 configuration); Type V: A single canal leaving the chamber and dividing into two separate canals at the apex (1-2 configuration); Type VI: Two separate canals leaving the pulp chamber, merging in the body of the root, and dividing again into two distinct canals short from the apex (2-1-2 configuration); Type VII: A single canal that divides, merges, and exits into two distinct canals short from the apex (1-2-1-2 configuration); Type VIII: Three distinct canals within one root from pulp chamber to the apex (3-3 configuration). (**c**) Thirty-seven most common anatomical configurations possible to be observed in a single root reported by Versiani and Ordinola-Zapata [18, 25]

on the radiographic evaluation of 7,275 extracted teeth, highlighted that single roots may contain multiple canal systems that are not usually seen in the clinical setting. Some years later, Vertucci et al. [24] developed a classification system based on the evaluation of 200 cleared maxillary second premolars, wherein the pulp cavities were stained with dye. They found eight canal systems (Fig. 8.4b) that were more complex than those described by Weine et al. [22]. Essentially, these configuration systems were based on the number of root canals that begin at the pulp chamber floor, arise along the course of the canal, and open through an apical foramen. More recently, Versiani and Ordinola-Zapata [25] expanded and adapted these classifications to 3D tomographic descriptions of at least 37 complex canal systems possible to be observed in a single root (Fig. 8.4c). Another important concept is that when two or more canals exist within the same root, communications in the form of fins or isthmuses can occur between them. Unless this concept of a root canal as a system is clearly recognized, and a proper method for shaping and cleaning is employed to address both the main canal and the anastomoses, infection will remain and treatment may fail. So, to the clinicians, it is important to know that success in root canal therapy can be achieved by first knowing the normal canal anatomy and then by being aware of the many variations that the path of the canal system can follow within the root. In addition, it should be remembered that while the following descriptions are the norm, occasionally other teeth may be encountered with unusual or even bizarre anatomy.

8.2.3 Anterior Teeth: Are They the Easiest Teeth to Treat?

It has been common knowledge that treating incisors and canines is an easy task. And sometimes it is. However, how can it be explained that the highest number of apical surgeries is performed in these groups of teeth [26] as a result of failure in the orthograde treatment? An acceptable answer would be because most people think that they are easy to treat and, therefore, they neglect to follow the basic treatment principles, such as the use of rubber dam, proper irrigation procedures, precise determination of the apical limit for preparation and filling, among others. Besides, sometimes these teeth also present anatomical anomalies or pathological conditions, such as calcifications, which increase the challenge for an adequate treatment. Anterior teeth are usually single-rooted teeth with a single canal and a relatively straight root. However, some important anatomical details and variations must be considered [27].

Maxillary central incisors usually have one root and one root canal despite the fact that multiple canals and some anomalies have been reported in the literature. Their pulp cavity usually follows the general outline of the crown and root, but the pulp chamber is very narrow at the incisal region and wider in the mesiodistal dimension than in the labiolingual dimension (Fig. 8.5a). The maxillary lateral incisor supplements the central incisor in function, and the crowns bear a close resemblance. However, the lateral incisor is smaller in all dimensions except root length. Several anomalies have been reported in this tooth group, including the presence of

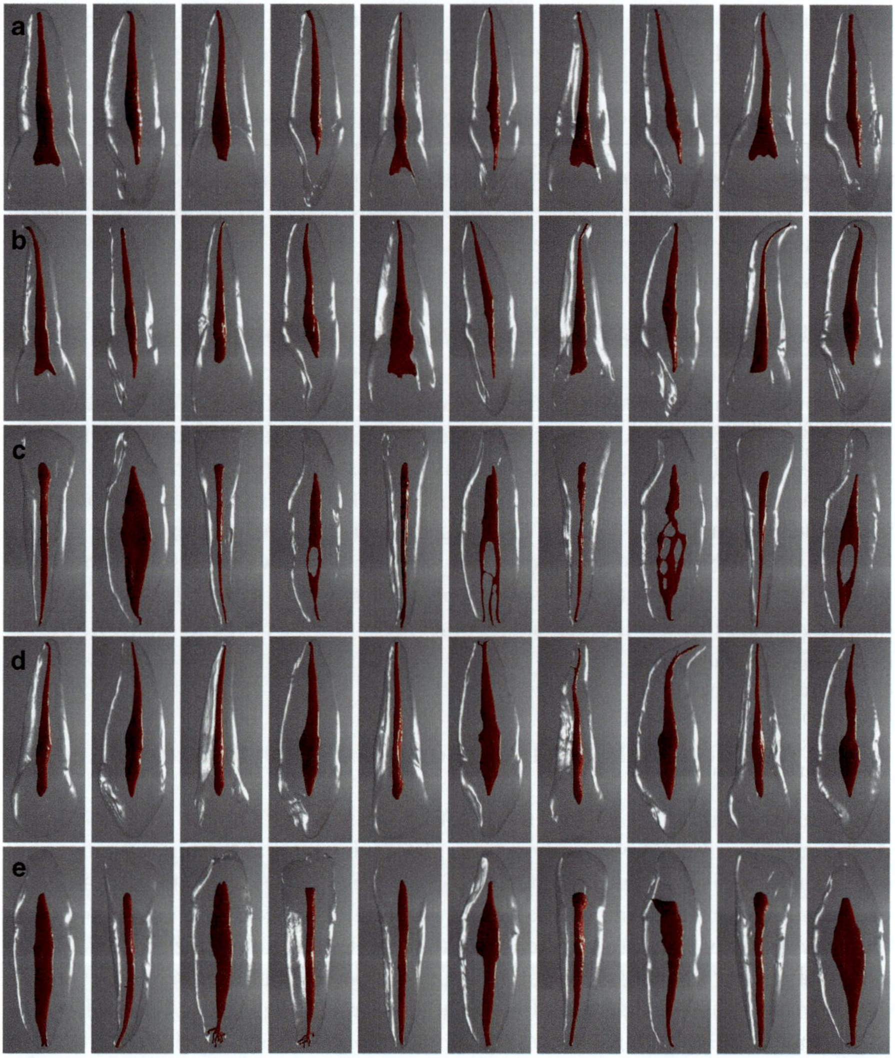

Fig. 8.5 Morphological aspects of the root canal system of anterior teeth (frontal and lateral views). (**a**) Maxillary central incisor. (**b**) Maxillary lateral incisor. (**c**) Mandibular central and lateral incisors. (**d**) Maxillary canine. (**e**) Mandibular canine

multiple canals, radicular groove, fusion/gemination, *dens invaginatus*, and *dens evaginatus*. The root of the maxillary lateral incisor is frequently curved apically, often in a palatal direction so that the curve may not be immediately apparent in a radiograph (Fig. 8.5b).

The mandibular central and lateral incisors are single-rooted teeth that have the smallest mesiodistal dimensions compared to any other teeth, with the central incisor being somewhat smaller than the lateral incisor. Mandibular incisors are usually single-rooted teeth; however, the root canal system of this group is unpredictable not only regarding its configuration among the same population, but also when compared with different populations [28]. So, although most of the time these teeth have only one canal, two ribbon-shaped canals may be found with relatively high frequency. When this happens, these canals generally join at the apical third and exit in a single foramen (Fig. 8.5c). The lingual canal, however, is often missed because of an inadequate access cavity preparation.

Maxillary canines are the longest teeth in the mouth. Their single roots are longer than those of any of the other teeth, and root canals normally have a larger labiolingual dimension than any tooth. Their length can be difficult to determine on radiographs as the apex tends to curve labially, and the tooth will appear to be shorter than it actually is. Although some rare anomalies have been reported, this is probably the tooth group with the least anatomical variations in the mouth. From a clinical perspective, however, their long size and thin apex may also represent a challenge during endodontic treatment. The oval canal of maxillary canines often seems large during instrumentation, but there is often a sudden narrowing at the apical third which may lead to an overinstrumentation if large instruments are used at this level (Fig. 8.5d). The mandibular canine is usually narrower although its root may be as long as that of the maxillary canine. Mandibular canines are commonly presented as having a single canal, but the presence of a second canal cannot be ignored. Its prevalence in some studies has been shown to vary from 10.3 to 31.8%, while the percentage frequency of a two-rooted configuration has been reported to range from 0.7 to 11.7% [29]. Because the presence of two canals cannot be easily detected radiographically, their presence must be ruled out clinically as well. Some mandibular canines demonstrate an abrupt narrowing of the pulp cavity when passing from the pulp chamber to the pulp canal, but others can demonstrate an abrupt narrowing of the pulp canal at the apical region (Fig. 8.5e).

In modern endodontics, straight-line access in anterior teeth has been achieved through a conservative cavity made closer to the incisal edge than to the cingulum, allowing the preservation of the tooth structure and facilitating the location and negotiation of extra root canals (Fig. 8.6). More details about other morphological aspects of the root and root canal anatomy of anterior teeth can be found in Table 8.1.

8.2.4 The Hidden Secrets of Premolars

Treating premolars without a previous and detailed evaluation of radiographic images may be sometimes surprising, mostly when dealing with the mandibular ones, considering the number of anatomical variations reported in this group of teeth.

Except for the mandibular molars, maxillary first premolars are the teeth more prone to display a two-rooted configuration, a clinical condition that varies according to the geographic region [2]. This tooth usually has two well-developed roots, two root projections that are not fully separated, or one broad root. Its roots are often very delicate and may curve quite sharply at the apical third, so canal enlargement

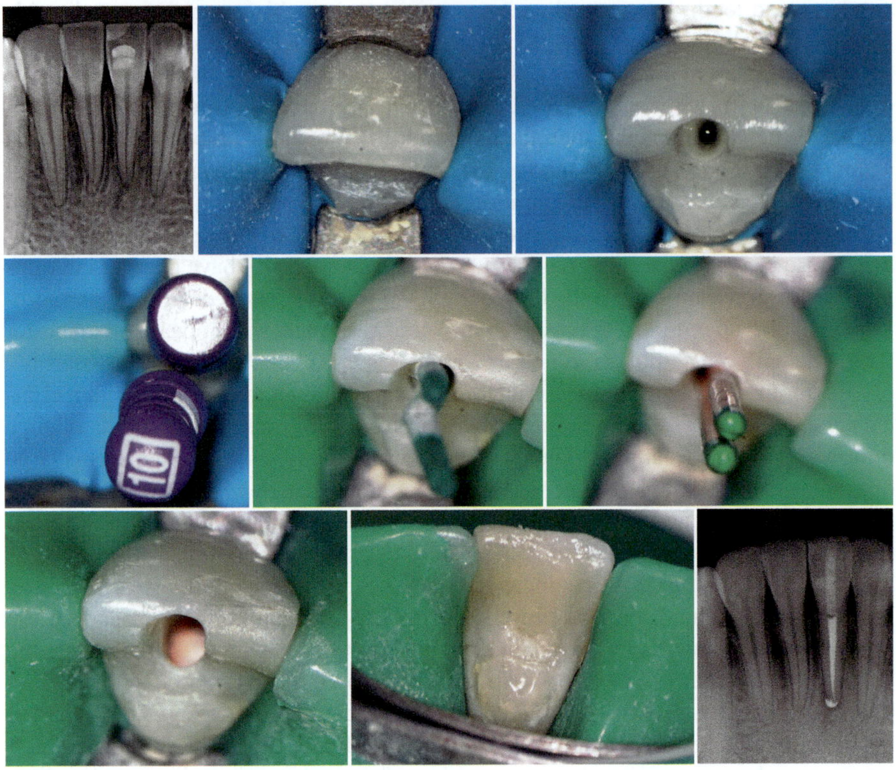

Fig. 8.6 Access cavity preparation in a mandibular anterior teeth using a current endodontic approach showing that straight-line access is achieved through a cavity made closer to the incisal edge than to the cingulum, allowing the preservation of tooth structure and facilitating the location and negotiation of extra root canals

needs to be carried out with caution. In addition, most of them have a distinct concavity in the mesial root surface, increasing the risk of perforation during access preparation. The majority of maxillary first premolars have two root canals, but a small percentage may present three roots and three canals that may at times be either difficult to see or almost undetectable radiographically. An important anatomical aspect that may compromise the identification of these extra canal orifices in clinics is the position of the pulp chamber floor, normally below the cementoenamel junction (Fig. 8.7a). The maxillary second premolar supplements the maxillary first premolar in function and closely resembles it in shape; however, in almost 50% of the cases, it has only one root and one broad oval-shaped canal. Two roots are possible, although two canals within a single root is more frequent (Fig. 8.7a) [27].

Mandibular premolars are more predictable than maxillary premolars regarding the number of roots, but not in terms of canal configuration, which can be highly complex. In the mandibular first premolar, the pulp chamber is usually large, and the pulp cavity may taper gently toward the apex or abruptly as the root canal starts. Its root usually shows a deep developmental groove often associated with complex

Table 8.1 Morphological aspects of the root and root canal anatomy of anterior teeth

	Maxillary central incisor	Maxillary lateral incisor	Mandibular incisors	Maxillary canine	Mandibular canine
Overall length	23.6 mm (16.5–32.6 mm)	22.5 mm (17.7–28.9 mm)	**C**: 20.8 mm (16.9–26.7 mm) **L**: 22.1 mm (18.5–26.6 mm)	26.4 mm (20.0–38.4 mm)	25.9 mm (16.1–34.5 mm)
Root length	13.0 mm (6.3–20.3 mm)	13.4 mm (9.6–19.4 mm)	**C**: 12.6 mm (7.7–17.9 mm) **L**: 13.5 mm (9.4–18.1 mm)	16.5 mm (10.8–28.5 mm)	15.9 mm (9.5–22.2 mm)
Number of roots	1 (99.94%); 2 (0.06%)	1 (99.94%); 2 (0.06%)	**C**: 1 (100%) **L**: 1 (99.92%); 2 (0.08%)	1 (100%)	1 (98.57%); 2 (1.43%)
Number of canals	1 (99.2%); 2 (0.8%)	1 (98.5%); 2 (1.5%)	**C**: 1 (86.5%); 2 (14.4%); other (0.1%) **L**: 1 (79.7%); 2 (20.2%); other (0.1%)	1 (97%); 2 (3%)	1 (92.4%); 2 (7.3%); other (0.3%)
Canal configuration	Types I (99.2%); IV (0.5%); II (0.1%); III (0.1%); V (0.1%)	Types I (98.5%); II (0.8%); V (0.4%); III (0.2%); IV (0.1%)	**C**: Types I (86.5%); III (8.1%); V (2.8%); II (2%); IV (1.4%); VII (0.1%); other (0.1%) **L**: Types I (79.7%); III (11.9%); V (3.8%); II (2.6%); IV (1.8%); VII (0.1%); other (0.1%)	Types I (98.5%); III (1.2%); II (0.8%); V (0.7%); IV (0.2%); other (0.1%)	Types I (92.4%); III (2.7%); II (1.9%); IV (1.5%); V (1.2%); other (0.3%)
Accessory canals	18.9–42.6% (coronal: 1%; middle: 6%; apical: 93%)	5.5–26% (coronal: 1%; middle: 8%; apical: 91%)	**C**: 0–20% (coronal: 3%; middle: 12%; apical: 85%) **L**: 0.9–18% (coronal: 2%; middle: 15%; apical: 83%)	3.4–30% (coronal: 0%; middle: 10%; apical: 90%)	4.5–30% (coronal: 4%; middle: 16%; apical: 80%)

(continued)

Table 8.1 (continued)

	Maxillary central incisor	Maxillary lateral incisor	Mandibular incisors	Maxillary canine	Mandibular canine
Apical curvature	Straight (75%); labial (9.3%); distal (7.8%); mesial (4.3%); palatal (3.6%)	Distal (49.2%); straight (29.7%); palatal (3.9%); labial (3.9%); mesial (3.1%); S-shaped (1.6%); other (8.6%)	**C**: Straight (66.7%); labial (18.8%); distal (12.5%); S-shaped (2%) **L**: Straight (54%); distal (33.3%); labial (10.7%); S-shaped (2%)	Straight (38.5%); distal (19.5%); labial (12.8%); mesial (12%); palatal (6.5%); other (10.7%)	Straight (68.2%); distal (19.6%); labial (6.8%); mesial (0.8%); S-shaped (1.5%); other (3.1%)
Anomalies	2 canals [175–177]; 3 canals [178]; 4 canals [179]; 2 roots [175–177]; radicular groove [180]; fusion/ gemination [181]	2 canals [182]; 3 canals [183]; 4 canals [184]; 2 roots [185]; radicular groove [180]; fusion/ gemination [186]; *Dens invaginatus* [187]; *Dens evaginatus* [188]; C-shaped [189]	3 canals [190]; fusion/ gemination [191]; *Dens invaginatus* [192]; 2 roots [193]	2 canals [194]; *Dens invaginatus* [195]	2 canals [29]; 3 canals [196]; 2 roots [29]

C central, *L* lateral. Root canal configurations are classified according to Vertucci [43]
Adapted from Versiani et al. [27]

anatomies, including C-shaped configuration or multiple canals (Fig. 8.7b). The occurrence of a split root canal is suggested radiographically when the image of the canal suddenly decreases dramatically in width or seemingly disappears. In the literature, there are also several reports of mandibular first premolars with three, four and even five root canals. The mandibular second premolar usually has a single root with one canal that may be curved, usually toward the distal direction. The pulp horns are prominent, and the pulp chamber and root canal gently taper toward the apex. The single root of the second premolar is larger and longer than that of the first premolar. The root is seldom, if ever, bifurcated, although some specimens show a deep developmental groove buccally (Fig. 8.7b). A split of the root canal can be seen, but less frequently than in the mandibular first premolar, and a three-rooted configuration is a rare occurrence. Overall, the complexity of the internal morphology of mandibular premolars can be determined by the severity of the radicular grooves, usually associated with the presence of multiple and complex canal systems, accessory canals at the furcation area, as well as the C-shaped configuration [27]. Additional morphological features of the root and root canal anatomy of premolar teeth can be found in Table 8.2.

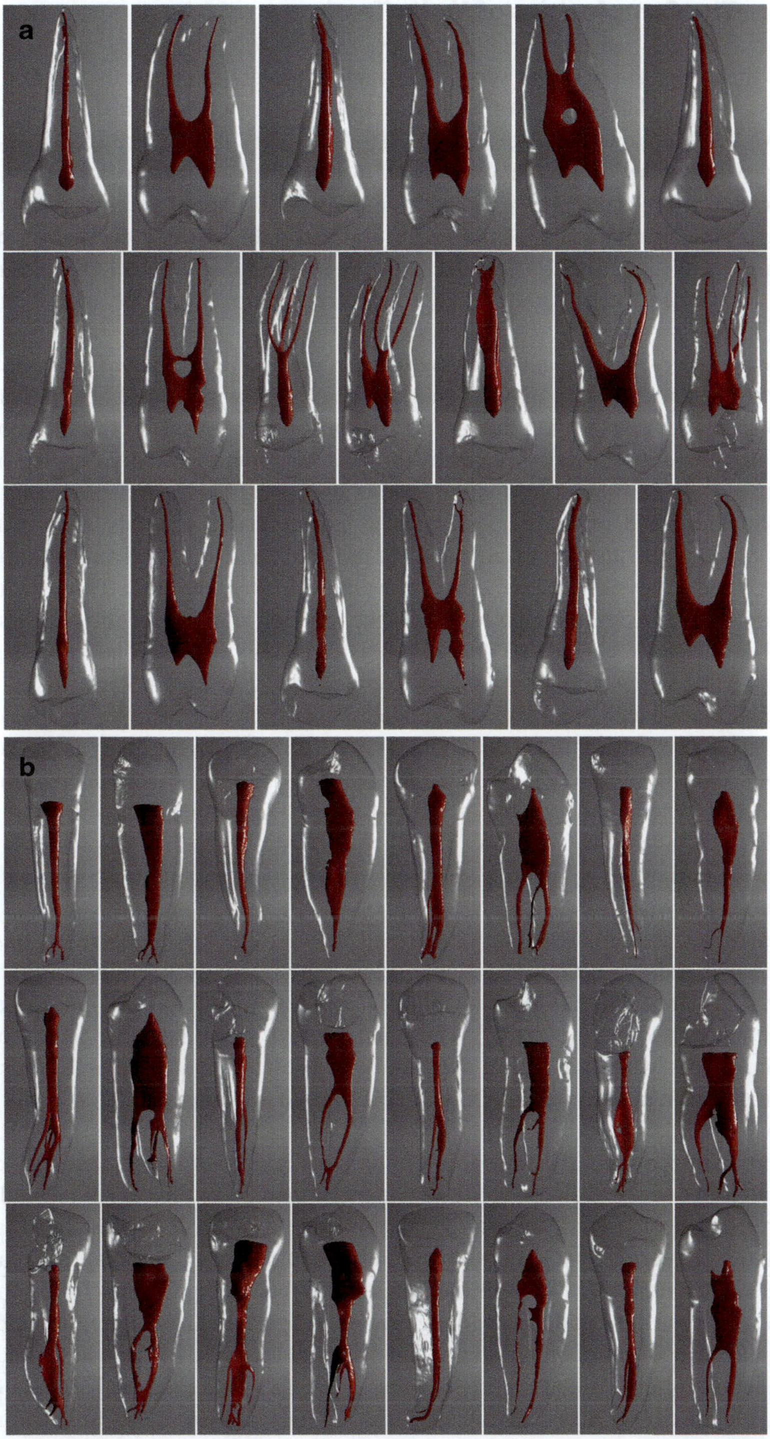

Fig. 8.7 Morphological aspects of the root canal system of premolar teeth (frontal and lateral views). (**a**) Maxillary first and second premolars. (**b**) Mandibular first and second premolars

8.2.5 The Complexities of Molar Teeth

In the literature, the first and second permanent molars are the most studied teeth because of the largest anatomical variations and morphological complexities observed in their internal anatomy [2]. The maxillary molars are the largest and strongest maxillary teeth. They are usually described as three-rooted teeth with three or four root canals; however, their anatomy may present distinct morphological aspects. Their palatal root is mostly often straight but may curve in a buccal direction in its apical part, a feature that may not be readily detected radiographically. Consequently, the apparent length on a radiograph would be shorter than its actual length.

The maxillary first molar usually has three roots and four canals. The complexity of their root canal system may surpass all other teeth within the human dentition. The palatal root usually has the largest dimensions, followed by the mesiobuccal (MB) and distobuccal roots, respectively. The MB root is usually curved, but its curvature can be difficult to visualize from radiographs. This root is often very wide buccolingually and normally possesses an extra canal commonly known as the MB2, which is the smallest of all canals in this tooth and almost always is superimposed by the other mesiobuccal canal in the radiography (Fig. 8.8). Thus, the use of magnification is recommended to enable the location not only of the MB2 orifice, but other additional canals that may also exist. The maxillary second molar supplements the first molar in function. Most often maxillary second molars possess three roots and three canals, and their mesiobuccal root is not as complex as that of the maxillary first molar. In the second molars, external root morphology is not so predictable, and the presence of a four-rooted configuration is not an uncommon finding. There is also a high tendency for root fusion, which often results in anatomical complexities, including unusual canal configurations with the presence of a C-shaped configuration, several intercanal connections, and multiple apical ramifications (Fig. 8.8).

Mandibular molars are usually described as two-rooted teeth; however, in Asian populations, there is a high prevalence of a second distal root in mandibular first molars (three-rooted configuration) and fused roots (single-rooted configuration) in mandibular second molars [2]. These anatomical variations have been reported as ethnic traits when analyzing the number of roots in mandibular molars. The mandibular first molar is usually the largest tooth in the mandibular arch and presents two well-developed and separated roots, one mesial and one distal, which are very broad buccolingually. This is often the most restored tooth in the adult dentition and a frequent candidate for root canal treatment. The mesial root usually has a more complicated canal system because of the presence of two or three canals, their interconnections, and accessory communication with the furcation area. The mesial canals are curved in both mesiodistal and buccolingual directions, and the curved furcation wall (named as 'danger zone') is particularly vulnerable to perforation during root canal preparation. The distal root usually has one large and oval canal, but two canals are often present. Occasionally, extra roots with an additional canal, the so-called *radix*, is present. The *radix paramolaris* is an uncommon

Table 8.2 Morphological aspects of the root and root canal anatomy of premolar teeth

	Maxillary first premolar	Maxillary second premolar	Mandibular first premolar	Mandibular second premolar
Overall length	21.5 mm (15.5–28.9 mm)	21.2 mm (15.2–28.4 mm)	22.4 mm (17.0–28.5 mm)	22.1 mm (16.8–28.1 mm)
Root length	13.4 mm (8.3–19.0 mm)	14.0 mm (8.0–20.6 mm)	14.4 mm (9.7–20.2 mm)	14.7 mm (9.2–21.2 mm)
Number of roots	2 (55.3%); 1 (43.1%); 3 (1.6%)	1 (86.2%); 2 (13.5%); 3 (0.3%)	1 (97.5%); 2 (2.5%)	1 (98.5%); 2 (1.5%)
Number of canals	2 (77.3%); 1 (20.1%); 3 (1.2%); other (1.3%)	2 (56.7%); 1 (42.7%); 3 (0.4%); other (0.3%)	1 (71.3%); 2 (27.9%); 3 (0.1%); other (0.7%)	1 (84.7%); 2 (15.05%); 3 (0.05%); other (0.2%)
Canal configuration	Types IV (50.1%); I (20.1%); II (17.4%); VI (4.9%); V (3%); III (1.5%); VIII (1.2%); VII (0.4%); other (1.3%)	Types I (42.7%); II (18.7%); IV (17.6%); V (9.6%); VI (6.3%); III (4%); VII (0.5%); VIII (0.4%); other (0.3%)	Types I (71.3%); V (18.7%); IV (3.5%); III (2.8%); II (2.3%); VI (0.5%); VII (0.1%); VIII (0.1%); other (0.7%)	Types I (84.7%); V (13.44%); II (0.7%); III (0.5%); IV (0.3%); VI (0.07%); VIII (0.05); VII (0.04%); other (0.2%)
Accessory canals	17.8–49.5% (coronal: 4.7%; middle: 10.3%; apical: 74%)	12.9–59.5% (coronal: 4%; middle: 16.2%; apical: 78.2%)	8.8–44.3% (coronal: 4.3%; middle: 16.1%; apical: 78.9%)	4–48.3% (coronal: 3.2%; middle: 16.4%; apical: 80.1%)
Apical curvature	**B**: Palatal (36.2%); straight (27.8%); distal (14%); buccal (14%); S-shaped (8%) **P**: Straight (44.4%); buccal (27.8%); distal (14%); palatal (8.3%); S-shaped (5.5%)	Straight (37.4%); distal (29.5%); buccal (15.7%); S-shaped (13%); distal (4.4%)	Straight (47.5%); distal (34.8%); lingual (7.1%); buccal (2.1%); S-shaped (6.4%); other (2.1%)	Distal (39.8%); straight (38.5%); buccal (10.1%); lingual (3.4%); S-shaped (6.8%); other (1.4%)
Anomalies	3 canals [197]; radicular groove [198]; fusion/gemination [199]; *Dens evaginatus* [200]	3 canals [197]; *Dens invaginatus* [201]	3 canals [159]; 4 canals [202]; radicular groove [203]; C-shaped [204]; *Dens evaginatus* [205]; *Dens invaginatus* [206]; fusion/gemination [207]	3 canals [208]; 4 canals [209]; 5 canals [210]; 2 roots [211]; C-shaped [212]; *Dens evaginatus* [213]; taurodontism [210]; fusion/gemination [214]

B buccal root/canal, *P* palatal root/canal. Root canal configurations are classified according to Vertucci [43]

Adapted from Versiani et al. [27]

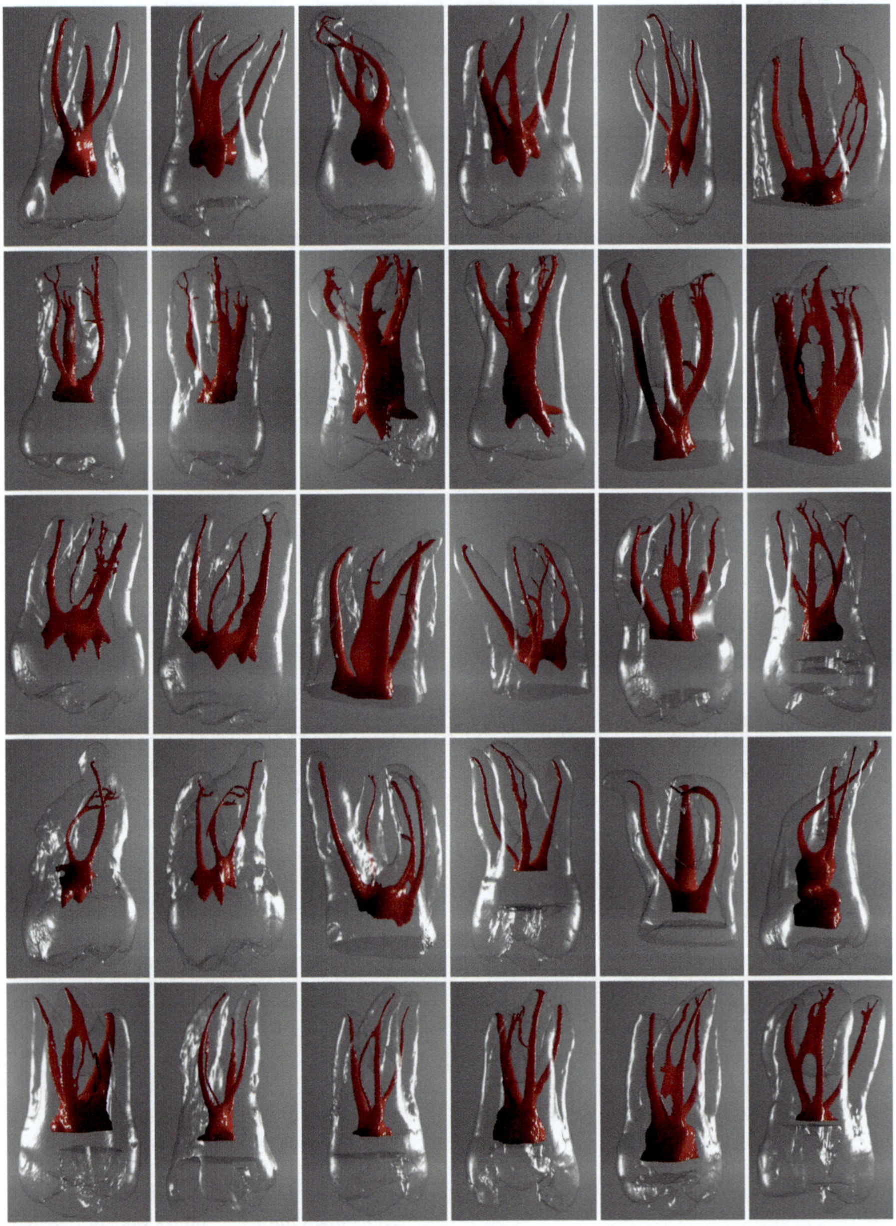

Fig. 8.8 Morphological aspects of the root canal system of maxillary molar teeth (frontal and lateral views)

finding, with a prevalence that varies from 1.2 to 1.6% for the mandibular first and second molars, respectively. On the other hand, *radix entomolaris* is more common, mainly in the mandibular first molars of Asian populations, where its prevalence can be as high as 22%, while in non-Asian populations, it is reported as under 7% (Fig. 8.9) [2]. The mandibular second molar usually has two well-developed roots, one mesial and one distal, that are not widely separated as in the mandibular first molar. Its buccolingual section demonstrates a pulp chamber and root canals that tend to be more variable and complex than those found in the mandibular first molar, such as the C-shaped configuration. C-shaped canals may exhibit a very complex system with a deep pulp chamber floor, a high incidence of accessory canals and isthmuses, as well as many canals ending in multiple foramens. Among other anatomical variations, the presence of a third root canal in the mesial root, the so-called middle mesial canal has also been reported as an uncommon finding in 2.2–5.5% of the mandibular second and first molars, respectively. Another important anatomical aspect in mandibular molar teeth is the high incidence of isthmus. This anatomical structure, also called transverse anastomosis, is defined as a narrow, ribbon-shaped communication between two root canals that may contain vital tissue, necrotic pulp, and/or biofilms. Isthmuses (or isthmi) may present with different configurations (Fig. 8.9) [2]. Experimental studies demonstrated the impossibility of obtaining a complete mechanical debridement or chemical disinfection of isthmuses with the current technology, mostly because of the presence of hard tissue debris packed into these areas during the mechanical canal preparation [30–33]. Clinical studies have also shown that unfilled isthmuses can be commonly observed after root-end resection in cases referred for apical surgery [34, 35].

The maxillary and mandibular third molars can be considered a separate group. Their morphology varies considerably and is rather unpredictable. However, if these teeth are well developed and appear clinically and radiographically as a first or second molar, root canal can be performed to keep them in function. But, if they present an extremely irregular form, it may or may not be possible to perform adequate root canal treatment and the final decision of saving or extraction must be made based on clinical and radiographic findings of each tooth [36].

Additional morphological aspects of the root and root canal anatomy of molar teeth are depicted in Table 8.3, while Table 8.4 shows the outcomes of epidemiological studies of all groups of teeth using CBCT in large populations, in which both root and root canal anatomy results are combined, offering an overview of the percentage frequencies of different numbers of roots and root canal configuration types.

8.2.6 The "Critical Apical Zone": Is It Really Critical?

The anatomical complexity of the root canal system, and particularly of the apical third, has been discussed in the dental literature for more than a century. The apical portion of the root canal system is characterized by a very complex and variable

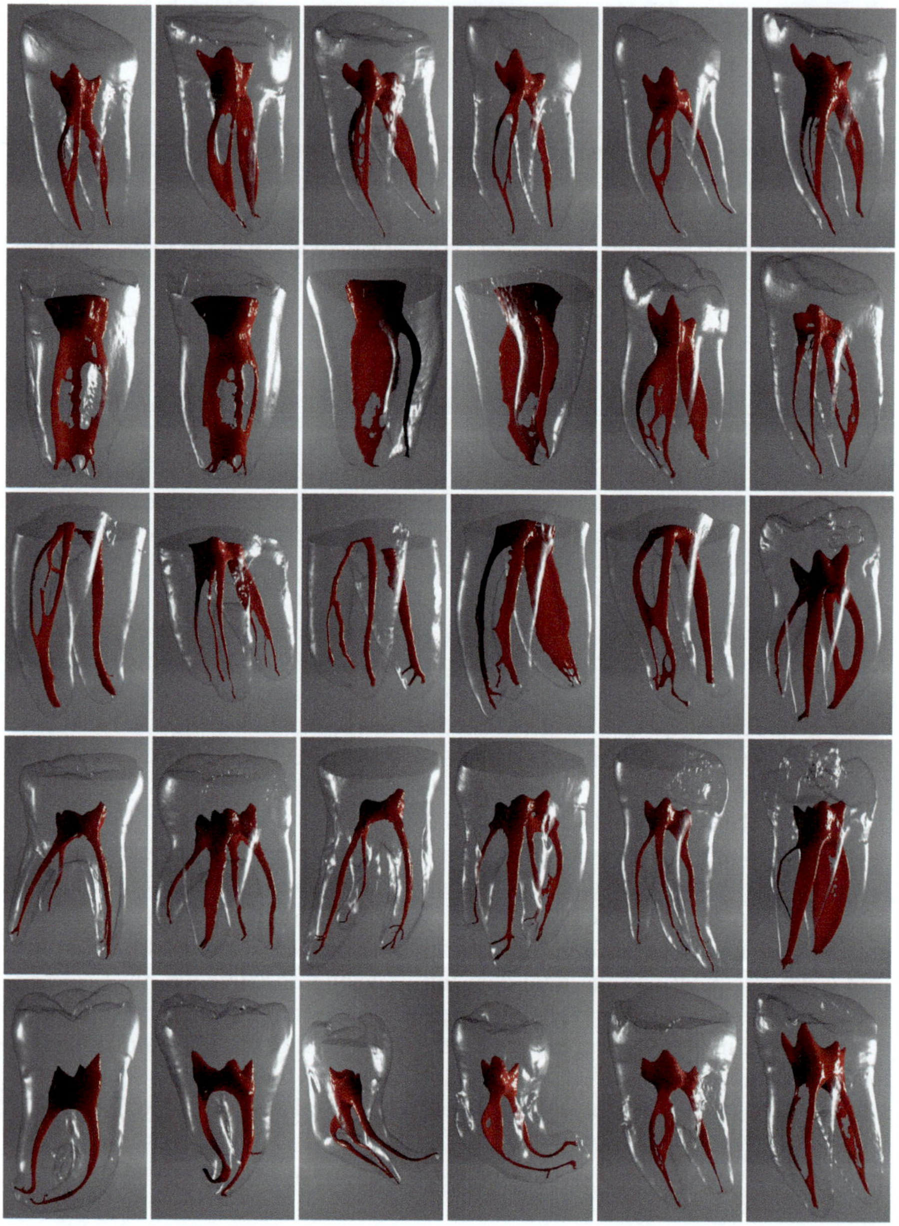

Fig. 8.9 Morphological aspects of the root canal system of mandibular molar teeth

Table 8.3 Morphological aspects of the root and root canal anatomy of molar teeth

	Maxillary first molar	Maxillary second molar	Mandibular first molar	Mandibular second molar
Overall length	20.1 mm (17.0–27.4 mm)	20.0 mm (16.0–26.2 mm)	20.9 mm (17.0–27.7 mm)	20.6 mm (15.5–25.5 mm)
Root length	**MB**:12.9 mm (8.5–18.8 mm) **DB**: 12.2 mm (8.9–15.5 mm) **P**: 13.7 mm (10.6–17.5 mm)	**MB**: 12.9 mm (9.0–18.2 mm) **DB**: 12.1 mm (9.0–16.3 mm) **P**: 13.5 mm (9.8–18.8 mm)	**M**: 14.0 mm (10.6–20.0 mm) **D**: 13.0 mm (8.1–17.7 mm)	**M**: 13.9 mm (9.3–18.3 mm) **D**: 13.0 mm (8.5–18.3 mm)
Number of roots	3 (97.7%); 2 (1.8%); 4 (0.3%); 1 (0.2%)	3 (73.7%); 2 (14.9%); 1 (10.7%); 4 (0.7%)	2 (86.9%); 3 (12.5%); 1 (0.55%); 4 (0.05%)	2 (78.6%); 1 (19%); 3 (2.2%); 4 (0.2%)
Number of canals	**MB**: 2 (60.4%); 1 (29.3%); 3 (0.1%); Other (0.4%) **DB**: 1 (98.6%); 2 (1.4%) **P**: 1 (99.26%); 2 (0.7%); other (0.04%)	**MB**: 1 (66.1%); 2 (33.7%); 3 (0.05%); Other (0.2%) **DB**: 1 (99.6%); 2 (0.4%) **P**: 1 (99.67%); 2 (0.35%); 3 (0.01%); Other (0.01%)	**M**: 1 (2.37%); 2 (96.59%); 3 (0.03%); Other (1.01%) **D**: 1 (70.3%); 2 (29.56%); other (0.14%)	**M**: 2 (87.1%); 1 (12.5%) **D**: 1 (92.56%); 2 (7.44%)
Canal configuration	**MB**: Types I (39.1%); II (29.3%); IV (26%); V (2%); III (1.6%); VI (1.4%); VII (0.1%); VIII (0.1%); other (0.4%) **DB**: Types I (98.6%), II (0.4%), 5 (0.4%); III (0.3%); IV (0.2%); VI (0.1%) **P**: Types I (99.26%); II (0.3%); III (0.2%); IV (0.1%); V (0.1%); other (0.04%)	**MB**: Types I (39.1%); II (29.3%); IV (26%); V (2%); III (1.6%); VI (1.4%); VII (0.1%); VIII (0.1%); other (0.4%) **DB**. Types I (98.6%); II (0.4%); V (0.4%); III (0.3%); IV (0.2%); VI (0.1%) **P**: Types I (99.26%); II (0.3%); III (0.2%); IV (0.1%); V (0.1%); other (0.04%)	**M**: Types IV (71.3%); II (19.9%); III (2.9%); I (2.37%); V (2.1%); VI (0.3%); VII (0.09%); VIII (0.03%); other (1.01%) **D**: Types I (70.3%); II (13%); IV (10.1%), III (3.6%), V (2.7%); VI (0.08%); VII (0.08%); other (0.14%)	**M**: Types IV (47.8%); II (32.8%); I (12.5%); III (3.27%); V (3%); VI (0.2%); VII (0.1%); other (0.33%) **D**. Types I (92.56%); II (4.4%); IV (2%); III (0.5%); V (0.5%); VI (0.04%)

(continued)

Table 8.3 (continued)

	Maxillary first molar	Maxillary second molar	Mandibular first molar	Mandibular second molar
Accessory canals	**MB**: 51% (coronal: 10.7%; middle: 13.1%; apical: 58.2%) **DB**: 36% (coronal: 10.1%; middle: 12.3%; apical: 59.6%) **P**: 48% (coronal: 9.4%; middle: 11.3%; apical: 61.3%)	**MB**: 50% (coronal: 10.1%; middle: 14.1%; apical: 65.8%) **DB**: 29% (coronal: 9.1%; middle: 13.3%; apical: 67.6%) **P**: 42% (coronal: 8.7%; middle: 11.2%; apical: 70.1%)	**M**: 45% (coronal: 10.4%; middle: 12.2%; apical: 54.4%) **D**: 30% (coronal: 8.7%; middle: 10.4%; apical: 57.9%)	**M**: 49% (coronal: 10.1%; middle: 13.1%; apical: 65.8%) **D**: 34% (coronal: 9.1%; middle: 11.6%; apical: 68.3%)
Apical curvature	**MB**: Distal (78%); straight (21%); S-shaped (1%) **DB**: Straight (54%); mesial (19%); distal (17%); S-shaped (10%) **P**: Buccal (55%); straight (40.7%); mesial (3.2%); distal (1.1%)	**MB**: Distal (54%); straight (22%); others (24%) **DB**: Straight (54%); mesial (17%); others (29%) **P**: Straight (63%); buccal (37%)	**M**: Distal (84%); straight (16%) **D**: Straight (73.5%); distal (18%); mesial (8.5%)	**M**: Distal (60.8%); straight (27.2%); buccal (4%); S-shaped (8%) **D**: Straight (57.6%); distal (18.4%); mesial (13.6%); buccal (4%); S-shaped (6.4%)
Anomalies	1 canal [215]; 5 canals [216]; 6 canals [217]; 7 canals [218]; 8 canals [219]; C-shaped [220]; 4 roots [221]; taurodontism [222]	1 or 2 canals [223]; 5 canals [224]; fusion/ gemination [225]; taurodontism [226]	5 canals [227]; 6 canals [228]; 7 canals [229]; *Radix* [165]; taurodontism [230]; fusion/gemination [231]; isthmus [232]; 3 roots [233]; C-shaped [234]; 3 canals in the distal root [235]	1 canal [236]; 2 canals [237]; 5 canals [238]; fusion/ gemination [239]; isthmus [232]; C-shaped [155]

MB mesiobuccal root/canal, *DB* distobuccal root/canal, *P* palatal root/canal, *M* mesial root/canal, *D* distal root/canal. Root canal configurations are classified according to Vertucci [43]
Adapted from Versiani et al. [27]

anatomy (Fig. 8.10), which can rarely be fully anticipated on the basis of conventional radiograph or even cone beam computed tomography. These complexities include ramifications, accessory canals, fine variations in the topography of the foramina, as well as, the sequelae of pathologic changes, such as resorption of the apical root structure and canal calcification, which may compromise the establishment of an adequate working length during shaping procedures [37]. The complexity of the root canal anatomy at the apical third and the preoperative histologic and microbiologic conditions of the pulp and periapical tissues can be regarded as the two major factors affecting the success rate of the endodontic treatment.

Table 8.4 Combined data from CBCT studies on root and root canal morphology of maxillary and mandibular permanent teeth

		Number of roots (%)				Root canal configuration (%)								
Maxillary teeth	Number of teeth	1	2	3	4	I	II	III	IV	V	VI	VII	VIII	Other
Central incisor	3125	**99.94**	0.06	0	0	**99.20**	0.1	0.1	0.5	0.1	0	0	0	0
Lateral incisor	3068	**99.94**	0.06	0	0	**98.50**	0.8	0.2	0.1	0.4	0	0	0	0
Canine	3148	**100**	0	0	0	**97.0**	0.8	1.2	0.2	0.7	0	0	0	0.1
1st premolar	2575	43.1	**55.3**	1.6	0	20.10	17.4	1.5	**50.1**	3.0	4.9	0.4	1.2	1.3
2nd premolar	2345	**86.2**	13.5	0.3	0	**42.70**	**18.7**	4.0	**17.6**	9.6	6.3	0.5	0.4	0.3
1st molar	8934	0.2	1.8	**97.7**	0.3									
MB root	8934					**39.10**	**29.3**	1.6	**26.0**	2.0	1.4	0.1	0.1	0.4
DB root	7473					**98.60**	0.4	0.3	0.2	0.4	0.01	0	0	0
P root	8445					**99.26**	0.3	0.2	0.1	0.1	0	0	0	0.04
2nd molar	9570	10.7	14.9	**73.7**	0.7									
MB root	9353					**66.10**	**15.3**	2.8	13.0	1.9	0.6	0.1	0.05	0.2
DB root	9570					**99.60**	0.2	0.07	0.1	0.03	0	0	0	0
P root	9570					**99.67**	0.1	0.1	0.1	0.05	0	0	0.01	0.01
Mandibular teeth		1	2	3	4	I	II	III	IV	V	VI	VII	VIII	Other
Central incisor	11,860	**100**	0	0	0	**86.5**	2.0	**8.1**	1.4	2.8	0	0.1	0	0.1
Lateral incisor	11,805	**99.92**	0.08	0	0	**79.7**	2.6	**11.9**	1.8	3.8	0	0.1	0	0.1
Canine	10,009	**98.57**	1.43	0	0	**92.4**	1.9	2.7	1.5	1.2	0	0	0	0.3
1st premolar	6043	**97.5**	2.5	0	0	**71.3**	2.3	2.8	3.5	**18.7**	0.5	0.1	0.1	0.7
2nd premolar	6350	**98.5**	1.5	0	0	**84.7**	0.7	0.5	0.3	**13.4**	0.07	0.04	0.05	0.2
1st molar	7388	0.55	**86.9**	**12.5**	0.05									
Mesial root	7388					2.37	**19.9**	2.9	**71.3**	2.1	0.3	0.09	0.03	1.01
Distal root	6712					**70.3**	**13.0**	3.6	10.1	2.7	0.08	0.08	0	0.14
2nd molar	7439	**19.0**	**78.6**	2.2	0.2									
Mesial root	6734					12.5	**32.8**	3.27	**47.8**	3.0	0.2	0.1	0	0.33
Distal root	7439					**92.56**	4.4	0.5	2.0	0.5	0.04	0	0	0

In bold letters, the highest percentage frequency is highlighted regarding the number of roots and canal configuration in each group of teeth
MB mesiobuccal, *DB* distobuccal, *P* palatal. Root canal configurations are classified according to Vertucci [43]
Adapted from Versiani et al. [27]

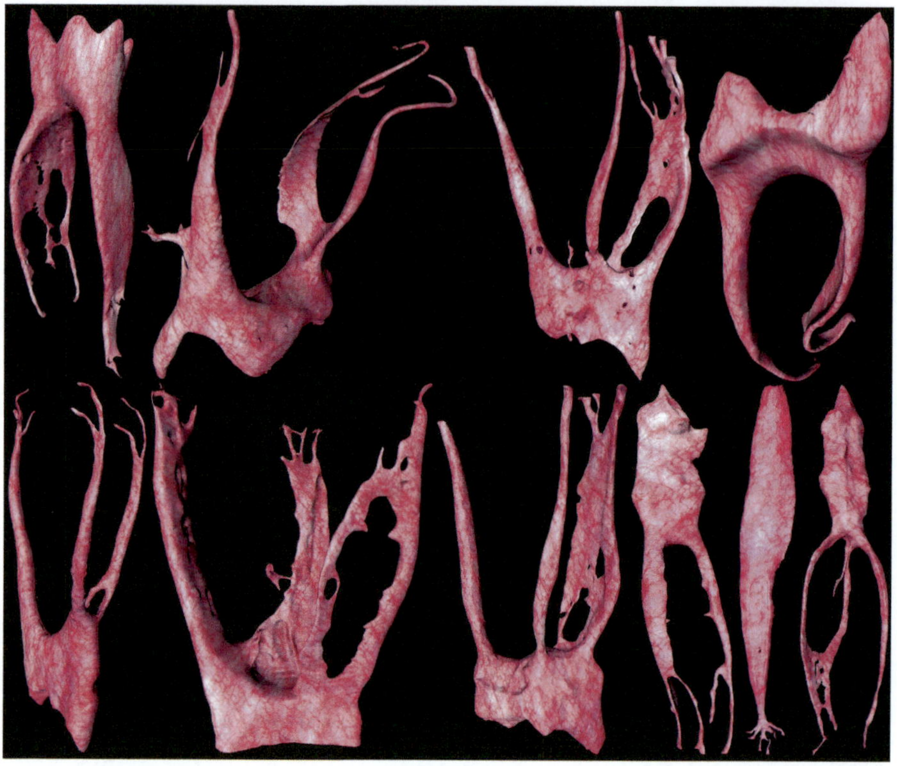

Fig. 8.10 3D models obtained by micro-CT scanning and texturized by means of advanced computational graphic techniques showing the complexities of the apical portion of the root canal system in different groups of teeth

In the absence of pathology, the root canal usually narrows toward the apex and ends at the apical foramen (major foramen). The narrowest apical portion of the root canal is called the "apical constriction" or "minor foramen," and from this anatomical landmark the canal widens as it approaches to the main foramen. The topography of the apical constriction is not constant and, when present, is usually located 0.5–1.5 mm from the center of the apical foramen [38]. The foramen diameter has been described as between 0.21 and 0.39 mm [39] and frequently opens laterally on the root surface, at a mean distance of 0.2 to 3.8 mm from the anatomic apex [40], despite larger distances having been also reported [41]. The anatomic apex is the tip or the end of the root, as determined morphologically. Depending on the type of tooth, the apical foramen can coincide with the anatomic apex in a percentage frequency ranging from 6.7 to 46% of cases [42–46], while a single canal configuration with no ramifications and terminating at the geometrical top of the root is relatively uncommon. The fact that the main foramen frequently ends at a location short of the root apex represents a problem for the clinician, because this condition can only be recognized in the radiographs when the foramen exits on the mesial or distal aspect of the root. The mesial roots of mandibular molars, the maxillary premolars and the mesiobuccal roots of maxillary molars show the highest percentage of multiple apical foramina [39]. A previous study on root apexes of all groups of permanent teeth showed that the number of foramina on each root may vary from 1 to 16 [40].

The analysis of the mineralized tissue topography forming the apical structure and its interrelationship with the surrounding structures deserves particular attention. The cementum layering the external apical surface folds into the foraminal opening, extending to varying distances to the coronal direction. The area where the cementum ends at the apical canal is called the cementum–dentin junction (CDJ), and at this histological landmark, pulp tissue ends and periodontal tissues begin. Actually, at the very end of the canal, the tissue should not be called "pulp tissue," as it is indistinguishable from the adjacent periodontal ligament. In fact, it is constituted mainly by fibroblasts and collagen bundles, and it is crossed by numerous vessels and nerves entering the pulp space. In the past, it was believed that the CDJ coincided with the apical constriction and this point was recommended as the apical limit of root canal preparation and filling. However, histologic observations demonstrated that the CDJ rarely coincides with the apical constriction. In longitudinal sections cut through the apical canal, the CDJ is frequently observed to be several millimeters higher on one wall than on the opposite wall [37].

In the presence of pathology, the clinical control of the infection at the apical third becomes critical. It is interesting for the clinician, however, to understand the dynamic involved in the spread of bacteria throughout the root canal space from their penetration into the pulp chamber, in order to make treatment as effective as possible [37]. When the pulp is exposed by caries, acute inflammation usually takes place and leads to the formation of necrotic areas in the coronal pulp. The advance of inflammation, necrosis, and infection through the pulp tissue to the apical direction is usually slow, but it progressively and gradually advances toward the apex. Contrary to common sense, early inflammatory changes can be observed in the apical periodontal tissues even when necrosis is still confined to the pulp chamber. At this stage, however, tissue present in lateral canals and apical ramifications is still vital and free from bacterial colonization. In later stages, as necrosis and bacterial infection are progressing to the apical direction, a distinct area of transition between necrotic and viable pulp tissue is present, and, although inflamed, vital tissue can be observed at the apical canal even in the presence of a periapical radiolucency. This happens because bacterial virulence factors may diffuse through the tissues and cause inflammation in a large area and are not only restricted to the narrow area immediately in contact with the most advanced bacteria. The diagnosis at this stage is referred to as "partial necrosis" and the inflamed connective tissue remaining at the most apical portion may not be colonized by bacteria [37].

If no treatment is provided, it is highly likely that the last portion of the apical tissue, including the tissue in ramifications, will be inevitably affected by necrosis and infection. Apical ramifications are defined as a morphology in which the main canal divides into multiple accessory canals, with the main canal becoming indistinguishable. In maxillary teeth, the percentage frequency of apical ramifications has been reported to range from 1% (central incisors) to 15.1% (second premolars), while in mandibular teeth, their frequency varies from 5% (central incisors) to 14% (distal root of first molars) [37]. Ricucci and Siqueira [47] reported a high prevalence of lateral canals and/or apical ramifications in approximately 75% of 493 human teeth investigated under light microscopy, mostly at the apical portion of posterior teeth. Gao et al. [48] also investigated the apical morphology of 1,400 extracted permanent human teeth from a Chinese subpopulation using micro-CT and reported a total of 634 apical branches (ranging from 3 to 18 per tooth), distributed in 6.3%, 8.8%, and 15.8% of anterior, premolar, and molar teeth, respectively. These branches started from 0.62 to 5.08 mm from the apex, and, in only 13% of these teeth (18 out of 136), this vertical distance was higher than 3 mm. It is important to notice that when infection reaches the entire extent of the root canal system up to the apical foramen, possibly affecting apical ramifications, complete disinfection becomes a significant challenge for clinicians and it is an important etiologic factor of nonsurgical failures. So, based on these findings, if 3 mm of the apical structure is resected during surgical procedures, the apical deltas with infecting bacterial biofilms will be fully removed in 87% of the cases, while 13% will harbor exposed biofilm-infected ramifications [37]. Therefore, a valid practical recommendation is to meticulously observe the resected surface under surgical microscope with dyes for remaining ramifications and eventually properly extend the resection length [35].

8.3 Anatomical Factors and Their Impact on the Prognosis of Root Canal Treatment

Prognosis and outcome are two terms routinely used in medicine and dentistry to predict and assess the treatment of a disease. Prognosis is a practitioner's assessment of how a patient will recover from an illness or injury. It is a forecast of the probable course of recovery for any particular disease, taking into consideration the assessment of the case. Outcome, on the other hand, is a measure of the success of the treatment, as a result of an activity or a process, and is a consequence of the decisions made during the course of treatment. Applied to endodontics, prognosis is a prediction of the resolution of the apical periodontitis, while outcome is the end result that follows as a consequence of endodontic treatment [49]. Prognosis is a critically important element in clinical decision-making, particularly when different alternatives are available for a treatment of a given disease. However, dentistry is not an art like painting, neither is it a science like physics. It is an applied science, and since each patient is a unique being, it can be very tricky to decide how to apply science and evidence to each individual case and situation [50], without proper knowledge.

In the literature, information about prognosis of endodontic treatment, retreatment, and apical surgery are available from several studies (Figs. 8.11, 8.12, and 8.13). However, the scientific evidence behind these results has been highly inconsistent, with a wide range of reported success rates because of methodologic and

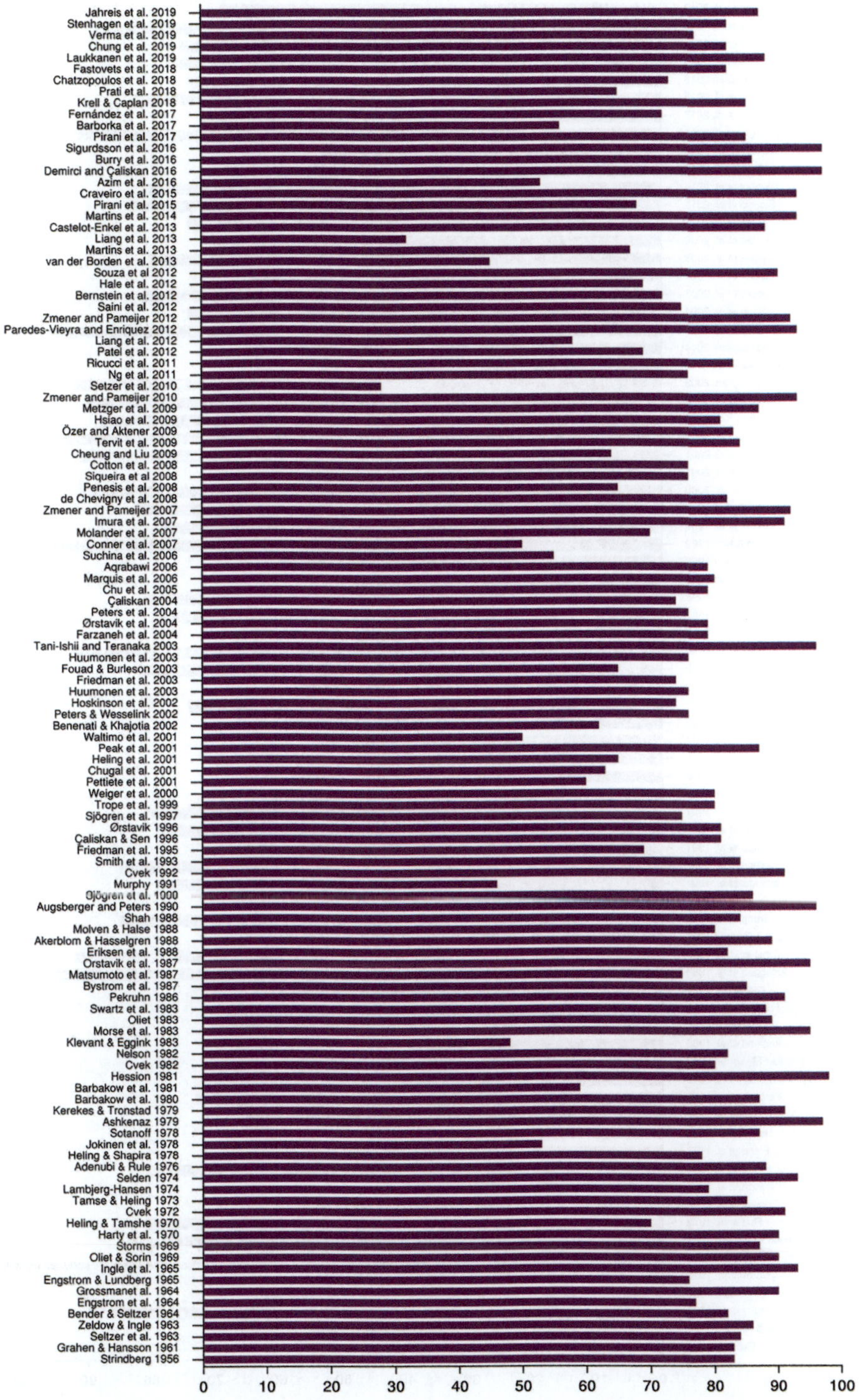

Fig. 8.11 Outcome of studies reporting the success rate of non-surgical endodontic treatment

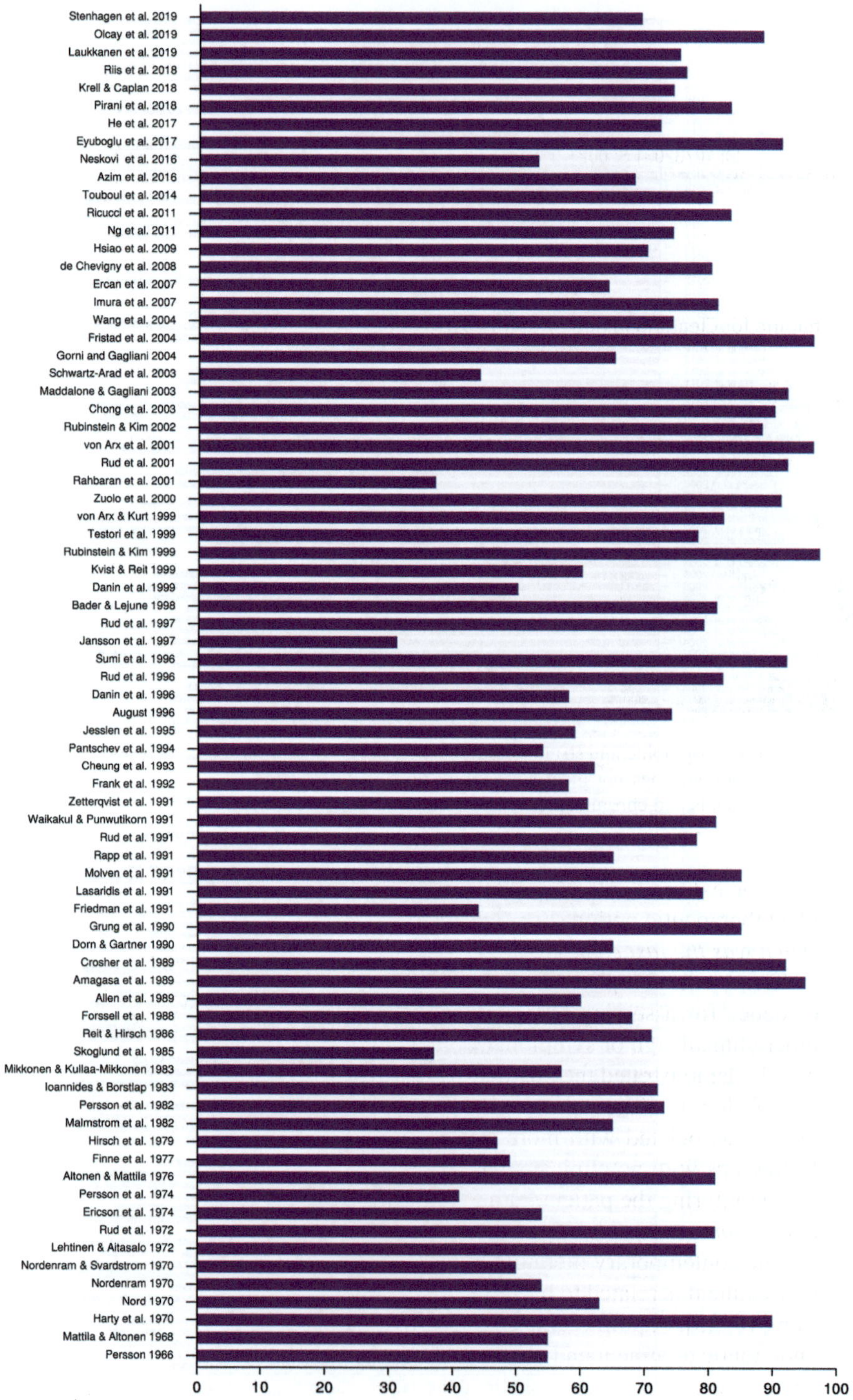

Fig. 8.12 Outcome of studies reporting the success rate of endodontic retreatment

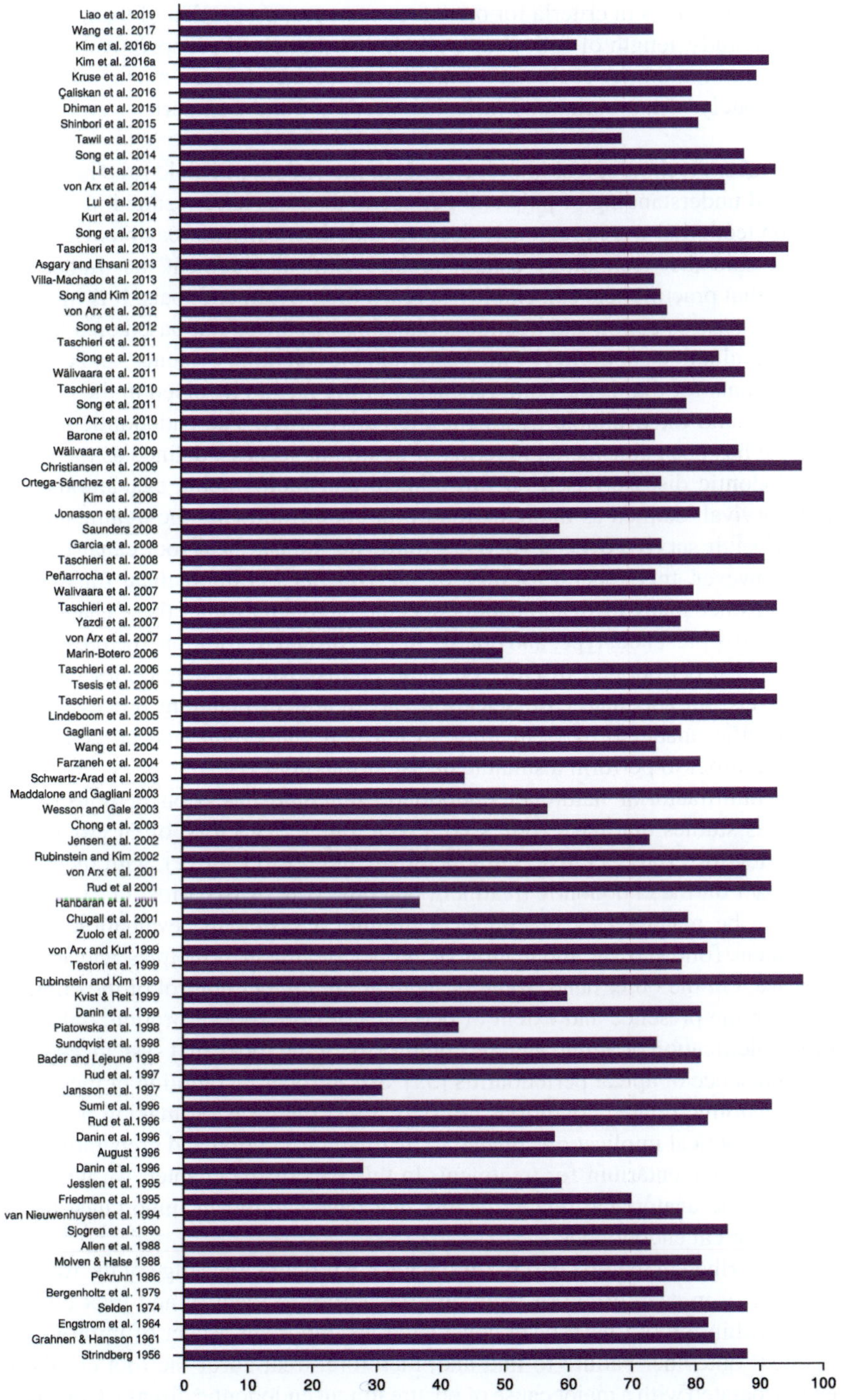

Fig. 8.13 Outcome of studies reporting the success rate of surgical endodontic treatment

technical variations in criteria for outcome measures, proportion of teeth of a given type in a study, length of follow-up period, distribution of preoperative diagnoses, inter-operator and inter-evaluator variability, associated factors, among others [49]. Unfortunately, these variations have hampered a valid comparison among these findings.

The recent technological improvements in the endodontic field together with the increased understanding of pulp and periapical diseases have resulted in the ability to retain teeth that were previously deemed endodontically untreatable. However, it may be said that technology cannot replace clinical judgment, but rather be an adjunct that practitioners can employ to reach their treatment goals. It is imperative that strict case selection and treatment planning be carried out based on a thorough clinical evaluation supported by the best available scientific evidence, and one of the key elements for that is the comprehension of the factors involved in the long-term prognosis and the available treatment alternatives [51]. The endodontic treatment outcome has been considered in terms of treatment success, defined as the absence of endodontic disease based on full clinical and radiographic evaluations, or by tooth survival, defined as the retention of the tooth following the treatment. About 90% of teeth survive over 2–10 years following nonsurgical root canal treatment [52]. However, this general average of survival rates is impractical for treatment planning since many teeth and patient-specific factors may alter these chances—for example, the presence, type, and quality of the coronal restoration, the presence and severity of a periodontal disease, or some predisposing systemic medical conditions. Thus, an adequate case selection and treatment planning process must be case-specific, made so by evaluating all relevant endodontic and non-endodontic factors in order to perform a suitable decision-making [51].

The multifactorial nature of endodontic outcome has been demonstrated in numerous studies that have addressed a wide range of factors, often grouped into three categories (preoperative, intraoperative, and postoperative), with their potential impact on the endodontic treatment outcome (Fig. 8.14). Most of these conditions can be managed by practitioners through a systematic evaluation and risk assessment followed by application of proper treatment principles and technical expertise. On the other hand, some of them are not under control of the clinicians, including the presence and extent of periapical lesion, root resorption, obliteration due to calcification or aging, and the complexity of the root canal system, especially in the presence of apical periodontitis [53]. So, a proper recognition of these preexisting anatomic-related conditions not only assist the decision-making process but also has practical implications related to treatment execution and preparation of the required armamentarium for treatment. In this part of the chapter, we will briefly discuss some anatomical-related factors that have significant importance for successful clinical endodontics.

As described in the first part of this chapter, a proper knowledge of the root canal morphology in each group of teeth and the ability to identify and treat all of the canals within a tooth have been considered an important aspect of improving the treatment outcome. Failure to find and, therefore, treat all of the root canals have been associated with a major cause of posttreatment endodontic disease. Considering

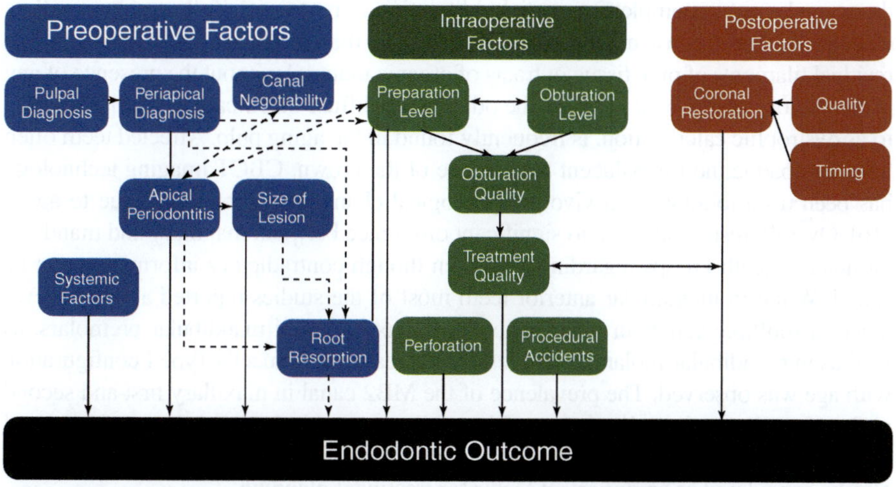

Fig. 8.14 Relationships among the prognostic factors that may affect the outcome of endodontic treatment. (Adapted from Chugal et al. [49, 53]. Published with permission)

that the literature is unequivocal in regarding preoperative periradicular osteolysis as one major indicator of postoperative healing or failure, teeth with this condition have poorer outcome after nonsurgical root canal treatment than teeth without periapical lesion [52]. Therefore, if disinfection of the root canal system is one of the main objectives to improve outcome, when infected canals are missed, remaining bacteria may maintain or cause disease, compromising the prognosis of the treatment. This means that difficulties in locating extra canals in multirooted teeth may predispose the patient to persistent symptoms and/or a decrease in the expected treatment outcome. Indeed, it has been reported that root-filled teeth with missed canals are 4.38 [54] to 6.25 [55] times more likely to be associated with apical periodontitis. Therefore, considering that complex morphologies, such as a single root with multiple canal systems, are challenging to debride effectively, knowledge of the prevalence of additional canals in each tooth group may help clinicians to anticipate their presence in clinical practice.

The root canal anatomy is also susceptible to changes overtime because of physiological or pathological events. Natural physiological aging tends to modify the root canal system morphology due to the deposition of secondary dentin, which starts to form once the tooth erupts and is in occlusion. Consequently, young patients tend to present large single canals and pulp chambers, while older patients tend to present more sharply defined and narrow root canals. Other pathological or iatrogenic factors can also modify the deposition of dentin, including occlusal trauma, periodontal disease, carious lesions, or deep restorative procedures. A pulpal response to trauma is characterized by a rapid deposition of hard tissue, and the entire canal space may appear obliterated radiographically. This phenomenon is called "calcific metamorphosis" and is commonly observed following traumatic injuries like concussion, subluxation, and luxation [56]. Depending on the severity of the injury and the developmental stage of the tooth, there can be either complete or partial obliteration of root canals followed by a yellow discoloration of the crown. However, histologically, there is always a persistence of fine residual filaments of pulp tissue or tracts of organic material without the presence of any inflammatory component [47]. On the other hand, diffuse calcification, usually referred to as dystrophic calcification, is frequently found in the aging pulp. Affected teeth often have an opaque, non-translucent appearance of the crown. CBCT imaging technology has been used to address in vivo morphological changes on root canals due to aging [16]. Overall, results showed no significant difference between maxillary and mandibular anterior teeth groups regarding age, even though contradictory information can be found. While in mandibular anterior teeth most of the studies reported a lower prevalence of multiple canals in older patients, in maxillary and mandibular premolars, as well as in mandibular molars, a progressive decrease of Vertucci's Type I configuration with age was observed. The prevalence of the MB2 canal in maxillary first and second molars was also evaluated and most of the studies reported a low prevalence of this canal in older patients. Therefore, aging may affect the original anatomy of teeth and must also be considered as an important factor for treatment planning.

8.4 Anatomical Factors in Practice for Treating Complex Anatomies

Root canal treatment is essentially directed toward the prevention or cure of apical periodontitis, maintaining or restoring the health of periapical tissues, and maintaining teeth in function. Consequently, the outcome of treatment is linked directly not only to effective canal debridement and disinfection through chemomechanical canal preparation, but also to the prevention of the ingress of new microorganisms into the root canal system by filling the root canal space and restoring teeth with high-quality materials. In this way, endodontic treatment can be performed in one or multiple visits and involves a sequence of steps including diagnosis, access preparation, orifice location, shaping, cleaning, filling, and restorative procedures.

8.4.1 Diagnostic Tools to Identify Anatomical Complexities: 2D × 3D

Most of the time in the clinical practice, two or more angled periapical radiographs together with a thorough clinical examination may provide the required information on tooth anatomy, as well as, the presence of pathologies that may go unnoticed by a single exam. By changing the horizontal angulation of periapical radiographs by 20–40°, the exact number of roots in maxillary and mandibular molars can be detected. However, radiography often fails to provide accurate information on root canal configuration when compared to CBCT examination, which has been proven to capture information in a more precise way than would be possible with two-dimensional radiographs for both diagnosis and treatment planning [57]. Actually, CBCT imaging overcomes several limitations found in conventional radiographic methods, allowing accurate image acquisition, a view in all three spatial planes eliminating the superimposition of multiple roots and/or surrounding anatomic structures, more sensitivity with regard to the detection of periradicular pathosis, root resorption and root fractures, visualization of multidimensional root curvatures, accurate determination of root length, precise intra- and inter-canal distance relationships, improved diagnostic capabilities for treatment planning, precision vertical depth measurements determined from the occlusal plane to multiple levels within the pulp chamber, and the identification of more complex anatomical root forms and root canal configurations, such as multiple canals in one root, isthmuses, canal confluences, accessory canals, position of the main foramen, C-shaped canals, and other aberrant canal configurations [58]. Furthermore, the collective information gained from numerous anatomic studies using CBCT can be applied clinically by establishing a through knowledge of commonly known root variations and average statistics for permanent human teeth with respect to type and location, as well as, common canal configurations, as depicted in this chapter (Table 8.4). However, studies that attempted to categorize anatomy and morphology can only provide treatment recommendations and guidelines in general circumstances since they are based on weighted averages and common observations. Although averages are useful when studying characteristics of populations, they are of limited predictive value for treatment of individual patients. Accordingly, in certain cases, a preoperative CBCT scan is mandatory for treatment planning and decision-making [51, 58].

8.4.2 Planning a Case: Armamentarium for a 3D Approach

As previously stated, one of the main objectives of endodontic treatment in infected teeth is the removal of necrotic tissues, microorganisms, and microbial by-products from the root canal space. Among the treatment steps to achieve these goals, chemomechanical procedures play a pivotal role in eliminating or reducing bacterial populations from the main root canal, but the disinfecting effects of instruments and irrigants may be somewhat hampered in cases of complex anatomy. Thus, a thorough understanding of the canal morphology and its variations and a high level comprehension skills regarding the armamentarium needed to manage these complexities are basic requirements for a predictable approach. The development of new instruments and techniques for diagnosis and treatment in endodontics has been a predominant aspect over the last few decades, and, because of that, endodontics has become a feasible and attractive discipline for many practitioners. As a collateral damage, however, many clinicians find it hard to resist purchasing the growing number of new devices and instruments frequently launched on the market and commonly advertised with the promise of simplifying procedures by shortening the working time or even influencing the success rate. Unfortunately, these guarantees are often not met, and, as a result, shelves full of unwanted gadgets may accumulate in our practices. It is beyond the scope of this chapter to cover all instruments, materials, or devices commonly used in endodontics, but it is important to comment about some of them together with basic requirements for performing modern endodontic therapy (Fig. 8.15), mostly when dealing with complex anatomies.

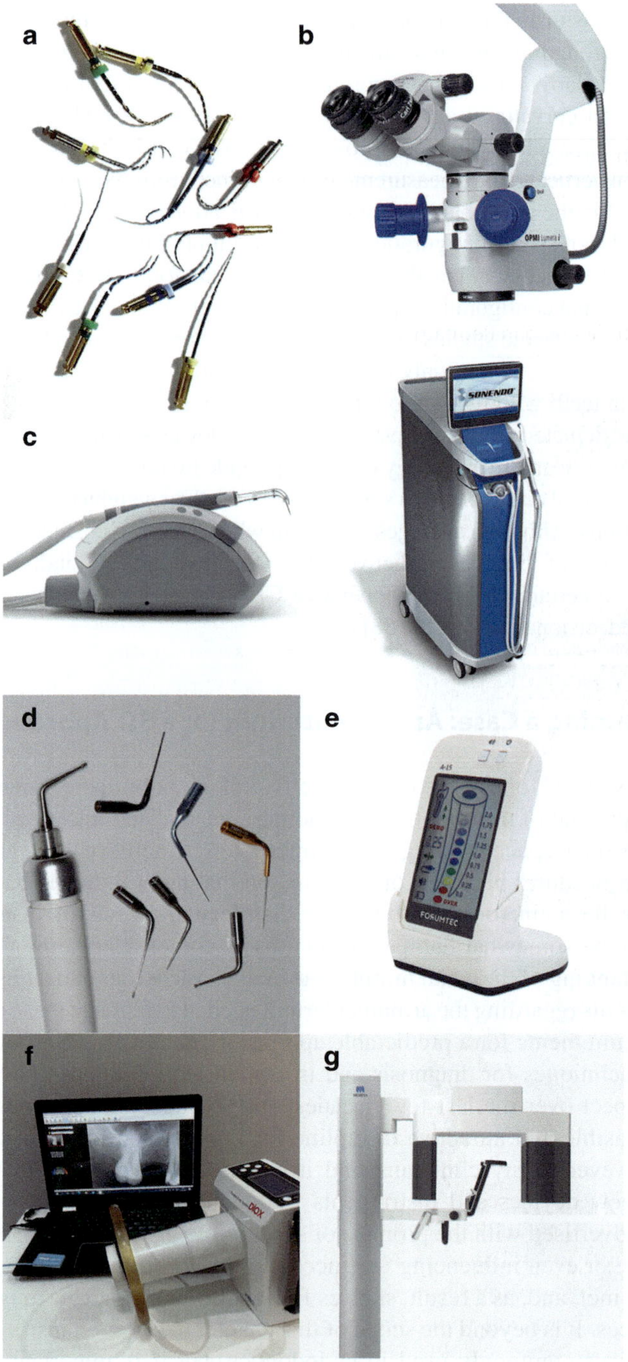

Fig. 8.15 Basic armamentarium to deal with complex anatomies in modern endodontic therapy. (**a**) Ultra-flexible instruments. (**b**) Visual magnification and superior illumination. (**c**) Enhanced root canal irrigation systems. (**d**) Ultrasonic instruments. (**e**) Electronic apex locator. (**f**) Digital imaging systems. (**g**) Three-dimensional imaging technology

Currently, technological advancements in the field of endodontics offer new possibilities for treating root canals with complex morphologies, including the use of:

- Ultra-flexible instruments. Over the years, several changes have been introduced by manufacturers to improve the flexibility and resistance to fracture of endodontic instruments, including different thermomechanical treatments of the nickel-titanium alloy. The use of flexible instruments also reduces the risk of iatrogenic complications when dealing with canal curvatures as they follow the original anatomy, decrease operator fatigue, and produce good-quality shape preparations (Fig. 8.15a).
- Visual magnification and superior illumination. The small dimensions of root canals make it extremely difficult to perform precise clinical procedures. The use of operating microscopes or loupes at increased light levels results in improvements in the precision routinely required for endodontic procedures. Loupes are available in many configurations and use convergent lenses to form a magnified image, but operating microscope is superior to loupes because of its continuous zoom and magnification steps in different depths of field. The benefits of using magnification devices for endodontic treatment include the improved visualization of the operating field, enhanced possibilities in locating canal orifices, aid in the removal of separated instruments, diagnosis of root fracture, perforation repair, as well as, case documentation. However, high-quality microscopes are expensive, and, thus far, the technology has met with limited adoption by general dentists [51] (Fig. 8.15b).
- Enhanced irrigation systems. The mechanical and chemical effects of irrigation play a crucial role in root canal cleaning and disinfection. Mechanical effects of irrigation are related to the flow of the irrigants in the root canal, either under a positive or negative apical pressure. Approaches for optimized disinfection include new systems and substances that either replace conventional chemomechanical procedures or supplement their effects, including negative pressure irrigation, sonic or ultrasonic activation of the irrigant solution, photodynamic therapy, photon-induced photoacoustic streaming using Er:YAG laser energy at subablative power levels, and the multisonic wave system (Fig. 8.15c).
- Ultrasonic instruments. The use of thin ultrasonic tips has been recommended to locate hidden canal orifices, to agitate the irrigant solutions, and for the management of complex anatomies, such as isthmuses, fins, and recesses (Fig. 8.15d).
- Electronic determination of the main foramen. The maintenance of a correct working length during root canal treatment is expected to positively influence the outcome and to prevent postoperative symptoms. However, variations in the apical anatomy render the identification of the correct working length by two-dimensional radiographs or other clinical means practically impossible. Therefore, modern electronic apex locators that use alternating electric current with various frequencies are recommended to determine the most appropriate endpoint for root canal preparation and filling (Fig. 8.15e).

- Digital imaging systems. Direct digital radiographic modalities that were introduced into modern endodontic practice have a number of advantages over conventional radiographs, such as immediate availability of the image for evaluation, lower radiation dosage required for the image acquisition, superior archiving and sharing capabilities, and easier manipulation of several radiographic properties, such as image contrast, brightness, and sharpness [51] (Fig. 8.15f).
- Three-dimensional imaging technology (CBCT). The combination of clinical examination and diagnostic imaging is the basis for endodontic preoperative diagnosis and clinical decision-making. CBCT has been suggested to be used for complicated diagnostic demands in endodontics, such as the identification of periapical periodontitis, the diagnosis of vertical root fractures and resorption, the management of dentoalveolar traumatic injuries, and, of course, the assessment of root canal anatomy (Fig. 8.15g).

Interestingly, in the midst of this technological development, these huge efforts would be futile if measures were not undertaken to prevent oral contaminants from entering the root canal space during the procedure. In light of this, although protecting the operating field with a rubber dam is the oldest and the most effective way to ensure proper infection control, it is worrying to think that, in several countries, the majority of clinicians seldom or never use rubber dam for endodontic treatment [59–65]. The use of rubber dam is mandatory in modern endodontic practice. Like any other treatment modality, endodontic treatment is exposed to the risk of complications that may raise additional dilemmas during the decision-making process. Using modern treatment techniques and adequate case selection, teeth that were traditionally planned for extraction can be successfully treated. Modern endodontic treatment also results in a predictably favorable long-term outcome and allows the retention of the natural dentition [51]. However, all of these technological advancements are meaningless if basic requirements for root canal treatment are not properly followed.

8.4.3 Access Preparation: To Open or Not to Open?

After diagnosis and treatment planning, the next step of endodontic treatment is access preparation. An adequate access cavity is necessary to uncover and locate all canal orifices, allowing the removal of infected tissues, the disinfection of the remaining tooth structure, and the complete filling of the root canal space. In essence, a proper access cavity preparation is considered a basic requirement for achieving the goals of high-quality endodontic treatment since it may impact on the subsequent treatment procedures. Indeed, inadequate access cavities may prevent the detection of caries, tooth fractures, and deficient/leaking restorations, as well as, the proper manipulation of instruments and irrigants. At the same time, it may lead to the creation of iatrogenic errors such as deviations from the original anatomy (canal transportation, ledges, zips), perforations, and instrument fractures, all of which can result in immediate or delayed posttreatment complications and/or disease [66].

Traditionally, endodontic access cavity preparation involves the complete removal of the pulp chamber roof, providing straight-line access to the canal orifices and ultimately to the canal terminus, followed by the removal of overhanging cervical dentin and enlargement of the canal orifice [67]. More recently, the emerged concept of minimally invasive access cavity preparation in endodontics aimed to preserve sound dentin by maintaining as much of the pulp chamber roof as possible, based on the assumption that retaining this structure would preserve the fracture resistance of teeth after root canal treatment [68]. The minimally invasive concept started as an empirical theory based on a series of cases [68] and evolved over time to a more structured concept requiring the use of ultra-flexible instruments, visual magnification, superior illumination, enhanced irrigation procedures, and three-dimensional imaging technology [69] (Fig. 8.16). However, making the access too small may

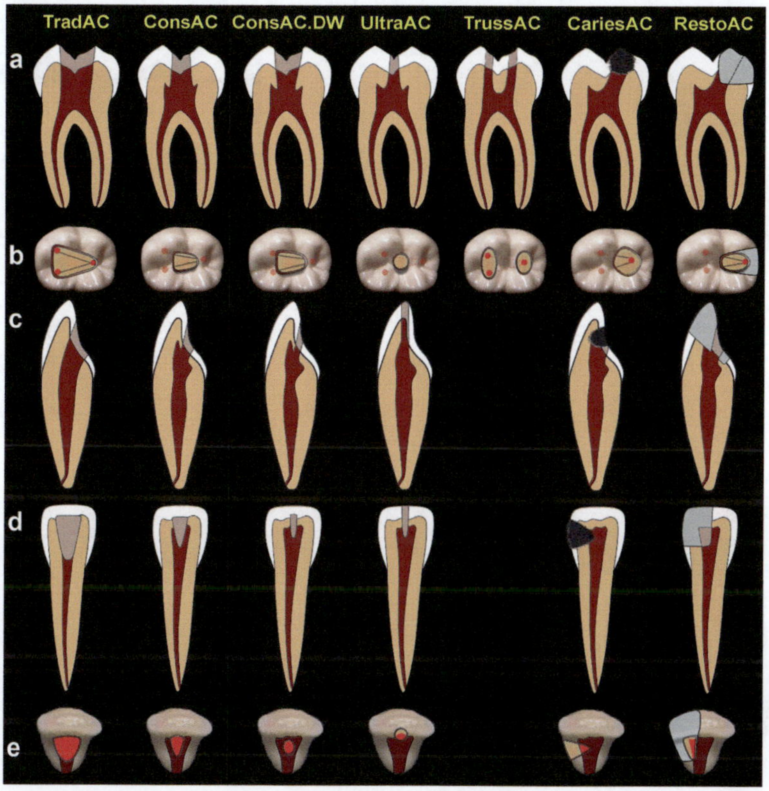

Fig. 8.16 Schematic illustration showing the different types of access cavity designs in posterior and anterior teeth. (**a–b**) Buccal and occlusal views of a mandibular molar. (**c–e**) Lateral, lingual and incisal views of a mandibular incisor. Traditional Access Cavity (**TradAC**): complete removal of the pulp chamber roof followed by achieving straight-line access to the canal orifices. Conservative Access Cavity (**ConsAC**): preparation with smoothly convergent axial walls, as far as necessary to detect the canal orifices, preserving part of the pulp chamber roof. Conservative Access Cavity with Divergent Walls (**ConsAC.DW**): A ConsAC with divergent walls. Ultra-Conservative Access Cavity (**UltraAC** or "ninja" access): cavity starts as the ConsAC, but maintains as much of the pulp chamber roof as possible. Truss Access Cavity (**TrussAC**): it aims to preserve the dentinal bridge between two or more small cavities prepared to access the canal orifice(s) in each root of multi-rooted teeth. Caries-Driven Access Cavity (**CariesAC**): it is performed by removing caries and preserving all remaining tooth structures. Restorative-Driven Access Cavity (**RestoAC**): it is performed by totally or partially removing existing restorations and by preserving all remaining tooth structures. (Adapted from Silva et al. [90])

affect the subsequent stages of root canal treatment by preventing the location of canal orifices or compromising the canal cleaning, shaping, and filling procedures (Fig. 8.17). Concurrently, it may also increase the potential for iatrogenic complications, including missed canals, deviations, and/or instrument fracture [66, 70, 71], often responsible for the perpetuation or development of periradicular pathosis [54, 55]. In addition, the residual roof of the pulp chamber may make it difficult to remove

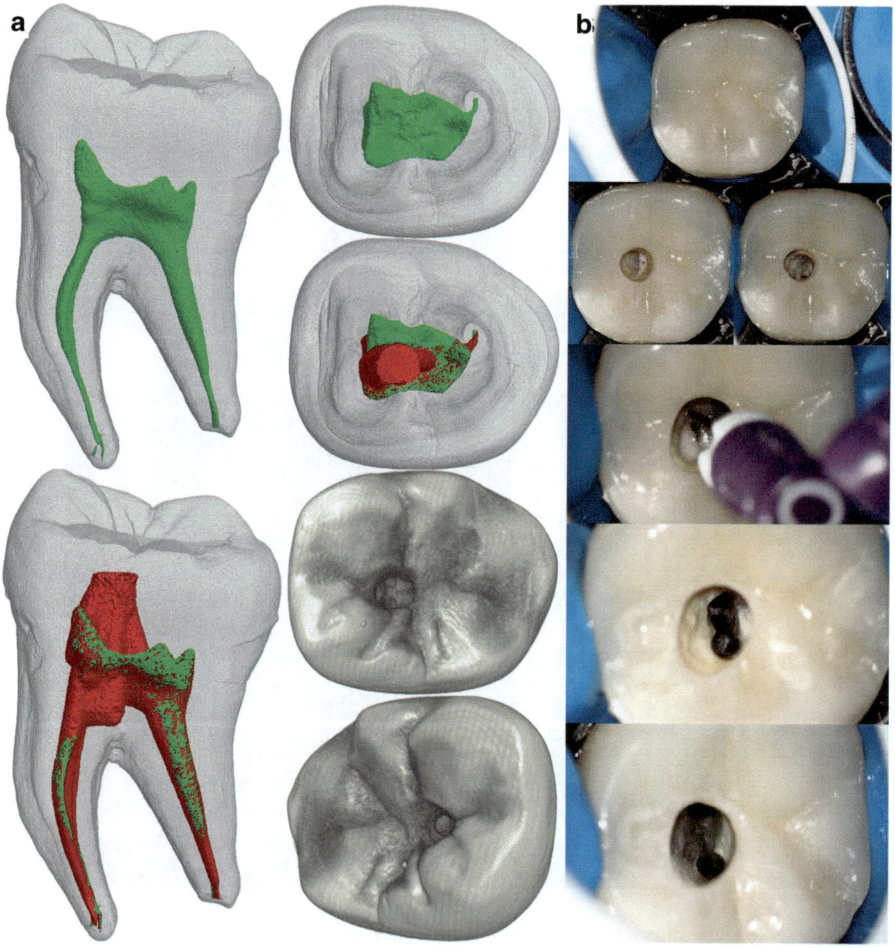

Fig. 8.17 (**a**) 3D images acquired by means of micro-CT technology showing the root canal system of a mandibular molar before (in green) and after (in red) the mechanical preparation with a reciprocating system depicting a conservative access cavity preparation. (**b**) Clinical case demonstrating a conservative access cavity preparation in a mandibular molar similar to (**a**). (Courtesy of Dr. Leandro Pereira, Brazil). It is important to notice that making access too small can compromise the subsequent stages of root canal treatment by preventing and/or complicating the location of canal orifices and the cleaning, shaping, and filling procedures. Although nowadays technological advancements allow clinicians to perform root canal treatment even under extremely conservative access cavities, treating infected teeth must demand a clinical decision based on the best cost-benefit balance for infection control

pulp remnants, dentinal debris, blood, filling materials, and other residues, which may cause tooth discoloration, support microbial growth, and have a negative impact on filling materials, particularly root canal sealers [70, 72]. In summary, at the present moment, there is a lack of supporting evidence for the introduction of minimally invasive access cavity preparation into routine clinical practice and/or the training of undergraduate and postgraduate students, mostly because anatomical complexities of the root canal is more the rule than the exception.

8.4.3.1 Minimally Invasive Endodontics: A Cost–Benefit Rationale

Every treatment in the health field needs to equalize its biological cost with the expected benefit. For instance, when taking a medication, the disease is treated under the expense of side effects that can be expressive or neglectable depending on the best balance of benefits and costs for such treatment. Several physicians believe that the more aggressive is a treatment, the better would be its benefit for the patient, a rational called "the more, the better," a mechanistic paradigm supported on biological plausibility toward the benefit [73]. However, the increase in treatment aggressiveness may lead to more undesired side effects (high biological cost), with no or neglectable increase in benefit.

In endodontics, as in medicine, dentists are always challenged for clinical decision-making under the rule of the cost–benefit dichotomy, which may be critical when balancing the amount of dental tissue that should be removed (biological cost) in order to reach an appropriate disinfection level (benefit). In the literature, laboratorial [74, 75] and clinical [76] studies have corroborated "the more, the better" paradigm toward the improvement of disinfection by applying concepts such as straight-line access, apical canal enlargement, large-tapered instruments, profuse irrigation with high concentrated solutions, among others, implying in more biological cost to the dental tissues, which ultimately may act as the major cause of tooth loss by root fracture [68, 77–79]. From an epidemiological perspective, root fracture is more prevalent in endodontically treated teeth [68, 77–79], an evidence that makes room for a counter theorization toward dentin preservation as a token for reducing the fracture rate, the so-called Minimally Invasive Endodontics (MIE) concept [66, 68, 80, 81]. The rationale behind it is quite simple: by reducing the amount of removed dentin, it is plausible that teeth become less brittle, consequently reducing the fracture rate. Nonetheless, a relevant question arises: how much would it be possible to reduce the biological cost (dental tissue removal) without hashing the benefits (disinfection and apical healing)? There is no simple answer for that, but a straightforward thought would believe that if being more aggressive does not increase the benefit of the therapy proportionally, the contrary would be also valid, i.e., being less aggressive may not consistently reduce the biological cost (fracture rate).

Most of clinicians that advocated MIE support their argument on saving dentin without giving much attention to disinfection control. It happens because the metrics of disinfection is surrogated by the achievement of specific technical landmarks giving the false impression of an adequate disinfection. In other words, dentists judge much higher risk of healing failure if the root canal filling is too short from the apex, than if the preparation is parallel, non-tapered, and narrow. Since the technological advancements in instruments allow the clinicians to reliably reach and fill the root canals up to the apex even under extremely conservative access cavities, the discussion on disinfection control is shaded. In this sense, the interplay between the argument of reducing the fracture risk of endodontically treated teeth, the current relative easiness to obtain certain technical parameters, and the blindness to an infection control, result in the rationale that day-after-day is backing up the MIE concept. However, treating infected teeth demands a clinical decision based on the best cost–benefit balance for infection control. Therefore, considering the current available concepts in endodontology, three treatment options can be drawn based on the asymmetrical principle [73], a concept in which the clinical evidence is balanced with plausibility evidence (given by in vitro studies) under a cost–benefit rationale (Table 8.5). From this table, it can depict that the MIE approach presents the weakest level of evidence coming from in vitro research with negative results for both cost and benefit [82–88], which means that nowadays MIE is not grounded on solid evidence.

Nevertheless, even though no randomized study has been published yet, several cases treated under the MIE concept are popping up in the social media and dental meetings demonstrating, by radiographic or even tomographic images, healed lesions in infected cases. As healing is possible to be considered in individual cases, it remains to be investigated whether these positive results are prevalent in the population, not only by providing similar or superior apical healing rates, but also on

Table 8.5 Cost–benefit for an evidence-based decision toward access preparation and root canal enlargement

	Treatment A Conservative	Treatment B Standard	Treatment C Aggressive
Preparation technique	Conservative or ultraconservative access cavity and an apical final size below 25, taper 0.02	Straight-line access cavity and apical final size 25 taper 0.04 or 0.06	Straight-line access cavity and apical final size 30 (or more) and taper 0.06 or 0.08
Cost (dentin removal, fracture resistance)	Similar dentin removal to standard (in vitro) [82] No superior fracture resistance in some tooth (in vitro) [82–84, 86, 87] No clinical data	Lower fracture resistance than no treatment (in vitro) [82–84, 86, 87] Observational data suggesting association of endodontic treatment and fracture rate [240]	More dentin removed and lower fracture resistance (in vitro) [87] No clinical data for fracture rate
Benefit (disinfection, healing rate)	Compromised disinfection (in vitro) [83, 85, 88] No clinical data	Superior disinfection than conservative (in vitro) [83, 85, 88] Longitudinal data on success rate over 75% [241]	Superior disinfection than standard (in vitro) [74, 75] Similar healing rate than standard [76]
Overall quality of evidence	Weak (negative in vitro effect for cost and benefit)	Strong (negative observational for cost and positive clinical for benefit)	Moderate (negative in vitro for cost and similar clinical for benefit)

reducing the fracture rate of endodontically treated teeth compared to standard and/or more aggressive treatments. It is crux that the MIE approach passes through the populational validation, otherwise its clinical application is inadequate. A usual mistake is to think that until there is no negative clinical proof of a new technique, it can be freely used and advocated. In science, however, the burden of the proof is to demonstrate efficacy (benefit). The inexistence of such effect is the basal concept given by the null hypothesis in a scientific study [89]. The science is not responsible to demonstrate that a treatment does not work, which would be considered the reversal of the burden of the proof, i.e., people advocating the treatment, while scientists try to disproof it. While the positive effect of a therapy is not demonstrated, the uncertainty about the treatment remains, leaving no room for its promotion. Another important point is that the MIE rationale is primarily grounded on the biological cost reduction (less dentin removed) and secondarily on the benefit (no reduction in disinfection ability) [81]. Placing cost prior to the benefit is not uncommon in the health field, even though it is wrong from a scientific perspective. First, a technique should prove its benefit; further comes the safety. One shall not propose a technique based only on its safeness or biological cost reduction, as it makes little sense. Imagine, for instance, to reduce the dose of a drug focusing on reducing its side effects. The therapy may become useless if this reduction compromises the benefit. That is the case for MIE, mostly considering that no significant increase in fracture resistance of teeth was reported so far in most of in vitro assays [90].

The inception of MIE [68] follows the natural footsteps of medical care that has massively moved toward minimally invasive treatments based on the wake of the strong advancements in the field of microsystems engineering, required to miniaturize high-tech devices, as well as, nanotechnology and high-resolution imaging tools for diagnostics and guidance of surgical instruments. It resulted in an unprecedent improvement in the capacity to access difficult-to-reach areas of the human body while reducing the injury to adjacent tissues and the surgical risks involved while, at the same time, improving the healing rate [91]. Several surgical protocols have moved from standard open access into minimally invasive techniques and currently became the gold standard in many areas [92–95]. Interestingly, for instance, the minimal invasion provided by laparoscopic-guided surgeries in medicine does not compromise the visual accuracy and accessibility to the operated area. Instead, the use of micro-systems, miniaturized cameras, and microtools provide a full adequate vision and access to the operative field (Fig. 8.18). This is a typical example where the biological cost is reduced without hashing the benefit or compromising the professional ability to adequately execute the procedure. Opposite to that, in MIE, an immediate consequence of reduced access cavities is a significant drop in the intra-canal visualization and location. No wonder literature points to various negative effects of MIE related to canal orifice location, iatrogenic deviations, instrument fractures, and tooth discoloration as consequences of over-contracted access preparations [90].

Undeniably, performing endodontic treatment through reduced cavities is densely dependent on a labor-intensive training and expanded chair time ultimately requesting a longer learning curve, which, from an educational standpoint, seems unwise considering the risk of potentially raising the incidence of procedural

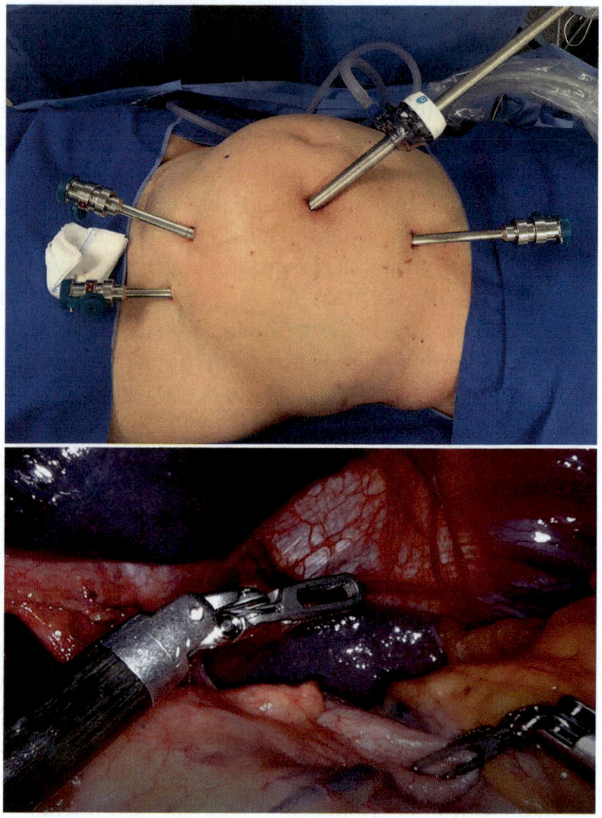

Fig. 8.18 External (top) and internal (bottom) views of an abdominal laparoscopic surgery illustrating that, although the abdominal incision is conservative, following the minimally invasive concept, the internal visualization of the operation field is fully granted and not compromised by the constricted access (Courtesy of Dr. Roclides Castro de Lima, Brazil), which contrasts with the minimally invasive access cavities in endodontics, as the visualization of the pulp chamber and canals location is invariably compromised

accidents and complications with no significant increase in tooth strengthening. These consistently place MIE in the opposite side compared to minimally invasive treatments in the medical field.

8.4.4 Cleaning and Shaping or Shaping for Cleaning?

Root canal preparation is considered the most important step of the endodontic treatment and is achieved simultaneously by the mechanical action of instruments and the mechanical and chemical effects of irrigation [37]. This procedure is of utmost importance for cleaning and disinfection, because instruments and irrigants act primarily in the main canal. Numerous studies have shown that instrumentation and irrigation are highly effective in reducing the intracanal bacterial populations [96–102]. Clinical [97, 103] and in vitro studies [104–106] have clearly demonstrated that (1) preparation using an antibacterial irrigating solution, such as NaOCl, significantly enhances disinfection compared with irrigation with saline or water; (2) most canals instrumented and irrigated with 2.5% NaOCl have the number of bacteria reduced 102- to 105-fold, resulting in an overall reduction of bacterial counts of 95–99% [104,

107–109]; (3) regular exchange and the use of large volumes of irrigants should maintain the optimum antibacterial effectiveness of the NaOCl solution, compensating for the effects of concentration [104]; and (4) the beneficial effects of using NaOCl when compared to saline are only observed after significant apical enlargement [97, 103]. Additionally, other studies support that supplementary irrigation methods, such as laser- or ultrasonic-activated irrigation and positive-pressure pulsed-delivery systems, perform better than syringe irrigation in the removal of dentin debris or soft-tissue remnants from fins and non-instrumented oval extensions; however the relative effectiveness of each method in terms of prognosis is still unclear [110].

Regarding the anatomy, accessory canals and dentinal tubules present similar challenges for root canal irrigation but at a different length scale [110]. Accessory canals (10–200 μm) are perceived to be smaller than the main canal but larger than dentinal tubules (0.5–3.2 μm) [111]. Irrigant flow in accessory canals and dentinal tubules is driven by the flow in the main canal and appears to be limited to a depth that is approximately twice their diameter, whereas diffusion dominates irrigant transport beyond that point. Therefore, optimum irrigant refreshment in the main canal to maintain a favorable concentration gradient, any increase in the temperature of the irrigants, and a longer application period could enhance particle transport. The disinfection of accessory canals are influenced by irrigants and antiseptics and only in rare instances will the outcome of the treatment depend on whether an accessory canal is actually obturated or not [110]. This is the case even if an endodontic lesion clearly originates from a lateral root canal. If adequate chemomechanical instrumentation and disinfection are carried out and the main root canal is filled, the lateral periodontitis will heal even if the lateral canal is not filled [36]. Nevertheless, the importance of cleaning accessory canal and the whole length of dentinal tubules for the success of root canal treatment is still a matter of debate.

Despite the optimal antibacterial effect obtained by chemomechanical preparation, clinical bacteriologic studies have demonstrated that 30–60% of previously infected root canals still have detectable levels of bacteria after instrumentation [37]. The main reasons for bacteria to persist after chemomechanical procedures is that they are resistant to treatment or they are unaffected by instruments/irrigants. Although some microorganisms have been shown to be resistant to some endodontic antimicrobial agents, resistance to both debridement and irrigant solution is highly unlikely to occur. Bacteria usually survive after treatment procedures not because they are more resistant but because they were not affected by instruments and irrigants. Bacteria remain unaffected because treatment was inadequately carried out (small instrumentation, too short of the apex, poor irrigation, etc.) or because bacteria were located in difficult-to-reach anatomic areas. In fact, the latter is the main reason for bacterial persistence even after diligent endodontic treatment. Canals that are flattened or oval-shaped are often not properly cleaned and disinfected by current hand or mechanical instrumentation even using reaming motion. Recesses are commonly left untouched at the extremities of the largest diameter of the canal. In addition to harboring remnants of pulp tissue or bacterial biofilms, such recesses may also be packed with dentin chips generated and pushed therein by mechanical instruments. Packed debris can interfere with the quality of the canal filling and, in infected root canals, can harbor bacteria to serve as a potential source of persistent infection. In recent years, instruments with different asymmetrical designs and concepts have been devised to deal with oval and flattened canals [37]; however, so far, improvements in the mechanical preparation have not been so significant. In summary, anatomic complexities represent physical constraints that pose a serious challenge to adequate disinfection. The main root canal lumen and minor anatomic irregularities are usually incorporated into preparation and affected by the irrigant solution, but bacteria and organic tissue may remain in areas not reached by instruments and irrigants [112–116]. Unaffected areas include root canal walls untouched by instruments, recesses, dentinal tubules, isthmuses, lateral canals, and apical ramifications [47, 114, 116–121]. These areas are usually not affected because of the inherent physical limitations of instruments and the short retention time of irrigants within the root canal. If bacterial biofilms remain in untouched and unaffected canal areas, the treatment outcome is put at risk [122].

Regarding the main question in this subsection (cleaning and shaping or Shaping for Cleaning?), it is important to highlight that the concept of cleaning and shaping in endodontics was introduced by Schilder in his classic article of 1974 [123] and refers to the removal of all organic substrate from the root canal system together with the development of a purposeful form within each canal for the reception of a dense and permanent filling, based on specific mechanical objectives that can be summarized as: root canal preparation should develop a continuously tapering cone, decreasing its cross-sectional diameters at every point apically and increasing at each point as the access cavity is approached, i.e., in multiple planes, without transportation of the foramen and keeping the apical opening as small as possible. This concept has influenced many dental schools worldwide and it is still applied by several clinicians. However, with the development of new instruments and techniques, the dynamic of root canal preparation has changed completely. Nowadays, with rotary and reciprocating flexible NiTi systems, it is possible to mechanically prepare even complex anatomies in a relatively safe and fast way, following all of Schilder's recommendations. This means that root canal treatment can be properly done in a single short-time session, which is great for both clinicians and patients. On the other hand, in the presence of infection, fast sessions may also become a problem since the retention time of the irrigant solution within the anatomical complexities of the root canal system may not be adequate to provide a proper disinfection. To overcome this limitation, several adjunctive steps or supplementary procedures have been recommended to be applied during and after the mechanical preparation with these mechanical systems. Based on these assumptions, in modern endodontic treatment, it would be more appropriate to change the classical concept of "cleaning and shaping" to "Shaping for Cleaning", as proposed in this book.

8.4.5 3D or 4D Canal Filling?

The ultimate objective of endodontic treatment is to fill the root canal space after it has been completely shaped, cleaned, and disinfected. In modern endodontic treatment, strong emphasis has been placed on the root canal shaping and cleaning rather than filling. Although this does not mean that filling is less important, the success rate of endodontic treatment is mostly dependent on the proper chemomechanical preparation of the root canal system. In the past, attention has been focused on the importance of obtaining a hermetic seal using 3D filling techniques. This statement, however, is based on two misconceptions. The first one is related to the term "hermetic." In science, a hermetic seal ensures a perfect waterproofing, allowing no air to escape or pass through, which, as we know, it is impossible to achieve considering that humans do not live in an air-free environment and 60% of the adult body is made of water. The second is the so-called 3D filling. In endodontics, this term has been used for a long time as part of everyday practice, but its real definition has been missed throughout the years. The term three-dimensional is related to the three spatial dimensions, i.e., length, width, and height. Thus, whether the canal filling is well performed or not, this procedure in the real world is always in the three dimensions. More recently, clinicians in social networks and meeting are replacing the classic 3D filling proposal with the '4D filling' concept, based on the idea that the mechanics behind this procedure can be viewed as operating not only in the three spatial dimensions (length, width, and height), but also in an extra fourth dimension, that is time. Sadly, this is another marketing strategy used to sell products and courses, as time is also part of the world we are living in.

For several years, filling techniques and the apical level of filling procedures have been considered significant outcome predictors of the endodontic treatment. However, it is important to understand that a short or long root filling, for instance, may be related to an unsatisfactory preparation or an apical canal blockage, which, ultimately, can compromise the treatment outcome, mostly when considering an infected canal. Thus, in terms of underfilling or overfilling, a distinction should be made between adequate/inadequate instrumentation/disinfection and its apical level. The former has a better outcome than the latter because of the elimination of intracanal bacteria. Another important condition that may compromise treatment outcome is an inadequate filling with voids, which would allow leakage of oral bacteria to reach the periapical tissues over time, and the presence of separated instrument or root perforation, which prevent an adequate sealing of the canal space, thus failing to achieve the effective elimination of bacteria [49].

In terms of filling techniques, the literature basically reports on cold or warm methods. The latter has been recommended in the presence of canal irregularities, being particularly useful in the presence of internal resorption, C-shaped canals, isthmuses, fins, or webs. Nonetheless, with the advent of single-file systems with tapered instruments for root canal preparation, a cold filling technique using only one gutta-percha point of matching taper and a sealer, the so-called single-cone technique, has also emerged. In canals with fewer irregularities, this technique has a clear advantage of simplicity and efficiency, mostly when associated with non-soluble sealers. In the last years, with the introduction of calcium silicate-based sealers or bioceramics, manufacturers have recommended the use of single-cone technique even in canals with anatomical complexities, mostly because of their high flowability. But the main disadvantage of the majority of current brands is their high solubility. So, it is still unknown whether tissue fluids may leach out of the sealer over time, compromising the treatment outcome, as lately reported with regard to the Resilon-based filling system [124, 125]. So this remains an issue to be solved with time.

8.5 Dealing with Complex Cases

Anomalous roots and canal morphologies can be found associated to any tooth in variable degrees and frequency in human dentition. Dental anomalies are formative defects caused by genetic disturbances during the morphogenesis of teeth. Anomalies may occur during the developmental stages of the tooth, which are manifested clinically later in life once the tooth is fully formed. Clinical management of complex canal anatomies is a challenging procedure that depends on special armamentarium, individual proficiency to master specific techniques and technological devices and, sometimes, multiple appointments. Once an anomaly is identified preoperatively, another challenging step must be made toward properly negotiating the canal anatomy. Obviously, some canal anatomies are more challenging than others, such as the presence of multiple canals in a single root and, in these cases, dealing with such complexities also increases the risk of iatrogenic events. Therefore, these situations must be studied preoperatively and should include root length and thickness, curvature, calcification, number of roots and canals, accessibility of the tooth, patient cooperation, canal diameter, root concavities (grooves), isthmuses, periodontal status, restorability, among others. Once these anatomical and clinical issues are considered, a multitude of possible scenarios can be made, and a proper treatment planned. Failure to diagnose teeth with an anomalous anatomy may lead to misdiagnosis and a treatment plan that could cause permanent irreversible damage and loss of the tooth. Thus, clinicians must be aware of the existence of these anatomical complexities in order to implement an appropriate treatment plan. Major anomalies that usually affect the endodontic practice include root curvature, narrow roots, C-shaped canals, taurodontism, extra roots (*radix*), *dens invaginatus*, and multiple canals in a single root.

8.5.1 Multiplanar Curvatures: What You See Is Not What You Get!

Preoperative knowledge of root curvature is an important factor in choosing the appropriate chemomechanical protocol to prepare the canal system. In the past, because of the physical limitations of stainless steel instruments, the common recommendation was that curved canals had to be enlarged to small apical diameters in order to avoid iatrogenic events such as zips, instrument fracture, ledges or perforations. However, the greatest problem with small preparation size is that, in the presence of infection, it may compromise the cleaning and disinfecting efficacy of chemomechanical procedures, as well as, the quality of the root canal filling. Nowadays, with advances in instrument manufacturing, design, and techniques, shaping curved canals is more predictable and safer and these iatrogenic complications are no longer a problem, except for instrument separation. Therefore, considering that curvature is one of the factors determining the difficulty of a treatment and the likelihood of iatrogenic errors, its preoperative recognition is of utmost importance [126].

Nearly all root canals are curved at the apical third, particularly in the buccolingual direction, which is not evident on standard radiography [38]. In general, curvatures may vary from gradual curvature of the entire canal, sharp curvature of the canal near the apex, or a gradual curvature of the canal with a straight apical ending. Numerous methods have been proposed to determine root canal curvature [127], but Schneider method has been the most widely used. Schneider [128] classified single-rooted permanent teeth according to the degree of curvature of the root, which was determined by first drawing a line parallel to the long axis of the canal and then a second line connecting the apical foramen to the point in the first line where the canal began to leave the long axis of the tooth. The angle formed by these two lines was the angle of curvature, and its degree was classified as straight (≤5°), moderate (10–20°), or severe (25–70°). Another method was introduced by Weine [129] and also relied on the definition of two straight lines, but it reflected the root canal curvature more accurately than Schneider's method, especially at the apical part. A third proposal, geometrically equivalent to Weine method, was introduced by Pruett et al. [130]. Its major innovation was the concurrent measurement of the radius of curvature by the superimposition of a circular arc on the curved part of the root canal [131].

In clinics, the most commonly used diagnostic method is periapical radiographs, and a combination of the Schneider angle, the radius and length of the curve has been recommended to provide a more precise estimation of the canal curvature. However, a radiograph is a two-dimensional representation of a 3D structure that usually allows visualization of curvatures only in the mesiodistal direction, a clear limitation of most techniques proposed for clinical use. On the other hand, in a laboratory research, it may be very useful. Schäfer et al. [132], for example, evaluated radiographically the curvature degree of 1,163 root canals from all groups of teeth. The degree of curvature ranged from 0° to 75° and from 0° to 69° in clinical (mesiodistal direction) and proximal (buccolingual direction) views, respectively. The highest degree of curvature was observed in the clinical view of the mesiobuccal canal of maxillary molars and in the mesial canals of mandibular molars. In several cases, the angles of proximal curvatures were higher than those of the clinical view. Additionally, a secondary curvature (S-shaped canal) was observed in 12.3% and 23.3% of the maxillary and mandibular teeth, respectively. Taken together, these results suggest that, in posterior teeth, canal curvature is almost always multiplanar, i.e., it can be observed in multiple planes and only different angled views could determine its presence, direction and severity (Figs. 8.19 and 8.20). Nowadays, limitations of the conventional radiography were overcome by CBCT imaging, which allows the visualization of the canal curvature in any plane. However, because radiography, and not CBCT, is readily available in endodontic practice, most of studies have suggested its use for the assessment of canal curvature [127].

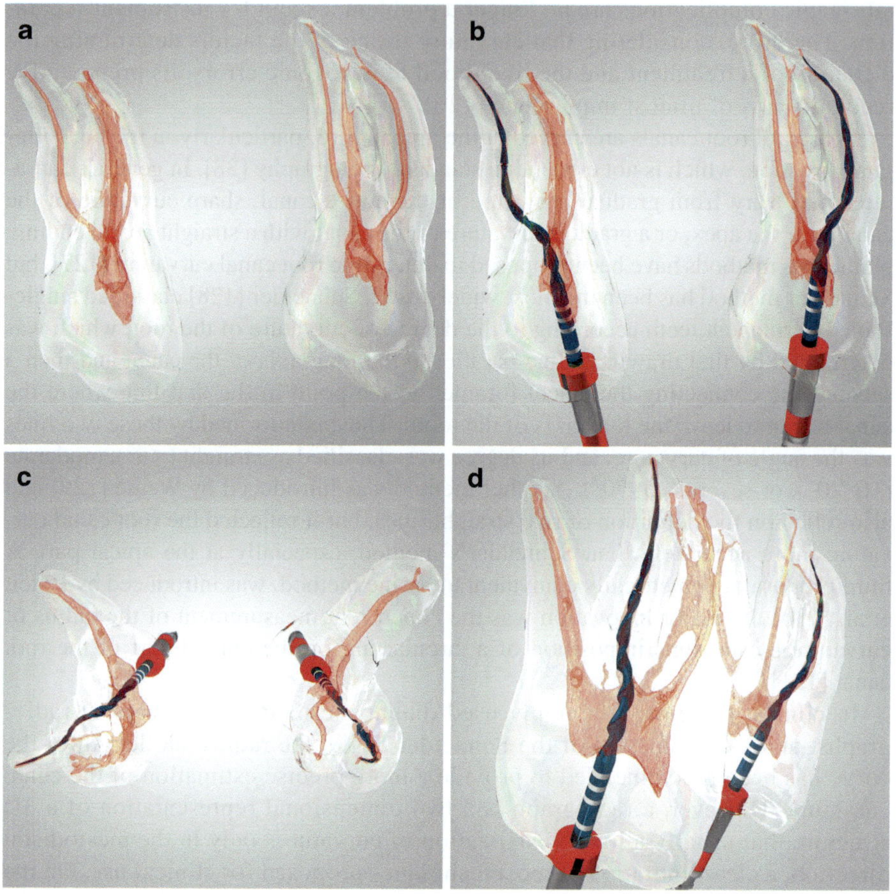

Fig. 8.19 (**a**) Transparent 3D reconstructions of two maxillary molars acquired by means of micro-CT technology in which (**b–d**) reciprocating instruments were digitally inserted into their mesial root canals to show, in different angles, the three-dimensional aspect of the canal curvature

8.5.2 Overcoming Preparation of Multiple Canals in Narrow Roots

Anatomic variations, including accessory canals and apical ramifications, isthmuses, curvatures, and oval-shaped or flattened canals, present a significant challenge for adequate cleaning and disinfection of the root canal system. In the literature, a great emphasis has been placed on the limitations of mechanical preparation of oval and flattened canals. The geometric cross-sectional shape of root canals has been classified by calculating the mean aspect ratio, defined as the ratio of the major to the minor canal diameters. The major diameter is the distance between the two most distant points of the canal in the buccolingual direction, while the minor diameter is the longest chord through the root canal that could be drawn

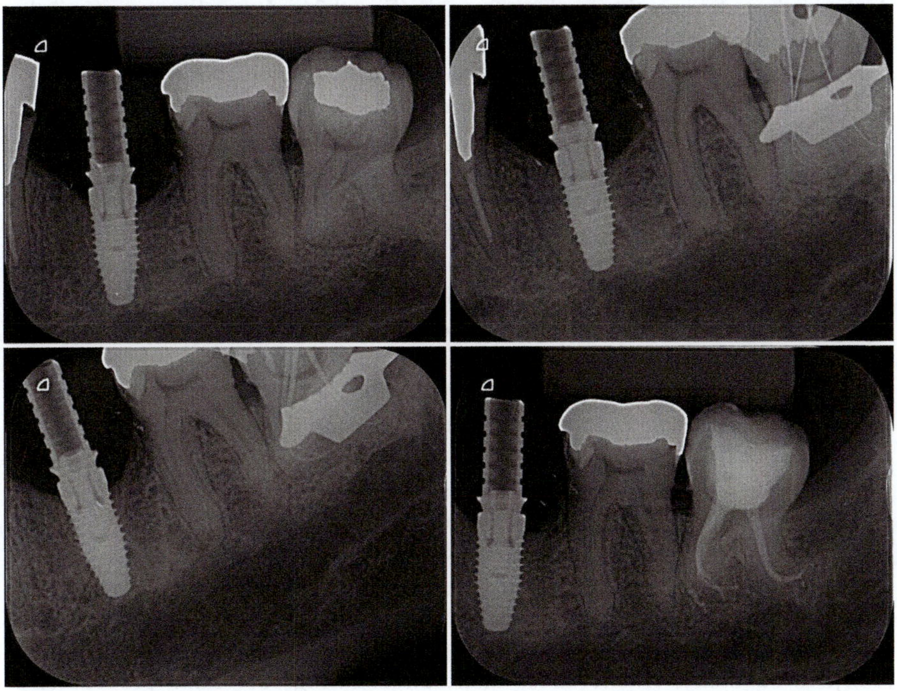

Fig. 8.20 Root canal treatment of a mandibular third left molar showing multiplanar curvatures in both mesial and distal roots. (Courtesy of Dr. Iracema Ehrhardt, Brazil)

in the orthogonal direction to that of the major diameter. Accordingly, an oval-shaped canal has an aspect ratio of between 1 and 2, a long oval canal higher than 2 but lower than 4, and a flattened canal higher than 4 [56]. This emphasis is somewhat logical given that mechanical preparation is done with rotary and/or recipro cating instruments made to cut in a round shape, and residual bacteria and debris may remain unaffected in unprepared canal walls of recesses. On the other hand, less attention has been given to the preparation of multiple canals in narrow roots. Treatment of narrow canals can be very challenging and has been associated with a high technical failure rate of 71% in the presence of pulp calcification [133]. In a retrospective prevalence study of fractured roots, Tamse et al. [134] also found that the most frequently fractured teeth were those with narrow roots (79%). Additionally, according to some authors, the roots most susceptible to fracture are those in which the mesiodistal diameter is narrow compared to the buccolingual dimension (oval, triangular, kidney-shaped, or ribbon-shaped) [135, 136] such as maxillary and mandibular premolars, mesial roots of mandibular molars, mandibular incisors, and the mesiobuccal root of maxillary molars [135].

In narrow roots with multiple canals, tissue removal and bacterial elimination become critical not only because difficulties in locating all canals but also to the fact that the overzealous canal enlargement may lead to excessive removal of dentin and predispose the tooth to fracture (Fig. 8.21). It has been reported that most vertical root fracture cases are related to teeth with roots presenting a cross-sectional mesiodistal dimension narrower than its buccolingual dimension [134, 137], indicating that this specific anatomy may be a significant risk factor that predisposes such teeth to fracture. For the same reason, vertical root fracture is among the primary causes of loss of endodontically treated mandibular molars, with extraction rates ranging from 51.8% [79] to 67% [138]. Recently, a micro-CT study [139] reported that preparation of middle mesial canals significantly reduced the fracture resistance of the mesial root of mandibular molars. Mesial roots of mandibular molars and mesiobuccal roots of maxillary molars display asymmetrical root shape in their cross section, with a deep developmental distal groove [140, 141] that commonly results in dentin thickness of 0.5–1 mm [142]. Root depression in the interproximal aspect of the mesial root of the mandibular molars and in the buccal root of the bifurcated maxillary premolar is also an anatomical entity that can lead to a predisposition to fractures and root perforations when excessive removal of dentin occurs [135]. Therefore, the increased susceptibility to fracture and perforation of narrow roots could be attributed to the combined effect of (1) reduced dentin thickness, (2) irregular canal shape, and (3) asymmetric root cross-section [143]. Additionally, it is important to note that these anatomical features can predispose narrow roots to fracture and/or perforation [134] mostly when the canals are prepared with large-tapered instruments [144]. In summary, tensile stress distribution during root canal procedures is affected by the combination of root shape and dentin thickness [143, 145]. Root

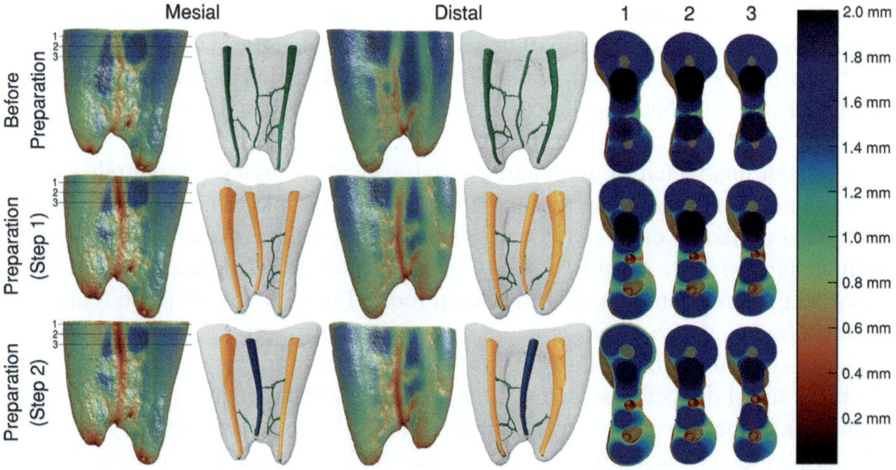

Fig. 8.21 Color-coded models of the mesial root of a mandibular molar acquired by micro-CT technology showing the dentin thickness at the furcation area (cross-sections) before and after preparation of the mesiobuccal, middle mesial, and mesiolingual canals with ProTaper Next X1 (Step 1) and X2 (Step 2) rotary instruments. Thick structures are in blue and green colors, while red color represents areas of thin dentin

canal shape, however, is the most important factor of the two since the area of reduced curvature radius (the buccal and lingual root aspects) is strongly influenced by stress concentrations, which explains the reason why roots usually fracture in a buccolingual direction and not mesiodistally, although more dentin is usually removed from the mesial and distal aspects of the root [135]. Furthermore, the mesial and distal aspects of the root are more calcified and harder than the buccolingual aspect, which is represented by the "butterfly effect" [145–147], which also explains the high prevalence of vertical root fractures in the buccolingual direction [135]. Thus, to minimize the risk of fracture, familiarity with the root anatomy and morphology is essential for appropriate instrumentation, filling, and restoration of these teeth [135], and specific approaches, including the use of low-tapered instruments and improved irrigation devices are recommended for the successful clinical management of narrow roots (Figs. 8.22, 8.23 and 8.24).

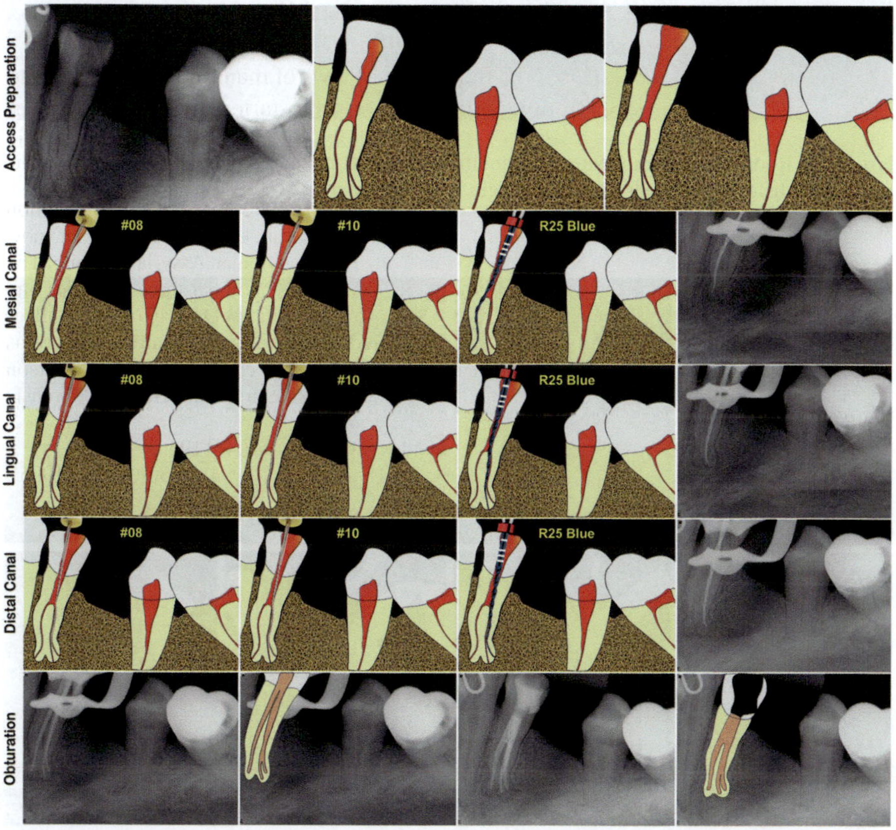

Fig. 8.22 Sequential steps for root canal treatment of a mandibular first left premolar with three root canals using hand scouting, preparation with a reciprocating instrument (Reciproc Blue R25), and single-cone filling technique. (Courtesy of Dr. José Eduardo de Mello Jr, Brazil)

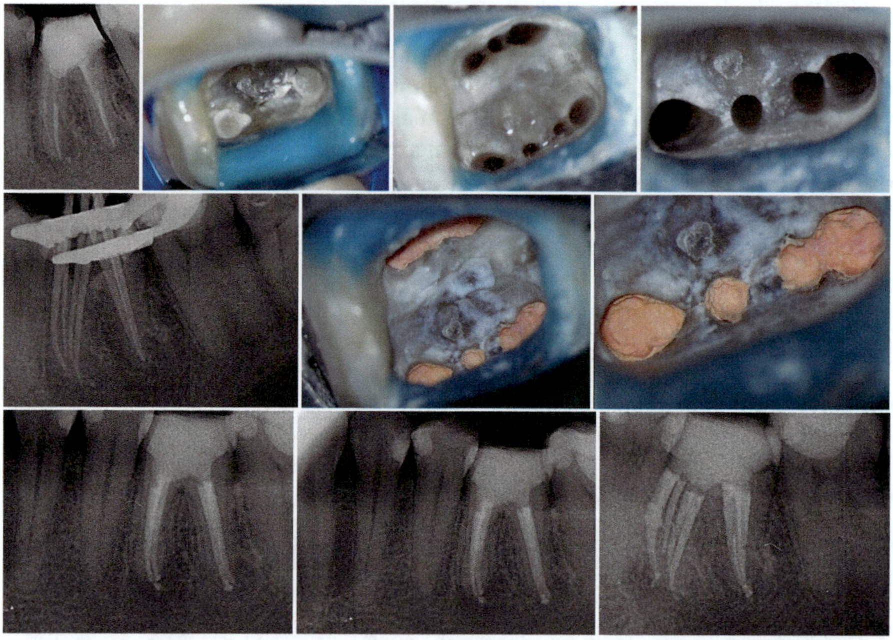

Fig. 8.23 Root canal retreatment of a mandibular first left molar having multiple canals in the mesial and distal roots. (Courtesy of Dr Sergiu Nicola, Romenia)

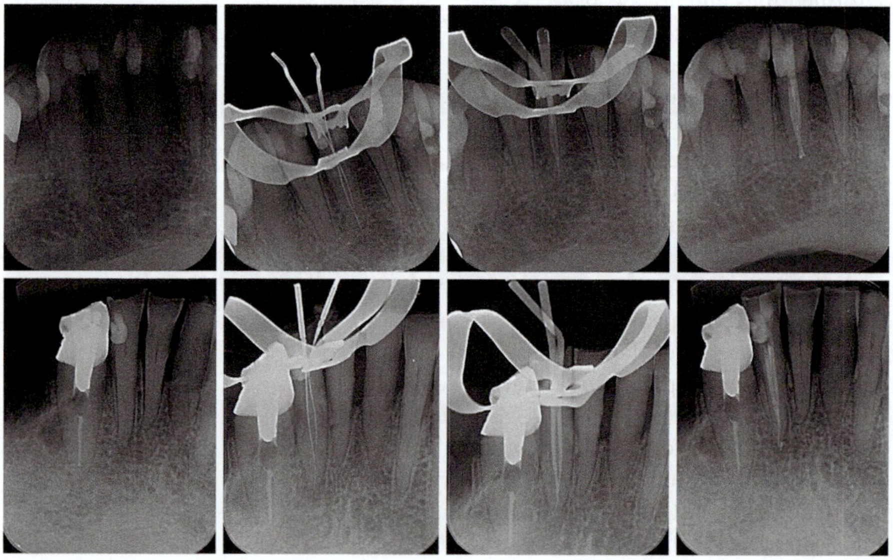

Fig. 8.24 Root canal treatment of mandibular central (top; courtesy of Dr. Iracema Ehrhardt, Brazil) and lateral (bottom; courtesy of Dr. Cristiane Prado Galdeano, Brazil) incisors having Vertucci Type II canal configuration (2-1)

8.5.3 The Challenge of C-Shaped Canal Management

The first systematic report of C-shaped configuration in the endodontic literature was done by Cooke and Cox [148], but this anatomical variation was recognized as early as the eighteenth century [149]. This anatomic variation is so named for the root and root canal cross-sectional shape of the capital letter "C." Its main anatomic feature is the presence of one or more isthmuses connecting individual canals, which can change the cross-sectional canal shape along the root. Typically, this configuration is found in teeth with fused roots either on their buccal or lingual aspect and results from the failure of Hertwig's epithelial root sheath to develop or fuse in the furcation area during the developing stage of teeth. In such teeth, the pulp chamber floor is frequently situated deeply and may assume an unusual anatomic appearance. Below the orifice level, the root structure of a C-shaped tooth can harbor a wide range of anatomic variations, which makes it a challenge with regard to disinfection. The C-shaped canal configuration may occur in different types of teeth; however, it is most commonly found in mandibular second molars, with a reported prevalence ranging from 2.7 to 44.5% [56]. There is significant ethnic variation in the frequency of C-shaped molar teeth, which are much more common in Asian than in Caucasian populations. In population-based studies, the reported prevalence was 10.6% in Saudi Arabians, 19.14% in Lebanese, 31.5% in Chinese, and 44.5% in Koreans [150]. To date, only a few studies have addressed the efficacy of different protocols in the preparation of C-shaped canals and reported a significant percentage of canal area unaffected by the mechanical procedures [151–153].

In 1991, Melton et al. [154] proposed a classification for C-shaped canals into three categories, according to the cross-sectional shape: Category I—a continuous C-shaped canal running from the pulp chamber to the apex; Category II—a semicolon-shaped orifice in which dentin separates a main C-shaped canal from one mesial distinct canal; and Category III—two or more discrete and separate canals, which could join in the apical (subdivision I), middle (subdivision II), or coronal (subdivision III) thirds. Melton's classification stated that categories II and III have separated canals, but no description was provided to differentiate them. Considering that C-shaped teeth present irregularities in their canal systems throughout the root, and these categories may vary from the pulp chamber to the apex, Fan et al. [155] modified Melton's method and recommended to classify each portion of the root using five categories: Category I—the shape is an uninterrupted "C" with no separation or division; Category II—the canal shape resembles a semicolon resulting from a discontinuation of the "C" outline; Category III—two or three separate canals; Category IV—only one round or oval canal in the cross-section (normally found near the apex); and Category V—no canal lumen (usually seen near the apex only). In this modified classification, one of the canals in Category II would appear as an arc and would be more likely to extend into the "fused" area of the root where the dentin wall may be quite thin.

C-shaped canal anatomy has been also reported in third molars, lateral incisors, mandibular first premolars, mandibular first molars, and maxillary first and second molars [150]. The prevalence of a C-shaped canal configuration in maxillary molars with fused roots was reported to be as high as 15% [156]. Mandibular first premolars also present a variety of root canal configurations that include the presence of two or three root canals and the C-shaped configuration. As in mandibular molars, C-shaped canal systems in the mandibular first premolars vary amongst different ethnic groups, with their prevalence ranging from 1 to 18% in different ethnic populations [150]. In premolars, this configuration has been strongly associated with Vertucci's type-V configuration with the presence of a groove or concavity on the external root surface (that usually begins 3 mm from the cementoenamel junction) and presents frequently on the proximal lingual area of the middle root, not always extending to the root apex [157–159] (Figs. 8.25 and 8.26).

Preoperative diagnosis of C-shaped canals is complex, mainly because these unique anatomic features are not easily recognized on conventional radiography. With the increased use of CBCT scanning, clinicians are able to detect this variation before the endodontic treatment. Nevertheless, even when recognized, the disinfection procedure still remains a challenge, mostly because of

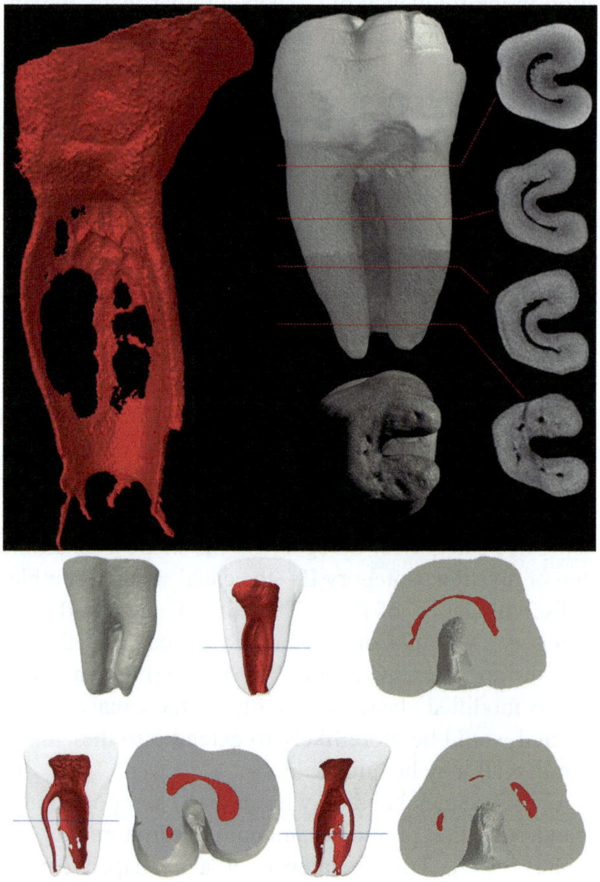

Fig. 8.25 3D models and root cross-sections of a mandibular second molar acquired by micro-CT technology showing different morphological aspects of the C-shaped canal

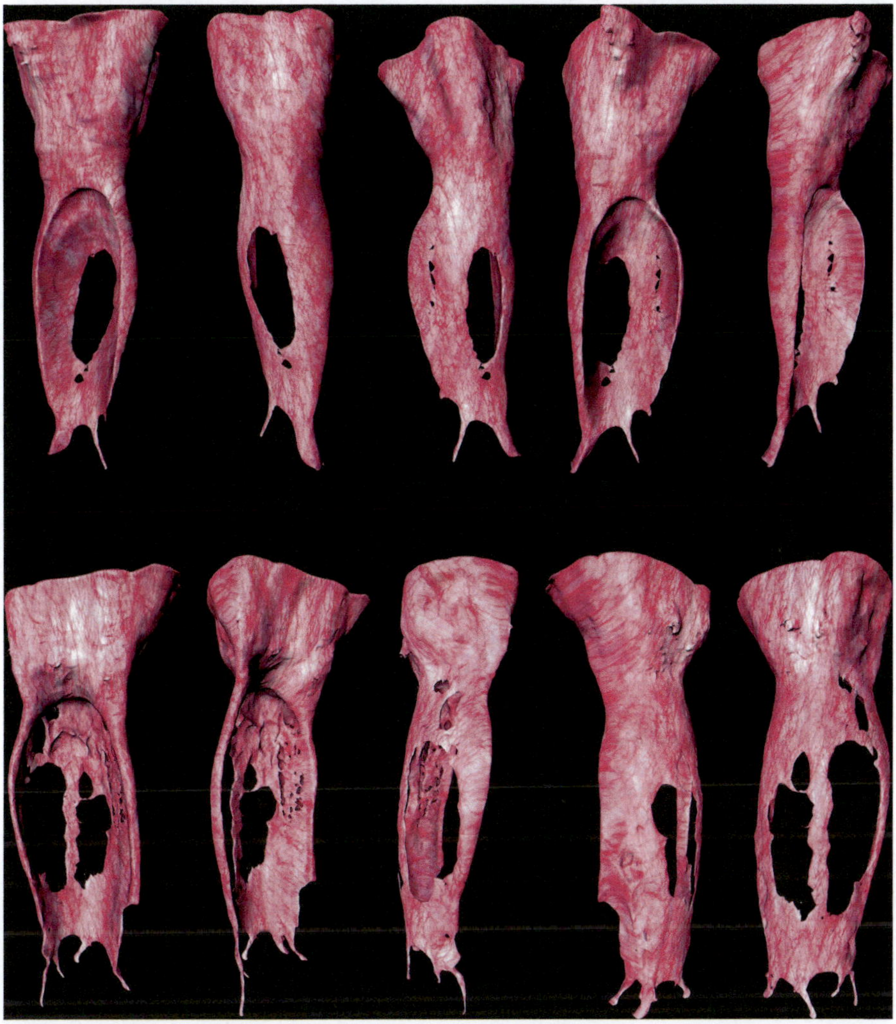

Fig. 8.26 Different views of 3D micro-CT models of the root canal system of two mandibular second molars showing the C-shaped configuration especially texturized using advanced computational graphic techniques

the thin isthmuses connecting the main canal areas. These anatomical complexities may house soft tissue remnants or infected debris that may escape thorough cleaning and may be a source of bleeding and severe pain. The use of a dental microscope associated with sonic or ultrasonic instrumentation techniques may make treatment outcome more predictable (Figs. 8.27 and 8.28). Because of its challenging morphology, the C-shaped canal anatomy increases the difficulty in root canal therapy and may account for the frequent occurrence of endodontic failure.

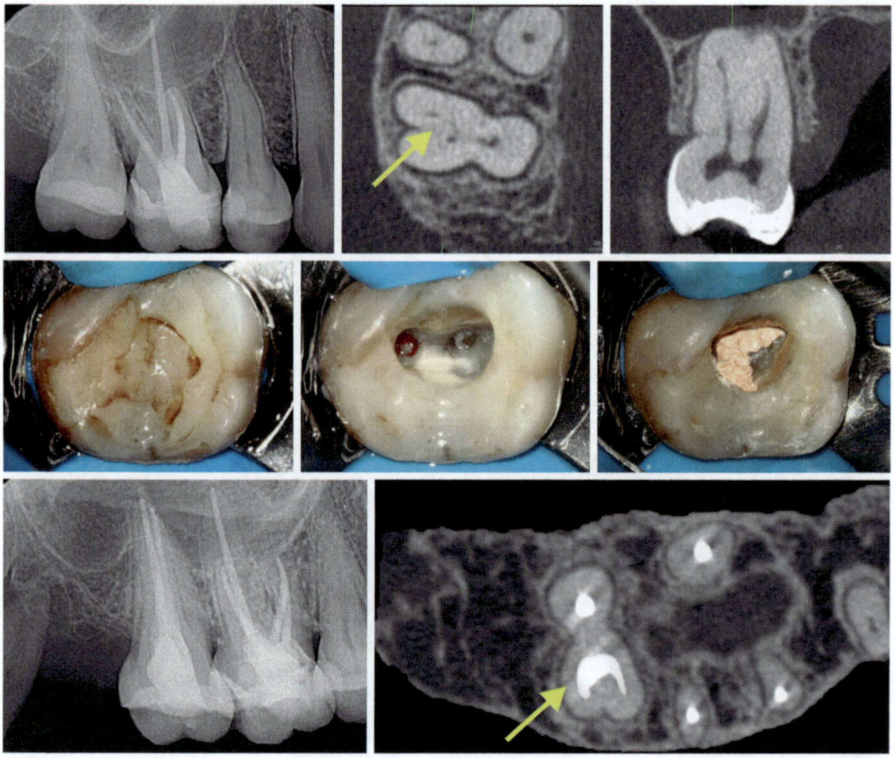

Fig. 8.27 Root canal treatment of a maxillary right second molar having a C-shaped configuration in the buccal root (arrow). (Courtesy of Dr Leandro Pereira, Brazil)

8.5.4 Taurodontism: Expanding the Pulp Chamber Size

Taurodontism is a morphologic variation in which the body of the tooth is enlarged, and the root is reduced in length. The oldest case of taurodontism was reported by Keith in 1913, as found in *Homo neanderthal* from the Krapina archeologic site [160]. A taurodont tooth presents a large pulp chamber with apical displacement of the pulpal floor and furcation of the roots. The etiology of taurodontism is still unclear, but it has been associated to certain genetic syndromes. It is thought to be caused by the failure of Hertwig's epithelial root sheath diaphragm to invaginate at the proper horizontal level, resulting in a tooth with normal dentin, short roots, elongated body, and enlarged pulp. The teeth involved are almost invariably molars or, rarely, premolars. Taurodontism can be uni- or bilateral, may affect single or multiple teeth, and was classified earlier by Shaw [161] according to its severity as normal (cynodontism), least pronounced (hypotaurodontism), moderate (mesotaurodontism), and severe (hypertaurodontism). Clinically, the crowns of these teeth usually have normal characteristics, and, therefore, the diagnosis is entirely radiologic. Owing to the complexity of the root canal anatomy and the

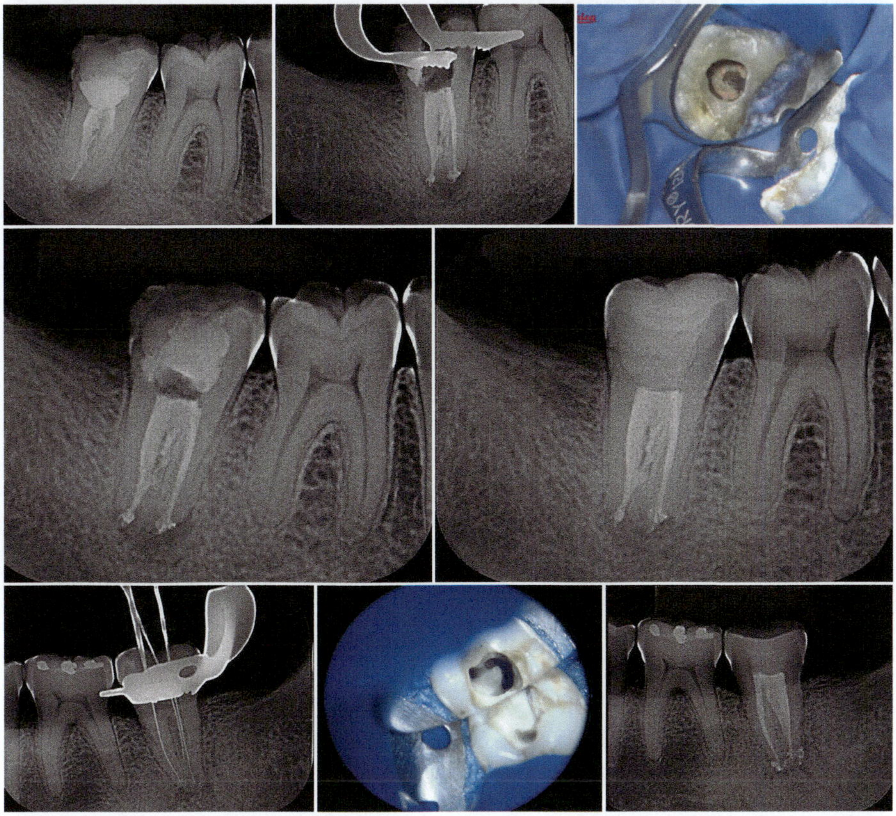

Fig. 8.28 Clinical cases showing pre-, post-operative, and follow-up images of a root canal retreatment in a mandibular second right molar (top) and (bottom) a canal treatment of a mandibular second left molar both with C-shaped canal configuration. (Courtesy of Dr. Daniel Kherlakian, Brazil)

proximity of the canal orifices to the root apex, complete filling of the apical third in taurodont teeth is challenging (Figs. 8.29 and 8.30). Because the pulp is usually voluminous, control of bleeding in cases of pulpitis may take additional time. Further efforts, such as the application of ultrasonic instrumentation combined with sodium hypochlorite (NaOCl), should be made to dissolve as much of organic materials as possible.

8.5.5 Extra Roots in Maxillary and Mandibular Molars: The Radix

Radix is a Latin word for root and refers to additional roots of teeth, mostly molars. In radix molars, each root usually contains a single root canal.

In four-rooted maxillary molars, the palatal part of the root complex is made up of two macrostructures located mesially and distally, which are in principle

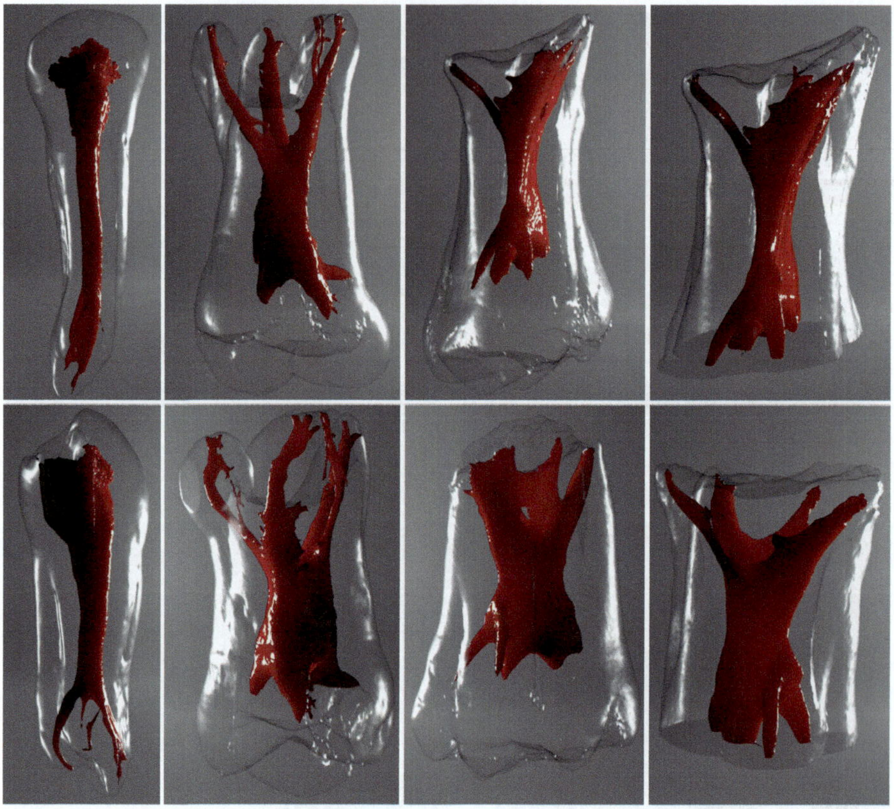

Fig. 8.29 Frontal and lateral views of 4 micro-CT 3D models of taurodont premolars and molars

cone-shaped and either separate or nonseparate in relation to each other. If the mesial of the two palatal root structures has direct affinity to the mesiolingual part of the crown, which is more pronounced, the mesial root structure is identified as *radix mesiolingualis*, whereas the distal structure is identical with the palatal root component. If the distal of the two palatal root structures has direct affinity with the distopalatal part of the crown, the distal root structure is identified as *radix distolingualis*, whereas the mesial structure is identical with the palatal root component [162] (Fig. 8.31a).

In mandibular molars, additional roots have been identified as *radix entomolaris* and *radix paramolaris*. *Radix entomolaris* has been defined as a supernumerary root located distolingually, whereas *radix paramolaris* is an extra root located mesiobuccally [163]. The presence of these anatomic anomalies has been associated with certain ethnic groups, such as Chinese, Inuit, and American Indians [164, 165]. *Radix paramolaris* is a very rare structure, and its prevalence was found to be 0%, 0.5%, and 2.0% for the mandibular first, second, and third molars, respectively, whereas *radix entomolaris* occurs with a higher frequency, ranging from 0.2 to 32% [166].

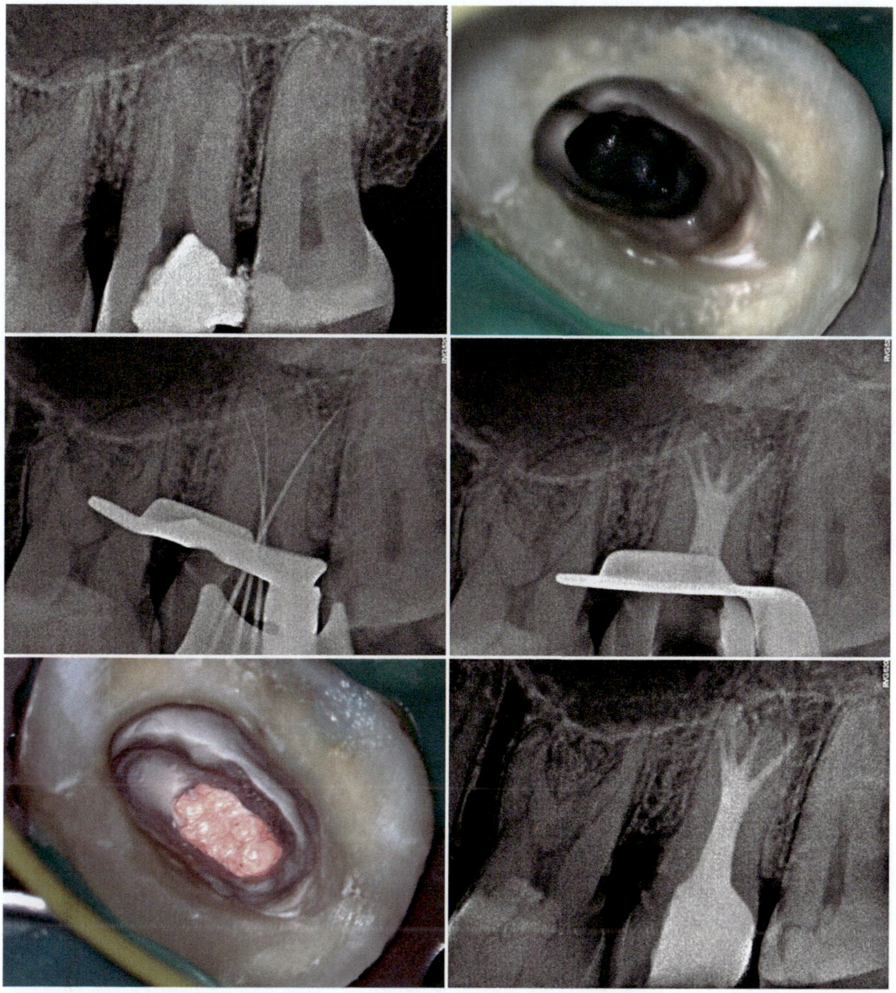

Fig. 8.30 Root canal treatment of a maxillary left second molar with hypertaurodontism. (Courtesy of Dr Jojo Kottoor, India)

The canal orifice of the *radix entomolaris* is located disto- to mesiolingually from the main canal or canals of the distal root, whereas the orifice of the *radix paramolaris* is located mesio- to distobuccally from the main mesial canals. A dark line or groove from the main root canal on the pulp chamber floor leads to these orifices. These anatomic variations are challenging because of their orifice inclination and root canal curvature (Fig. 8.31b). An accurate diagnosis of these anatomic variations is important to avoid missed canals. Therefore, preoperative periapical radiographs at different horizontal angles or a CBCT examination are required to identify this additional root. In addition, its management demands a modified access cavity (Fig. 8.32).

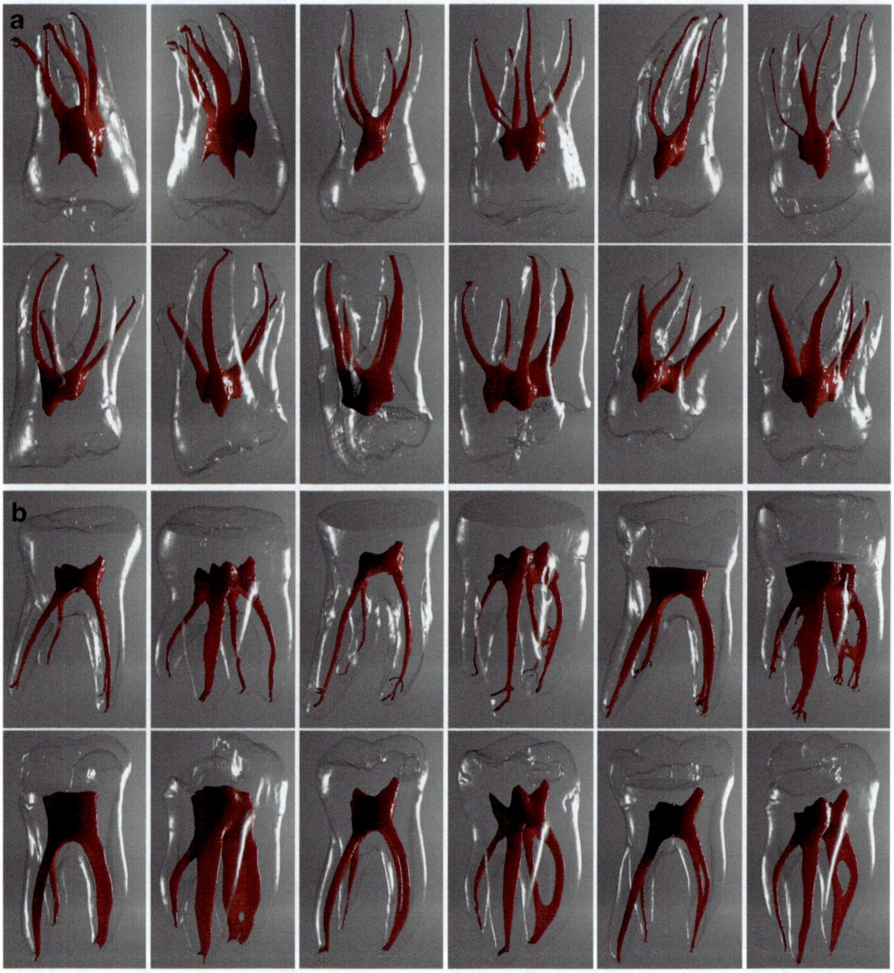

Fig. 8.31 Frontal and lateral views of 3D models acquired by micro-CT technology showing the presence of an extra root in (**a**) maxillary molars and (**b**) mandibular molars

8.5.6 The Dens Invaginatus Dilemma: Conservative and/or Surgical Approach?

Dens invaginatus, also known as *dens in dente*, dilated composite odontome, dilated odontome, gestant anomaly, invaginated odontome, dilated gestant odontome, tooth inclusion, and *dentoid in dente*, is a developmental defect resulting from invagination in the surface of the tooth crown before calcification has occurred [56]. Clinically, it may appear as an accentuation of the lingual pit in anterior teeth and, in its more severe form, gives a radiographic appearance of a tooth within a tooth, hence the term *dens in dente*. Its etiology is controversial and

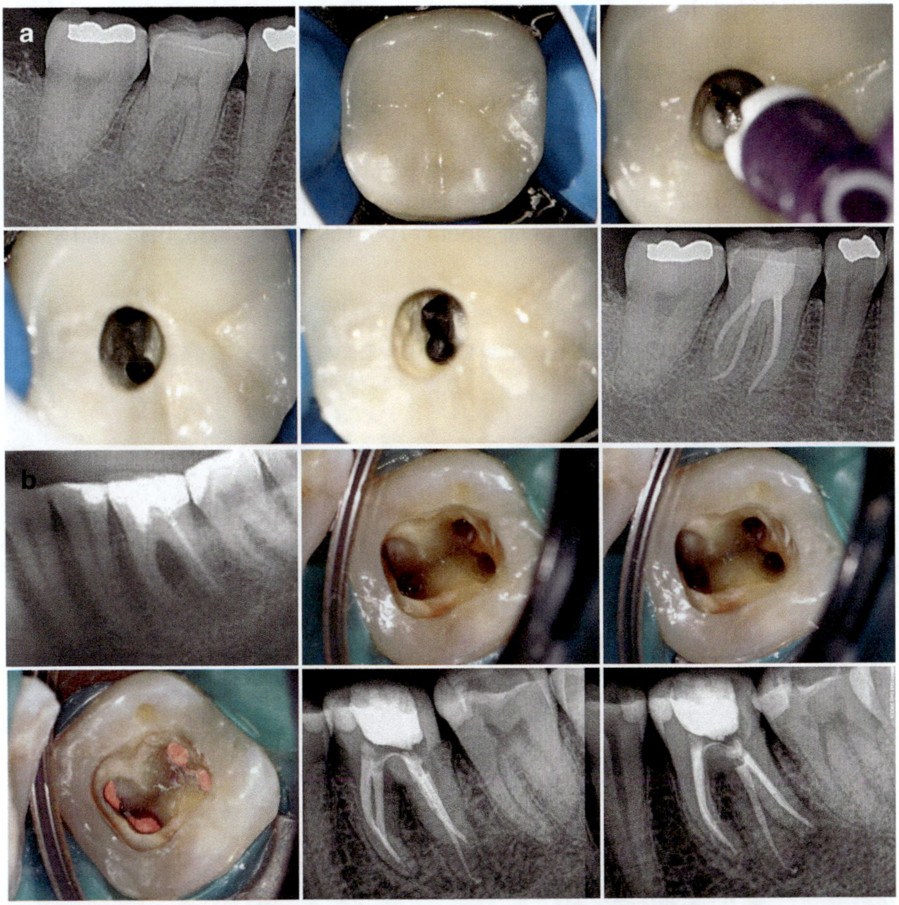

Fig. 8.32 Root canal treatment of (**a**) a mandibular first right molar (Courtesy of Dr Leandro Pereira, Brazil) and (**b**) a mandibular first left molar (Courtesy of Dr Jorge Martins, Portugal) having an extra root at the distolingual aspect of the tooth, the so-called *radix entomolarix*

remains unclear. The affected teeth radiographically show an in-folding of enamel and dentin that may extend deep into the pulp cavity and into the root and sometimes even reach the root apex. The most common associated clinical finding is an early pulpal involvement, explained by the existence of a canal extending from the invagination into the pulp. The invagination also allows the entry of irritants into an area that is separated from pulpal tissue by only a thin layer of enamel and dentin and presents a predisposition for the development of dental caries. Therefore, this condition must be recognized early and the tooth prophylactically restored. The variability of its root canal system configuration is unlimited. Clinically, however, it can only be speculated upon from radiographs. In light of this, the most commonly referred classification was proposed by Oehlers [167], who categorized this condition into three types: Type 1—the invagination is confined to the crown and does not extend beyond the CEJ; Type 2—the invagination extends past the CEJ and does not involve the peri-radicular tissues, but may communicate with the dental pulp; and Type 3—the invagination extends beyond the CEJ and may present a second apical foramen, with no immediate communication with the pulp. In the literature, the reported prevalence of this anomaly varies from 0.25% to 10%, and the most affected teeth are permanent maxillary lateral incisors, although it may occur in any tooth [168, 169] (Figs. 8.33, 8.34, and 8.35).

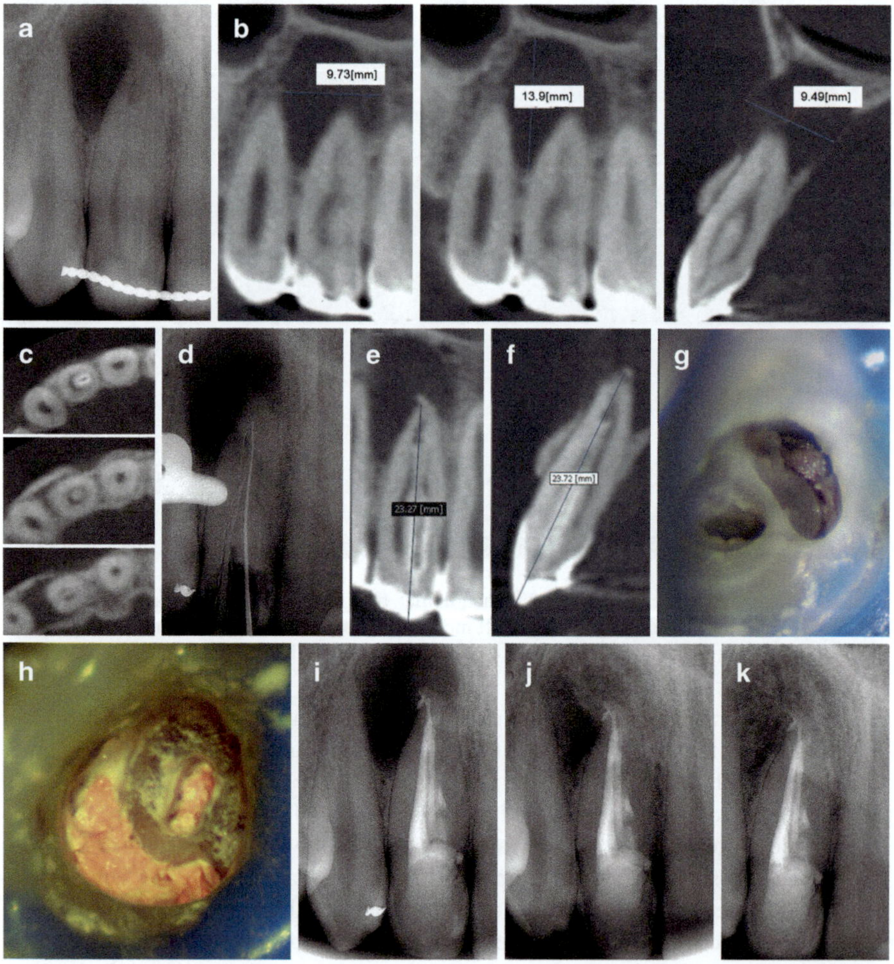

Fig. 8.33 (**a**–**j**) Radiographic, tomographic, and clinical images of the root canal treatment performed in a maxillary right lateral incisor with *dens invaginatus* Type III associated with a large periapical lesion using manual instruments and the Self-Adjusting File. (**k**) 2-year follow-up showing the repair of the apical bone. (Courtesy of Dr Michael Solomonov, Israel)

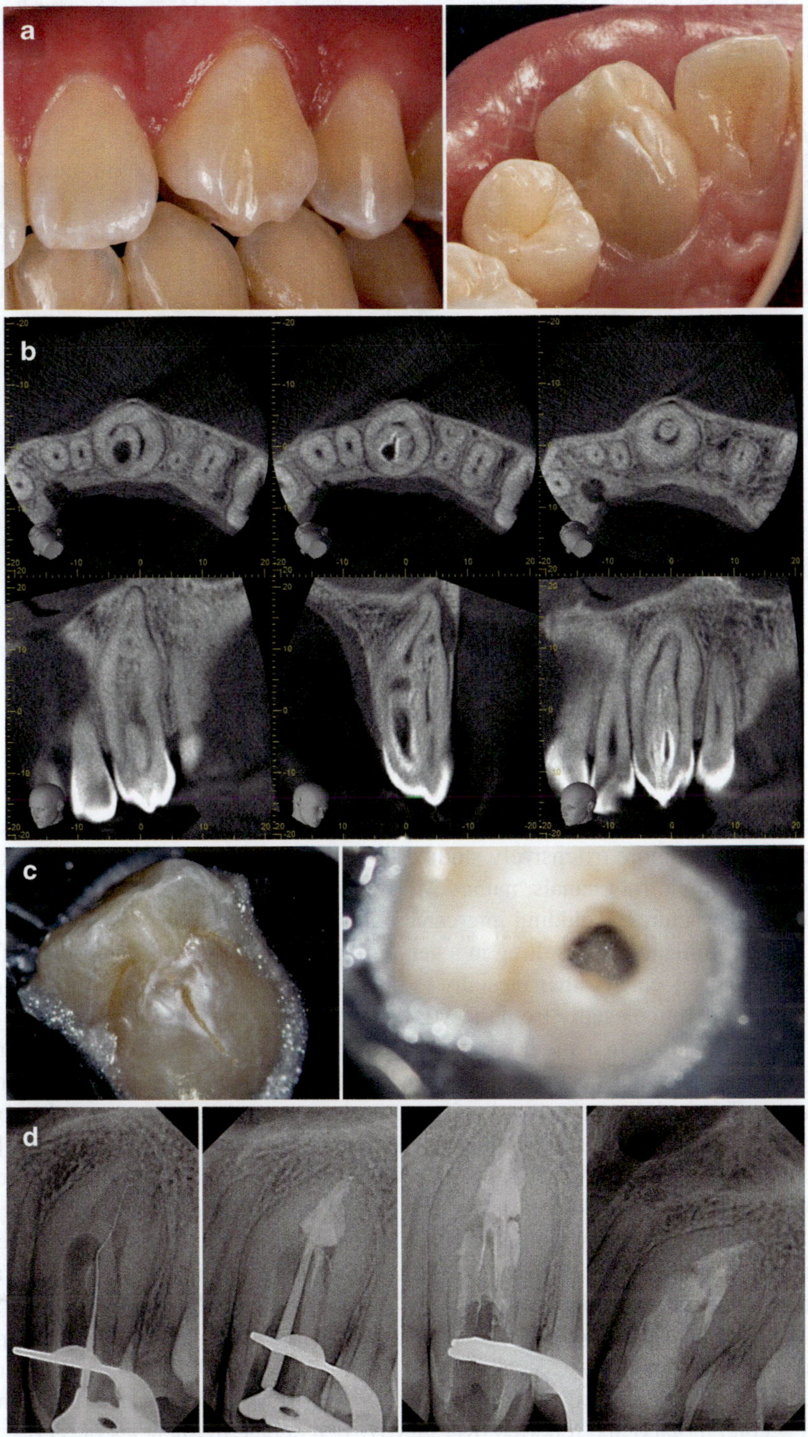

Fig. 8.34 (**a–d**) Clinical and tomographic images of the root canal treatment of a rare case of *dens invaginatus* Type III in a maxillary left canine. (Courtesy of Dr Oscar von Stetten, Germany)

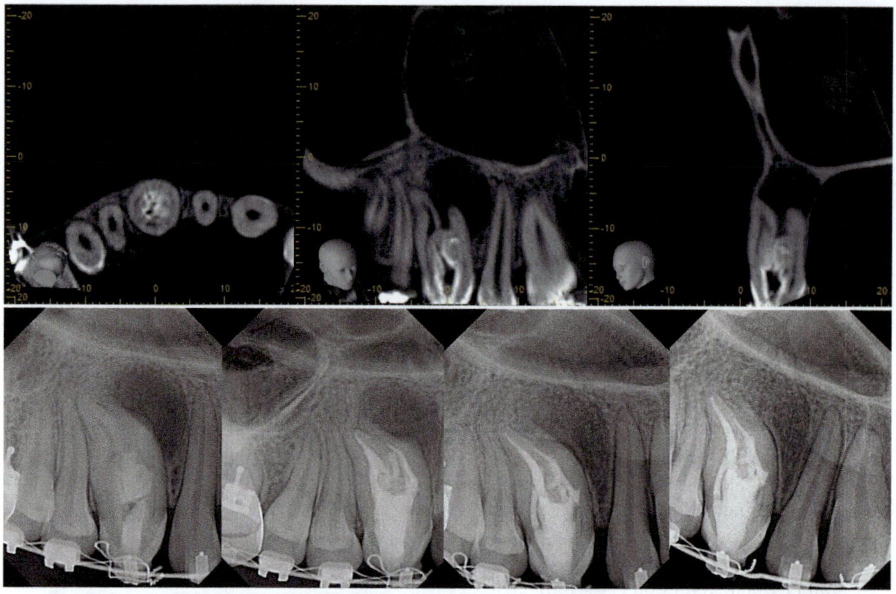

Fig. 8.35 Tomographic and radiographic images of a well succeeded root canal treatment of a rare case of *dens invaginatus* Type III in a maxillary right canine. (Courtesy of Dr Oscar von Stetten, Germany)

8.5.7 MB2 Again? Yes, But Let's Also Talk About the MB3!

In the last few decades, the morphology of the mesiobuccal (MB) root of maxillary molars has been more extensively studied than any other root. This root commonly presents two main root canals, named MB1 and MB2, and a high incidence of fine anatomical structures, including intercanal communications, loops, accessory canals and apical ramifications, resulting in a very complex canal system. The orifice of the MB2 is usually located either mesially to or in the subpulpal groove within 3.5 mm palatally and 2 mm mesially from the MB1, often hidden under the shelf of the dentin wall or calcifications in a small groove [170]. Consequently, it can be missed in routine clinical practice, especially when magnification or special lighting equipment is not used. This inability to recognize its presence and to adequately treat it has been considered the major cause of failure in root canal therapy of maxillary molars [54, 171, 172]. Clinicians, therefore, must be aware of MB2 prevalence and adopt procedural steps to locate and prepare it properly. In the literature, the percentage frequency of MB2 canal in maxillary molars has been reported to vary from 10 to 95%, depending not only on the method used in the study, such as sectioning, dye injection, radiography, scanning electron microscopy, or micro-CT, but also on ethnic and demographic factors related to the studied population, which may include geographic region, age, and gender. A recent analysis of prevalence studies using CBCT comprised data of 23,926 maxillary molars (15,285 maxillary first molars and 8,641 maxillary second molars) and reported overall MB2 percentage frequencies of 69.6% and

39.0% in maxillary first and second molars, respectively. Additionally, a meta-analysis of data demonstrated not only that males had higher odds of having MB2 canal than females in both maxillary molars, but also significant differences among geographic region, while age could not be associated with possible sources of heterogeneity [170] (Fig. 8.36a).

The impact of missed canals in the outcome of endodontic treatment has already been established in the literature and can be applied to all groups of teeth. This includes a few common anatomies such as the presence of a middle mesial canal in mandibular molars, lingual canals in mandibular incisors and mandibular premolars, and two palatal canals or the MB2 canal in the maxillary molars, but also a third root canal in the MB root of maxillary molars, the so-called MB3 [173]. The

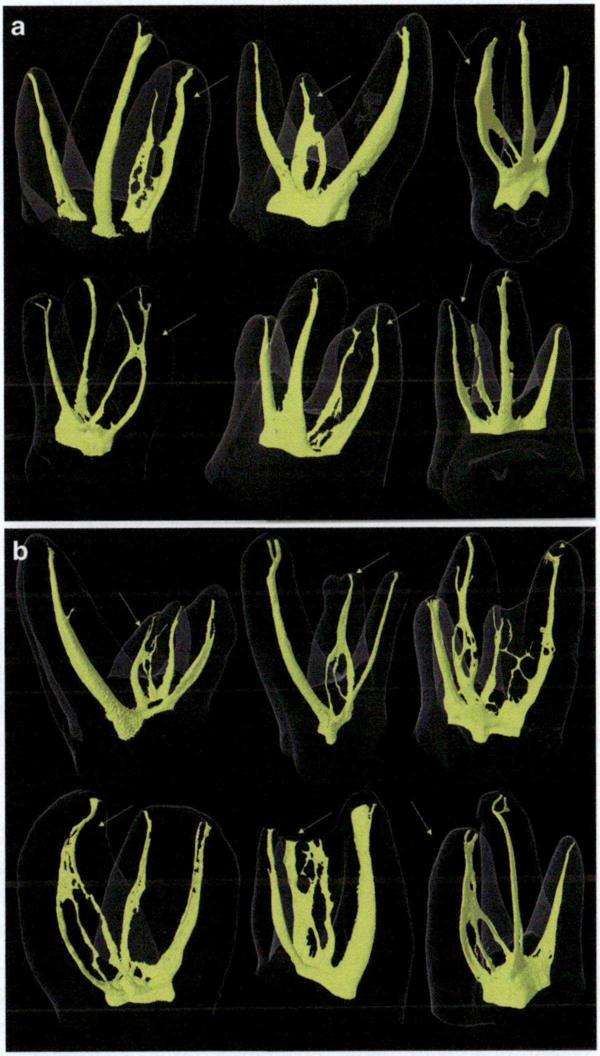

Fig. 8.36 3D models acquired by micro-CT technology showing the presence of (**a**) two or (**b**) three root canals in the mesiobuccal (MB) root of maxillary molars. These extra root canals are named as MB1, MB2, and MB3

MB3 canal can be defined as a third main root canal located in between the MB1 and MB2 main canals of the MB root of maxillary molars. As an analogy, it can be considered the middle mesial canal of the MB root of maxillary molars. Literature regarding the morphological description of the MB3 canal is scarce and most of the information comes in the form of clinical reports or incidental findings from laboratorial studies, but not as the main topic of research. A recent review of the internal anatomy of maxillary molars [174] reported a global proportion of MB3 in 0.5% of 12,200 maxillary first molars and 0.3% of 4,090 maxillary second molars. However, ex vivo studies using micro-CT imaging systems reported a higher percentage frequency of MB3 canals (4.9–10.0%) when compared with in vivo studies using the CBCT method (0.1–1.8%) or clinical studies that only inspected the pulp chamber floor (3.1%) [173]. These contradictory results can be explained by the obvious methodological differences between clinical reports and anatomical ex vivo research findings. The presence of the MB3 canal has also been related to a high complexity on the root canal system configuration, including confluent anatomy (such as isthmuses), accessory canals, and foramina (Fig. 8.36b). Furthermore, once the MB3 canal is identified in clinics, special attention is required to perform its enlargement because of the thinnest dentin thickness observed near the furcation aspect of the MB root. So, the use of less tapered instruments is recommended during its shaping (Fig. 8.37). If surgery becomes necessary, the natural anatomy of the MB root is altered, and these additional anatomic features must also be addressed. To date, it is still unclear whether the complexity of the MB3 root anatomy is being underestimated in the clinical scenario and what would be the real impact of a missed MB3 canal on the outcome of endodontic treatment.

8.6 Concluding Remarks

In daily practice, clinicians routinely face three situations when performing root canal treatment: (1) teeth with vital and irreversibly inflamed pulps; (2) teeth with necrotic pulps with or without primary apical periodontitis; and (3) retreatment cases with posttreatment apical periodontitis. In teeth with irreversible pulpitis, infection is usually restricted to the coronal parts of the canal and is easily controlled by abundant irrigation of the pulp chamber with an antimicrobial solution after access cavity preparation. In necrotic untreated or treated teeth, an infection is established in the root canal system, and, in addition to shaping and cleaning the canal, the clinician also needs to control infection. However, the outcomes of nonsurgical and surgical endodontic procedures are highly influenced by variations in canal configuration and cross-sectional shapes and by the presence of canal irregularities and curvatures. The high frequency of fins and communications between canals within the same root make it impossible for any mechanical or chemical technique to completely disinfect the root canal system. It is worth pointing out that some factors, such as physiologic aging, pathology, occlusion, and the secondary deposition of dentin, can increase these complexities, making shaping and cleaning the root canals a real challenge. Clinicians ought, therefore, to be aware of complex root canal structures, cross-sectional dimensions, and iatrogenic

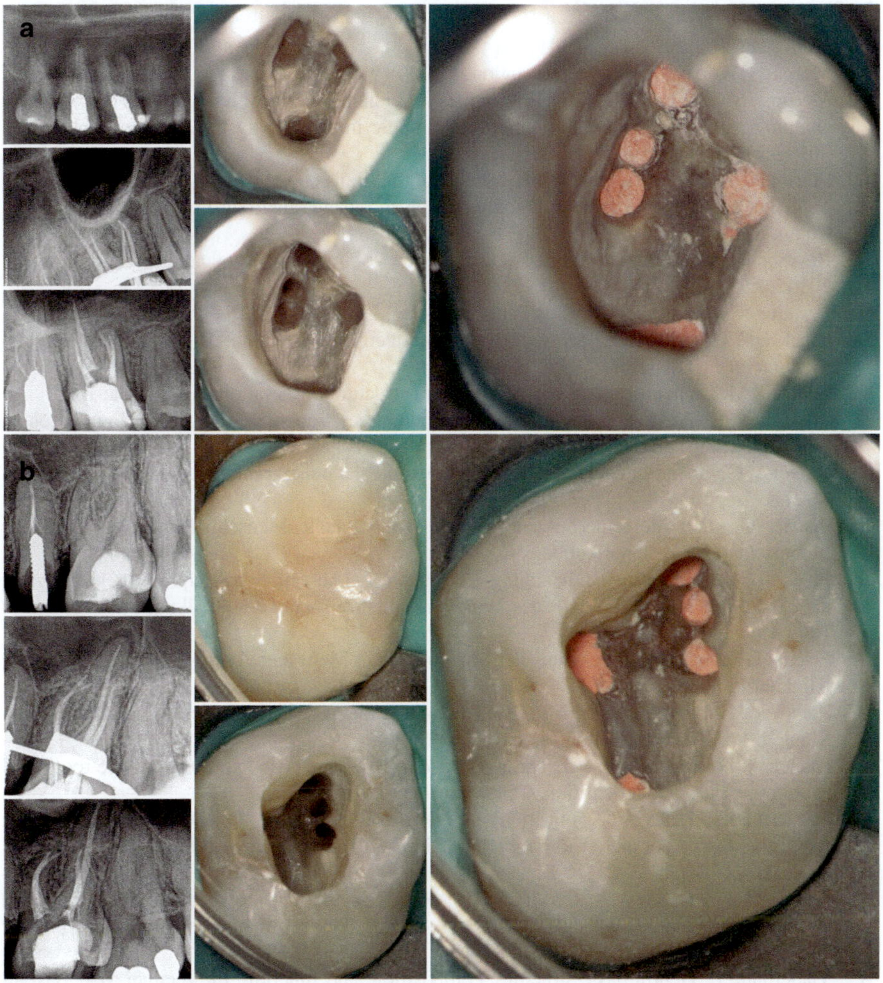

Fig. 8.37 Two clinical cases showing (**a**) the root canal retreatment of a maxillary first right molar and (**b**) the canal treatment a maxillary first left molar. These teeth had three root canals in the mesiobuccal root, the so-called MB1, MB2, and MB3. In both cases, the canals had independent orifices, but the MB3 canal merges with the other mesiobuccal canals in their trajectory to the apex. (Courtesy of Dr Jorge Martins, Portugal)

alterations of canal anatomy. It is advisable to make a careful diagnostic interpretation based on angled radiographs or tomographic examinations, proper access preparation, and a detailed inspection of the pulp chamber floor. Ideally, the search for root canal orifices should be done under magnification with high-intensity lighting, aiming to improve the treatment outcome. The successful treatment outcome will depend on how effective the clinician is in achieving these goals and the Shaping for Cleaning protocol presented in this book can be a valuable approach to overcome these challenges.

References

1. Morgan HW. Anatomy—the foundation. JADA. 1919;6:801–5.
2. Martins JNR, Marques D, Silva E, Carames J, Versiani MA. Prevalence studies on root canal anatomy using cone-beam computed tomographic imaging: a systematic review. J Endod. 2019;45:372–86.e4.
3. Perrini N, Versiani MA. Historical overview of the studies on root canal anatomy. In: Versiani MA, Basrani B, Sousa Neto MD, editors. The root canal anatomy in permanent dentition. Cham: Springer; 2018. p. 3–16.
4. Reveron RR. Herophilus and Erasistratus, pioneers of human anatomical dissection. Vesalius. 2014;20:55–8.
5. Vesalius A. De Humani Corporis Fabrica Basilea: Libri Septem; 1543.
6. Black GV. Descriptive anatomy of the human teeth. Philadelphia: The Wilmington Dental Manufacturing Co.; 1890.
7. Fraenkel M. De penitiori dentium humanorum structura observations. Bratislava; 1835.
8. Mühlreiter E. Anatomie des menschlichen Gebisses von med. Th. E. de Jonge Cohen. Leipzig: Arthur Felix; 1870.
9. Witzel A. Compendium der pathologie und therapie der pulpakrankheiten des zahnes. Hagen: Risel & Co.; 1886.
10. Fischer G. Über die feinere Anatomie der Wurzelkanäle Menschlicher Zähne. Deutsche Monatschrift fur Zahnheilkunde. 1907.
11. Fischer G. Beitrage zur Behandlung Erkrankter Zahne mit besonderer Berucksichtigung der Anatomie und Pathologie der Wurzelkanale. Deutsche Zahnheilkunde in Vortragen. 1908:4–5.
12. Fischer G. Bau und Entwickelung der Mundhohle des Menschen. Leipzig: Verlag von Werner Klinkhardt; 1909.
13. Preiswerk G. Leherbuch und Atlas der Zahnheilkunde mit Einschlu*β* der Mund-Krankheiten. Munich: J. F. Lehmann; 1903.
14. Kishen A. Foreword I. In: Versiani MA, Basrani B, Sousa Neto MD, editors. The root canal anatomy in permanent dentition. Cham: Springer; 2018. p. vii.
15. Versiani MA, Keles A. Applications of micro-CT technology in endodontics. In: Orhan K, editor. Micro-computed tomography (micro-CT) in medicine and engineering. Cham: Springer; 2020. p. 183–211.
16. Martins JN, Versiani MA. CBCT and micro-CT on the study of root canal anatomy. In: Versiani MA, Basrani B, Sousa Neto MD, editors. The root canal anatomy in permanent dentition. Cham: Springer; 2018. p. 89–180.
17. Tjäderhane L. Dentin basic structure, composition, and function. In: Versiani MA, Basrani B, Sousa Neto MD, editors. The root canal anatomy in permanent dentition. Cham: Springer; 2018. p. 17–30.
18. Ordinola-Zapata R, Versiani MA, Bramante CM. Root canal components. In: Versiani MA, Basrani B, Sousa Neto MD, editors. The root canal anatomy in permanent dentition. Cham: Springer; 2018. p. 31–46.
19. Hess W. Die pulpaamputation als selbstandige wurzelbehandlungsmethod. Leipzig: Georg Thiéme; 1917.
20. Hess W, Zürcher E. The anatomy of the root canals of the teeth of the permanent and deciduous dentitions. London: John Bale, Sons & Danielsson, Ltd.; 1925.
21. Zürcher E. Zur Anatomie der Wurzelkanale des menschliches Milchgebisses und der 6 Jahr-Molaren. Zurich; 1922.
22. Weine FS, Healey HJ, Gerstein H, Evanson L. Canal configuration in the mesiobuccal root of the maxillary first molar and its endodontic significance. Oral Surg Oral Med Oral Pathol. 1969;28:419–25.
23. Pineda F, Kuttler Y. Mesiodistal and buccolingual roentgenographic investigation of 7,275 root canals. Oral Surg Oral Med Oral Pathol. 1972;33:101–10.

24. Vertucci F, Seelig A, Gillis R. Root canal morphology of the human maxillary second premolar. Oral Surg Oral Med Oral Pathol. 1974;38:456–64.
25. Versiani MA, Ordinola-Zapata R. Root canal anatomy: implications in biofilm disinfection. In: Chavez de Paz L, Sedgley C, Kishen A, editors. Root canal biofilms. Toronto: Springer; 2015.
26. Salehrabi R, Rotstein I. Endodontic treatment outcomes in a large patient population in the USA: an epidemiological study. J Endod. 2004;30:846–50.
27. Versiani MA, Pereira MR, Pécora JD, Sousa Neto MD. Root canal anatomy of maxillary and mandibular teeth. In: Versiani MA, Basrani B, Sousa Neto MD, editors. The root canal anatomy in permanent dentition. Cham: Springer; 2018. p. 181–240.
28. Martins JNR, Marques D, Leal Silva EJN, Carames J, Mata A, Versiani MA. Influence of demographic factors on the prevalence of a second root canal in mandibular anterior teeth—a systematic review and meta-analysis of cross-sectional studies using cone beam computed tomography. Arch Oral Biol. 2020;116:104749.
29. Versiani MA, Pécora JD, Sousa-Neto MD. The anatomy of two-rooted mandibular canines determined using micro-computed tomography. Int Endod J. 2011;44:682–7.
30. Chan R, Versiani MA, Friedman S, Malkhassian G, Sousa-Neto MD, Leoni GB, et al. Efficacy of 3 supplementary irrigation protocols in the removal of hard tissue debris from the mesial root canal system of mandibular molars. J Endod. 2019;45:923–9.
31. Leoni GB, Versiani MA, Silva-Sousa YT, Bruniera JF, Pécora JD, Sousa-Neto MD. Ex vivo evaluation of four final irrigation protocols on the removal of hard-tissue debris from the mesial root canal system of mandibular first molars. Int Endod J. 2017;50:398–406.
32. Versiani MA, Alves FR, Andrade-Junior CV, Marceliano-Alves MF, Provenzano JC, Rocas IN, et al. Micro-CT evaluation of the efficacy of hard-tissue removal from the root canal and isthmus area by positive and negative pressure irrigation systems. Int Endod J. 2016;49:1079–87.
33. Keleş A, Alcin H, Sousa-Neto MD, Versiani MA. Supplementary steps for removing hard tissue debris from isthmus-containing canal systems. J Endod. 2016;42:1677–82.
34. von Arx T. Frequency and type of canal isthmuses in first molars detected by endoscopic inspection during periradicular surgery. Int Endod J. 2005;38:160–8.
35. von Arx T, Steiner RG, Tay FR. Apical surgery: endoscopic findings at the resection level of 168 consecutively treated roots. Int Endod J. 2011;44:290–302.
36. Tronstad L. Clinical endodontics: a textbook. 3rd rev. ed. Stuttgart. New York: Thieme; 2009.
37. Siqueira JF Jr, Roças IN, Ricucci D. Internal tooth anatomy and root canal instrumentation. In: Versiani MA, Basrani B, Sousa Neto MD, editors. The root canal anatomy in permanent dentition. Cham: Springer; 2018. p. 277–302.
38. Vertucci FJ. Root canal morphology and its relationship to endodontic procedures. Endod Topics. 2005;10:3–29.
39. Morfis A, Sylaras SN, Georgopoulou M, Kernani M, Prountzos F. Study of the apices of human permanent teeth with the use of a scanning electron microscope. Oral Surg Oral Med Oral Pathol. 1994;77:172–6.
40. Gutierrez JH, Aguayo P. Apical foraminal openings in human teeth. Number and location. Oral Surg Oral Med Oral Pathol Oral Radiol Endod. 1995;79:769–77.
41. Versiani MA, Ahmed HM, Sousa-Neto MD, De-Deus G, Dummer PM. Unusual deviation of the main foramen from the root apex. Braz Dent J. 2016;27:589–91.
42. Burch JG, Hulen S. The relationship of the apical foramen to the anatomic apex of the tooth root. Oral Surg Oral Med Oral Pathol. 1972;34:262–8.
43. Vertucci FJ. Root canal anatomy of the human permanent teeth. Oral Surg Oral Med Oral Pathol. 1984;58:589–99.
44. Green D. A stereomicroscopic study of the root apices of 400 maxillary and mandibular anterior teeth. Oral Surg Oral Med Oral Pathol. 1956;9:1224–32.
45. Piñeda F, Kuttler Y. Mesiodistal and buccolingual roentgenographic investigation of 7,275 root canals. Oral Surg Oral Med Oral Pathol. 1972;33:101–10.

46. Mizutani T, Ohno N, Nakamura H. Anatomical study of the root apex in the maxillary anterior teeth. J Endod. 1992;18:344–7.
47. Ricucci D, Siqueira JF Jr. Fate of the tissue in lateral canals and apical ramifications in response to pathologic conditions and treatment procedures. J Endod. 2010;36:1–15.
48. Gao X, Tay FR, Gutmann JL, Fan W, Xu T, Fan B. Micro-CT evaluation of apical delta morphologies in human teeth. Sci Rep. 2016;6:36501.
49. Chugal NM, Lin ML, Kahler B. Introduction: endodontic prognosis and outcome. In: Chugal NM, Lin ML, editors. Endodontic prognosis—clinical guide for optimal treatment outcome. Cham: Springer; 2017. p. 1–12.
50. Kvist T. Apical periodontitis in root-filled teeth. 1st ed. Cham: Springer; 2018.
51. Rosen E, Russell P, Tsesis I. Evidence-based decision making in dentistry: the endodontic perspective. In: Rosen E, Nemcovsky CE, Tsesis I, editors. Evidence-based decision making in dentistry: multidisciplinary management of the natural dentition. Cham: Springer; 2017. p. 19–38.
52. Friedman S. Prognosis of healing in treated teeth with endodontic infections. In: Fouad AF, editor. Endodontic microbiology. Ames, IA: Wiley; 2017. p. 341–84.
53. Chugal NM, Clive JM, Spangberg LS. A prognostic model for assessment of the outcome of endodontic treatment: effect of biologic and diagnostic variables. Oral Surg Oral Med Oral Pathol Oral Radiol Endod. 2001;91:342–52.
54. Karabucak B, Bunes A, Chehoud C, Kohli M, Setzer F. Prevalence of apical periodontitis in endodontically treated premolars and molars with untreated canal: a cone-beam computed tomography study. J Endod. 2016;42:538–41.
55. Costa FFNP, Pacheco-Yanes J, Siqueira JF Jr, Oliveira ACS, Gazzaneo I, Amorim CA, et al. Association between missed canals and apical periodontitis. Int Endod J. 2019;52:400–6.
56. Versiani MA, Martins JN, Basrani B. 3D visual glossary of terminology in root and root canal anatomy. In: Versiani MA, Basrani B, Sousa Neto MD, editors. The root canal anatomy in permanent dentition. Cham: Springer; 2018. p. 391–422.
57. Barnett F. Anatomy, access, and length determination. In: Chugal NM, Lin ML, editors. Endodontic prognosis—clinical guide for optimal treatment outcome. Cham: Springer; 2017. p. 115–30.
58. Fayad M, Johnson BR. 3D imaging in endodontics: a new era in diagnosis and treatment. Cham: Springer; 2016.
59. Al-Nahlawi T, Doumani M, Alalo HA, Habib A. Dentists' knowledge, attitude and practice of root canal treatment procedure: survey-based research. J Contemp Dent Pract. 2019;20:347–54.
60. Madarati AA. Why dentists don't use rubber dam during endodontics and how to promote its usage? BMC Oral Health. 2016;16:24.
61. Kapitan M, Hodacova L, Jagelska J, Kaplan J, Ivancakova R, Sustova Z. The attitude of Czech dental patients to the use of rubber dam. Health Expect. 2015;18:1282–90.
62. Gaikwad A, Jain D, Rane P, Bhondwe S, Taur S, Doshi S. Attitude of general dental practitioners toward root canal treatment procedures in India. J Contemp Dent Pract. 2013;14:528–31.
63. Kapitan M, Sustova Z. The use of rubber dam among Czech dental practitioners. Acta Medica (Hradec Kralove). 2011;54:144–8.
64. Slaus G, Bottenberg P. A survey of endodontic practice amongst Flemish dentists. Int Endod J. 2002;35:759–67.
65. Whitworth JM, Seccombe GV, Shoker K, Steele JG. Use of rubber dam and irrigant selection in UK general dental practice. Int Endod J. 2000;33:435–41.
66. Gluskin AH, Peters CI, Peters OA. Minimally invasive endodontics: challenging prevailing paradigms. Br Dent J. 2014;216:347–53.
67. Levin HJ. Access cavities. Dent Clin North Am. 1967:701–10.
68. Clark D, Khademi J. Modern molar endodontic access and directed dentin conservation. Dent Clin North Am. 2010;54:249–73.
69. Bóveda C, Kishen A. Contracted endodontic cavities: the foundation for less invasive alternatives in the management of apical periodontitis. Endod Topics. 2015;33:169–86.

70. Silva EJNL, Rover G, Belladonna FG, De-Deus G, Teixeira CS, FIdalgo TKS. Impact of contracted endodontic cavities on fracture resistance of endodontically treated teeth: a systematic review of in vitro studies. Clin Oral Investig. 2017;22:109–18.
71. Krishan R, Paqué F, Ossareh A, Kishen A, Dao T, Friedman S. Impacts of conservative endodontic cavity on root canal instrumentation efficacy and resistance to fracture assessed in incisors, premolars, and molars. J Endod. 2014;40:1160–6.
72. Neelakantan P, Khan K, Hei Ng GP, Yip CY, Zhang C, Pan Cheung GS. Does the orifice-directed dentin conservation access design debride pulp chamber and mesial root canal systems of mandibular molars similar to a traditional access design? J Endod. 2018;44:274–9.
73. Correia LC. O Princípio da Assimetria: uso de máscaras e aquecimento global. http://medicinabaseadaemevidencias.blogspot.com/2011/03/. Accessed 24 Mar 2011.
74. Bürklein S, Hinschitza K, Dammaschke T, Schäfer E. Shaping ability and cleaning effectiveness of two single-file systems in severely curved root canals of extracted teeth: Reciproc and WaveOne versus Mtwo and ProTaper. Int Endod J. 2012;45:449–61.
75. Paqué F, Musch U, Hülsmann M. Comparison of root canal preparation using RaCe and ProTaper rotary Ni-Ti instruments. Int Endod J. 2005;38:8–16.
76. Saini HR, Tewari S, Sangwan P, Duhan J, Gupta A. Effect of different apical preparation sizes on outcome of primary endodontic treatment: a randomized controlled trial. J Endod. 2012;38:1309–15.
77. Garcia-Guerrero C, Parra-Junco C, Quijano-Guauque S, Molano N, Pineda GA, Marin-Zuluaga DJ. Vertical root fractures in endodontically-treated teeth: a retrospective analysis of possible risk factors. J Investig Clin Dent. 2018;9.
78. Haueisen H, Gartner K, Kaiser L, Trohorsch D, Heidemann D. Vertical root fracture: prevalence, etiology, and diagnosis. Quintessence Int. 2013;44:467–74.
79. Yoshino K, Ito K, Kuroda M, Sugihara N. Prevalence of vertical root fracture as the reason for tooth extraction in dental clinics. Clin Oral Investig. 2015;19:1405–9.
80. Bürklein S, Schäfer E. Minimally invasive endodontics. Quintessence Int. 2015;46:119–24.
81. Ruddle CJ. FOCUS on: minimally invasive endodontics. Dent Today. 2014;33:14.
82. Augusto CM, Barbosa AFA, Guimaraes CC, Lima CO, Ferreira CM, Sassone LM, et al. A laboratory study of the impact of ultraconservative access cavities and minimal root canal tapers on the ability to shape canals in extracted mandibular molars and their fracture resistance. Int Endod J. 2020;53(11):1516–29. https://doi.org/10.1111/iej.13369.
83. Barbosa AFA, Lima CO, Coelho BP, Ferreira CM, Sassone LM, Silva E. The influence of endodontic access cavity design on the efficacy of canal instrumentation, microbial reduction, root canal filling and fracture resistance in mandibular molars. Int Endod J. 2020;53(12):1666–79. https://doi.org/10.1111/iej.13383.
84. Corsentino G, Pedulla E, Castelli L, Liguori M, Spicciarelli V, Martignoni M, et al. Influence of access cavity preparation and remaining tooth substance on fracture strength of endodontically treated teeth. J Endod. 2018;44:1416–21.
85. Moore B, Verdelis K, Kishen A, Dao T, Friedman S. Impacts of contracted endodontic cavities on instrumentation efficacy and biomechanical responses in maxillary molars. J Endod. 2016;42:1779–83.
86. Özyürek T, Ülker Ö, Demiryürek EÖ, Yilmaz F. The effects of endodontic access cavity preparation design on the fracture strength of endodontically treated teeth: traditional versus conservative preparation. J Endod. 2018;44:800–5.
87. Sabeti M, Kazem M, Dianat O, Bahrololumi N, Beglou A, Rahimipour K, et al. Impact of access cavity design and root canal taper on fracture resistance of endodontically treated teeth: an ex vivo investigation. J Endod. 2018;44:1402–6.
88. Vieira GCS, Perez AR, Alves FRF, Provenzano JC, Mdala I, Siqueira JF Jr, et al. Impact of contracted endodontic cavities on root canal disinfection and shaping. J Endod. 2020;46:655–61.
89. Montgomery DC. Design and analysis of experiments. 10th ed. New York: Wiley; 2019.
90. Silva E, Pinto KP, Ferreira CM, Belladonna FG, De-Deus G, Dummer PMH, et al. Current status on minimal access cavity preparations: a critical analysis and a proposal for a universal nomenclature. Int Endod J. 2020;53:1618–35.

91. Pache B, Hubner M, Jurt J, Demartines N, Grass F. Minimally invasive surgery and enhanced recovery after surgery: the ideal combination? J Surg Oncol. 2017;116:613–6.
92. AlAsseri N, Swennen G. Minimally invasive orthognathic surgery: a systematic review. Int J Oral Maxillofac Surg. 2018;47:1299–310.
93. Cloyd JM. Minimally invasive surgery for palliation. Surg Oncol Clin N Am. 2019;28:79–88.
94. Costantino CL, Mullen JT. Minimally invasive gastric cancer surgery. Surg Oncol Clin N Am. 2019;28:201–13.
95. Garmpis N, Dimitroulis D, Garmpi A, Diamantis E, Spartalis E, Schizas D, et al. Enhanced recovery after surgery: is it time to change our strategy regarding laparoscopic colectomy? In Vivo. 2019;33:669–74.
96. McGurkin-Smith R, Trope M, Caplan D, Sigurdsson A. Reduction of intracanal bacteria using GT rotary instrumentation, 5.25% NaOCl, EDTA, and $Ca(OH)_2$. J Endod. 2005;31:359–63.
97. Shuping GB, Ørstavik D, Sigurdsson A, Trope M. Reduction of intracanal bacteria using nickel-titanium rotary instrumentation and various medications. J Endod. 2000;26:751–5.
98. Sakamoto M, Siqueira JF Jr, Rôças IN, Benno Y. Bacterial reduction and persistence after endodontic treatment procedures. Oral Microbiol Immunol. 2007;22:19–23.
99. Siqueira JF Jr, Paiva SS, Rôças IN. Reduction in the cultivable bacterial populations in infected root canals by a chlorhexidine-based antimicrobial protocol. J Endod. 2007;33:541–7.
100. Neves MA, Rôças IN, Siqueira JF Jr. Clinical antibacterial effectiveness of the self-adjusting file system. Int Endod J. 2014;47:356–65.
101. Rôças IN, Lima KC, Siqueira JF Jr. Reduction in bacterial counts in infected root canals after rotary or hand nickel-titanium instrumentation—a clinical study. Int Endod J. 2013;46:681–7.
102. Zandi H, Rodrigues RC, Kristoffersen AK, Enersen M, Mdala I, Orstavik D, et al. Antibacterial effectiveness of 2 root canal irrigants in root-filled teeth with infection: a randomized clinical trial. J Endod. 2016;42:1307–13.
103. Rodrigues RCV, Zandi H, Kristoffersen AK, Enersen M, Mdala I, Ørstavik D, et al. Influence of the apical preparation size and the irrigant type on bacterial reduction in root canal–treated teeth with apical periodontitis. J Endod. 2017;43(7):1058–63.
104. Siqueira JF Jr, Rôças IN, Favieri A, Lima KC. Chemomechanical reduction of the bacterial population in the root canal after instrumentation and irrigation with 1%, 2.5%, and 5.25% sodium hypochlorite. J Endod. 2000;26:331–4.
105. Siqueira JF Jr, Rôças IN, Santos SR, Lima KC, Magalhães FA, de Uzeda M. Efficacy of instrumentation techniques and irrigation regimens in reducing the bacterial population within root canals. J Endod. 2002;28:181–4.
106. Brito PR, Souza LC, Machado de Oliveira JC, Alves FR, De-Deus G, Lopes HP, et al. Comparison of the effectiveness of three irrigation techniques in reducing intracanal Enterococcus faecalis populations: an in vitro study. J Endod. 2009;35:1422–7.
107. Neves MA, Provenzano JC, Rôças IN, Siqueira JF Jr. Clinical antibacterial effectiveness of root canal preparation with reciprocating single-instrument or continuously rotating multi-instrument systems. J Endod. 2016;42:25–9.
108. Rôças IN, Provenzano JC, Neves MA, Siqueira JF Jr. Disinfecting effects of rotary instrumentation with either 2.5% sodium hypochlorite or 2% chlorhexidine as the main irrigant: a randomized clinical study. J Endod. 2016;42:943–7.
109. Siqueira JF Jr, Guimarães-Pinto T, Rôças IN. Effects of chemomechanical preparation with 2.5% sodium hypochlorite and intracanal medication with calcium hydroxide on cultivable bacteria in infected root canals. J Endod. 2007;33:800–5.
110. Boutsioukis C. Internal tooth anatomy and root canal irrigation. In: Versiani MA, Basrani B, Sousa Neto MD, editors. The root canal anatomy in permanent dentition. Cham: Springer; 2018. p. 303–22.
111. Garberoglio R, Brännström M. Scanning electron microscopic investigation of human dentinal tubules. Arch Oral Biol. 1976;21:355–62.
112. Siqueira JF Jr, Araujo MC, Garcia PF, Fraga RC, Dantas CJ. Histological evaluation of the effectiveness of five instrumentation techniques for cleaning the apical third of root canals. J Endod. 1997;23:499–502.

113. Walton RE. Histologic evaluation of different methods of enlarging the pulp canal space. J Endod. 1976;2:304–11.
114. Nair PN, Henry S, Cano V, Vera J. Microbial status of apical root canal system of human mandibular first molars with primary apical periodontitis after "one-visit" endodontic treatment. Oral Surg Oral Med Oral Pathol Oral Radiol Endod. 2005;99:231–52.
115. Ricucci D, Siqueira JF Jr, Bate AL, Pitt Ford TR. Histologic investigation of root canal-treated teeth with apical periodontitis: a retrospective study from twenty-four patients. J Endod. 2009;35:493–502.
116. Vera J, Siqueira JF Jr, Ricucci D, Loghin S, Fernandez N, Flores B, et al. One- versus two-visit endodontic treatment of teeth with apical periodontitis: a histobacteriologic study. J Endod. 2012;38:1040–52.
117. Peters OA, Schönenberger K, Laib A. Effects of four Ni-Ti preparation techniques on root canal geometry assessed by micro computed tomography. Int Endod J. 2001;34:221–30.
118. Siqueira JF Jr, Alves FR, Versiani MA, Rôças IN, Almeida BM, Neves MA, et al. Correlative bacteriologic and micro-computed tomographic analysis of mandibular molar mesial canals prepared by self-adjusting file, Reciproc, and Twisted File systems. J Endod. 2013;39:1044–50.
119. Paqué F, Balmer M, Attin T, Peters OA. Preparation of oval-shaped root canals in mandibular molars using nickel-titanium rotary instruments: a micro-computed tomography study. J Endod. 2010;36:703–7.
120. Ricucci D, Siqueira JF Jr. Apical actinomycosis as a continuum of intraradicular and extraradicular infection: case report and critical review on its involvement with treatment failure. J Endod. 2008;34:1124–9.
121. Vieira AR, Siqueira JF Jr, Ricucci D, Lopes WS. Dentinal tubule infection as the cause of recurrent disease and late endodontic treatment failure: a case report. J Endod. 2012;38:250–4.
122. Siqueira JF Jr, Rôças IN. Clinical implications and microbiology of bacterial persistence after treatment procedures. J Endod. 2008;34:1291–301.e3.
123. Schilder H. Cleaning and shaping the root canal. Dent Clin North Am. 1974;18:269–96.
124. Barborka BJ, Woodmansey KF, Glickman GN, Schneiderman E, He J. Long-term clinical outcome of teeth obturated with Resilon. J Endod. 2017;43:556–60.
125. Strange KA, Tawil PZ, Phillips C, Walia HD, Fouad AF. Long-term outcomes of endodontic treatment performed with Resilon/Epiphany. J Endod. 2019;45:507–12.
126. Faraj S, Boutsioukis C. Observer variation in the assessment of root canal curvature. Int Endod J. 2017;50:167–76.
127. Hartmann RC, Fensterseifer M, Peters OA, de Figueiredo JAP, Gomes MS, Rossi-Fedele G. Methods for measurement of root canal curvature: a systematic and critical review. Int Endod J. 2019;52:169–80.
128. Schneider SW. A comparison of canal preparations in straight and curved root canals. Oral Surg Oral Med Oral Pathol. 1971;32:271–5.
129. Weine F. Endodontic therapy. 3rd ed. St. Louis: Mosby; 1982.
130. Pruett JP, Clement DJ, Carnes DL Jr. Cyclic fatigue testing of nickel-titanium endodontic instruments. J Endod. 1997;23:77–85.
131. Gunday M, Sazak H, Garip Y. A comparative study of three different root canal curvature measurement techniques and measuring the canal access angle in curved canals. J Endod. 2005;31:796–8.
132. Schäfer E, Diez C, Hoppe W, Tepel J. Roentgenographic investigation of frequency and degree of canal curvatures in human permanent teeth. J Endod. 2002;28:211–6.
133. Cvek M, Granath L, Lundberg M. Failures and healing in endodontically treated non-vital anterior teeth with posttraumatically reduced pulpal lumen. Acta Odontol Scand. 1982;40:223–8.
134. Tamse A, Fuss Z, Lustig J, Kaplavi J. An evaluation of endodontically treated vertically fractured teeth. J Endod. 1999;25:506–8.
135. Tamse A. Vertical root fractures in endodontically treated teeth: diagnostic signs and clinical management. Endod Topics. 2006;13:84–94.

136. Gutmann JL. The dentin-root complex: anatomic and biologic considerations in restoring endodontically treated teeth. J Prosthet Dent. 1992;67:458–67.
137. Rundquist BD, Versluis A. How does canal taper affect root stresses? Int Endod J. 2006;39:226–37.
138. Gher ME Jr, Dunlap RM, Anderson MH, Kuhl LV. Clinical survey of fractured teeth. J Am Dent Assoc. 1987;114:174–7.
139. Keleş A, Keskin C, Karataslioglu E, Kishen A, Versiani MA. Middle mesial canal preparation enhances the risk of fracture in mesial root of mandibular molars. J Endod. 2020;46(9):1323–9. https://doi.org/10.1016/j.joen.2020.05.019.
140. De-Deus G, Rodrigues EA, Belladonna FG, Simoes-Carvalho M, Cavalcante DM, Oliveira DS, et al. Anatomical danger zone reconsidered: a micro-CT study on dentine thickness in mandibular molars. Int Endod J. 2019;52:1501–7.
141. Versiani MA, Ordinola-Zapata R, Keleş A, Alcin H, Bramante CM, Pécora JD, et al. Middle mesial canals in mandibular first molars: a micro-CT study in different populations. Arch Oral Biol. 2016;61:130–7.
142. Keleş A, Keskin C, Alqawasmi R, Versiani MA. Evaluation of dentine thickness of middle mesial canals of mandibular molars prepared with rotary instruments: a micro-CT study. Int Endod J. 2019;53(4):519–28.
143. Lertchirakarn V, Palamara JEA, Messer HH. Patterns of vertical root fracture: factors affecting stress distribution in the root canal. J Endod. 2003;29:523–8.
144. Lim SS, Stock CJ. The risk of perforation in the curved canal: anticurvature filing compared with the stepback technique. Int Endod J. 1987;20:33–9.
145. Russell AA, Chris He LH, Chandler NP. Investigation of dentin hardness in roots exhibiting the butterfly effect. J Endod. 2014;40:842–4.
146. Russell AA, Chandler NP, Hauman C, Siddiqui AY, Tompkins GR. The butterfly effect: an investigation of sectioned roots. J Endod. 2013;39:208–10.
147. Vasiliadis L, Darling AI, Levers BG. The amount and distribution of sclerotic human root dentine. Arch Oral Biol. 1983;28:645–9.
148. Cooke HG 3rd, Cox FL. C-shaped canal configurations in mandibular molars. J Am Dent Assoc. 1979;99:836–9.
149. Malpighi M. Observationes de dentibus: Manoscritto 936 Busta II D; 1690.
150. Martins JNR, Marques D, Silva E, Carames J, Mata A, Versiani MA. Prevalence of C-shaped canal morphology using cone beam computed tomography—a systematic review with meta-analysis. Int Endod J. 2019;52:1556–72.
151. Solomonov M, Paque F, Fan B, Eilat Y, Berman LH. The challenge of C-shaped canal systems: a comparative study of the Self-Adjusting File and ProTaper. J Endod. 2012;38:209–14.
152. Yin X, Cheung GS, Zhang C, Masuda YM, Kimura Y, Matsumoto K. Micro-computed tomographic comparison of nickel-titanium rotary versus traditional instruments in C-shaped root canal system. J Endod. 2010;36:708–12.
153. Fan B, Min Y, Lu G, Yang J, Cheung GS, Gutmann JL. Negotiation of C-shaped canal systems in mandibular second molars. J Endod. 2009;35:1003–8.
154. Melton DC, Krell KV, Fuller MW. Anatomical and histological features of C-shaped canals in mandibular second molars. J Endod. 1991;17:384–8.
155. Fan B, Cheung GS, Fan M, Gutmann JL, Bian Z. C-shaped canal system in mandibular second molars: part I—anatomical features. J Endod. 2004;30:899–903.
156. Ordinola-Zapata R, Martins JN, Bramante CM, Villas-Boas MH, Duarte MH, Versiani MA. Morphological evaluation of maxillary second molars with fused roots: a micro-CT study. Int Endod J. 2017;50:1192–200.
157. Boschetti E, Silva-Sousa YTC, Mazzi-Chaves JF, Leoni GB, Versiani MA, Pecora JD, et al. Micro-CT evaluation of root and canal morphology of mandibular first premolars with radicular grooves. Braz Dent J. 2017;28:597–603.
158. Ordinola-Zapata R, Monteiro Bramante C, Gagliardi Minotti P, Cavalini Cavenago B, Gutmann JL, Moldauer BI, et al. Micro-CT evaluation of C-shaped mandibular first premolars in a Brazilian subpopulation. Int Endod J. 2015;48:807–13.

159. Ordinola-Zapata R, Bramante CM, Villas-Boas MH, Cavenago BC, Duarte MH, Versiani MA. Morphologic micro-computed tomography analysis of mandibular premolars with three root canals. J Endod. 2013;39:1130–5.
160. Keith A. Problems relating to the teeth of the earlier forms of prehistoric man. Proc R Soc Med. 1913;6:103–24.
161. Shaw JC. Taurodont teeth in South African races. J Anat. 1928;62:476–98.
162. Carlsen O, Alexandersen V. Radix mesiolingualis and radix distolingualis in a collection of permanent maxillary molars. Acta Odontol Scand. 2000;58:229–36.
163. AAE. Glossary of endodontics terms. 9th ed. Chicago: American Association of Endodontists; 2016.
164. Calberson FL, De Moor RJ, Deroose CA. The radix entomolaris and paramolaris: clinical approach in endodontics. J Endod. 2007;33:58–63.
165. De Moor RJ, Deroose CA, Calberson FL. The radix entomolaris in mandibular first molars: an endodontic challenge. Int Endod J. 2004;37:789–99.
166. Turner CG. Three-rooted mandibular first permanent molars and the question of American Indian origins. Am J Phys Anthropol. 1971;34:229–41.
167. Oehlers FA. Dens invaginatus (dilated composite odontome). I. Variations of the invagination process and associated anterior crown forms. Oral Surg Oral Med Oral Pathol. 1957;10:1204–18 contd.
168. Hülsmann M. Dens invaginatus: aetiology, classification, prevalence, diagnosis, and treatment considerations. Int Endod J. 1997;30:79–90.
169. Oehlers FA. Dens invaginatus (dilated composite odontome). II. Associated posterior crown forms and pathogenesis. Oral Surg Oral Med Oral Pathol. 1957;10:1302–16.
170. Martins JNR, Marques D, Silva E, Carames J, Mata A, Versiani MA. Second mesiobuccal root canal in maxillary molars—a systematic review and meta-analysis of prevalence studies using cone beam computed tomography. Arch Oral Biol. 2020;113:104589.
171. Huumonen S, Kvist T, Grondahl K, Molander A. Diagnostic value of computed tomography in re-treatment of root fillings in maxillary molars. Int Endod J. 2006;39:827–33.
172. Wolcott J, Ishley D, Kennedy W, Johnson S, Minnich S. Clinical investigation of second mesiobuccal canals in endodontically treated and retreated maxillary molars. J Endod. 2002;28:477–9.
173. Ordinola-Zapata R, Martins JNR, Plascencia H, Versiani MA, Bramante CM. The MB3 canal in maxillary molars: a micro-CT study. Clin Oral Investig. 2020;24(11):4109–21. https://doi.org/10.1007/s00784-020-3284-7.
174. Tomaszewska IM, Skinningsrud B, Jarzebska A, Pekala JR, Tarasiuk J, Iwanaga J. Internal and external morphology of mandibular molars: an original micro-CT study and meta-analysis with review of implications for endodontic therapy. Clin Anat. 2018;31:797–811.
175. Gonzalez-Plata RR, Gonzalez-Plata EW. Conventional and surgical treatment of a two-rooted maxillary central incisor. J Endod. 2003;29:422–4.
176. Lambruschini GM, Camps J. A two-rooted maxillary central incisor with a normal clinical crown. J Endod. 1993;19:95–6.
177. Lin WC, Yang SF, Pai SF. Nonsurgical endodontic treatment of a two-rooted maxillary central incisor. J Endod. 2006;32:478–81.
178. Gondim E Jr, Setzer F, Zingg P, Karabucak B. A maxillary central incisor with three root canals: a case report. J Endod. 2009;35:1445–7.
179. Mangani F, Ruddle CJ. Endodontic treatment of a "very particular" maxillary central incisor. J Endod. 1994;20:560–1.
180. Pécora JD, da Cruz Filho AM. Study of the incidence of radicular grooves in maxillary incisors. Braz Dent J. 1992;3:11–6.
181. Libfeld H, Stabholz A, Friedman S. Endodontic therapy of bilaterally geminated permanent maxillary central incisors. J Endod. 1986;12:214–6.
182. Pécora JD, Santana SV. Maxillary lateral incisor with two roots—case report. Braz Dent J. 1992;2:151–3.

183. Peix-Sanchez M, Minana-Laliga R. A case of unusual anatomy: a maxillary lateral incisor with three canals. Int Endod J. 1999;32:236–40.
184. Kottoor J, Murugesan R, Albuquerque DV. A maxillary lateral incisor with four root canals. Int Endod J. 2012;45:393–7.
185. Fried IL, Winter AA. Diagnosis and treatment of a two-rooted maxillary lateral incisor. Periodontal Case Rep. 1984;6:40–4.
186. Wong M. Treatment considerations in a geminated maxillary lateral incisor. J Endod. 1991;17:179–81.
187. Pécora JD, Saquy PC, de Souza JE, Sousa-Neto MD. Endodontic treatment of a maxillary lateral incisor presenting dens invaginatus and transposition to the region of the canine—case report. Braz Dent J. 1991;2:5–8.
188. Mupparapu M, Singer SR, Goodchild JH. Dens evaginatus and dens invaginatus in a maxillary lateral incisor: report of a rare occurrence and review of literature. Aust Dent J. 2004;49:201–3.
189. Boveda C, Fajardo M, Millan B. Root canal treatment of an invaginated maxillary lateral incisor with a C-shaped canal. Quintessence Int. 1999;30:707–11.
190. Leoni GB, Versiani MA, Pécora JD, Sousa-Neto MD. Micro–computed tomographic analysis of the root canal morphology of mandibular incisors. J Endod. 2013;40:710–6.
191. Sachdeva GS, Malhotra D, Sachdeva LT, Sharma N, Negi A. Endodontic management of mandibular central incisor fused to a supernumerary tooth associated with a talon cusp: a case report. Int Endod J. 2012;45:590–6.
192. Khabbaz MG, Konstantaki MN, Sykaras SN. Dens invaginatus in a mandibular lateral incisor. Int Endod J. 1995;28:303–5.
193. Loushine RJ, Jurcak JJ, Jeffalone DM. A two-rooted mandibular incisor. J Endod. 1993;19:250–1.
194. Barkhordar RA, Nguyen NT. Maxillary canine with two roots. J Endod. 1985;11:224–7.
195. Sousa Neto MD, Zuccolotto WG, Saquy PC, Grandini SA, Pécora JD. Treatment of dens invaginatus in a maxillary canine case report. Braz Dent J. 1992;2:147–50.
196. Orguneser A, Kartal N. Three canals and two foramina in a mandibular canine. J Endod. 1998;24:444–5.
197. Soares JA, Leonardo RT. Root canal treatment of three-rooted maxillary first and second premolars—a case report. Int Endod J. 2003;36:705–10.
198. Lammertyn PA, Rodrigo SB, Brunotto M, Crosa M. Furcation groove of maxillary first premolar, thickness, and dentin structures. J Endod. 2009;35:814–7.
199. Nahmias Y, Rampado ME. Root-canal treatment of a trifid crown premolar. Int Endod J. 2002;35:390–4.
200. Colak H, Aylikci BU, Keklik H. Dens evaginatus on maxillary first premolar: report of a rare clinical case. J Nat Sci Biol Med. 2012;3:192–4.
201. Rotstein I, Stabholz A, Friedman S. Endodontic therapy for dens invaginatus in a maxillary second premolar. Oral Surg Oral Med Oral Pathol. 1987;63:237–40.
202. Vaghela DJ, Sinha AA. Endodontic management of four rooted mandibular first premolar. J Conserv Dent. 2013;16:87–9.
203. Gu Y, Zhang Y, Liao Z. Root and canal morphology of mandibular first premolars with radicular grooves. Arch Oral Biol. 2013;58:1609–17.
204. Fan B, Yang J, Gutmann JL, Fan M. Root canal systems in mandibular first premolars with C-shaped root configurations. Part I: microcomputed tomography mapping of the radicular groove and associated root canal cross-sections. J Endod. 2008;34:1337–41.
205. Stecker S, DiAngelis AJ. Dens evaginatus: a diagnostic and treatment challenge. J Am Dent Assoc. 2002;133:190–3.
206. Tavano SM, de Sousa SM, Bramante CM. Dens invaginatus in first mandibular premolar. Endod Dent Traumatol. 1994;10:27–9.
207. Aryanpour S, Bercy P, Van Nieuwenhuysen JP. Endodontic and periodontal treatments of a geminated mandibular first premolar. Int Endod J. 2002;35:209–14.

208. De Moor RJ, Calberson FL. Root canal treatment in a mandibular second premolar with three root canals. J Endod. 2005;31:310–3.
209. Farmakis ET. Four-rooted mandibular second premolar. Aust Endod J. 2008;34:126–8.
210. Demiryürek EO, Gönülol N, Bulucu B. Endodontic treatment of a taurodontic premolar with five canals. Aust Endod J. 2013;39:81–4.
211. Goswami M, Chandra S, Chandra S, Singh S. Mandibular premolar with two roots. J Endod. 1997;23:187.
212. Cleghorn BM, Christie WH, Dong CC. Anomalous mandibular premolars: a mandibular first premolar with three roots and a mandibular second premolar with a C-shaped canal system. Int Endod J. 2008;41:1005–14.
213. Koh ET, Ford TR, Kariyawasam SP, Chen NN, Torabinejad M. Prophylactic treatment of dens evaginatus using mineral trioxide aggregate. J Endod. 2001;27:540–2.
214. Muthukumar RS, Arunkumar S, Sadasiva K. Bilateral fusion of mandibular second premolar and supernumerary tooth: a rare case report. J Oral Maxillofac Pathol. 2012;16:128–30.
215. Gopikrishna V, Bhargavi N, Kandaswamy D. Endodontic management of a maxillary first molar with a single root and a single canal diagnosed with the aid of spiral CT: a case report. J Endod. 2006;32:687–91.
216. Beatty RG. A five-canal maxillary first molar. J Endod. 1984;10:156–7.
217. Albuquerque DV, Kottoor J, Dham S, Velmurugan N, Abarajithan M, Sudha R. Endodontic management of maxillary permanent first molar with 6 root canals: 3 case reports. Oral Surg Oral Med Oral Pathol Oral Radiol Endod. 2010;110:e79–83.
218. Kottoor J, Velmurugan N, Sudha R, Hemamalathi S. Maxillary first molar with seven root canals diagnosed with cone-beam computed tomography scanning: a case report. J Endod. 2010;36:915–21.
219. Kottoor J, Velmurugan N, Surendran S. Endodontic management of a maxillary first molar with eight root canal systems evaluated using cone-beam computed tomography scanning: a case report. J Endod. 2011;37:715–9.
220. De Moor RJ. C-shaped root canal configuration in maxillary first molars. Int Endod J. 2002;35:200–8.
221. Versiani MA, Pécora JD, Sousa-Neto MD. Root and root canal morphology of four-rooted maxillary second molars: a micro-computed tomography study. J Endod. 2012;38:977–82.
222. Sert S, Bayrl G. Taurodontism in six molars: a case report. J Endod. 2004;30:601–2.
223. Peikoff MD, Christie WH, Fogel HM. The maxillary second molar: variations in the number of roots and canals. Int Endod J. 1996;29:365–9.
224. Kottoor J, Hemamalathi S, Sudha R, Velmurugan N. Maxillary second molar with 5 roots and 5 canals evaluated using cone beam computerized tomography: a case report. Oral Surg Oral Med Oral Pathol Oral Radiol Endod. 2010;109:e162–5.
225. Koenen DJ, Pahncke D. Gemination or fusion: use of a CT scan to assist in diagnosis and endodontic treatment of a maxillary second molar—a case report. ENDO. 2008;2:145–51.
226. Radwan A, Kim SG. Treatment of a hypertaurodontic maxillary second molar in a patient with 10 taurodonts: a case report. J Endod. 2013;40:140–4.
227. Friedman S, Moshonov J, Stabholz A. Five root canals in a mandibular first molar. Endod Dent Traumatol. 1986;2:226–8.
228. Ryan JL, Bowles WR, Baisden MK, McClanahan SB. Mandibular first molar with six separate canals. J Endod. 2011;37:878–80.
229. Reeh ES. Seven canals in a lower first molar. J Endod. 1998;24:497–9.
230. Ashwin R, Arathi R. Taurodontism of deciduous and permanent molars: report of two cases. J Indian Soc Pedod Prev Dent. 2006;24:42–4.
231. Tsesis I, Steinbock N, Rosenberg E, Kaufman AY. Endodontic treatment of developmental anomalies in posterior teeth: treatment of geminated/fused teeth—report of two cases. Int Endod J. 2003;36:372–9.
232. Fan B, Pan Y, Gao Y, Fang F, Wu Q, Gutmann JL. Three-dimensional morphologic analysis of isthmuses in the mesial roots of mandibular molars. J Endod. 2010;36:1866–9.